Injectable biomaterials

Related titles:

Cellular response to biomaterials
(ISBN 978-1-84569-358-9)
The response of cells to biomaterials is critical in medical devices. It has been realised that specific cell responses may be beneficial – encouraging adhesion, healing or cell multiplication. *Cellular response to biomaterials* will examine the response of cells with a wide range of materials, targeted at specific medical applications. Chapters in the first section review cellular response to polymers and ceramics. A second group of chapters discuss cell responses and regenerative medicine for nerves, muscles and orthopaedic materials. The final set of chapters analyse the effect of surface chemistry and how it can be manipulated to provoke a useful cell response.

Drug–device combination products
(ISBN 978-1-84569-470-8)
Drug delivery systems represent a vast area of research and development within biomaterials and medicine and the demand for sophisticated drug delivery devices continues to drive developments. Advanced drug delivery devices can offer significant advantages to conventional drugs, such as increased efficiency and convenience. Chapters in Part I discuss specific applications such as drug eluting stents and antimicrobial cements. Part II covers the development of drug–device combination products with such topics as preclinical testing and regulation of products. This book will provide a thorough analysis of the fundamentals, applications and new technologies of drug–device combination products for use throughout the human body.

Tissue engineering using ceramics and polymers
(ISBN 978-1-84569-176-9)
Tissue engineering is rapidly developing as a technique for the repair and regeneration of diseased tissue in the body. This authoritative and wide-ranging book reviews how ceramic and polymeric biomaterials are being used in tissue engineering. The first part of the book reviews the nature of ceramics and polymers as biomaterials together with techniques for using them such as building tissue scaffolds, transplantation techniques, surface modification and ways of combining tissue engineering with drug delivery and biosensor systems. The second part of the book discusses the regeneration of particular types of tissue from bone, cardiac and intervertebral disc tissue to skin, liver, kidney and lung tissue.

Details of these and other Woodhead Publishing materials books can be obtained by:

- visiting our web site at www.woodheadpublishing.com
- contacting Customer Services (e-mail: sales@woodheadpublishing.com; fax: +44 (0) 1223 832819; tel.: +44 (0) 1223 499140 ext. 130; address: Woodhead Publishing Limited, 80 High Street, Sawston, Cambridge CB22 3HJ, UK)

If you would like to receive information on forthcoming titles, please send your address details to: Francis Dodds (address, tel. and fax as above; email: francis.dodds@woodheadpublishing.com). Please confirm which subject areas you are interested in.

Injectable biomaterials

Science and applications

Edited by
Brent Vernon

WOODHEAD PUBLISHING

Oxford Cambridge Philadelphia New Delhi

Published by Woodhead Publishing Limited,
80 High Street, Sawston, Cambridge CB22 3HJ, UK
www.woodheadpublishing.com

Woodhead Publishing, 1518 Walnut Street, Suite 1100, Philadelphia, PA 19102-3406, USA

Woodhead Publishing India Private Limited, G-2, Vardaan House,
7/28 Ansari Road, Daryaganj, New Delhi – 110002, India
www.woodheadpublishingindia.com

First published 2011, Woodhead Publishing Limited

British Library Cataloguing in Publication Data
A catalogue record for this book is available from the British Library.

ISBN 978-0-08-101493-6 (print)
ISBN 978-0-85709-137-6 (online)

The publisher's policy is to use permanent paper from mills that operate a sustainable forestry policy, and which has been manufactured from pulp which is processed using acid-free and elemental chlorine-free practices. Furthermore, the publisher ensures that the text paper and cover board used have met acceptable environmental accreditation standards.

Typeset by Godiva Publishing Services Limited, Coventry, West Midlands, UK

Contents

Contributor contact details

(* = main contact)

Editor

B. Vernon
Harrington Department of Bioengineering
Arizona State University
ECG Room 334
P.O. Box 879709
Tempe, AZ 85287
USA
E-mail: brent.vernon@asu.edu

Chapter 1

R. Condie and G. D. Prestwich*
Department of Bioengineering
The University of Utah
50 Central Campus Drive
Room 2480
Salt Lake City, UT 84112
USA
E-mail: gprestwich@pharm.utah.edu

Chapter 2

M. Bohner
RMS Foundation
Bischmattstrasse 12
CH-2544 Bettlach
Switzerland
E-mail: marc.bohner@rms-foundation.ch

Chapter 3

R. McLemore
Banner Good Samaritan Medical Center
1300 N 12th Street, Suite 620
Phoenix, AZ 85006
USA
E-mail: ryan.mclemore@gmail.com

Chapter 4

Y. Qiu, S. K. Hamilton, and J. S. Temenoff*
Coulter Department of Biomedical Engineering
Georgia Tech/Emory University
313 Ferst Drive
Room 2112
Atlanta, GA 30332
E-mail: johnna.temenoff@bme.gatech.edu

Chapter 5

D. J. Overstreet* and B. L. Vernon
Harrington Department of Bioengineering
Arizona State University
ECG Room 334
Tempe, AZ 85287
USA
E-mail: derek.overstreet@asu.edu

H. A. von Recum
Case Western Reserve University
Cleveland, OH
USA

Chapter 6

S. Kona, A. S. Wadajkar and K. T. Nguyen*
501 West First Street
ELB 220
Arlington, TX 76019
USA
E-mail: knguyen@uta.edu

Chapter 7

B. L. Vernon* and C. Riley
School of Biological and Health Systems Engineering
Arizona State University
ECG 334
P.O. Box 879709
Tempe, AZ 85287
USA
email: brent.vernon@asu.edu

Chapter 8

A. C. McLaren* and C. S. Estes
Banner Good Samaritan Medical Center
1300 N 12th Street, Suite 620
Phoenix, AZ 85006
USA
E-mail: alex.mclaren@bannerhealth.com

Chapter 9

R. W. Hasel*
Division of Anatomy
Stanford University School of Medicine
269 Campus Drive, CCSR Building Room 0135
Stanford, CA 94305
USA
E-mail: rhasel@stanford.edu

E. Combe
Division of Biomaterials
Department of Restorative Sciences
University of Minnesota School of Dentistry
16-212 Moos Tower
515 Delaware Street SE
Minneapolis, MN 55455-0348
E-mail: combe001@umn.edu

Chapter 10

R. B. Arote*
School of Dentistry
Seoul National University
Seoul 110-749
South Korea
E-mail: arote.rohidas@gmail.com

C.-S. Cho*, D. Jere, Y.-K. Kim and Y.-J. Choi
Department of Agricultural Biotechnology
Seoul National University
Seoul 151-921
South Korea
E-mail: chocs@plaza.snu.ac.kr

M.-H. Cho and H.-L. Jiang
College of Veterinary Medicine
Seoul National University
Seoul 151-742
South Korea

Chapter 11

H. H. Bearat* and B. L. Vernon
Harrington Department of Bioengineering
Arizona State University
ECG Room 334
Tempe, AZ 85287
USA
E-mail: hanin.bearat@asu.edu

Chapter 12

F. Cellesi* and N. Tirelli
School of Pharmacy and Pharmaceutical Sciences
University of Manchester
Stopford Building
Oxford Road
Manchester M13 9PT
UK
E-mail: f.cellesi@manchester.ac.uk
nicola.tirelli@manchester.ac.uk

Chapter 13

B. Jeong
Department of Chemistry and Nano Science
Department of Bioinspired Science
Ewha Womans University
Daehyun-Dong
Seodaemun-Ku
Seoul, 120-750
Korea
E-mail: bjeong@ewha.ac.kr

Chapter 14

T. A. Becker
Independent Medical Device Consultant
3361 South Walkup Drive
Flagstaff, AZ 86001
USA
E-mail: becker.tim@att.net

Chapter 15

S. A. Guelcher
Department of Chemical and Biomolecular Engineering
Vanderbilt University
PMB 351604
2301 Vanderbilt Place
Nashville, TN 37235-1604
USA
E-mail:
scott.guelcher@Vanderbilt.Edu

Chapter 16

R. Scott
Department of Biomedical Engineering
Saint Louis University
St. Louis, MO 63103
USA

R. Kuntz Willits*
Department of Biomedical Engineering
University of Akron
185 East Mill Street
Akron, OH 44325-0302
USA
E-mail: willits@uakron.edu

Part I

Materials and properties

1

Designing clinically useful substitutes for the extracellular matrix

R. CONDIE and G. D. PRESTWICH,
The University of Utah, USA

Abstract: This chapter focuses on design criteria for FDA-approvable and affordable matrices for cell delivery. We first describe the challenges for translational biomaterials; next, we define the scientific and real-world design criteria to be considered. Most important is to use a material that allows seamless transition from preclinical studies to use in human clinical trials. Next, we focus on chemically modified hyaluronic acid as a building block for creating semi-synthetic ECMs. Finally, we describe the use of the sECMs to incorporate biological cues and accomplish the delivery of cells and growth factors *in vivo*.

Key words: hyaluronic acid, translational research, chemical modification, cell therapy, practical design criteria.

1.1 Introduction: the translational challenge

As regenerative medicine matures from research projects to clinical products, market forces intervene. The traditional paradigm of innovation that focuses on elegant technology and reductionist research has generally failed to deliver products to the market. Many a well-constructed ship has been sunk on her maiden voyage by the icebergs of unconvincing clinical outcomes, faulty business models, shortage of investor funding, unmet manufacturing requirements, ever-moving regulatory hurdles, lack of physician acceptance, or the absence of a reimbursement code. Nonetheless, funding programs are calling for a new generation of translational approaches that can navigate to the clinic, avoiding the Scylla of technological and regulatory complexity and the Charybdis of inadequate funding. One new approach integrates market research into the design criteria for engineering a solution to a given problem. In this approach, one designs products to meet the needs of the end users – patients and physicians – and thoroughly considers the pathway to those users from the very beginning (Prestwich, 2007).

The developing field of tissue engineering (TE) is rife with cautionary tales of over-promising and under-delivering. The promise of rebuilding organs originally attracted enthusiastic attention and investment in the 1990s, but the early companies met with disappointment in the market. R&D funding dropped 50% in 2002 from a value of US$580 million only two years earlier. Organogenesis and Advanced Tissue Sciences filed bankruptcy that same year. Expectations and strategies were adjusted, and incremental progress was gained. The autologous cartilage implant Carticel became profitable in 2005, eight years after its FDA approval. By 2007 TE engineering sales from ~170 companies reached US$1.3 billion (Place *et al.*, 2009).

Still, cell-based therapies have the potential to harness the complex power of biology to address clinical needs in ways that no human-engineered device could: enhancing wound healing, restoring lost organ function, integrating naturally with the host. However, as cell behavior is highly dependent upon the biochemical and mechanical environment (Place *et al.*, 2009), there is an urgent need for biomimetic materials with sufficient instructive potential to appropriately guide cell phenotype and function. Lacking the knowledge and synthetic methods to fully replicate the complexity of biology (Brigham *et al.*, 2009), we must simplify our synthetic strategies. These simplifications of the cellular environment, which aim to balance an appropriate degree of biological complexity with manageable chemistry, have been described as synthetic extracellular matrices (sECMs). The biomimetic, 3-dimensional (3-D) environment that they provide can be far superior to traditional tissue culture in 2-D on a polystyrene surface (Serban *et al.*, 2008a). The scope of this review is limited to a selection of sECMs based on hydrogel derivatives of the particularly promising material: hyaluronic acid (HA). A variety of innovative and promising materials of other composition or intended use must regrettably be excluded.

1.2 Design criteria for extracellular matrix (ECM) mimetics

The design of successful products is driven by end user needs (i.e. patients and physicians) and regulatory and commercial factors in addition to function (Prestwich, 2007). Commercialization demands a simple, affordable product, easy for physicians to handle, manufacturable, and reimbursable. For regulatory approval, the material must be chemically defined and of controllable and reproducible composition. This can be a challenge for naturally derived materials, which are otherwise desirable for improved cell behavior and integration with host tissue. For example, Matrigel is unsuitable for use in humans despite its extensive use in research because it is derived from murine sarcoma. Synthetic materials are typically more reproducible and defined, but nearly always elicit some degree of inflammatory response. This can potentially be limited to the acute phase in the case of biodegradable materials, which may be remodeled by host tissue at a tuned rate given the right stimuli. Their cell and tissue interactions may be enhanced with biomimetic moieties, including conjugated biomolecules and controlled-release growth factors, for example to maintain cell phenotype, recruit host cells, or induce vascularization. Toxicity of components must be eliminated as well as that of reaction or degradation products, heat or acidity generated in the oxygen and enzyme rich host environment (Shu *et al.*, 2004b). Simple, cost-effective, biomimetic materials are more likely to clear regulatory and commercial hurdles than many innovative but over-engineered solutions so prevalent in research.

Further design criteria are required for injectable hydrogel cell delivery vehicles. For ease of administration, gel precursors may be injected and allowed to crosslink or polymerize *in situ*. The sol to gel transition may be induced by body temperature, pH, ionic strength, presence of biomolecules, or other gentle environmental conditions (Haines-Butterick *et al.*, 2007). Photopolymerization or photocrosslinking may be applied to exposed tissues if photoinitiator toxicity and excess heat can be avoided. The gelation rate must be slow enough to permit the encapsulation and injection of cells but fast enough to prevent their settling or leaking from the site (Haines-Butterick *et al.*, 2007). Alternatively, thixotropic or shear thinning gels become temporarily liquid under pressure and shear of injection and recover their gel condition *in vivo*. These strategies allow the gel to conform to tissue geometry and adhere by binding to the tissues by adhesion and microscopic interlocking. Material stiffness should ideally be tuned to that of the target tissue to avoid the deformation or loosening associated with modulus mismatch (Khetan *et al.*, 2009). *In situ* swelling or contraction should usually be minimized.

1.3 Single-module semi-synthetic extracellular matrices (sECMs) based on hyaluronic acid (HA)

Soft, three-dimensional hydrogel derived from natural materials can provide excellent *in vitro* environments for cell culture. HA, an unbranched chain of the repeating disaccharide units β-1,4-D-glucuronic acid and α-1,3-N-acetyl-D-glucosamine, is a non-sulfated glycosaminoglycan (GAG) prevalent in all connective tissue, where it is noncovalently bound to core proteins and a variety of proteoglycans (Fraser *et al.*, 1997). These heterogeneous networks, together with a milieu of other biomolecules, comprise the native extracellular matrix (ECM). The ECM provides a dynamic mechanical and biochemical environment to support cellular function. HA plays a significant role in early development, cell motility proliferation and differentiation, morphogenesis, wound healing, inflammation, joint lubrication, and hydration (Fraser *et al.*, 1997; Gerecht *et al.*, 2007; Allison and Grande-Allen, 2006). As an *in vitro* cellular environment, the material contributes to angiogenesis, osteointegration, and phenotype preservation. HA is a highly hydrated, polyanionic macromolecule that is rapidly turned over by hyaluronidase, with a tissue half life of several hours to several days (Laurent and Fraser, 1986).

1.3.1 Chemical modifications of HA

Chemical processing of HA is challenged by its low solubility in organic solvents, sensitivity to degradation, and multifunctionality. Modifications of HA often target carboxyl or hydroxyl groups to add functionality or decrease degradation rate. Polymerized or crosslinked HA derivatives have been used in viscosurgery, viscosupplementation, ophthalmic surgery, prevention of post-surgical adhesions, and as a cell scaffolding material (Prestwich and Kuo, 2008). Chemical modifications of HA and its uses in tissue engineering and regenerative medicine have been described in several recent reviews (Allison and Grande-Allen, 2006; Prestwich and Kuo, 2008; Schiller *et al.*, 2010; Kuo and Prestwich, 2010) and can be divided into two types: monolithic and living (Prestwich and Kuo, 2008). The vast array of chemical derivatives will not be described in detail here. Rather, this chapter will focus on the use of living HA derivatives as the basis for injectable sECMs, and Table 1.1 summarizes (i) the ECM or sECM components and chemistry used, (ii) the properties of the biomaterials, (iii) selected uses for each sECM, and (iv) the literature citations for each example.

1.3.2 Chemical crosslinking of HA

Thiol modification of HA is a living chemistry, and thiol-mediated crosslinking provides the basis for a portfolio of modular sECMs that can be used for cell delivery and retention (Serban and Prestwich, 2008). Reaction of the carboxylic acid groups of HA with di(thiopropionyl) bishydrazide (DTPH) incorporates a disulfide linkage that can be converted to a free thiol using dithiothreitol (DTT) as a reducing agent (Shu *et al.*, 2002). The thiol groups can be autocrosslinked by oxidation overnight in air, or more rapidly with oxidants such as peroxide. These disulfide cross-linked hyaluronan hydrogels (Shu *et al.*, 2002) can be dried in air to give rehydratable films (Liu *et al.*, 2005b) or lyophilized to produce macroporous sponges (Liu *et al.*, 2004). Alternatively, polyethylene glycol diacrylate (PEGDA) can be used as a cytocompatible bivalent electrophile to produce crosslinked hydrogels (Shu *et al.*, 2004b), for which the gelation time can be tuned from 10 to 120 min with a slight adjustment of pH. Partial carboxymethylation of the HA at the C-6 hydroxyl groups gives provides more sites for thiol modification and further decreases degradation rate without diminishing biological performance (Prestwich, 2007). The resulting thiolated carboxylmethyl HA, or CMHA-S, has been shown to promote scar-free wound healing and prevents adhesions in several surgical applications (Kirker *et al.*, 2004; Proctor *et al.*, 2006; Sondrup *et al.*, 2006; Liu *et al.*, 2007b; Prestwich, 2010), in part by acting as a non-inflammatory barrier to cell migration. Electrophilic, thiol-reactive hyaluronan haloacetates can be mixed with CHMA-S to yield cross-linker-free sECMs (Serban and Prestwich, 2007). Other homo-

Table 1.1 Living HA hydrogels

Materials	Properties	Applications	References
Chemically crosslinked HA			
Thiolated HA, PEGDA	Rapid XL, non-inflammatory cell barrier	Scar-free wound healing	Shu *et al.* (2004b), Kirker *et al.* (2004)
Disulfide crosslinked HA	Slow XL, non-inflammatory cell barrier	Post-surgical adhesion prevention	Serban *et al.* (2008b), Shu *et al.* (2002), Liu *et al.* (2004, 2005a)
Carboxymethylated, thiolated HA (CMHA-S), PEGDA	Rapid XL, non-inflammatory cell barrier	Post-surgical adhesion prevention	Liu *et al.* (2005b, 2007a), Sondrup *et al.* (2006), Connors *et al.* (2007), Park *et al.* (2006)
CMHA-S, PEGDA	Rapid XL, non-inflammatory cell barrier	Scar-free wound healing	Proctor *et al.* (2006), Prestwich *et al.* (2010), Vanderhooft *et al.* (2007), Kirker *et al.* (2002), Yang *et al.* (2010), Chung and Burdick (2009)
Hyaluronan haloacetate (HAHA)	Crosslinker-free gelation	3D cell culture	Serban and Prestwich (2007)
CMHA-S, TetraPAcs	Rapid XL, robust	Bioprinting	Skardal *et al.* (2010a)
Tyramine crosslinked HA	Enzymatic crosslinking	3D cell culture	Darr and Calabro (2009)
Click chemistry crosslinked HA	Azide/alkyne crosslinking	3D cell culture	Crescenzi *et al.* (2007)
Ugi condensation crosslinked HA	Anticoagulant	Blood-contacting materials	Crescenzi *et al.* (2002)
Photochemically crosslinked HA			
Methacrylated HA	Photocrosslinkable, robust	3D cell culture	Burdick *et al.* (2005), Prata *et al.* (2010)
HA, PEODA	Photocrosslinkable, robust	Chondrogenesis	Sharma *et al.* (2007)
Glycidyl methacrylate-HA, PEG-peptides	Bioactive	Soft tissue engineering	Leach *et al.* (2004)
Methacrylated HA and gelatin	Photocrosslinkable, robust	Bioprinting	Skardal *et al.* (2010b)

Table 1.1 Continued

Materials	Properties	Applications	References
Dynamic and reversibly crosslinked HA			
Disulfide PEGDA	Dissolves in NAcCys or glutathione	Cell recovery	Zhang *et al.* (2008)
Polymer silica nanocomposite	Thixotropic, shear thinning	Cell recovery	Pek *et al.* (2008)
Gold nanoparticles, CMHA-S, gelatin-DTPH	Thioxotropic, shear thinning	Bioprinting, cell recovery	Skardal *et al.* (2010c)
Adding cell attachment factors			
CMHA-S, PEGDA, RGD peptide	Rapid XL, cell attachment	3D cell culture	Shu *et al.* (2004a)
CMHA-S, PEGDA, fibronectin	Rapid XL, cell attachment	3D cell culture	Ghosh *et al.* (2006)
CMHA-S, gelatin-DTPH, PEGDA	Rapid XL, cell attachment	3D cell culture, tissue engineering	Shu *et al.* (2004b), Vanderhooft *et al.* (2008), Prestwich *et al.* (2006)
Controlled release of growth factors			
HP-DTPH, CS-DTPH	Growth factor sequestration	Controlled growth factor release	Liu *et al.* (2007a)
CMHA-S, gelatin-DTPH, PEGDA, heparin-DTPH	Growth factor sequestration	Controlled growth factor release	Liu *et al.* (2007a), Pike *et al.* (2006), Peattie *et al.* (2004, 2006, 2008), Riley *et al.* (2006), Hosack *et al.* (2008), Elia *et al.* (2010), Zhao *et al.* (2008)
HA, PEGDA, BSA-PLGA microspheres	Growth factor sequestration	Controlled growth factor release	Leach and Schmidt (2005)
Cell differentiation factors			
HA, optional ECM components	Phenotype maintenance	Stem cell culture	Turner *et al.* (2008)
Matrigel, CMHA-S, gelatin-DTPH, heparin-DTPH	Phenotype maintenance	Stem cell culture	Van Hoof *et al.* (2008)
HA, poly(NiPAAm-co-AAc)	Growth factor sequestration	Chondrogenesis	Choi *et al.* (2007)

Methacrylated HA	Phenotype maintenance	Stem cell culture	Proctor *et al.* (2006)
Tuning mechanics and adding patterns			
HA, fibronectin	Tunable stiffness	3D cell culture	Ghosh *et al.* (2007)
CMHA-S, gelatin-DTPH, PEGDA, heparin-DTPH	Tunable stiffness	Stem cell culture	Seib *et al.* (2009)
CMHA-S, gelatin-DTPH, PEGDA	Centrifugal casting	Tubular tissue constructs	Mironov *et al.* (2005, 2008)
HA, collagen	Photocrosslinkable, robust	Photopatterned	Suri and Schmidt (2009)
Methacrylated HA	Photocrosslinkable, robust	Patterned by soft-lithography	Khademhosseini *et al.* (2006)
HA	Hydrogel beads	Suspension culture	Bae *et al.* (2006)
Collagen-coated dextran	Microcarriers	Suspension culture	Hjelm *et al.* (2002)
CMHA-S, gelatin-DTPH, PEGDA microcarriers	Porous sponges for cell attachment	Suspension culture	Skardal *et al.* (2010d)
Using injectable sECMs *in vivo*			
CMHA-S, gelatin-DTPH, heparin-DTPH	Growth factor sequestration	Neural tissue filler	Zhong *et al.* (2010)
HA, IKVAV peptides or laminin	Neural outgrowth	Brain lesion repair	Wei *et al.* (2007), Hou *et al.* (2005)
CMHA-S, gelatin-DTPH, PEGDA	Rapid XL, cell attachment	Adipose tissue engineering	Flynn *et al.* (2008)
CMHA-S, gelatin-DTPH, PEGDA	Rapid XL, cell attachment	Drug testing	Prestwich *et al.* (2007), Zhang *et al.* (2009), Xu *et al.* (2009)
CMHA-S, gelatin-DTPH, PEGDA	Rapid XL, cell attachment	Cell delivery	Liu *et al.* (2006), Serban *et al.* (2008c)
CMHA-S, gelatin-DTPH, PEGDA	Rapid XL, cell attachment	Tumor xenograft	Serban *et al.* (2008b), Liu *et al.* (2007c), Scaife *et al.* (2008), Zhang *et al.* (2009), Xu *et al.* (2009)
HA- based sECM	Stem cell culture and injection	Therapeutic MSC delivery	Compte *et al.* (2009)
CMHA-S, PEGDA	Rapid XL, non-inflammatory cell barrier	Vocal fold repair	Hansen *et al.* (2005), (Duflo *et al.* (2006a, 2006b)
CMHA-S, gelatin-DTPH, PEGDA	Rapid XL, cell attachment	Vocal fold repair	Thibeault *et al.* (2009)
HA microgels	Dual crosslinked networks	Vocal fold repair	Jia *et al.* (2006)

bifunctional PEG derivatives have also been used as crosslinkers, including PEG di-maleimide which led to gelation of CMHA-S in less than 1 min (Vanderhooft *et al.*, 2007).

Moving beyond bifunctional crosslinkers to polyvalent crosslinkers can have surprising outcomes in forming HA hydrogels. We recently described the synthesis of two new four-armed polyethylene glycol (PEG) acrylate derivatives, the TetraPAcs. These novel linkers were used to co-crosslink thiolated hyaluronic acid and gelatin derivatives into extrudable sECM hydrogels containing up to 25 million cells/mL. After optimization of the composition, rheology, biocompatibility, and physical handling characteristics, the TetraPAc sECMs were used to bioprint a proof-of-concept tubular construct using an open-source rapid prototyping device (Skardal *et al.*, 2010d).

Double crosslinked networks with enhanced mechanical strength have been designed by embedding sub-micron HA hydrogel particles within a second covalently crosslinked network. The particles were functionalized with aldehydes by sodium periodate oxidation and covalently linked to the surrounding network composed of a hydrazide derivative of HA (Jha *et al.*, 2009). Tyramine-based HA gels are an example of enzymatic crosslinking that shows potential utility for cell encapsulation (Darr *et al.*, 2009). Peroxidase catalyzes the formation of stable amide bonds between the free carboxyl groups on HA and the free amine groups on tyramine under cytocompatible conditions. Click chemistry has also been used to form gels by mixing solutions of HA with alkyne or azide functionalized side chains (Crescenzi *et al.*, 2007). The dipolar cycloaddition reaction occurs rapidly enough to ensure homogenous distribution of yeast cells, but currently requires catalysis by copper, which may not be compatible with all cell types. Gels with excellent anticoagulant properties have been prepared from partially deacetylated HA with minimal chain degradation using a Ugi multicomponent condensation reaction (Crescenzi *et al.*, 2002). A recent review tabulates a series of bifunctional crosslinkers and their reaction conditions (Schiller *et al.*, 2010).

1.3.3 Photochemical crosslinking of HA

In addition to providing a rapid homogenous gelation mechanism for mechanically robust materials, photochemical crosslinking permits spatiotemporal patterning of scaffold cellular environments in an early step toward fabrication of constructs with tissue-level organization. The process can be limited by the depth of light penetration, the resolution of refracted incident light and chemical reaction, and by toxicity of photoinitiators. An excellent review describes photopolymerizable and degradable biomaterials for tissue engineering applications (Ifkovits and Burdick, 2007). A few noteworthy examples are summarized here.

A series of photopolymerized HA networks was characterized over a range of molecular weights, concentrations, swelling ratios, compressive moduli, and degradation times and evaluated for the formation of neocartilage from cultured chondroctyes *in vitro* (Burdick *et al.*, 2005). Analogous methyacrylated HA hydrogels proved to be an effective environment for maintaining long-term self-renewal of human embryonic stem cells (hESCs), maintaining an undifferentiated state, and formation of embryoid bodies with full differentiation capacity (Gerecht *et al.*, 2007). Photocrosslinkable and slow-degrading glycidyl methacrylate-HA (GMHA), which are themselves bioactive and appropriate for soft tissue scaffolding, have been functionalized by conjugation with acrylated PEG and PEG-peptide complexes (Leach *et al.*, 2004). In a new application, a methacrylated ethanolamide derivative of gelatin was combined with methacrylated HA and partially crosslinked to give an extrudable gel-like fluid. Cell-containing and acellular gels were printed through a needle in robust structures, followed by a second photocrosslinking to create a bioprinted tubular construct (Skardal *et al.*, 2010c). The viscoelasticity of methacrylated HA gels can be varied by adjusting the degree of methacrylation and by post-processing. Lightly crosslinked near-gels and emulsion-crosslinked-microspheres are strongly viscoelastic, while centrifuged microspheres formed elastic microgels (Prata *et al.*, 2010).

1.3.4 Dynamic and reversible crosslinking of HA

In many cases, it is desirable to recover cells for analysis or subsequent culture following encapsulation and expansion in sECMs. Incorporating disulfide groups within PEGDA crosslinkers allows the use of *N*-acetyl-cysteine (NAcCys) or glutathione to induce a thiol-disulfide which dissolves the gel, permitting cell recovery under non-enzymatic conditions (Zhang *et al.*, 2008). Shear thinning gels exhibit the unique property of transient network disruption upon the application of shear force, resulting in a large decrease in viscosity. One example is a thixotropic polymer-silica nanocomposite which can be loaded with cells after vortexing, allowed to resolidify, and vortexed again for cell recovery (Pek *et al.*, 2008). The network recovers and viscosity is restored upon removal of shear force. Shear thinning also holds promise for cell delivery by injection and for bioprinting. One such shear thinning gel was formed by the lateral self assembly of amphiphilic hair-pin peptides (Haines-Butterick *et al.*, 2007). Network formation was triggered by charge-screening with salts such as those found in culture medium (Haines-Butterick *et al.*, 2007). Most recently, gold nanoparticles were employed as nanomeric, multifunctional crosslinkers for the thiol-modified macromonomers comprising the sECM described above. These AuNP-crosslinked HA-gelatin sECM hydrogels exhibited the unique property of dynamic crosslinking. That is, initially formed bioprinted hydrogel macrofilaments held together by intragel crosslinks could, within hours, form intergel crosslinks. This led to fusion of the cellularized macrofilaments and facilitated cell growth and maturation within the printed constructs. Moreover, addition of

NAcCys effectively dissolved the hydrogel, releasing any encapsulated cells (Skardal *et al.*, 2010b).

1.4 Adding function to hyaluronic acid (HA) matrices

1.4.1 Cell attachment factors

Even lacking appropriate cell attachment factors, HA-only gels have important uses in tissue engineering and regenerative medicine. In preclinical and clinical settings, crosslinked CMHA gels can promote wound repair for cutaneous wounds (Kirker *et al.*, 2002, 2004; Prestwich, 2010), sinus surgery (Proctor *et al.*, 2006), and ophthalmic injuries (Yang *et al.*, 2010), relieve joint pain (Bellamy *et al.*, 2006), and serve as cell barriers for adhesion prevention in abdominal (Liu *et al.*, 2005a), tracheal (Sondrup *et al.*, 2006), pericardial (Connors *et al.*, 2007), and otological (Park *et al.*, 2006) surgical interventions (Liu *et al.*, 2007b). Selected cell types, including chondrocytes (Chung *et al.*, 2009, Burdick *et al.*, 2005) and embryonic stem cells (Gerecht *et al.*, 2007) also grow and proliferate in HA-only environments. However for most adherent cells, cell attachment factors are required. The signals required for engaging integrin interactions necessary for tissue culture and cell delivery applications can be provided by RGD peptides (Shu *et al.*, 2004a), fibronectin domains (Ghosh *et al.*, 2006), laminin peptides, or by co-gelation with gelatin-DTPH (Shu *et al.*, 2004b). Gelatin-DTPH, a thiol modified denatured collagen, was developed for use with CMHA-S and an appropriate crosslinker. Gelatin content reduces both gel stiffness and degradation rate (Vanderhooft *et al.*, 2008). This soft matrix provides a biomimetic three-dimensional environment for culture of a variety of cell lines with good preservation of phenotype and superior cell proliferation and matrix remodeling compared to Matrigel (Serban *et al.*, 2008a). The following cell lines have been encapsulated and cultured in these modified HA/gelatin materials with good attachment, proliferation, and tissue-like morphology: neonatal human dermal fibroblasts, T31 human tracheal scar fibroblasts, L929 and NIH 3T3 murine fibroblasts, MCF10A human breast cells, human breast epithelial cells, human adipose-derived stem cells, HEPG2-C3A human hepatic cells, rat primary hepatocytes, Int 407 human intestinal cells, human mesenchymal stem cells, rat primary bone marrow stromal cells, and pig primary chondrocytes (Prestwich *et al.*, 2006; Serban *et al.*, 2008a).

1.4.2 Controlled release of growth factors with proteoglycan mimetics

Incorporation and slow release of growth factors from thiol-modified hydrogels can be accomplished by incorporation with thiol-modified heparin (HP-DTPH) or chondroitin sulfate (CS-DTPH) (Liu *et al.*, 2007a). This formulation creates in effect a CS or HS proteoglycan (PG) mimetic sECM, since the sulfated GAG is covalently bound to the sECM in the same way that a PG has covalenty linked GAG chains to non-covalently immobilize growth factors *in vivo*. For example, 0.03% w/w HP-DTPH reduced vascular endothelial growth factor (VEGF) release from 30% to 21% over the course of 42 days, while gelatin increased augmented release rate (Pike *et al.*, 2006; Peattie *et al.*, 2008). Growth factors can be incorporated in Heprasil, in which thiolated heparin is covalently linked into the HA-gelatin sECM. VEGF, basic fibroblast growth factor (bFGF), angiopoietin-1 (Ang-1), and keratinocyte growth factor (KGF) individually increased microvessel density and maturity and showed synergistic effects in Heprasil films implanted in mouse ear pinnae (Peattie *et al.*, 2004, 2006, 2008; Riley *et al.*, 2006; Hosack *et al.*, 2008; Elia *et al.*, 2010). Schmidt *et al.* extended the release profile from photocrosslinked HA/PEGDA gels by embedding drug-loaded BSA-poly(lactic-co-glycolic acid) microspheres within the hydrogel (Leach and Schmidt, 2005).

An alternative to cell delivery *per se* is to attract endogenous stem cells and precursor cells to the defect site for *de novo* tissue regeneration. Hepatocyte growth factor (HGF) induces migration of MSCs *in vitro* but is rapidly degraded by proteolysis *in vivo*. Extended, localized delivery of HGF was achieved with Heprasil sECM hydrogels, and the sECM composition could be optimized for controlled release of HGF that resulted in recruitment of human bone marrow MSCs into the scaffold *in vitro* (Zhao *et al.*, 2008).

1.4.3 Cell differentiation factors and other effectors

Whether in development or culture, cells depend not only on soluble biomolecules but also upon the surrounding ECM for differentiation cues or phenotype maintenance. While engineering a complete recapitulation of the developmental process remains a lofty and perhaps unrealistic goal, considerable progress has been made in preventing and directing stem cell differentiation with both soluble and matrix differentiation factors. Design criteria have been established for bioartificial stem cell niches intended to provide micro-environments for expansion of stem cells and maintenance of their undifferentiated phenotype (Prestwich *et al.*, 2010). This also includes providing mechanical and biochemical cues for cell survival, proliferation, migration, and invasion, as well as we practical considerations for biological, regulatory, commercial, and clinical success. The essential roles of HA in embryonic development makes it a natural candidate for such applications (Fraser *et al.*, 1997). In fact, advanced non-invasive NMR metabolomic profiling techniques showed that soft, HA-only hydrogels were able to maintain hepatic stem cell and hepatoblast lineages, while incorporation of other ECM components varied the expression of the key metabolites studied (Turner *et al.*, 2008). Soft hydrogels were also able to maintain proteomic and morphological indicators characteristic of 3D Matrigel culture conditions superior to that of feeder layers (Van Hoof *et al.*, 2008).

In vitro and *in vivo* studies showed that embedding mesenchymal stem cells (MSC) in photocrosslinked PEGDA/HA hydrogels with and without TGF-β3 resulted in many-fold upregulation of chondrogenesis (Chung *et al.*, 2009). Furthermore, bone marrow-derived mesenchymal stem cells encapsulated in photopolymerized PEGDA with HA and TGF-β3 and implanted subcutaneously in nude mice produced higher quality cartilage than groups with either additive or the control (Sharma *et al.*, 2007), though another *in vitro* study showed stronger cartilage expression with chondroitin sulfate than with HA (Hwang *et al.*, 2007). Embedding rabbit chondrocytes in an injectable poly(NiPAAm-co-AAc)/HA loaded with dexamethasone and TGF-β-3 greatly increased the cell number, maintained their phenotype, and resulted in cartilage production (Choi *et al.*, 2007).

1.4.4 Tuning mechanics and adding patterns

Attempts to engineer the cellular microenvironment would be wholly inadequate without careful attention to the mechanical properties upon which cellular behavior is so dependent. For example, human dermal fibroblasts cultured on stiffer substrates exhibit a more stretched morphology, proliferated more abundantly, and migrated more slowly than on softer surfaces (Ghosh *et al.*, 2007). Proteomic screens revealed that compliance affects not only the phenotype and differentiation state of MSCs, but also their paracrine secretion. IL-8, in particular, was upregulated in substrates with compliance relevant to muscle tissue as compared to softer substrates comparable to brain tissue (Seib *et al.*, 2009). Stiffness is represented by Young's modulus (E) or shear modulus (G) and can be adjusted with composition. For example, thiol-modified gel stiffness can be tuned from 10 to 3500 Pa by varying concentration of CMHA-S, Gelatin-DTPH, and PEGDA, molecular weight, and degree of thiol substitution (Liu *et al.*, 2005b; Vanderhooft *et al.*, 2008). The elastic modulus for an equal mixture of components at 0.8% w/V each is 800 Pa, a value comparable to the stiffness of adipose or hepatic tissue (Vanderhooft *et al.*, 2008). Stiffer hydrogels can be achieved by increasing concentration and incorporating other macromers or crosslinking agents, such as photopolymerized methacrylic anhydride, which attained a modulus of ~100 kPa (Burdick *et al.*, 2005).

However biochemically relevant, a homogenous matrix system cannot fully replicate the diverse microenvironment of tissues. Ideally, mechanical and other matrix cues should be differentially defined in three dimensions to encourage the organization of encapsulated cells into functional biological tissues. Photo-patterning techniques can control stiffness and swelling with high spatial resolution in two or three dimensions by exposing photoactive crosslinkers to light, especially through patterned masks (Suri and Schmidt, 2009). These patterned crosslinks can be incorporated within existing gels as an interpenetrating network. Robust materials can be combined with soft-lithography techniques to micromold gels, creating microchannels and other structures (Khademhosseini *et al.*, 2006). Providing microchannels or another form of perfusable vessel network will be critical for culturing tissues thicker than the 200–400 μm oxygen diffusion limit which holds back the field of tissue engineering at present. Centrifugal casting (Mironov *et al.*, 2005; 2008) of gel-encapsulated cells can created tubular constructs. For example, 5 mm vessels with high viable cell densities were created from small intestine submucosa tubular scaffolds with laser-machined micropores (Kasyanov *et al.*, 2008). Bioprinting efforts are beginning to take another approach at providing 3D organization: printing out encapsulated cells line by line and layer upon layer (Mironov *et al.*, 2007). The delivery matrix may be gel precursors to be chemically or photocrosslinked after printing (Skardal *et al.*, 2010c) or shear-thinning gels which become liquid under shear stress and subsequently recover their viscosity (Skardal *et al.*, 2010b). Porous beads and other microcarriers (Hjelm *et al.*, 2002) suspended in culture media can also serve as injectable cell or organoid substrates.

Recently, microcarrier beads were coated with the Extracel (HA-gelatin) sECM using disulfide chemistry to allow enzyme-free cell detachment after cell proliferation in 3-D in a rotating wall vessel (RWV) bioreactor designed to mimic the low fluid shear stress environments in the body. Human intestinal epithelial cells (Int 407) formed multilayered cell aggregates on the sECM beads, which could be harvested using *N*-acetyl cysteine to dissolve the gel and release the cell clusters. The clusters could be further expanded in a scaffold-free state in the RWV bioreactor to produce spheroidal microtissues that have utility for studying host-pathogen interactions, evaluating new therapeutic agents, and creating clusters for bioprinting and cell therapy (Skardal *et al.*, 2010a).

1.5 Using injectable synthetic extracellular matrices (sECMs) *in vivo*

The success of cell therapies has been limited by poor cell retention at the site of injection, poor cell survival, inadequate phenotype maintenance, and incomplete cellular integration with existing tissues (Yeo *et al.*, 2007; Burst *et al.*, 2010). Improved delivery matrices have shown recent promise in addressing these challenges. In one example, the covalent heparin-gelatin-HA sECM hydrogel described above (HyStem-HP) promoted the survival of neuroprogenitors cells injected into necrotic stroke cavities and reduced inflammatory infiltration (Zhong *et al.*, 2010). Second, permissive HA matrices with IKVAV peptides (Wei *et al.*, 2007) or laminin (Hou *et al.*, 2005) aided repair of rat brain lesions and recruited axons, supporting glial cells, and blood vessels. Third, in a new approach to adipose tissue engineering, a scaffold was combined with cells and an HA-derived hydrogel (Flynn *et al.*, 2008). Thus subcutaneous implantation of primary human adipose-derived stem cells in placental decellularized matrix with crosslinked HA into athymic mice led to the production of human adipose tissue. The implants retained their volume, supported adipogenesis and angiogenesis, and displayed evidence of host integration (Flynn *et al.*, 2008). Fourth, human hepatoblasts and hepatic stem cells have been maintained and expanded in an sECM hydrogels. Primary rat hepatocytes cultured in thiol-modified HA and gelatin retained cytochrome P-450 activity, a key metabolic function for drug testing models (Prestwich *et al.*, 2007). Finally, the same versatile sECM has also been used to deliver mesenchymal stem cells to full-thickness defects in the patellar groove of femoral articular cartilage in rabbits, resulting in repaired defects filled with well-integrated, translucent cartilage after 12 weeks (Liu *et al.*, 2006).

The thiol-modified macromolecular components of the sECM hydrogels can be conveniently prepared for cell encapsulation and injection. Cells can be incorporated into a non-viscous medium, and the cell suspension precursor can be injected during gelation, which continues *in situ* to retain the encapsulated cells at the site of injection (Serban *et al.*, 2008b). This strategy has been particularly useful in developing orthotopic tumor models in mice useful for drug development, cancer research, and potential applications in personalized medicine. The resulting tumor xenografts exhibited improved cancer incidence, growth, consistency of size, tissue integration, localization, vascularization (and reduced necrosis), and general animal health compared with cell injection in serum free medium (Liu *et al.*, 2007c). Tumor growth and metastasis were also enhanced in a pancreatic adenocarcinoma model (Scaife *et al.*, 2008). The following human cancer lines have been injected in CMHA-S with gelatin: colon (HCT-116, Caco-2), breast (MCF-7, Sk-Br-3, MDA-MB-231, MDA-MB-468), ovarian (OVCAR-3, SK-OV-3, and pancreatic (MiaPaCa-2) (Prestwich *et al.*, 2006). Notably, breast cancer (Zhang *et al.*, 2009, Xu *et al.*, 2009) and non-small cell lung carcinoma (Xu and Prestwich, 2010) xenograft models have proven effective for evaluating promising new cancer drugs that inhibit oncogenic lipid signaling pathways. Analogous materials have been used to confine MSCs expressing luciferase or secreting bispecific αCEA/αCD3 diabody (MSCdAb) in tumor xenografts. The latter application resulted in activation of transplanted human lymphocytes and tumor regression over the course of 6 weeks of diabody release (Compte *et al.*, 2009).

HA-derived sECM injections also show promise in vocal fold repair, reducing fibrosis and improving elasticity and viscosity (Hansen *et al.*, 2005). Analysis of ECM production genes indicated an enhanced the short-term wound healing response (Duflo *et al.*, 2006a). Including gelatin with the HA network further improved wound tissue biomechanics (Duflo *et al.*, 2006b). Implanting autologous fibroblasts in scarred rabbit vocal folds two months after injury improved elasticity and viscosity while inclusion of sECMs accelerated matrix production (Thibeault *et al.*, 2009). Doubly crosslinked networks composed of HA microgels and crosslinked hydrogels with tunable viscoelasticity in the relevant frequency range have also been proposed for vocal fold healing (Jia *et al.*, 2006).

1.6 Conclusions and future trends

The vast complexity of developmental biology defies attempts to recapitulate its intricacies by precisely engineering the desired outcome. Tissues emerge *in vivo* from the dynamic interactions of a host of differentiating cells, biochemical signaling gradients, mechanical stimuli, and matrix cues that are coordinated in space and time (Burdick and Vunjak-Novakovic, 2009). Lacking both the information and capacity to adequately manipulate this environment, we have selected a permissive strategy, in which a modular, simplified mimic of the ECM allows the rich interactive capacity of cells to remodel the environment (Prestwich, 2007). Remarkable results can be achieved with biologically relevant synthetic, semi-synthetic, and naturally derived materials. The platforms can be modular and versatile, incorporating various ECM and biochemical components for diverse applications (Serban and Prestwich, 2008b). Materials that cannot overcome biological, regulatory, and commercial hurdles will be of limited use in the clinic. The ongoing quest will be to achieve optimal reductions to the minimum essential cell-instructive cues with simple biomimetic materials, and to 'let biology do the heavy lifting' (Prestwich, 2007).

1.7 References

Allison D D and Grande-Allen K J (2006), 'Review. Hyaluronan: a powerful tissue engineering tool', *Tissue Eng*, 12, 2131–40.

Bae K H, Yoon J J and Park T G (2006), 'Fabrication of hyaluronic acid hydrogel beads for cell encapsulation', *Biotechnol Prog*, 22, 297–302.

Bellamy N, Campbell J, Robinson V, Gee T, Bourne R and Wells G (2006), 'Viscosupplementation for the treatment of osteoarthritis of the knee', *Cochrane Database Syst Rev*, CD005321.

Brigham M D, Bick A, Lo E, Bendali A, Burdick J A and Khademhosseini A (2009), 'Mechanically robust and bioadhesive collagen and photocrosslinkable hyaluronic acid semi-interpenetrating networks', *Tissue Eng Part A*, 15, 1645–53.

Burdick J A, Chung C, Jia X, Randolph M A and Langer R (2005), 'Controlled degradation and mechanical behavior of photopolymerized hyaluronic acid networks', *Biomacromolecules*, 6, 386–91.

Burdick J A and Vunjak-Novakovic G (2009), 'Engineered microenvironments for controlled stem cell differentiation', *Tissue Eng Part A*, 15, 205–19.

Burst V R, Gillis M, Putsch F, Herzog R, Fischer J H, Heid P, Muller-Ehmsen J, Schenk K, Fries J W, Baldamus C A and Benzing T (2010), 'Poor cell survival limits the beneficial impact of mesenchymal stem cell transplantation on acute kidney injury', *Nephron Exp Nephrol*, 114, e107–16.

Choi S J, Na K, Kim S, Woo D G, Sun B K, Chung H M and Park K H (2007), 'Combination of ascorbate and growth factor (tgf beta-3) in thermo-reversible hydrogel constructs embedded with rabbit chondrocytes for neocartilage formation', *J Biomed Mater Res A*, 83, 897–905.

Chung C and Burdick J A (2009), 'Influence of three-dimensional hyaluronic acid microenvironments on mesenchymal stem cell chondrogenesis', *Tissue Eng Part A*, 15, 243–54.

Compte M, Cuesta A M, Sanchez-Martin D, Alonso-Camino V, Vicario J L, Sanz L and Alvarez-Vallina L (2009), 'Tumor immunotherapy using gene-modified human mesenchymal stem cells loaded into synthetic extracellular matrix scaffolds', *Stem Cells*, 27, 753–60.

Connors R C, Muir J J, Liu Y, Reiss G R, Kouretas P C, Whitten M G, Sorenson T K, Prestwich G D and Bull D A (2007), 'Postoperative pericardial adhesion prevention using carbylan-sx in a rabbit model', *J Surg Res*, 140, 237–42.

Crescenzi V, Francescangeli A, Renier D and Bellini D (2002), 'New cross-linked and sulfated derivatives of partially deacetylated hyaluronan: synthesis and preliminary characterization', *Biopolymers*, 64, 86–94.

Crescenzi V, Cornelio L, Di Meo C, Nardecchia S and Lamanna R (2007), 'Novel hydrogels via click chemistry: synthesis and potential biomedical applications', *Biomacromolecules*, 8, 1844–50.

Darr A and Calabro A (2009), 'Synthesis and characterization of tyramine-based hyaluronan hydrogels', *J Mater Sci Mater Med*, 20, 33–44.

Duflo S, Thibeault S L, Li W, Shu X Z and Prestwich G (2006a), 'Effect of a synthetic extracellular matrix on vocal fold lamina propria gene expression in early wound healing', *Tissue Eng*, 12, 3201–7.

Duflo S, Thibeault S L, Li W, Shu X Z and Prestwich G D (2006b), 'Vocal fold tissue repair *in vivo* using a synthetic extracellular matrix', *Tissue Eng*, 12, 2171–80.

Elia R, Fuegy P W, VanDelden A, Firpo M A, Prestwich G D and Peattie R A (2010), 'Stimulation of *in vivo* angiogenesis by *in situ* crosslinked, dual growth factor-loaded, glycosaminoglycan hydrogels', *Biomaterials*, 31, 4630–8.

Flynn L, Prestwich G D, Semple J L and Woodhouse K A (2008), 'Adipose tissue engineering *in vivo* with adipose-derived stem cells on naturally derived scaffolds', *J Biomed Mater Res A*, 89, 929–41.

Fraser J R, Laurent T C and Laurent U B (1997), 'Hyaluronan: its nature, distribution, functions and turnover', *J Intern Med*, 242, 27–33.

Gerecht S, Burdick J A, Ferreira L S, Townsend S A, Langer R and Vunjak-Novakovic G (2007), 'Hyaluronic acid hydrogel for controlled self-renewal and differentiation of human embryonic stem cells', *Proc Natl Acad Sci USA*, 104, 11298–303.

Ghosh K, Ren X D, Shu X Z, Prestwich G D and Clark R A (2006), 'Fibronectin functional domains coupled to hyaluronan stimulate adult human dermal fibroblast responses critical for wound healing', *Tissue Eng*, 12, 601–13.

Ghosh K, Pan Z, Guan E, Ge S, Liu Y, Nakamura T, Ren X D, Rafailovich M and Clark R A (2007), 'Cell adaptation to a physiologically relevant ECM mimic with different viscoelastic properties', *Biomaterials*, 28, 671–9.

Haines-Butterick L, Rajagopal K, Branco M, Salick D, Rughani R, Pilarz M, Lamm M S, Pochan D J and Schneider J P (2007), 'Controlling hydrogelation kinetics by peptide design for three-dimensional encapsulation and injectable delivery of cells', *Proc Natl Acad Sci USA*, 104, 7791–6.

Hansen J K, Thibeault S L, Walsh J F, Shu X Z and Prestwich G D (2005), '*In vivo* engineering of the vocal fold extracellular matrix with injectable hyaluronic acid

hydrogels: early effects on tissue repair and biomechanics in a rabbit model', *Ann Otol Rhinol Laryngol*, 114, 662–70.
Hjelm B E, Berta A N, Nickerson C A, Arntzen C J and Herbst-Kralovetz M M (2002), 'Development and characterization of a three-dimensional organotypic human vaginal epithelial cell model', *Biol Reprod*, 82, 617–27.
Hosack L W, Firpo M A, Scott J A, Prestwich G D and Peattie R A (2008), 'Microvascular maturity elicited in tissue treated with cytokine-loaded hyaluronan-based hydrogels', *Biomaterials*, 29, 2336–47.
Hou S, Xu Q, Tian W, Cui F, Cai Q, Ma J and Lee I S (2005), 'The repair of brain lesion by implantation of hyaluronic acid hydrogels modified with laminin', *J Neurosci Methods*, 148, 60–70.
Hwang N S, Varghese S, Lee H J, Theprungsirikul P, Canver A, Sharma B and Elisseeff J (2007), 'Response of zonal chondrocytes to extracellular matrix-hydrogels', *FEBS Lett*, 581, 4172–8.
Ifkovits J L and Burdick J A (2007), 'Review: photopolymerizable and degradable biomaterials for tissue engineering applications', *Tissue Eng*, 13, 2369–85.
Jha A K, Hule R A, Jiao T, Teller S S, Clifton R J, Duncan R L, Pochan D J and Jia X (2009), 'Structural analysis and mechanical characterization of hyaluronic acid-based doubly cross-linked networks', *Macromolecules*, 42, 537–546.
Jia X, Yeo Y, Clifton R J, Jiao T, Kohane D S, Kobler J B, Zeitels S M and Langer R (2006), 'Hyaluronic acid-based microgels and microgel networks for vocal fold regeneration', *Biomacromolecules*, 7, 3336–44.
Kasyanov V A, Hodde J, Hiles M C, Eisenberg C, Eisenberg L, De Castro L E F, Ozolanta I, Murovska M, Fraughn R A, Prestwich G D R, Markwald R, Mironov V (2008), 'Rapid biofabrication of tubular tissue construct by centrifugal casting in a decellularized natural scaffold with laser-machined icropores', *J Mater Sci Mater Med*, 20, 329–37.
Khademhosseini A, Eng G, Yeh J, Fukuda J, Blumling J, 3rd, Langer R and Burdick J A (2006), 'Micromolding of photocrosslinkable hyaluronic acid for cell encapsulation and entrapment', *J Biomed Mater Res A*, 79, 522–32.
Khetan S, Chung C and Burdick J A (2009), 'Tuning hydrogel properties for applications in tissue engineering', *Conf Proc IEEE Eng Med Biol Soc*, 1, 2094–6.
Kirker K R, Luo Y, Nielson J H, Shelby J and Prestwich G D (2002), 'Glycosaminoglycan hydrogel films as bio-interactive dressings for wound healing', *Biomaterials*, 23, 3661–71.
Kirker K R, Luo Y, Morris S E, Shelby J and Prestwich G D (2004), 'Glycosaminoglycan hydrogels as supplemental wound dressings for donor sites', *J Burn Care Rehabil*, 25, 276–86.
Kuo J W and Prestwich G D (2010), 'Hyaluronic acid', in Ducheyne P, Healy K, Hutmacher D and Kirkpatrick J (Eds.) *Materials of biological origin – materials analysis and implant uses, comprehensive biomaterials*. Elsevier.
Laurent T C and Fraser J R (1986), 'The properties and turnover of hyaluronan', *Ciba Found Symp*, 124, 9–29.
Leach J B and Schmidt C E (2005), 'Characterization of protein release from photocrosslinkable hyaluronic acid-polyethylene glycol hydrogel tissue engineering scaffolds', *Biomaterials*, 26, 125–35.
Leach J B, Bivens K A, Collins C N and Schmidt C E (2004), 'Development of photocrosslinkable hyaluronic acid-polyethylene glycol-peptide composite hydrogels for soft tissue engineering', *J Biomed Mater Res A*, 70, 74–82.
Liu Y, Shu X Z, Gray S D and Prestwich G D (2004), 'Disulfide-crosslinked

hyaluronan-gelatin sponge: growth of fibrous tissue *in vivo*', *J Biomed Mater Res A*, 68, 142–9.
Liu Y, Li H, Shu X Z, Gray S D and Prestwich G D (2005a), 'Crosslinked hyaluronan hydrogels containing mitomycin c reduce postoperative abdominal adhesions', *Fertil Steril*, 83 Suppl 1, 1275–83.
Liu Y, Shu X Z and Prestwich G D (2005b), 'Biocompatibility and stability of disulfide-crosslinked hyaluronan films', *Biomaterials*, 26, 4737–46.
Liu Y, Shu X Z and Prestwich G D (2006), 'Osteochondral defect repair with autologous bone marrow-derived mesenchymal stem cells in an injectable, *in situ*, cross-linked synthetic extracellular matrix', *Tissue Eng*, 12, 3405–16.
Liu Y, Cai S, Shu X Z, Shelby J and Prestwich G D (2007a), 'Release of basic fibroblast growth factor from a crosslinked glycosaminoglycan hydrogel promotes wound healing', *Wound Repair Regen*, 15, 245–51.
Liu Y, Shu X Z and Prestwich G D (2007b), 'Reduced postoperative intra-abdominal adhesions using carbylan-sx, a semisynthetic glycosaminoglycan hydrogel', *Fertil Steril*, 87, 940–8.
Liu Y, Shu X Z and Prestwich G D (2007c), 'Tumor engineering: orthotopic cancer models in mice using cell-loaded, injectable, cross-linked hyaluronan-derived hydrogels', *Tissue Eng*, 13, 1091–101.
Mironov V, Kasyanov V, Shu X Z, Eisenberg C, Eisenberg L, Gonda S, Trusk T, Markwald R R and Prestwich G D (2005), 'Fabrication of tubular tissue constructs by centrifugal casting of cells suspended in an *in situ* crosslinkable hyaluronan-gelatin hydrogel', *Biomaterials*, 26, 7628–35.
Mironov V, Prestwich G D and Forgacs G (2007), 'Bioprinting living structures', *J Mater Chem*, 17, 2054–60.
Mironov V, Kasyanov V, Markwald R R and Prestwich G D (2008), 'Bioreactor-free tissue engineering: directed tissue assembly by centrifugal casting', *Expert Opin Biol Ther*, 8, 143–52.
Park A H, Hughes C W, Jackson A, Hunter L, McGill L, Simonsen S E, Alder S C, Shu X Z and Prestwich G D (2006), 'Crosslinked hydrogels for tympanic membrane repair', *Otolaryngol Head Neck Surg*, 135, 877–83.
Peattie R A, Nayate A P, Firpo M A, Shelby J, Fisher R J and Prestwich G D (2004), 'Stimulation of *in vivo* angiogenesis by cytokine-loaded hyaluronic acid hydrogel implants', *Biomaterials*, 25, 2789–98.
Peattie R A, Rieke E R, Hewett E M, Fisher R J, Shu X Z and Prestwich G D (2006), 'Dual growth factor-induced angiogenesis *in vivo* using hyaluronan hydrogel implants', *Biomaterials*, 27, 1868–75.
Peattie R A, Pike D B, Yu B, Cai S, Shu X Z, Prestwich G D, Firpo M A and Fisher R J (2008), 'Effect of gelatin on heparin regulation of cytokine release from hyaluronan-based hydrogels', *Drug Deliv*, 15, 389–97.
Pek Y S, Wan A C, Shekaran A, Zhuo L and Ying J Y (2008), 'A thixotropic nanocomposite gel for three-dimensional cell culture', *Nat Nanotechnol*, 3, 671–5.
Pike D B, Cai S, Pomraning K R, Firpo M A, Fisher R J, Shu X Z, Prestwich G D and Peattie R A (2006), 'Heparin-regulated release of growth factors *in vitro* and angiogenic response *in vivo* to implanted hyaluronan hydrogels containing vegf and bfgf', *Biomaterials*, 27, 5242–51.
Place E S, Evans N D and Stevens M M (2009), 'Complexity in biomaterials for tissue engineering', *Nat Mater*, 8, 457–70.
Prata J E, Barth T A, Bencherif S A and Washburn N R (2010), 'Complex fluids based on methacrylated hyaluronic acid', *Biomacromolecules*, 11, 769–75.

Prestwich G D (2007), 'Simplifying the extracellular matrix for 3-D cell culture and tissue engineering: a pragmatic approach', *J Cell Biochem*, 101, 1370–83.
Prestwich G D (2010), 'Clinical biomaterials for scar-free healing and localized delivery of cells and growth factors', *Wound Healing Society Yearbook (WHSYB) – Advances in Wound Care*, 1, 394–9.
Prestwich G D and Kuo J W (2008), 'Chemically-modified ha for therapy and regenerative medicine', *Curr Pharm Biotechnol*, 9, 242–5.
Prestwich G D, Shu X Z, Liu Y, Cai S, Walsh J F, Hughes C W, Ahmad S, Kirker K R, Yu B, Orlandi R R, Park A H, Thibeault S L, Duflo S and Smith M E (2006), 'Injectable synthetic extracellular matrices for tissue engineering and repair', *Adv Exp Med Biol*, 585, 125–33.
Prestwich G D, Liu Y, Yu B, Shu X Z and Scott A (2007), '3-D culture in synthetic extracellular matrices: new tissue models for drug toxicology and cancer drug discovery', *Adv Enzyme Regul*, 47, 196–207.
Prestwich G D, Ghaly T, Brudnicki P, Ratliff B and Goligorsky M S (2010), 'Bioartificial stem cell niches: engineering a regenerative microenvironment', in Goligorsky M S (Ed.) *Renegerative nephrology*. Elsevier, in press.
Proctor M, Proctor K, Shu X Z, McGill L D, Prestwich G D and Orlandi R R (2006), 'Composition of hyaluronan affects wound healing in the rabbit maxillary sinus', *Am J Rhinol*, 20, 206–11.
Riley C M, Fuegy P W, Firpo M A, Shu X Z, Prestwich G D and Peattie R A (2006), 'Stimulation of *in vivo* angiogenesis using dual growth factor-loaded crosslinked glycosaminoglycan hydrogels', *Biomaterials*, 27, 5935–43.
Scaife C L, Shea J E, Dai Q, Firpo M A, Prestwich G D and Mulvihill S J (2008), 'Synthetic extracellular matrix enhances tumor growth and metastasis in an orthotopic mouse model of pancreatic adenocarcinoma', *J Gastrointest Surg*, 12, 1074–80.
Schiller J, Becher J, Moller S, Nimptzsch K, Riemer T and Schnabelrauch M (2010), 'Synthesis and characterization of chemically modified glycosaminoglycans of the extracellular matrix', *Mini Reviews in Organic Chemistry*, in press.
Seib F P, Prewitz M, Werner C and Bornhauser M (2009), 'Matrix elasticity regulates the secretory profile of human bone marrow-derived multipotent mesenchymal stromal cells (mscs)', *Biochem Biophys Res Commun*, 389, 663–7.
Serban M A and Prestwich G D (2007), 'Synthesis of hyaluronan haloacetates and biology of novel cross-linker-free synthetic extracellular matrix hydrogels', *Biomacromolecules*, 8, 2821–8.
Serban M A and Prestwich G D (2008), 'Modular extracellular matrices: solutions for the puzzle', *Methods*, 45, 93–8.
Serban M A, Liu Y and Prestwich G D (2008a), 'Effects of extracellular matrix analogues on primary human fibroblast behavior', *Acta Biomater*, 4, 67–75.
Serban M A, Scott A and Prestwich G D (2008b), 'Use of hyaluronan-derived hydrogels for three-dimensional cell culture and tumor xenografts', *Curr Protoc Cell Biol*, Chapter 10, Unit 10 14.
Sharma B, Williams C G, Khan M, Manson P and Elisseeff J H (2007), '*In vivo* chondrogenesis of mesenchymal stem cells in a photopolymerized hydrogel', *Plast Reconstr Surg*, 119, 112–20.
Shu X Z, Liu Y, Luo Y, Roberts M C and Prestwich G D (2002), 'Disulfide cross-linked hyaluronan hydrogels', *Biomacromolecules*, 3, 1304–11.
Shu X Z, Ghosh K, Liu Y, Palumbo F S, Luo Y, Clark R A and Prestwich G D (2004a), 'Attachment and spreading of fibroblasts on an RGD peptide-modified injectable hyaluronan hydrogel', *J Biomed Mater Res A*, 68, 365–75.

Shu X Z, Liu Y, Palumbo F S, Luo Y and Prestwich G D (2004b), '*In situ* crosslinkable hyaluronan hydrogels for tissue engineering', *Biomaterials*, 25, 1339–48.

Skardal A, Sarker S, Crabbe A, Nickerson C A and Prestwich G D (2010a), 'Hyaluronan-gelatin coated microcarriers for spherical microtissue culture and recovery', *Biomaterials*, 31, 8426–35.

Skardal A, Zhang H, McCoard L, Oottamasathien S and Prestwich G D (2010b), 'Dynamically crosslinked gold nanoparticle – hyaluronan hydrogels', *Adv Mater*, doi:10.102.adma.201001436.

Skardal A, Zhang H, McCoard L, Xu X, Oottamasathien S and Prestwich G D (2010c), 'Photocrosslinkable hyaluronan-gelatin hydrogels for two-step bioprinting', *Tissue Eng Part A*, 16, 2675–85.

Skardal A, Zhang J and Prestwich G D (2010d), 'Bioprinting vessel-like constructs using hyaluronan hydrogels crosslinked with tetrahedral polyethylene glycol tetracrylates', *Biomaterials*, 31, 6173–81.

Sondrup C, Liu Y, Shu X Z, Prestwich G D and Smith M E (2006), 'Cross-linked hyaluronan-coated stents in the prevention of airway stenosis', *Otolaryngol Head Neck Surg*, 135, 28–35.

Suri S and Schmidt C E (2009), 'Photopatterned collagen-hyaluronic acid interpenetrating polymer network hydrogels', *Acta Biomater*, 5, 2385–97.

Thibeault S L, Klemuk S A, Smith M E, Leugers C and Prestwich G (2009), '*In vivo* comparison of biomimetic approaches for tissue regeneration of the scarred vocal fold', *Tissue Eng Part A*, 15, 1481–7.

Turner W S, Seagle C, Galanko J A, Favorov O, Prestwich G D, Macdonald J M and Reid L M (2008), 'Nuclear magnetic resonance metabolomic footprinting of human hepatic stem cells and hepatoblasts cultured in hyaluronan-matrix hydrogels', *Stem Cells*, 26, 1547–55.

Van Hoof D, Braam S R, Dormeyer W, Ward-van Oostwaard D, Heck A J, Krijgsveld J and Mummery C L (2008), 'Feeder-free monolayer cultures of human embryonic stem cells express an epithelial plasma membrane protein profile', *Stem Cells*, 26, 2777–81.

Vanderhooft J L, Mann B K and Prestwich G D (2007), 'Synthesis and characterization of novel thiol-reactive poly(ethylene glycol) cross-linkers for extracellular-matrix-mimetic biomaterials', *Biomacromolecules*, 8, 2883–9.

Vanderhooft J L, Alcoutlabi M, Magda J J and Prestwich G D (2008), 'Rheological properties of cross-linked hyaluronan-gelatin hydrogels for tissue engineering', *Macromol Biosci*, 9, 20–28.

Wei Y T, Tian W M, Yu X, Cui F Z, Hou S P, Xu Q Y and Lee I S (2007), 'Hyaluronic acid hydrogels with ikvav peptides for tissue repair and axonal regeneration in an injured rat brain', *Biomed Mater*, 2, S142–6.

Xu X and Prestwich G D (2010) 'Inhibition of tumor growth and angiogenesis by a lysophosphatidic acid antagonist in an engineered three-dimensional lung cancer xenograft model', *Cancer*, 116, 1739–50.

Xu X, Yang G, Zhang H and Prestwich G D (2009), 'Evaluating dual activity lpa receptor pan-antagonist/autotaxin inhibitors as anti-cancer agents *in vivo* using engineered human tumors', *Prostaglandins Other Lipid Mediat*, 89, 140–6.

Yang G, Espandar L, Mamalis N and Prestwich G D (2010), 'Accelerated repair of corneal epithelial abrasion and alkali burn injuries in rabbits with a crosslinked hyaluronan derivative', *Vet. Ophthalmology*, 13, 144–50.

Yeo Y, Geng W, Ito T, Kohane D S, Burdick J A and Radisic M (2007), 'Photocrosslinkable hydrogel for myocyte cell culture and injection', *J Biomed Mater Res B Appl Biomater*, 81, 312–22.

Zhang H, Xu X, Gajewiak J, Tsukahara R, Fujiwara Y, Liu J, Fells J I, Perygin D, Parrill A L, Tigyi G and Prestwich G D (2009), 'Dual activity lysophosphatidic acid receptor pan-antagonist/autotaxin inhibitor reduces breast cancer cell migration *in vitro* and causes tumor regression *in vivo*', *Cancer Res*, 69, 5441–9.

Zhang J, Skardal A and Prestwich G D (2008), 'Engineered extracellular matrices with cleavable crosslinkers for cell expansion and easy cell recovery', *Biomaterials*, 29, 4521–31.

Zhao J, Zhang N, Prestwich G D and Wen X (2008), 'Recruitment of endogenous stem cells for tissue repair', *Macromol Biosci*, 8, 836–42.

Zhong J, Chan A, Morad L, Kornblum H, Fan G and Carmichael S T (2010), 'Hydrogel matrix to support stem cell survival after brain transplantation in stroke', *Neurorehabilitation & Neural Repair*, 24, 636–44.

2

Designing ceramics for injectable bone graft substitutes

M. BOHNER, RMS Foundation, Switzerland

Abstract: In the last 15 years, a large number of commercial cement and pasty bone graft substitutes have been introduced. As a result, great efforts have been made to improve our understanding of the specific properties of these materials, such as injectability, cohesion, setting time (for cements), and *in vivo* properties. The aim of this chapter is to summarize our present knowledge in the field. Instead of just looking at scientific aspects, industrial needs will also be considered, including mixing and delivery, sterilization, and shelf-life.

Key words: putty, cement, bone graft substitute, calcium phosphate, injectable.

2.1 Introduction

A few million patients every year need a bone graft or bone graft substitute to repair a bone defect resulting from an injury or a disease. A large number of bone graft substitutes can be used: unprocessed or processed allogenic bone, animal-derived bone substitutes and synthetic bone substitutes, mostly ceramics.[1]

Even though the first studies dealing with ceramic bone substitutes are more than 100 years old,[2,3] it was only in the 1970s that research soared.[4–11] In the early days, studies were focused mainly on porous blocks and granules.[4,6,8–11] However, the discovery of calcium phosphate cements (CPC) in 1982–1983[12,13] opened up a new era in which the handling properties of bone graft substitute became of paramount importance.

Several new approaches have been proposed to improve them. For example, in 1986 Hanker[14] combined plaster of Paris with calcium phosphate granules to obtain an injectable and setting biphasic paste. In 1987, Klein *et al.* proposed to mix a sodium alginate solution with β-tricalcium phosphate (β-TCP; $Ca_3(PO_4)_2$; see Table 2.1) granules (0.5–1.0 mm in diameter) to obtain an injectable and hardening paste (hardening of the alginate molecules through crosslinking with Ca ions).[15] Similarly, Gerhart *et al.*[16,17] presented in 1988 a system consisting of gelatine solution, β-TCP granules (0.355–0.60 mm) and a crosslinker. In the mid-1990s two commercial CPC formulations were introduced.[18–20] These were followed by more than a dozen other commercial CPC formulations (Table 2.2).

Table 2.1 Main calcium phosphate compounds. The first six compounds precipitate at room temperature in aqueous systems. The last six compounds are obtained by thermal decomposition or thermal synthesis. The five columns contain the name, the corresponding chemical formula, the Ca to P molar ratio, the mineral name, and the typical acronym, respectively. When $x > 0$ in the chemical composition of 'precipitated hydroxyapatite', one talks also about 'calcium-deficient hydroxyapatite' (CDHA). Generally, $x = 1$ so that in most cases CDHA has the composition $Ca_9(HPO_4)(PO_4)_5OH$

Name	Formula	Ca/P	Mineral	Symbol
Monocalcium phosphate monohydrate	$Ca(H_2PO_4)_2 \cdot H_2O$	0.50	–	MCPM
Dicalcium phosphate	$CaHPO_4$	1.00	Monetite	DCP
Dicalcium phosphate dihydrate	$CaHPO_4 \cdot 2H_2O$	1.00	Brushite	DCPD
Octocalcium phosphate	$Ca_8H_2(PO_4)_6 \cdot 5H_2O$	1.33	–	OCP
Precipitated hydroxyapatite[a]	$Ca_{10-x}(HPO_4)_x(PO_4)_{6-x}(OH)_{2-x}$	1.33–1.67	–	PHA
Precipitated amorphous calcium phosphate	$Ca_3(PO_4)_2 \cdot nH_2O$ where n = 3-4.5; 15–20% H_2O	1.50	–	ACP
Monocalcium phosphate	$Ca(H_2PO_4)_2$	0.50	–	MCP
α-Tricalcium phosphate	α-$Ca_3(PO_4)_2$	1.50	–	α-TCP
β-Tricalcium phosphate	β-$Ca_3(PO_4)_2$	1.50	–	β-TCP
Sintered hydroxyapatite	$Ca_{10}(PO_4)_6(OH)_2$	1.67	Hydroxyapatite	SHA
Oxyapatite	$Ca_{10}(PO_4)_6O$	1.67	--	OXA
Tetracalcium phosphate	$Ca_4(PO_4)_2O$	2.00	Hilgenstockite	TetCP

[a] x may vary between 0 and 2.

Table 2.2 List of commercial ceramic cements with the producer, product name, composition (when available) and main end-product. The main end-product of the reaction can be either an apatite (calcium-deficient, carbonated, etc.), brushite (= DCPD) or gypsum ($CaSO_4{\cdot}2H_2O$; CSD)

Producer	Product name	Composition	Product
Berkeley Advanced Biomaterials (US)	Cem-Ostetic™	Powder: calcium phosphates (details unknown); Solution: sterile water[f]	Apatite
	Tri-Ostetic™	Powder: calcium phosphates (details unknown); Solution: sterile water[f]	Apatite
Biocomposites Ltd (GB)	Genex®	Composition: could not be found[a]	Gypsum
Biomet (US) Interpore (US)	Calcibon®	Powder: α-TCP (61%), DCP (26%), $CaCO_3$ (10%), PHA (3%); Solution: H_2O, Na_2HPO_4[100]	Apatite
Walter Lorenz Surgical (GER)	Mimix™	Powder: TetCP, α-TCP, $C_6H_5O_7Na_32H_2O$; Solution: H_2O, $C_6H_8O_7$[f]	Apatite
	Quick Set Mimix™	Powder: calcium phosphate powders, $Na_3C_6H_5O_72H_2O$; Solution: citric acid aqueous solution[f]	Apatite
	Bone Plast® QS	Powder: $CaSO_4{\cdot}½H_2O$; Solution: sterile aqueous solution[f]	Gypsum
BoneSupport AB (SWE)	Cerament™	Powder: $CaSO_4{\cdot}½H_2O$ (60%), HA (40%); Solution: aqueous solution of an iodine radiopacifier (http://www.bonesupport.com/)	Gypsum
ETEX (US)	α-BSM; Embarc; Biobon	Powder: ACP (50%), DCPD (50%); Solution: unbuffered aqueous saline solution[101,102]	Apatite
	OssiPro	Composition: could not be found[a]	Apatite
Futura Biomedical (US)	OsteoCure	Powder: $CaSO_4{\cdot}½H_2O$; Solution: sterile mixing solution[f]	Gypsum
Graftys (FR)	Graftys® HBS	Composition: could not be found[a]	Apatite
Kasios (FR)	Jectos Eurobone®	Powder: β-TCP (98%), $Na_4P_2O_7$ (2%); Solution: H_2O, H_3PO_4 (3.0 M), H_2SO_4 (0.1 M)[103]	Brushite
	Jectos+	Composition: could not be found (likely to be close to that of Jectos)[a] (http://www.kasios.com/doc-pdf/JECTOS%2B699ed03-frgb.pdf)	Brushite

Kyphon (US)	KyphOs™	Powder: α-TCP (77%), $Mg_3(PO_4)_2$ (14%), $MgHPO_4$ (4.8%), $SrCO_3$ (3.6%); Solution: H_2O, $(NH_4)_2HPO_4$ (3.5M)[104]	Apatite
Lifecore (US)	CalMatrix	Powder: 90% $CaSO_4 \cdot ½H_2O$ and 10% carboxymethylcellulose[f]; Solution: unknown	Gypsum
Mitsubishi Materials (J)	Biopex®	Powder: α-TCP (75%), TetCP (18–20%), DCPD (5%), HA (0–2%) Solution: H_2O, Sodium succinate (12–13%), sodium chondroitin sulfate (5–5.4%) (when two values are indicated, the first value stems from reference (105) and the second value from reference (106))	Apatite
	Biopex®-R	Powder: α-TCP, TetCP, DCPD, HA, $Mg_3(PO_4)_2$, $NaHSO_3$ Solution: H_2O, Sodium succinate, sodium chondroitin sulfate[106]	Apatite
Orthogen Corporation	DentoGen	CSH powder and aqueous solution	Gypsum
Produits Dentaires SA (CH) CalciphOs (CH)	VitalOs[d]	Solution 1: β-TCP (1.34 g), $Na_2H_2P_2O_7$ (0.025 g), H_2O, salts (0.05 M pH 7.4 PBS solution); Solution 2: MCPM (0.78 g), $CaSO_42H_2O$ (0.39 g), H_2O, H_3PO_4 (0.05 M)[107]	Brushite
Shanghai Rebone Biomaterials Co (CN)	Rebone	Powder: TetCP, DCP; Solution: H_2O[108b]	Apatite
Skeletal Kinetics (US)	Callos™	Composition: α-TCP, $CaCO_3$, MCPM; Solution: sodium silicate[109]	Apatite
	Callos Inject™	Composition: α-tricalcium phosphate and unknown compounds (likely to be close to that of Callos™)[a]	Apatite
Stryker (US) Leibinger (GER)	BoneSource	Powder: TetCP (73%), DCPD (27%); Solution: H_2O, mixture of Na_2HPO_4 and NaH_2PO_4[12,86,110]	Apatite
	HydroSet™	Powder: TetCP, DCPD, trisodium citrate; Solution: H_2O, polyvynilpyrrolidone, sodium phosphate[111]	Apatite
Synthes (US)	Norian® SRS Norian® CRS	Powder: α-TCP (85%), $CaCO_3$ (12%) MCPM (3%); Solution: H_2O, Na_2HPO_4[18,112c]	Apatite
	Norian® SRS Fast Set Putty Norian® CRS Fast Set Putty	Composition: could not be found (likely to be close to that of Norian SRS/CRS)[a]	Apatite

Table 2.2 Continued

Producer	Product name	Composition	Product
	chronOS™ Inject	Powder: β-TCP (73%), MCPM (21%), $MgHPO_4 \cdot 3H_2O$ (5%), $MgSO_4$ (<1%), $Na_2H_2P_2O_7$ (<1%); Solution: H_2O, sodium hyaluronate (0.5%)[83]	Brushite
Teknimed (FR)	Cementek®	Powder: α-TCP, TetCP, Na Glycerophosphate; Solution: H_2O, $Ca(OH)_2$, H_3PO_4 (S. Goncalves, Teknimed, private communication)	Apatite
	Cementek® LV	Powder: α-TCP, TetCP, Na Glycerophosphate, dimethylsiloxane; Solution: H_2O, $Ca(OH)_2$, H_3PO_4 (S. Goncalves, Teknimed, private communication)	Apatite
Wright Medical (US)	MIIG™ 115	Powder: CSH; Solution: saline[113]	Gypsum
	MIIG® X3	Composition: CSH; Solution: sterile water (contains also traces of an accelerant)	Gypsum
	MIIG® X3 High-Visc	Composition: CSH; Solution: sterile water (less than in MIIG® X3; contains also traces of an accelerant)	Gypsum
	Pro-Dense®	Composition: 75% CSH, 25% brushite and granular β-TCP	Gypsum

[a] Not found in the literature or on the web.
[b] Assumed composition based on the scientific literature.
[c] Estimated composition.
[d] The cement consists of two liquids in which the various powder components are dispersed. Mixing occurs during delivery.
[e] To be used in combination with demineralised bone matrix.
[f] FDA website (http://www.fda.gov/search.html).

Recently, efforts towards composites of hydrogels and bone substitutes[21–28] have been intensified and several products have been launched (Table 2.3). These efforts are expressed by a rapid increase in the number of publications. For example, a search in 'Scopus' (www.scopus.com) using the two keywords 'Injectable' and 'Ceramic' (in 'all fields') shows that almost 350 publications were published in 2009 (Fig. 2.1).

The title of this chapter is 'Designing ceramics for injectable bone graft substitutes'. However, the injectability of a paste is a relative concept.[29] So, since all pastes have a certain degree of injectability, all types of pasty bone substitutes involving ceramics will be considered here. The spectrum goes from non-setting hydrogel-granule putties to CPCs. The term 'ceramic' refers generally to non-metallic inorganic materials obtained at high temperature. Here, a broader definition is used since cements are consolidated at or close to room temperature. Therefore, 'ceramic' here refers simply to non-metallic inorganic synthetic materials. As a result, all bone-derived pastes are excluded from this chapter.

The most important aspects of ceramic pastes will be addressed in this chapter: the rheological properties, the handling and delivery, the hardening (for cements), the mechanical properties, the biological properties, and finally some industrial requirements.

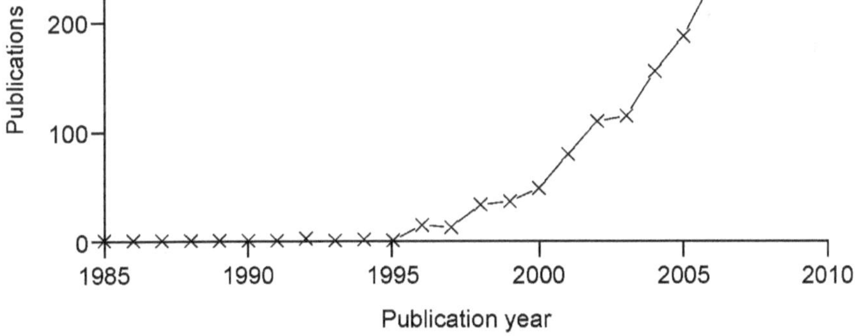

2.1 Number of articles cited per year in Scopus (www.scopus.com) when selecting 'Injectable' and 'Ceramic' as keywords (search in all fields). State on March 30, 2010.

Table 2.3 List of some non-setting non-allogenic pastes with indication of producer, product name, composition and form (pre-mixed or to be mixed). Denominations: HA = Hydroxyapatite; β-TCP = β-Tricalcium phosphate; BCP = biphasic calcium phosphate (composite between HA and β-TCP); CMC = carboxymethylcellulose; HPMC: hydroxypropylmethylcellulose

Producer	Product name	Composition	Form
ApaTech (UK)	Actifuse™ Actifuse™ Shape	HA, polymer and aqueous solution[a] Silicon-substituted calcium phosphate and polymer	Pre-mixed Pre-mixed
Baxter (US)	TricOs™	BCP (60% HA, 40% β-TCP) granules and Tissucol (fibrin glue)[a]	To be mixed
BioForm (US)	'Calcium hydroxylapatite implant'	HA powder embedded in a mixture of glycerine, water, and CMC[a]	Pre-mixed
Biomatlante (FR)	MBCP Gel®	BCP granules (60% HA, 40% β-TCP; 0.08–0.2 mm) and 2% HPMC[114,115]	Pre-mixed
Degradable Solutions (CH)	Easy graft™	β-TCP or BCP granules (0.45–1.00 mm) coated with 10 μm PLGA, N-methyl-2-pyrrolydone (K. Ruffieux, private communication)	To be mixed
Dentsply (US)	Pepgen P-15® flow	Hydroxyapatite (0.25–0.42 mm), P-15 peptide and aqueous sodium hyaluronate solution (product brochure)	To be mixed
DePuy Spine (US)	Healos® Fx	HA (20–30%) and collagen[a]	To be mixed
Fluidinova (P)	nanoXIM TCP nanoXIM HA	β-TCP (5 or 15%) and water (company website) HA (5, 15, 30, or 40%) and water (company website)	Pre-mixed Pre-mixed

Mathys Ltd (CH)	Ceros® Putty/cyclOS® Putty	β-TCP granules (0.125–0.71 mm; 94%) and recombinant sodium hyaluronate powder (6%)	To be mixed
Medtronic (US)	Mastergraft®	BCP (85% HA, 15% β-TCP) and bovine collagen[a]	To be mixed
NovaBone (US)	NovaBone® Putty	Bioglass and synthetic binder[a]	Pre-mixed
Orthovita (US)	Vitoss Flow	Contains at least bioactive glass and saline solution (or blood marrow aspirate, or blood)[a]	To be mixed
	Vitoss Pack	Contains at least bioactive glass and saline solution (or blood marrow aspirate, or blood)[a]	To be mixed
Osartis (GER)	Ostim®	Nanocrystalline HA (35%) and water (65%)[116]	Pre-mixed
Smith & Nephew (US)	JAX CS	CSD granules and an aqueous solution (http://global.smith-nephew.com/us/JAX.CS.OVERVIEW.7221.htm)	To be mixed
	JAX TCP	β-TCP granules and an aqueous solution of 1.75% CMC and 10% glycerol[117]	To be mixed
Stryker (US)	Calstrux™	β-TCP granules and CMC[a]	To be mixed
Therics (US)	Therigraft™ Putty	β-TCP granules and polymer[a]	Pre-mixed
Zimmer (US)	Collagraft	BCP granules (65% HA, 35% β-TCP; 0.5–1.0 mm), bovine collagen, and bone marrow aspirate[118]	To be mixed

[a] FDA website (http://www.fda.gov/search.html).

2.2 Rheological properties of bone substitute pastes

The rheological properties of a bone substitute paste are obviously very important. These include injectability, cohesion and viscosity. Regarding injectability, our understanding has improved markedly in recent years.[29,30] When a paste, which is a biphasic mixture of a finely divided solid (powder, granules) and a liquid, is submitted to a pressure gradient, the liquid may flow faster than the solid, resulting in local changes of paste composition. Specifically, the paste present in the region of the highest pressure (e.g. close to the plunger of a syringe) may become so depleted in liquid that the biphasic mixture in this zone is no longer a paste but a wet powder.[29,30] Conversely, the paste in the zone of the lowest pressure (e.g. at the cannula tip) is enriched in liquid. Since these effects are dynamic, the size of the zone depleted in liquid (wet powder) increases during injection, eventually reaching the tip of the injection device and plugging it. The effects described herein have been mostly called filter-pressing and phase migration.

Fortunately, filter-pressing can be reduced or even eliminated by decreasing the particle size of the finely divided solid (powder, granules),[29] using rounder particles,[31] using additives to increase the viscosity of the mixing liquid,[29,32] or manipulating the plastic limit and liquid-to-solid ratio (LSR) of the paste.[29] Concerning the latter strategy, it has been demonstrated that injectability increases when the difference between the paste LSR and the plastic limit (minimum amount of liquid to add to a solid to obtain a paste) increases.[29] This can either be achieved with an increase of the LSR,[29,33] or with a decrease in the plastic limit, for example by adding citrate ions or polyacrylic acid into the mixing liquid,[29,34] or by optimizing the particle size distribution of the solid.[35]

Importantly, there is presently no agreement in the scientific community about the meaning of injectability. For many authors, injectability is a concept related to the force that has to be applied to a syringe in order to inject the paste, independently of the fact that the force is a function of syringe size.[36] A paste is declared non-injectable if the paste cannot be injected with an arbitrary force (generally 100 N) using an arbitrary syringe geometry. In this chapter, injectability is related to the ability of a paste to remain homogeneous under pressure, since phase separation is the cause of filter-pressing. So, according to this definition, injectability is still related to a given geometry, but no longer to a force. In other words, an injectable paste, according to the definition used here, might be found non-injectable according to the definition of Khairoun *et al.*[36]

The second rheological property that should be carefully considered while designing a ceramic bone substitute is paste cohesion (= cohesiveness, 'non-decay'). Specifically, it is the ability of the paste to keep its geometrical integrity in an aqueous solution. For a cement, poor cohesion may prevent setting and may lead to negative *in vivo* reactions due to the release of microparticles.[37]

Since high cohesion is the result of strong attractive forces between particles, factors enhancing van der Waals forces (attractive) and decreasing electrostatic forces (repulsive) can be used to improve cohesion. These include a decrease of mean particle size and LSR, and an increase in ionic strength of the mixing solution.[38] Another approach is to increase the viscosity of the mixing liquid using hydrogels.[32,38,39]

To date, relatively little is known about ways to control the viscosity of cement pastes. In fact, to talk about viscosity is an approximation of reality: calcium phosphate pastes are generally non-Newtonian fluids and as a result, the viscosity is a function of shear forces (40). Furthermore, cements have transient properties meaning that the viscosity of a cement paste is a function of shear and time.[41] Generally, calcium phosphate pastes are thixotropic (shear-thinning).[40,41] Both an increase in LSR and an increase in particle size decrease paste viscosity.[40,41] Additives are also known to affect viscosity. For example, citrate ions or poly(acrylic acid) decrease particle interactions and hence decrease viscosity and cohesion.[40]

2.3 Handling and delivery

The handling of a product is of paramount importance for its commercial success. In the case of injectable ceramics, the following aspects have to be carefully looked at: mixing, transfer into a delivery system, and delivery. Besides, the product should be versatile. These various aspects are discussed hereafter.

There are three categories of products regarding mixing: pre-mixed (= ready-to-use) products (Table 2.3), products that are mixed during delivery (e.g. 'VitalOs' in Table 2.2), and products that have to be mixed prior to use (Tables 2.2–2.3). Even though pre-mixed products appear very attractive, each of the latter three categories has specific advantages and disadvantages. So, it is important to understand them during the design process of the product. Here is a quick review.

Pre-mixed products are the easiest to use because they do not require any mixing and any transfer into an appropriate delivery system. Moreover, there is no time constraint to use the product once it is open. However, pre-mixing is not a versatile approach to deliver a product, since the mixture composition is already pre-defined. Moreover, it is not adapted to CPC formulations. Presently, only two methods have been proposed to package ready-to-use cement formulations. First, the reactive cement components are combined with a non-aqueous liquid to form a non-reactive pasty mixture. Reaction then occurs *in vivo*, when the non-aqueous liquid is slowly replaced with physiological fluids. Unfortunately, the setting reaction is difficult to control and the mechanical properties are poor.[42] The second approach is to freeze down the cement components.[43] However, it is not clear how injectable such mixtures would be and how the storage and handling could be controlled (freezing at −80 °C). Another interesting approach consists of mixing two reactive liquids during their injection by means of a static mixer.[44] This approach has more time constraints than ready-to-use putties, but since mixing only occurs in the cannula (= static mixer), the cannula can be changed, for example after cement hardening, and more cement can be injected. However, such an approach is difficult to apply to highly viscous pastes (leads to syringe plugging). Moreover, it has only been described for brushite CPCs which are used much less than apatite CPCs. The third and last approach to mix the paste is to combine the powder(s) with the liquid(s) just before use. This approach is more cumbersome, but also more versatile than the other two since it allows the addition of various components (e.g. drug solution, platelet-rich plasma, etc.). Moreover, it is generally easier to have liquid and solid components as single components during production (e.g. for sterilization – see hereafter). However, as a change of cement composition affects the setting reaction, the modification of the composition by the user is not recommended with setting pastes. To conclude, mixing is not only defined by the possibilities offered by the chemical nature of the product (non-setting or setting paste, composition), but also by the versatility that the producers would like to offer to their customers, as well as the limitations set by the product manufacturing.

2.3.1 Hardening (for cements)

A very important handling property of cements is their hardening rate (= setting rate) because it directly affects the clinical procedure. Specifically, a too early setting reaction limits the period during which the surgeon can apply the cement, whereas a too late setting reaction prevents the surgeon to close the defect and hence extent the overall procedure duration. Generally, the setting rate is characterized by measuring the setting time, i.e. the time it takes to reach a certain mechanical stability, either using a Gillmore needle[45] or the Vicat test.[46] Unfortunately, the setting time is just one point along the curve relating compressive strength and reaction time. In other words, the setting time does not describe the shape of the curve, e.g. the presence of initial lag, or stepwise versus steady increase. Therefore, various authors have made efforts to not only better characterize the setting reaction but also to better understand the factors affecting it.[47–51]

A large number of strategies exist to modify the hardening rate of cements, for example changing the particle size of the reagents, adding a nucleating phase, or dissolving adequate additives (accelerators or retarders) into the mixing solution.[52] So, it is easy to modify the cement composition to reach a setting time that is clinically relevant, typically close to 10 min. Unfortunately, it is more difficult to simultaneously control the initial rate of the reaction and the overall cement reaction (for example, to shorten the overall duration of the setting reaction). Therefore, there is potential for improvement and efforts have been focused towards this goal. For instance, it was recently shown that a simple thermal treatment at 500 °C could extend the initial part of the setting reaction from a few minutes to a few hours.[53]

2.4 Mechanical and biological properties of bone substitute pastes

2.4.1 Mechanical properties

The compressive strength of CPCs and calcium sulphate cements is generally one of the properties presented in scientific publications. It is also often put forward by commercial organizations. Unfortunately, these values are close to be meaningless due to the inherent brittleness of ceramics: the indication of a mean compressive strength of, e.g., 50 MPa measured on perfectly shaped and perfectly prepared samples does not inform the reader with which probability this cement will fail *in situ* under a cyclic load of, e.g., 10 MPa. The comparison of the compressive strength of the cementitious bone substitute with that of cancellous bone is not very helpful either because cancellous bone is much less brittle than ceramic cements. In fact, the reader should get additional information regarding the strength distribution of the cementitious material (so-called Weibull distribution[54]). Moreover, since loads always contain shear or tensile components, the tensile or the shear properties should also be measured.[55] Typically, tensile strength is one order of magnitude lower than compressive strength. Last, but not least, loads are generally cyclic, which means that fatigue properties and fracture mechanics are aspects that should also be addressed.[54,56] When all these measurements are considered, it becomes very clear that CPCs and calcium sulphate cements can only be applied in non-load-bearing applications. The poor mechanical properties of CPCs explain why CPCs are not even performing well in applications where low load-bearing properties are required, for example in bone augmentation.[57–62]

Another important aspect to consider when looking at the mechanical properties of cementitious bone substitutes is that the mechanical properties may vary quite extensively upon implantation. For example, since gypsum and brushite are soluble in physiological conditions, the mechanical properties of these materials rapidly decrease upon implantation.[63] This spontaneous dissolution is also the reason why these materials are often combined with less soluble bone substitute such as β-TCP or HA.[14,64,65]

2.4.2 Biological properties

Since none of the bone substitutes proposed so far in the scientific world is load-bearing or even close to being load-bearing, the main strategy presently used to repair bone defects is to use a bone substitute that is rapidly resorbed and replaced by new mature bone. To reach this goal, not only the chemistry but also the geometry of the bone substitute has to be optimized.[66,67] For example, it is particularly important to use a bone substitute that can be easily invaded by cells and blood vessels. For that purpose, the bone substitute must have a fully interconnected porous structure with diameters of pores and pore interconnections larger than about 50 μm.[67–69] CPCs are highly porous materials but do not contain such macropores (here defined as pores with a diameter larger than 50 μm). To remedy to this problem, CPC pastes have been combined with highly soluble solids,[70–73] hydrophobic liquids,[74] and gas bubbles.[75–78] Unfortunately, the as-generated macropores are generally not interconnected, which limits the extent of this strategy. Another approach to obtain a macroporous pasty bone substitute is to combine granules with a hydrogel, for example, sodium alginate,[15] dextran,[21] sodium hyaluronate,[22] and hydroxypropylmethyl cellulose.[23,24] Since the solid content of hydrogels is generally very low (a few per cent), cells can easily penetrate the hydrogel-filled macroporous gaps present between granules. The size of the macroporous gaps is controlled by the hydrogel fraction and by the granule size distribution.

Another important aspect that should be addressed here is related to the size of the ceramic particles present in the bone substitute paste. It is indeed known that the *in vivo* response of particular bone substitutes is a function of their dimension and amount.[79,80] For example, Evans and Clarke-Smith[81] observed that 'only (HA) particles smaller than about 5 μm are able to cause damage'. So, the biological responses of pastes consisting of loose nano- or micro-sized particles might differ from pastes consisting of mm-sized particles. Since it is only recently that products consisting of densely packed but loose particles have been introduced, there is presently too little *in vivo* data to really assess the potential risks or benefits associated with loose nano- or micro-sized particles. Therefore, caution is required when designing a ceramic bone substitute consisting of loose nano- or micro-sized particles.

In the last decades, there has been a trend towards the use of highly resorbable bone substitutes. Whereas some of these materials, such as β-TCP, are resorbed by cells, others, such as gypsum and brushite, are resorbed by simple dissolution. At equilibrium, water in contact with gypsum has a calcium concentration roughly ten times higher than that of serum. Brushite is one order of magnitude less soluble than gypsum, but it is still slightly soluble in physiological conditions. As a result, it has been reported that gypsum dissolves more rapidly than bone grows, leading to the appearance of fibrous tissue in the defect centre.[82] Regarding brushite, brushite cements have been shown to rapidly lose their mechanical strength[63] and to transform in their centre into an apatite.[83–85] Also, a fibrous gap is observed between ingrowing bone front and resorbing cement front.[86,87] However, this gap disappears when only apatite remains in the CPC block.

In the original CPC formulation proposed by Brown and Chow,[12,88] no fibrous gap is observed between cement and bone, but physico-chemical changes also occur within the CPC paste due to the fact that the latter formulation sets in basic conditions:[89] apatite precipitates *in vivo*, hence leading to denser and stronger cements.[90] As apatite is a basic compound, the precipitation of apatite acidifies the surrounding medium. This is not a problem for an inherently basic cement such as the one proposed by Brown and Chow,[12,88] but has been thought to provoke negative *in vivo* reactions when large amounts of brushite cements are implanted.[83,91] To conclude, the use of fast resorbable cement may lead to a rapid transformation of a bone defect into mature bone, but bears the risk of negative biological reactions and/or too fast a disappearance leaving an empty defect.

2.5 Industrial design

When the composition of a bone graft substitute has been optimized to achieve adequate handling, physico-chemical, and biological properties, other problems might arise and render the project non-feasible: non-availability of raw materials, poor product shelf-life, or difficulty with sterilizing the product. These aspects are discussed in the next paragraphs.

Whereas in certain fields the specifications of a raw material can be freely chosen, restrictions often exist in the bone graft substitute field due to a small market size. For example, when purchasing calcium phosphates, it is of interest to get a high purity. Unfortunately, most commercially available calcium phosphates contain impurities in concentrations high enough to cause problems (e.g. Mg content in powders used for α-TCP synthesis[92,93]). Whereas the problem might not be too stringent for ceramic raw materials, more problems might arise when purchasing polymeric rheological additives. Currently, hyaluronates (acid or salt) have the highest availability among pharma-grade polymer additives. However, hyaluronates are generally sold as non-sterile powders and sterilization is complicated (ultra-filtration), particularly for highly concentrated solutions (>3%). Furthermore, when hyaluronates are sold as solution (e.g. for aesthetic surgery, arthrosis, ophtalmology), the concentration is generally too low (typically < 1%) and the volume is either too large (200–300 mL) or too small (0.2–1.0 mL). Finally, when all criteria are fulfilled, hyaluronates producers might not be willing to sell the material due to too small a need from the bone graft substitute producers.

Once the product is packaged, it must be sterilized. Unfortunately, polymers and ceramics may require different sterilization methods. For example, most polymers lose their integrity during gamma-sterilization and sometimes also during autoclaving. Alternatively, ceramics are often unstable during autoclaving (e.g. CSD). As a result, it might be impossible to find a way to sterilize a ceramic-polymer paste. In the latter case, the only solution is to purchase sterile products and to mix them under aseptic conditions. Unfortunately, as many products cannot be bought sterile and cannot be easily sterilized (e.g. sodium hyaluronate), it might be impossible to produce a product according to its initial design. Instead of offering a one-component product, pre-mixed and ready to be injected in their customers, companies might have to sell a two-component product that has to be mixed in the operating room.

Once packaged and sterilized, the product must be stable during storage, i.e. during the so-called shelf-life. Obviously, wet pastes are more likely to be unstable than dry mixtures. For example, calcium phosphates may dissolve and precipitate in the solution, leading to a change in the mean crystal/particle size or even to the formation of agglomerates. Since the rheological properties of a paste (e.g. injectability) depend on the mean particle size, rheological properties may be completely altered. Even the stability of dry mixtures is not a trivial problem. For example, Gbureck *et al.*[94] showed that extensive mixing of the dry components of a brushite CPC markedly decreased its shelf-life.

2.6 Future trends

The last decade has experienced a tremendous change in the bone graft substitute market due to rapidly rising sales: whereas most companies sold only granules and blocks in the 1980s and 1990s, practically all major companies are now offering cements and putties. Furthermore, there is a clear trend towards a specialization of the products: companies are now designing products for specific clinical indications. In other words, the bone graft substitute market has reached a critical size. Since the sales are still rising rapidly, this trend will go on in the future.

A particularly strong and recent trend is the introduction of non-setting pastes or putties. Presently, there are as many non-setting pastes as cements. Since their production is often less tricky than that of cements (no need to provide a paste with always the same setting time), and their biological response is often better, it is very likely that there will soon be more commercial formulations of non-setting pastes than cements. Interestingly, academic research is very limited in this field.

Another important trend in the future will be the improvement in the biological properties of bone substitutes, the aim being to transform a bone defect into new mature bone as fast as possible. This implies that the focus will be set on resorbable materials that possess an open-porous structure allowing cells to invade the structure. Another potential focus could be set on osteo-inductive ceramics.[95] A number of authors have indeed observed that ceramic bone graft substitutes implanted under the skin or in muscles are filled or coated with bone over time. However, despite very intensive research, there is only a poor understanding of the mechanisms leading to osteoinduction, and as a result, it is not possible at the moment to design an osteoinductive ceramic.

A last trend is to add minute amounts of foreign ions into ceramic bone graft substitutes to improve their biological behaviour. Most efforts have been set on Si, but other ions have been looked at such as Mg, Na, Sr, or Zn.[96–101] Even though effects can be anticipated, strong scientific evidence is still missing, partly because it is difficult to incorporate foreign ions without modifying other ceramic properties (e.g. solubility, grain size, pore size), and partly because it is difficult to synthesize truly pure ceramics. As a result, it is always difficult or even impossible to know whether the change of biological reaction is due to the release of the investigated ions or to a different factor. A way out of this problem might be to load or coat the bone graft substitutes with soluble salts of the considered ions.[102]

2.7 Sources of further information and advice

Dorozhkin SV. Calcium orthophosphate cements for biomedical application. *J Mater Sci.* 2008; 43: 3028–57.

Dorozhkin SV. Calcium orthophosphates. *J Mater Sci.* 2007; 42: 1061–95.

Elliott JC. Structure and chemistry of the apatites and other calcium orthophosphates. In *Studies in Inorganic Chemistry*, vol. 18, Elsevier, Amsterdam, 1994.

2.8 References

1. Bauer TW, Muschler GF. Bone graft materials. An overview of the basic science. *Clin Orthop.* 2000 Feb(371): 10–27.
2. Albee H, Morrison SJ. Studies in bone growth triple calcium phosphate as a stimulus to osteogenesis. *Annals of Surgery.* 1920; 71(1): 32–9.
3. Dreesmann H. *Ueber Knochenplombierung.* 1892: 804–10.
4. Cameron HU, Macnab I, Pilliar RM. Evaluation of a biodegradable ceramic. *J Biomed Mater Res.* 1977; 11: 179–86.
5. Hench LL. Biomaterials. *Science.* 1980 May 23; 208(4446): 826–31.
6. Hulbert SF, Young FA, Mathews RS, Klawitter JJ, Talbert CD, Stelling FH. Potential of ceramic materials as permanently implantable skeletal prostheses. *J Biomed Mater Res.* 1970 Sep; 4(3): 433–56.
7. Jarcho M, Bolen CH, Thomas MB, Bobick J, Kay JF, Doremus RH. Hydroxylapatite synthesis and characterization in dense polycrystalline form. *J Mater Sci Lett.* 1976; 11: 2027–35.
8. Klawitter JJ, Hulbert SF. Application of porous ceramics for the attachment of load bearing internal orthopedic applications. *J Biomed Mater Res Symp.* 1971; 2(1): 161–229.
9. Nery EB, Lynch KL, Rooney GE. Alveolar ridge augmentation with tricalcium phosphate ceramic. *J Prosthetic Dentistry.* 1978 Dec; 40(6): 668–75.
10. Roy DM, Linnehan SK. Hydroxyapatite formed from coral skeletal carbonate by hydrothermal exchange. *Nature.* 1974 Jan 25; 247(438): 220–2.
11. White RA, Weber JN, White EW. Replamineform: a new process for preparing porous ceramic, metal, and polymer prosthetic materials. *Science.* 1972 May 26; 176(37): 922–4.
12. Brown WE, Chow LC. A new calcium phosphate setting cement. *J Dental Res.*

1983; 62: 672.
13. LeGeros RZ, Chohayeb A, Shulman A. Apatitic calcium phosphates: possible dental restorative materials. *J Dental Res*. 1982; 1982(61): 343.
14. Hanker JS, Terry BC, Ambrose WW, Lupton CR, inventors; University of North Carolina, assignee. Plaster of paris as a bioresorbable scaffold in implants for bone repair. USA. 1986.
15. Klein CP, van der Lubbe HB, de Groot K. A plastic composite of alginate with calcium phosphate granulate as implant material: an *in vivo* study. *Biomaterials*. 1987 Jul; 8(4): 308–10.
16. Gerhart TN, Miller RL, Kleshinski SJ, Hayes WC. *In vitro* characterization and biomechanical optimization of a biodegradable particulate composite bone cement. *J Biomed Mater Res*. 1988 Nov; 22(11): 1071–82.
17. Gerhart TN, Renshaw AA, Miller RL, Noecker RJ, Hayes WC. *In vivo* histologic and biomechanical characterization of a biodegradable particulate composite bone cement. *J Biomed Mater Res*. 1989 Jan; 23(1): 1–16.
18. Constantz BR, Ison IC, Fulmer MT, Poser RD, Smith ST, VanWagoner M, *et al.* Skeletal repair by *in situ* formation of the mineral phase of bone. *Science*. 1995 Mar 24; 267(5205): 1796–9.
19. Kveton JF, Friedman CD, Costantino PD. Indications for hydroxyapatite cement reconstruction in lateral skull base surgery. *Am J Otol*. 1995 Jul; 16(4): 465–9.
20. Kveton JF, Friedman CD, Piepmeier JM, Costantino PD. Reconstruction of suboccipital craniectomy defects with hydroxyapatite cement: a preliminary report. *Laryngoscope*. 1995 Feb; 105(2): 156–9.
21. Chan C, Thompson I, Robinson P, Wilson J, Hench L. Evaluation of Bioglass/dextran composite as a bone graft substitute. *Int J Oral Maxillofac Surg*. 2002 Feb; 31(1): 73–7.
22. Chazono M, Tanaka T, Komaki H, Fujii K. Bone formation and bioresorption after implantation of injectable beta-tricalcium phosphate granules-hyaluronate complex in rabbit bone defects. *J Biomed Mater Res*. 2004 Sep 15; 70A(4): 542–9.
23. Dupraz A, Delecrin J, Moreau A, Pilet P, Passuti N. Long-term bone response to particulate injectable ceramic. *J Biomed Mater Res*. 1998 Dec 5; 42(3): 368–75.
24. Grimandi G, Weiss P, Millot F, Daculsi G. *In vitro* evaluation of a new injectable calcium phosphate material. *J Biomed Mater Res*. 1998 Mar 15; 39(4): 660–6.
25. Ito M. *In vitro* properties of a chitosan-bonded hydroxyapatite bone-filling paste. *Biomaterials*. 1991 Jan; 12(1): 41–5.
26. Maruyama M, Terayama K, Ito M, Takei T, Kitagawa E. Hydroxyapatite clay for gap filling and adequate bone ingrowth. *J Biomed Mater Res*. 1995 Mar; 29(3): 329–36.
27. Momota Y, Miyamoto Y, Ishikawa K, Takechi M, Yuasa T, Tatehara S, *et al.* Evaluation of feasibility of hydroxyapatite putty as a local hemostatic agent for bone. *J Biomed Mater Res*. 2002; 63(5): 542–7.
28. Pompili A, Caroli F, Carpanese L, Caterino M, Raus L, Sestili G, *et al.* Cranioplasty performed with a new osteoconductive osteoinducing hydroxyapatite-derived material. *J Neurosurg*. 1998 Aug; 89(2): 236–42.
29. Bohner M, Baroud G. Injectability of calcium phosphate pastes. *Biomaterials*. 2005 May; 26(13): 1553–63.
30. Habib M, Baroud G, Gitzhofer F, Bohner M. Mechanisms underlying the limited injectability of hydraulic calcium phosphate paste. *Acta Biomaterialia*. 2008; 4(5): 1465–71.
31. Ishikawa K. Effects of spherical tetracalcium phosphate on injectability and basic

properties of apatitic cement. *Key Eng Mat*. 2003; 240–2: 369–72.
32. Andrianjatovo H, Lemaitre J, Deramond H, Duquesnoy B, Hardouin P, Leclet H, *et al*. Effects of polysaccharides on the cement properties in the monocalcium phosphate/β-tricalcium phosphate system. *Innovation et technologie en biologie et médecine*. 1995; 16: 140–7.
33. Burguera EF, Xu HH, Sun L. Injectable calcium phosphate cement: effects of powder-to-liquid ratio and needle size. *J Biomed Mater Res B Appl Biomater*. 2008 Feb; 84(2): 493–502.
34. Barralet JE, Grover LM, Gbureck U. Ionic modification of calcium phosphate cement viscosity. Part II: hypodermic injection and strength improvement of brushite cement. *Biomaterials*. 2004 May; 25(11): 2197–203.
35. Gbureck U, Spatz K, Thull R, Barralet JE. Rheological enhancement of mechanically activated alpha-tricalcium phosphate cements. *J Biomed Mater Res B Appl Biomater*. 2005 Apr; 73(1): 1–6.
36. Khairoun I, Boltong MG, Driessens FCM, Planell JA. Some factors controlling the injectability of calcium phosphate bone cements. *J Mater Sci-Mater M*. 1998 Aug; 9(8): 425–8.
37. Miyamoto Y, Ishikawa K, Takechi M, Toh T, Yuasa T, Nagayama M, *et al*. Histological and compositional evaluations of three types of calcium phosphate cements when implanted in subcutaneous tissue immediately after mixing. *J Biomed Mater Res*. 1999 Spring; 48(1): 36–42.
38. Bohner M, Doebelin N, Baroud G. Theoretical and experimental approach to test the cohesion of calcium phosphate pastes. *Eur Cell Mater*. 2006; 12: 26–35.
39. Cherng A, Takagi S, Chow LC. Effects of hydroxypropyl methylcellulose and other gelling agents on the handling properties of calcium phosphate cement. *J Biomed Mater Res*. 1997 Jun 5; 35(3): 273–7.
40. Baroud G, Cayer E, Bohner M. Rheological characterization of concentrated aqueous β-tricalcium phosphate suspensions: the effect of liquid-to-powder ratio, milling time and additives. *Acta Biomaterialia*. 2005; 1(3): 357–63.
41. Liu C, Shao H, Chen F, Zheng H. Rheological properties of concentrated aqueous injectable calcium phosphate cement slurry. *Biomaterials*. 2006 Oct; 27(29): 5003–13.
42. Carey LE, Xu HH, Simon CG, Jr., Takagi S, Chow LC. Premixed rapid-setting calcium phosphate composites for bone repair. *Biomaterials*. 2005 Aug; 26(24): 5002–14.
43. Grover LM, Hofmann MP, Gbureck U, Kumarasami B, Barralet JE. Frozen delivery of brushite calcium phosphate cements. *Acta Biomaterialia*. 2008; 4(6): 1916–23.
44. Lemaitre J, Pittet C, Brendlen D, inventors; Pasty or liquid multiple constituent compositions for injectable calcium phosphate cements. 2003.
45. ASTM ASfTaM. Standard test method for time of setting of hydraulic-cement paste by gillmore needles. *ASTM standards*. 1999; C266-99: 1–3.
46. ASTM. Standard test method for time of setting of hydraulic cement by Vicat needle. *ASTM standards*. 2002; C191-01a: 1–6.
47. Bohner M, Malsy AK, Camire CL, Gbureck U. Combining particle size distribution and isothermal calorimetry data to determine the reaction kinetics of α-tricalcium phosphate-water mixtures. *Acta Biomaterialia*. 2006; 2(3): 343–8.
48. Fukase Y, Eanes ED, Takagi S, Chow LC, Brown WE. Setting reactions and compressive strengths of calcium phosphate cements. *J Dent Res*. 1990 Dec; 69(12): 1852–6.
49. Fulmer M, Brown PW. The effects of particle size and solution chemistry on the formation of hydroxyapatite. *Mat Res Soc Symp Proc*. 1990; 174: 39–44.

50. Ginebra MP, Fernandez E, Driessens FCM, Planell JA. Modeling of the hydrolysis of alpha-tricalcium phosphate. *J Am Ceram Soc.* 1999 Oct; 82(10): 2808–12.
51. Hofmann MP, Young AM, Gbureck U, Nazhat SN, Barralet JE. FTIR-monitoring of a fast setting brushite bone cement: effect of intermediate phases. *J Mater Chem.* 2006; 16: 3199–206.
52. Bohner M. Reactivity of calcium phosphate cements. *J Mater Chem.* 2007; 17: 3980–6.
53. Bohner M, Luginbühl R, Reber C. A physical approach to modify the hydraulic reactivity of α-tricalcium phosphate powder. *Acta Biomaterialia.* 2009; 5: 3524–35.
54. Morgan JP, Dauskardt RH. Notch strength insensitivity of self-setting hydroxyapatite bone cements. *J Mater Sci-Mater M.* 2003 Jul; 14(7): 647–53.
55. Charriere E, Terrazzoni S, Pittet C, Mordasini PH, Dutoit M, Lemaitre J, *et al.* Mechanical characterization of brushite and hydroxyapatite cements. *Biomaterials.* 2001 Nov; 22(21): 2937–45.
56. Gisep A, Kugler S, Wahl D, Rahn B. Mechanical characterisation of a bone defect model filled with ceramic cements. *J Mater Sci Mater Med.* 2004 Oct; 15(10): 1065–71.
57. Blattert TR, Katscher S, Weckbach A. Bone cements in balloon kyphoplasty – Requirements and clinical suitability. Zementwahl bei der ballonkyphoplastie – Anforderungsprofil und klinische Eignung. *Aktuelle Traumatologie.* 2006; 36(1): 18–22.
58. Libicher M, Hillmeier J, Liegibel U, Sommer U, Pyerin W, Vetter M, *et al.* Osseous integration of calcium phosphate in osteoporotic vertebral fractures after kyphoplasty: initial results from a clinical and experimental pilot study. *Osteoporos Int.* 2006; 17(8): 1208–15.
59. Libicher M, Vetter M, Wolf I, Noeldge G, Kasperk C, Grafe I, *et al.* CT volumetry of intravertebral cement after kyphoplasty. Comparison of polymethylmethacrylate and calcium phosphate in a 12-month follow-up. *Eur Radiol.* 2005 Aug; 15(8): 1544–9.
60. Maestretti G, Cremer C, Otten P, Jakob RP. Prospective study of standalone balloon kyphoplasty with calcium phosphate cement augmentation in traumatic fractures. *European Spine Journal.* 2007; 16: 601–10.
61. Nakano M, Hirano N, Ishihara H, Kawaguchi Y, Matsuura K. Calcium phosphate cement leakage after percutaneous vertebroplasty for osteoporotic vertebral fractures: risk factor analysis for cement leakage. *J Neurosurg Spine.* 2005 Jan; 2(1): 27–33.
62. Nakano M, Hirano N, Matsuura K, Watanabe H, Kitagawa H, Ishihara H, *et al.* Percutaneous transpedicular vertebroplasty with calcium phosphate cement in the treatment of osteoporotic vertebral compression and burst fractures. *J Neurosurg.* 2002 Oct; 97(3 Suppl): 287–93.
63. Ikenaga M, Hardouin P, Lemaitre J, Andrianjatovo H, Flautre B. Biomechanical characterization of a biodegradable calcium phosphate hydraulic cement: a comparison with porous biphasic calcium phosphate ceramics. *J Biomed Mater Res.* 1998 Apr; 40(1): 139–44.
64. Ohura K, Bohner M, Hardouin P, Lemaitre J, Pasquier G, Flautre B. Resorption of, and bone formation from, new beta-tricalcium phosphate-monocalcium phosphate cements: an *in vivo* study. *J Biomed Mater Res.* 1996 Feb; 30(2): 193–200.
65. Sato S, Koshino T, Saito T. Osteogenic response of rabbit tibia to hydroxyapatite particle-Plaster of Paris mixture. *Biomaterials.* 1998 Oct; 19(20): 1895–900.
66. Bohner M. Calcium orthophosphates in medicine: from ceramics to calcium

phosphate cements. *Injury*. 2000 Dec; 31 Suppl 4: 37–47.
67. Bohner M, Baumgart F. Theoretical model to determine the effects of geometrical factors on the resorption of calcium phosphate bone substitutes. *Biomaterials*. 2004 Aug; 25(17): 3569–82.
68. Lu JX, Flautre B, Anselme K, Hardouin P, Gallur A, Descamps M, *et al.* Role of interconnections in porous bioceramics on bone recolonization *in vitro* and *in vivo*. *J Mater Sci-Mater M*. 1999 Feb; 10(2): 111–20.
69. von Doernberg MC, von Rechenberg B, Bohner M, Grunenfelder S, van Lenthe GH, Muller R, *et al. In vivo* behavior of calcium phosphate scaffolds with four different pore sizes. *Biomaterials*. 2006 Oct; 27(30): 5186–98.
70. Barralet JE, Grover L, Gaunt T, Wright AJ, Gibson IR. Preparation of macroporous calcium phosphate cement tissue engineering scaffold. *Biomaterials*. 2002 Aug; 23(15): 3063–72.
71. Fernandez E, Vlad MD, Gel MM, Lopez J, Torres R, Cauich JV, *et al.* Modulation of porosity in apatitic cements by the use of alpha-tricalcium phosphate-calcium sulphate dihydrate mixtures. *Biomaterials*. 2005 Jun; 26(17): 3395–404.
72. Takagi S, Chow LC. Formation of macropores in calcium phosphate cement implants. *J Mater Sci-Mater M*. 2001 Feb; 12(2): 135–9.
73. Xu HH, Quinn JB, Takagi S, Chow LC, Eichmiller FC. Strong and macroporous calcium phosphate cement: effects of porosity and fiber reinforcement on mechanical properties. *J Biomed Mater Res*. 2001 Dec 5; 57(3): 457–66.
74. Bohner M. Calcium phosphate emulsions: possible applications. *Key Eng Mat*. 2001; 192–195: 765–8.
75. Almirall A, Larrecq G, Delgado JA, Martinez S, Planell JA, Ginebra MP. Fabrication of low temperature macroporous hydroxyapatite scaffolds by foaming and hydrolysis of an alpha-TCP paste. *Biomaterials*. 2004 Aug; 25(17): 3671–80.
76. del Valle S, Miño N, Muñoz F, González A, Planell JA, Ginebra MP. *In vivo* evaluation of an injectable macroporous calcium phosphate cement. *J Mater Sci: Mater M*. 2007; 18(2): 353–61.
77. Ginebra MP, Delgado JA, Harr I, Almirall A, Del Valle S, Planell JA. Factors affecting the structure and properties of an injectable self-setting calcium phosphate foam. *J Biomed Mater Res*. 2007; 80(2): 351–61.
78. Sarda S, Fernandez E, Nilsson M, Planell JA. Influence of air-entraining agent on bone cement macroporosity. *Key Eng Mat*. 2002; 218–2: 335–8.
79. Frank RM, Klewansky P, Hemmerle J, Tenenbaum H. Ultrastructural demonstration of the importance of crystal size of bioceramic powders implanted into human periodontal lesions. *J Clin Periodontol*. 1991 Oct; 18(9): 669–80.
80. Pioletti DP, Takei H, Lin T, Van Landuyt P, Ma QJ, Kwon SY, *et al.* The effects of calcium phosphate cement particles on osteoblast functions. *Biomaterials*. 2000 Jun; 21(11): 1103–14.
81. Evans EJ, Clarke-Smith EMH. Studies on the mechanism of cell damage by finely ground hydroxyapatite particles *in vitro*. *Clin Mater*. 1991; 7: 241–5.
82. Urban RM, Turner TM, Hall DJ, Infanger S, Cheema N, Lim TH. Healing of large defects treated with calcium sulfate pellets containing demineralized bone matrix particles. *Orthopedics*. 2003 May; 26(5 Suppl): s581–5.
83. Bohner M, Theiss F, Apelt D, Hirsiger W, Houriet R, Rizzoli G, *et al.* Compositional changes of a dicalcium phosphate dihydrate cement after implantation in sheep. *Biomaterials*. 2003 Sep; 24(20): 3463–74.
84. Constantz BR, Barr BM, Ison IC, Fulmer MT, Baker J, McKinney L, *et al.* Histological, chemical, and crystallographic analysis of four calcium phosphate

cements in different rabbit osseous sites. *J Biomed Mater Res.* 1998 Winter; 43(4): 451–61.
85. Penel G, Leroy N, Van Landuyt P, Flautre B, Hardouin P, Lemaitre J, *et al.* Raman microspectrometry studies of brushite cement: *in vivo* evolution in a sheep model. *Bone.* 1999 Aug; 25(2 Suppl): 81S–4S.
86. Brown WE, Chow LC, inventors; American Dental Association Health Foundation, assignee. Dental restorative cement pastes. USA. 1985.
87. Greish YE, Brown PW. Phase evolution during the formation of stoichiometric hydroxyapatite at 37.4 degrees C. *J Biomed Mater Res.* 2003 Oct 15; 67B(1): 632–7.
88. Ishikawa K, Takagi S, Chow LC, Ishikawa Y, Eanes ED, Asaoka K. Behavior of a calcium phosphate cement in simulated blood plasma *in vitro*. *Dent Mater.* 1994 Jan; 10(1): 26–32.
89. Flautre B, Delecourt C, Blary MC, Van Landuyt P, Lemaitre J, Hardouin P. Volume effect on biological properties of a calcium phosphate hydraulic cement: experimental study in sheep. *Bone.* 1999 Aug; 25(2 Suppl): 35S–9S.
90. Carrodeguas RG, De Aza AH, Turrillas X, Pena P, De Aza S. New approach to the beta-alpha polymorphic transformation in magnesium-substituted tricalcium phosphate and its practical implications. *J Am Ceram Soc.* 2008; 91(4): 1281–6.
91. Enderle R, Gotz-Neunhoeffer F, Gobbels M, Muller FA, Greil P. Influence of magnesium doping on the phase transformation temperature of beta-TCP ceramics examined by Rietveld refinement. *Biomaterials.* 2005 Jun; 26(17): 3379–84.
92. Gbureck U, Dembski S, Thull R, Barralet JE. Factors influencing calcium phosphate cement shelf-life. *Biomaterials.* 2005 Jun; 26(17): 3691–7.
93. Habibovic P, de Groot K. Osteoinductive biomaterials – properties and relevance in bone repair. *J Tissue Eng Regen Med.* 2007 Jan–Feb; 1(1): 25–32.
94. Yoshida K, Hyuga H, Kondo N, Kita H, Sasaki M, Mitamura M, *et al.* Substitution model of monovalent (Li, Na, and K), divalent (Mg), and trivalent (Al) metal ions for $\hat{I}^2$-tricalcium phosphate. *J Am Ceram Soc.* 2006; 89(2): 688–90.
95. Saint-Jean SJ, Camire CL, Nevsten P, Hansen S, Ginebra MP. Study of the reactivity and *in vitro* bioactivity of Sr-substituted alpha-TCP cements. *J Mater Sci Mater Med.* 2005 Nov; 16(11): 993–1001.
96. Ergun C, Webster TJ, Bizios R, Doremus RH. Hydroxylapatite with substituted magnesium, zinc, cadmium, and yttrium. I. Structure and microstructure. *J Biomed Mater Res.* 2002; 59(2): 305–11.
97. Gibson IR, Best SM, Bonfield W. Chemical characterization of silicon-substituted hydroxyapatite. *J Biomed Mater Res.* 1999; 44: 422–8.
98. Bigi A, Foresti E, Gandolfi M, Gazzano M, Roveri N. Isomorphous substitutions in β-tricalcium phosphate: the different effects of zinc and strontium. *J Inorg Biochem.* 1997; 66(4): 259–65.
99. LeGeros RZ, Daculsi G, Kijkowska R, Kerebel B, ed YI, J D, *et al.* The effect of magnesium on the formation of apatites and whitlockites. *Magnesium in Health and Disease.* 1989:11–9.
100. Khairoun I, Driessens FC, Boltong MG, Planell JA, Wenz R. Addition of cohesion promotors to calcium phosphate cements. *Biomaterials.* 1999 Feb; 20(4): 393–8.
101. Lee DD, Tofighi A, Aiolova M, Chakravarthy P, Catalano A, Majahad A, *et al.* alpha-BSM: a biomimetic bone substitute and drug delivery vehicle. *Clin Orthop.* 1999 Oct (367 Suppl): S396–405.
102. Tofighi A, Mounic S, Chakravarthy P, Rey C, Lee D. Setting reactions involved in injectable cements based on amorphous calcium phosphate. *Key Eng Mat.* 2001; 192–195: 769–72.

103. Frayssinet P, Roudier M, Lerch A, Ceolin JL, Depres E, Rouquet N. Tissue reaction against a self-setting calcium phosphate cement set in bone or outside the organism. *J Mater Sci-Mater M.* 2000 Dec; 11(12): 811–15.
104. Mulliez MA, Wenz R. Physical-chemical characterization of a new magnesium containing calcium phosphate cement SOPRIM. European Society for Biomaterials Annual Meeting (ESB 2002); 2002 Sept 11–14, 2002; Barcelona.
105. Kurashina K, Kurita H, Hirano M, Kotani A, Klein CP, de Groot K. *In vivo* study of calcium phosphate cements: implantation of an alpha-tricalcium phosphate/dicalcium phosphate dibasic/tetracalcium phosphate monoxide cement paste. *Biomaterials.* 1997 Apr; 18(7): 539–43.
106. Tanaka S, Kishi T, Shimogoryo R, Matsuya S, Ishikawa K. Biopex acquires anti-washout properties by adding sodium alginate into its liquid phase. *Dent Mater J.* 2003 Sep; 22(3): 301–12.
107. Brendlen D, Pittet C, Lemaitre J. Feasibility of a new dual-paste presentation of injectable brushite cement. *Proceedings of the 13th GRIBOI Meeting.* 2003 March 14–15, 2003; Baltimore (USA).
108. Liu C, Shen W, Gu Y, Hu L. Mechanism of the hardening process for a hydroxyapatite cement. *J Biomed Mater Res.* 1997 Apr; 35(1): 75–80.
109. Constantz BR, inventor Skeletal Kinetics, LLC, assignee. Calcium phosphate cements prepared from silicate solutions. USA 2002.
110. Chow LC. Development of self-setting calcium phosphate cements. *J Ceram Soc Jap.* 1991; 99(10): 954–64.
111. Hannink G, Wolke JGC, Schreurs BW, Buma P. *In vivo* behavior of a novel injectable calcium phosphate cement compared with two other commercially available calcium phosphate cements. *J Biomed Mater Res B Appl Biomater.* 2008; 85(2): 478–88.
112. Fernandez E, Planell JA, Best SM, Bonfield W. Synthesis of dahllite through a cement setting reaction. *J Mater Sci-Mater M.* 1998 Dec; 9(12): 789–92.
113. Turner TM, Urban RM, Gitelis S, Haggard WO, Richelsoph K. Resorption evaluation of a large bolus of calcium sulfate in a canine medullary defect. *Orthopedics.* 2003 May; 26(5 Suppl): s577–9.
114. Boix D, Weiss P, Gauthier O, Guicheux J, Bouler JM, Pilet P, *et al.* Injectable bone substitute to preserve alveolar ridge resorption after tooth extraction: a study in dog. *J Mater Sci Mater Med.* 2006 Nov; 17(11): 1145–52.
115. Gauthier O, Muller R, von Stechow D, Lamy B, Weiss P, Bouler JM, *et al. In vivo* bone regeneration with injectable calcium phosphate biomaterial: a three-dimensional micro-computed tomographic, biomechanical and SEM study. *Biomaterials.* 2005 Sep; 26(27): 5444–53.
116. Laschke MW, Witt K, Pohlemann T, Menger MD. Injectable nanocrystalline hydroxyapatite paste for bone substitution: *in vivo* analysis of biocompatibility and vascularization. *J Biomed Mater Res B Appl Biomater.* 2007 Aug; 82(2): 494–505.
117. Clarke SA, Hoskins NL, Jordan GR, Henderson SA, Marsh DR. *In vitro* testing of Advanced JAX Bone Void Filler System: species differences in the response of bone marrow stromal cells to beta tri-calcium phosphate and carboxymethylcellulose gel. *J Mater Sci Mater Med.* 2007 Dec; 18(12): 2283–90.
118. Bucholz RW. Nonallograft osteoconductive bone graft substitutes. *Clin Orthop.* 2002 Feb(395): 44–52.

3

Rheological properties of injectable biomaterials

R. McLEMORE, Banner Good Samaritan Medical Center, USA

Abstract: This chapter covers a basic introduction to rheology similar to that present in many introductory bioengineering texts. Additional attention is paid to examples of the use of rheology to characterize different types of *in situ* gelling systems currently being researched for medical applications. The discussion focuses on the differences between materials based on types and kinetics, and data that can be obtained from rheological measurements relevant to the development of procedures for the delivery of *in situ* gelling materials. Some tips are provided for overcoming common experimental difficulties that may arise during use of a rheometer to characterize materials that exhibit shrinkage or evaporation. Finally, the chapter closes with a discussion of future directions in *in situ* gelling materials, and the effects that rheology has in shaping those directions.

Key words: rheology, shrinkage, kinetics, swelling, evaporation, radio-opaque, solvent exchange, chemical gel.

3.1 Introduction

This chapter begins with a very brief primer on rheology for those who may be unfamiliar with the technique. The remainder is concerned with discussing techniques and observations useful for the rheology of hydrogels and other *in situ* gelling materials. This information is organized into the following sections, briefly summarized below:

- Basic introduction to rheology. This section provides a short description of the technology underlying a rheometer. Additionally, it includes some basic descriptions and characteristics of gel rheology.
- Types of *in situ* gelling materials: chemical gels, solvent exchange, physical gels. This section introduces the reader to selected examples of *in situ* hydrogels from the literature, and tries to clearly explain the differences between them. A discussion of frequency and creep measurements is included herein in reference to these different types of injectable materials.
- Shrinkage, swelling, and evaporation. This is a short discussion of environmental effects that one needs to be aware of and account for in rheological data of *in situ* forming hydrogels and other polymeric materials.
- Kinetics and injectability. This section discusses the additional application of rheology in helping to control the rate of transition of *in situ* gelling materials.

- The role of statistics and uncertainty in rheological characterization. This section very briefly presents some statistical tools which may be useful in the characterization of rheological data for *in situ* gelling materials.
- Future trends. This section presents a short discussion of the trends and future directions in the field.

3.1.1 Basic introduction to rheology

We begin the discussion by defining the technique itself. Rheology is a branch of science concerned with the characterization of viscoelastic fluids. A more scientific definition of rheology is the study of materials which are not completely described by either classic Hookean mechanics, which describe solids, or Newton's law of viscosity, which describe liquids, but instead fall somewhere in-between.[1] So, when we talk about the rheology of viscoelastic solids/liquids, what we mean is that we are monitoring the viscosity, elasticity, and other 'flow' properties, and the change in those properties over time in the presence of stimuli.

A basic discussion of rheology usually begins with a discussion of viscoelasticity, or a resistance of liquids to flow easily. Viscoelasticity commonly becomes an issue in solutions made up of molecules that are of a significant size in kDa (kilo Daltons). Examples from everyday experience might include foods like margarine and cheese or polymers like paints. Polymer and food science frequently handle samples in similar environments, either incorporating solvents to solubilize the high molecular weight components, or handling the materials in a semi-liquid state referred to as a 'melt'. The two simplest classical models for viscoelasticity are the Maxwell and the Kelvin-Voight models.[2] These simple models consist of a dashpot (mechanical device which consists of a weight which moves through a fluid that resists its movement due to drag and friction) and a spring, either in series or in parallel. Dashpots are commonly found on screen doors to prevent them from slamming shut. The spring describes the proportion of the load that behaves elastically, essentially following the following equation:

$$F = kx$$

The dashpot describes the behavior of the liquid portion, which classically follows the simple expression[3] (known as Newton's law of viscosity):

$$\tau = \eta \frac{\mathrm{d}\gamma}{\mathrm{d}t}$$

where τ is the shear stress, η is the viscosity of the fluid, and $\mathrm{d}\gamma/\mathrm{d}t$ represents the change in the strain rate of the fluid over time. There are several models of viscoelastic behavior more complicated than the Maxwell and Kelvin-Voight model, including the General Linear Model. These models essentially consist of combinations of dashpots and springs which are combined either in series or in parallel to produce a finite element structure, which provides responses in shear stress similar to those produced by the fluid under study. Rheological parameters are calculated as follows:[4]

$$G^* = \frac{\sigma_o}{\gamma_o} \qquad G' = G^* \cos\delta \qquad G'' = G^* \sin\delta$$

where σ is the stress exerted by the machine, γ is the strain exerted by the machine, G^* is the complex modulus, G' is the storage modulus, G'' is the loss modulus, and δ is the degree to which the measured strain is out of phase with the oscillating head, as discussed above. Readers with additional interest in this topic are encouraged to pursue reference number 4 above, which provides a much more detailed rheological discussion.

With a basic background in viscoelasticity, we can briefly discuss the basic parameters that a rheometer measures, and how they relate to the material that is under study. For the case of oscillatory flow, the rheometer will typically provide three basic parameters of interest in characterizing the properties of a gel under study. These parameters are:

- G': The storage modulus: The storage modulus is defined as the elastic component of the gel or liquid under study. Essentially, this represents the degree of in phase behavior that the gel provides, or describes the strength and degree to which the gel acts like a solid.
- G'': The loss modulus: The loss modulus basically defines the viscous component of the gel or liquid under study. This represents the degree of lagging, or out of phase behavior that the gel provides. A high G'' relative to G' describes a highly viscous material.
- δ: The phase angle: δ is defined as the arctangent of G''/G'. Essentially, when G'' is very large compared to G', δ will be near 90°, and when G' is very large relative to G'', δ will be very close to zero. The *gel point* is classically defined as the point where δ crosses 45° in time or temperature dependent experiments. Figure 3.1 illustrates these two cases:

Figure 3.1(a) shows the case where G'' is much larger than G'. The solid line represents the oscillation of the head of the rheometer, and the dotted line represents the strain response by the fluid. Figure 3.1(b) shows the opposite case, where G' is relatively high compared to G''.

These plots represent small time steps during the oscillatory motion the rheometer employs to monitor the sample. The above plot depicts the motion of the head of the rheometer as a black line, and illustrates the response of the sample with a grey dotted line. As a gel becomes more solid, the response of the material will move 'in phase' with the head of the rheometer, since the elastic modulus will be relatively stronger than the loss (viscous) modulus. During this time, both G' and G'' are growing as the crosslink density in the sample changes. The machine will report the data usually in the following manner.

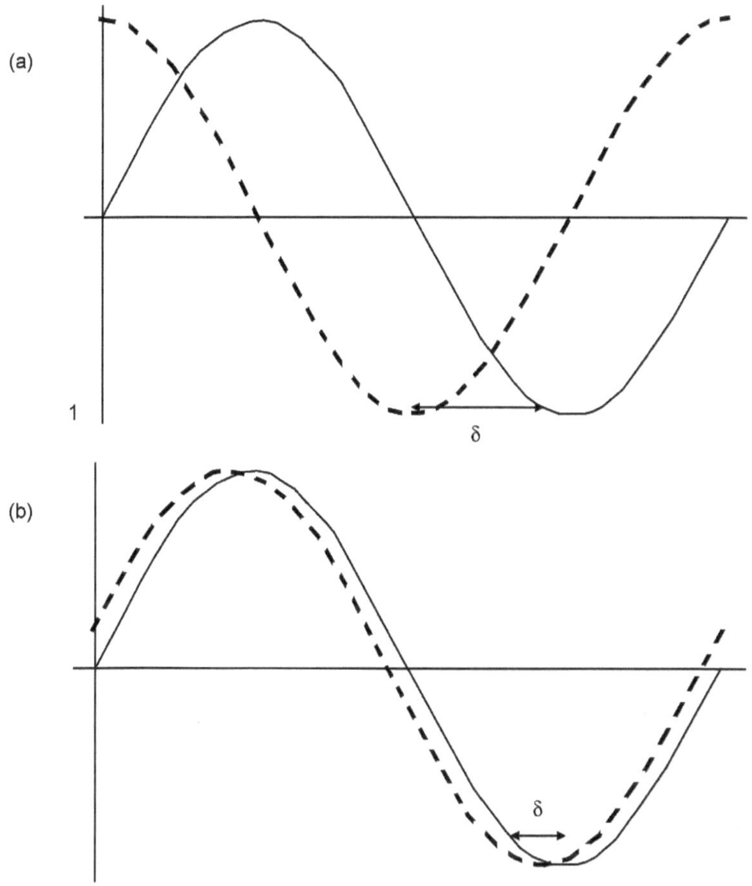

3.1 Relationship between shear stress, strain, and delta in an oscillatory experiment.

Figure 3.2 shows a theoretical trace as might be produced by a rheometer during the course of a chemical gelation experiment over time. The black solid line represents G', the grey dotted line represents G'', and the black dotted line represents δ. δ ranges from 90° to 0°, with 45° occurring at the gel point, when G'' and G' are equal. All three traces have been superimposed on this plot, but will usually be shown on split axes.

Finally, most rheometers will calculate the dynamic viscosity of the sample. This is a derived value which is related to G''. There is a difference between the dynamic and the kinematic viscosities, and several methods of estimating viscosity do not always agree with high precision as to the viscosities of fluids, but for the purposes of the discussion herein, we can use this value as a point estimator for the viscosity of the fluid under measurement for similar shear rates.

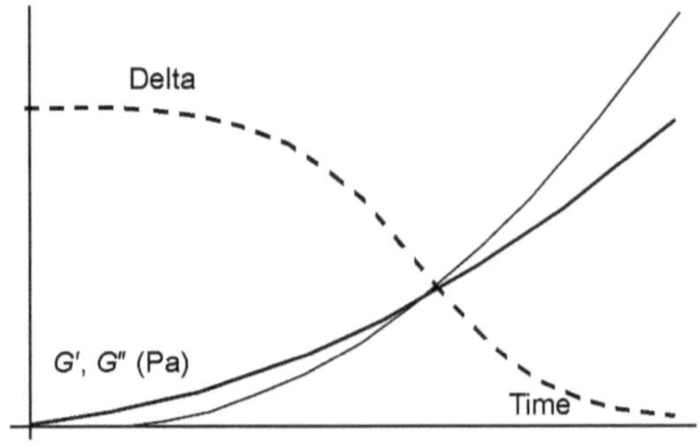

3.2 Relationship between G', G'', and delta during a chemical gelation.

For most oscillatory measurements, one has to control multiple variables, ramp (cover a range of values with a set rate of change) one variable, and measure several more variables. Classical oscillatory measurements included on most systems are stress sweeps, frequency sweeps, time sweeps, and temperature sweeps (if a peltier unit is included).

Some of the newer machines can perform constant flow experiments, and additionally may incorporate UV curing apparatus to enable the study of materials whose gelation is triggered by UV light. One complication that tends to occur with rheology includes discussion of the LVER (linear viscoelastic region). This refers to a region, usually identified in a strain sweep, where G' is independent of strain.[5,6] Another way of saying this is that the machine setup will affect the material's response to an increasing amplitude deformation at constant frequency. The reason for this caveat is that if one is not in the LVER, the relative contribution of G' to G^* will change at a constant frequency as a function of strain. The LVER is highly sample dependent and will be dependent on the frequency (strain rate) of the measurement. For *in situ* gelling hydrogels, there may in fact be reasons to measure systems outside of the LVER, if, for instance, particular strain rates are more in keeping with the application that the material may see in use, but in these cases, the experimenter should clearly note the frequency used, and be cognizant that the experiments are likely only comparable to gels run at similar frequency, as the estimated magnitude of G' and G'' is likely to change if one is outside the LVER.

3.2 Different types of *in situ* gelling materials: chemical gels, solvent exchange, and physical gels

In practice, most *in situ*-gelling polymers rely on one of four strategies:

1. *Chemical gelation*: Many of the original polymers developed for *in situ* gelation relied upon a chemical reaction in which monomers polymerize

upon some initiation. An example of a chemical gelation is two-part epoxies. These epoxies, when mixed, will form chemical bonds in a rapid fashion. This gelation reaction is commonly triggered by mixing a multipart system together or by exposure to air. Once the reaction is initiated, there is a window of available time to introduce the material before the polymer becomes solid and no longer useful.[7] Chemical gelation materials generally delivered in water have very high swelling, so instead of using a reaction initiator in water, it may be advantageous to use photopolymerization.

2. *Thermal gelation*: These materials rely upon a temperature induced phase change to initiate gel formation, usually an increase in environmental temperature. This behavior is unique from our common everyday experience in which higher temperatures melt solid materials into liquids. In this case, higher temperatures cause liquid solutions of polymer molecules to collapse into a solid block. This unusual behavior is because of the competing thermodynamic properties of enthalpy (energy) and entropy (disorder). These properties are used to describe a thermodynamic system, an arbitrary physical object or collection of objects to be studied (in this case, we are considering a solution of polymer chains as the system). Classically, at low temperatures, enthalpy is more important for determining the behavior of the system; essentially, the system will favor conformations that lower the energy (enthalpy). At higher temperatures, disorder is more important and systems will often change configurations with a greater amount of disorder.

   Polymer chains with both hydrophobic and hydrophilic groups interact with water to make organized structures of water molecules around the hydrophilic groups. This lowers the energy of the system, which is typical at lower temperatures. However, at higher temperatures, these water structures breakdown as the water molecules tumble more chaotically, and the polymer chains are forced together to make a solid material. The temperature at which the polymer chains precipitate out of the solution into a solid mass is the lower critical solution temperature (LCST).

   An application of polymers that exhibit this temperature behavior is the delivery of a cold polymer solution through a catheter into a patient's body. If the LCST is around body temperature, as the solution warms up, the material will become solid at the injection site. The distance that the polymer will travel before gelling depends upon the diameter of the induction device and the temperature of the original polymer, relative to the gelation temperature, or LCST of the material.[8]

3. *Solvent exchange*: Describes a specific set of materials that rely upon diffusion of an organic solvent and its replacement by an aqueous one. Practically, this process would be highly inefficient for injection into the blood stream, but can be used peritoneally or subcutaneously, where there is little threat of embolus, and a long time course for diffusion to occur. This technique has been employed with an ethylene vinyl alcohol embolization

system, termed Onyx™, but research indicates that filling aneurysms with this material is very slow, and requires a number of successive inflations of a surgical balloon to keep the material in place while the organic solvent dimethyl sulfoxide (DMSO) exchanges with water.[9]

4. *Mixing*: Although these polymers are similar to those that rely on chemical gelation strategies, I place these in a separate class because of the technique used to induce them. Owing to advances in catheter design, it is now possible to create dual-lumen catheters of a diameter capable of penetrating many of the smaller blood vessels in the body. Delivery usually involves taking two low viscosity fluids, and separately running them through much of the catheter in their respective lumens. Using a system with a very high reaction rate, it is then possible to mix the system shortly before injecting it into the target vacancy, generating a system with a very short range but a very quick reaction. This is common to many of the calcium alginate gels designed for *in situ* polymerization.[10]

For many of these types of materials, rheology can be a tremendously useful tool in their characterization. For chemical and thermal gelation, rheometers can commonly be configured to perform a temperature ramp to trigger the changes, or to simulate the environment the gel is intended for (traveling down a catheter at a given temperature, and then entering the body at another temperature, for instance). Rheology can additionally be used as a quality control technology to verify the consistency of the various components involved in mixing or solvent exchange type systems (ensuring the batch-to-batch viscosity is similar, for instance), but it is understandably more difficult to use it to monitor their gelation properties due to challenges in recreating the environmental triggers that lead to gelation in an area that the rheometer can measure, since there is frequently no good way with a cone and plate rheometer to create an external source of fluid for the system to equilibrate with.

3.2.1 Interpretation of frequency sweeps for different types of gels

Other chapters in this book describe differing applications of *in situ* gelling materials. In certain clinical applications, such as occlusion of arteriovenous malformation, the resistance of the final material to flow under pressure can be of significant clinical concern. In other applications, such as soft tissue replacement, these properties may be less of a concern.

One active area of research involves the generation of polymers that can form chemical crosslinks once delivered onsite. For applications where creep (slow, unrecoverable deformation of the material under stress) is a concern, a frequency sweep can be used to get an estimation of relative changes (increases in G' at a given frequency, for instance) over time with regards to viscous behavior

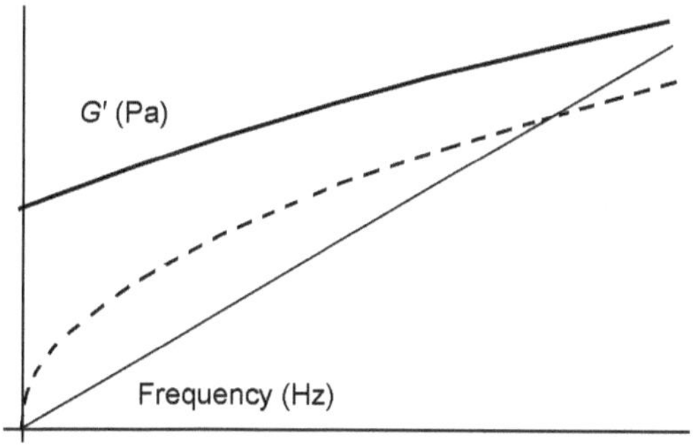

3.3 Frequency sweeps for Newtonian, low crosslink density, and high crosslink density fluids. The thin black line represents a Newtonian fluid, the dotted grey line represents a low chemical-crosslink density gel, the dotted black line represents a higher chemical-crosslink density gel, all measured over the same frequency range.

of the gel as a reaction occurs over time, but is often difficult to correlate exactly with an experimental environment.

An oscillatory rheometer will produce a plot of G' and G'' versus frequency of the rheometer head. This plot is analogous to the normal Newton's law of viscosity plot that one can generate for a newtonian or non-newtonian fluid. While the classical plots will show τ vs. $\dot{\gamma}$ (shear stress vs. strain rate), the rheometer plot of G' (Pa) vs. frequency (Hz) is dimensionally similar and highly comparable. Figure 3.3 explains the changes one might expect to see in a frequency plot as the degree of crosslinking in a chemical gel increases. The black line representing a Newtonian fluid is included for reference, and would be measured vs. shear stress, not G'. Most fluids that the rheometer can measure will not provide a Newtonian curve, and the magnitudes of the curves below are normalized so that the reader can appreciate the change in slope, most gels will have a significantly higher viscosity than water. Again, G' is not the same thing as viscosity.

This technique can be very useful in characterizing design changes (thickening of the material in response to low frequency stresses, for instance) and evaluating the properties of both the mix type, chemical gelation type, and thermal gelation type systems (although the peltier system needs to be on and the sample needs to be equilibrated prior to the measurement). For high throughput applications or for comparative measurements, this can often be more time efficient than a classic creep measurement, and can also allow the experimenter to view the behavior of the system at multiple frequencies, instead of the classic load relaxation seen in a creep experiment.

3.2.2 Creep measurements

Many oscillatory rheometers can also perform creep experiments. Essentially, these protocols will place the sample under a constant stress for a fixed amount of time, and then allow the sample to relax, and measure the amount of distention present. Such measurements can be useful in describing the amount of creep over time a gel might see at a given shear rate. Overall, these experiments are quite useful but tend to be very time consuming, owing to the inability to accelerate the elongation process.

3.3 Shrinkage, swelling, and evaporation

During the rheological measurement of gels, there are several significant processes that one needs to be aware of involving environmental changes and stability of the gel over the period of the experiment. Referring to Fig. 3.2, we see a normal curve that would represent the gelation of a multipart system that was left to gel on the rheometer. Now imagine that we run three replicates of that gel, and recover the following data for G' (Fig. 3.4).

This type of effect usually will occur in systems that undergo thermal gelation, and exhibit both fast and slow shrinkage. The particularly large deviation in the estimated G' post gelation arises from the averaging nature of the rheometer. As the gel shrinks, it forces water out of the body of the gel and into contact with the cone that the rheometer uses to measure the sample. The juxtaposition of water and the highly viscous gel leads the machine to measure a reduced viscosity because of reduced surface area coverage of the gel. Because of this effect, the range in observed G' in the plateau region of gels can vary significantly. Frequently, using a system with normal force control can help to compensate for this variability, as the system can push the water out of the way to maintain contact with the receding gel surface. Failing that, it is possible to dab away excess fluid with a chemwipe, and then replace the head of the geometry. This is frequently difficult to do consistently, however, as the shrinkage of thermal materials, for instance, can occur over several hours.

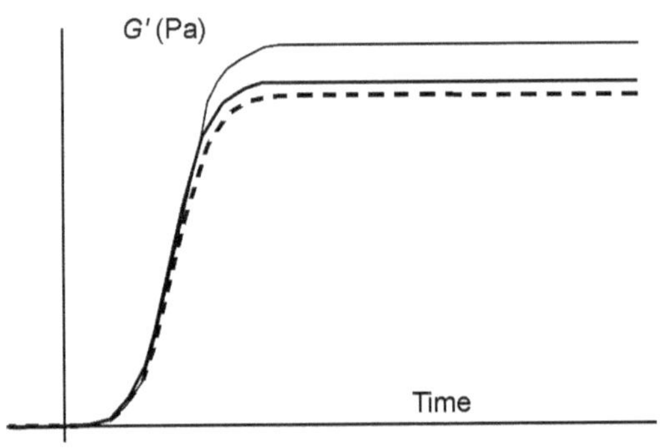

3.4 Traces showing typical behavior for G' in shrinking chemical gels. The three different traces show three different trials of the same material. Note that the G' data in most systems is displayed exponentially.

3.3.1 Swelling and evaporation

Swelling, the expansion of gel as it absorbs liquid, and evaporation (of the solvent that is absorbed in the gel) can be challenging with gel rheology, but, in general, are less of a problem than shrinkage when measuring hydrogels and similar materials. Most modern instruments will have an option to use an evaporation chamber. For most water-soluble materials, it is a good idea to put a thin bead of mineral oil around the top and the bottom of the environmental chamber to provide a barrier to evaporation, and if there is a recessed cavity on the plate, that area can be packed with moist tissue. In general, however, one needs to be aware of the effect of evaporation in experiments involving high molecular weight, high concentration, or long periods of time. Evaporation will occur from the edge of the sample in, and will show a drift in the sample towards higher viscosity and G'/G''.

3.4 Kinetics and injectability

As has been discussed briefly above, the main thing that separates *in situ* gelling systems from other polymeric systems is that they go through a transition on site, rather than being preformed and implanted. For systems that are delivered into relatively avascular areas, like the subcutaneous space, concerns over initial viscosity are fairly minimal. Solutions that are of low viscosity are likely to diffuse away prior to gelation without any consequences for the patients (assuming little to no reaction). However, solutions delivered into the blood stream are subject to the forces placed upon them during their transition, which may interfere in their gelation. This unique property means that one must be concerned about their properties prior to, during, and after delivery. Vernon,[11] Becker,[12] and others have published on the control of *in situ* forming gels, and examined the challenges inherent in their use. When delivering a gel near blood-flow, the main concerns that one faces are dissolution and stroke. Dissolution, the loss of the material as it dilutes in the blood, in most cases is less of a problem for the patient; if the material dissolves, there is unlikely to be an adverse reaction for the patient, as the materials will be highly dispersed and likely to clear through the kidney. However, if a material escapes the site of injection, but is partially reacted into a small solid structure, it is likely to form embolus. So, these small particles would travel through the vascular system and would be likely to cause stroke. Because of this concern, it is important to ensure that materials are viscoelastic enough to resist dispersion and flow before they are delivered. The level of viscoelasticity that would be safe is dependent on the blood-flow conditions in the area the gel is delivered, but in general blood flow in the extremities near aneurism or AVM is low-pressure flow. Previous publications,[13] including those cited above have begun to look at how to more closely model and understand the level of safety necessary for these injections in a clinical setting. The approach with the highest safety margin, however, is to formulate gels so that they have the highest viscosity possible while still being injectable. Practically, this will ensure that the risk of any embolus, separation, or other undesirable outcome is minimized. In the case of chemical gelation, especially, rheology can be used to simulate the environments in which the gelation occurs. The kinetics of the gel, measured from the increase in G' and decrease in δ over time with a time sweep, can then be correlated with separate delivery experiments, like flow chambers or animal models, in similar environmental conditions. This can also help to identify the viscoelasticity and time at which a material becomes too solid to inject. Refinement of injection procedures is usually a cyclical process, with changes being made both to the delivery protocol and to the chemistry and kinetics of the system one is studying, but the end result will be a better documented, safer, and more reliable gel.

To illustrate this concept, I will provide an example from my own graduate research. As part of my project, I needed to design a gel that would be able to travel down a three-foot long catheter, and be able to be injected into significant fluid flow at the other end without causing embolus, and without overfilling the site due to ballooning of the catheter under pressure. Prior to my discovery of rheology, initial attempts at this feat left me quite hopeless. Either the material would be too thin and runny, or it would gel long before it reached the appropriate length of the catheter. Overcoming this problem required an iterative approach coupling rheometry with successive attempts to move the gel down the catheter using a syringe pump at a constant volumetric rate. By making the volumetric rate fairly slow, it was possible to limit the expansion and contraction of the catheter, thus controlling the volumetric accuracy issue. By changing the initiator concentration and setting the rheometer to mimic the temperature conditions of the body, I was able to change the gelation curve by changing the initiator concentration as shown in Fig. 3.5.

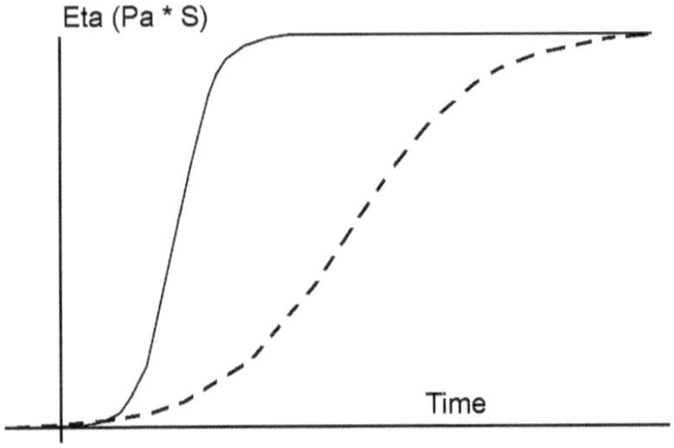

3.5 An example from research of the use of rheology to quantify gelation rates. The solid black line shows the original gelation rate, the dotted grey line shows the modified, slower gelation rate.

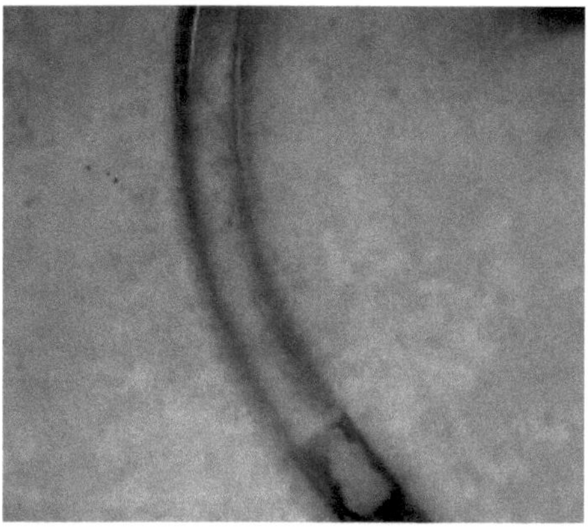

3.6 Image of successful injection of gel into a tube through a 3′ catheter at 37°C, into flowing water. This image shows the gel emerging from the catheter and gelling to the side of the tube wall in the laboratory.

By comparing the viscosity of the new formulations to the above data, I identified several likely candidates, which had a high viscosity for several minutes, but were below ~1000 Pa·s, which was approximately where I determined my gel to begin to become uninjectable. This allowed me to design a formulation of gel that was injectable for approximately 15 minutes, long enough to push it down the long catheter over 15 minutes, and yet have a gel that was still able to gel upon reaching the target location, despite significant cross flow with fluid. An image of the successful injection is shown in Fig. 3.6.

3.5 The role of statistics and uncertainty in rheological characterization

Statistics play a major role in most modern data analysis. Much of the discussion in this chapter has focused on techniques for using the rheometer to mock the environment one intends to deliver the gel to. It is tempting from this assertion to then state that such techniques give one pinpoint control over the behavior of the gel thus designed. It is vitally important to realize, however, that, for most of these applications, there will still be significant deviation in the gelation rate observed. Experimentally, three identical samples tested will give slightly variable measurements as to their gelation rates, and this difference in rate in many systems will approximately scale with increased gelation time. The simplest way to evaluate this difference is to run 3–5 samples, calculate the average and standard deviation in time of the gel point, and evaluate how critical that time range is to the application you are considering. For instance, if your application requires a gel time of 1 minute, and your rheology shows a gel time of 1 minute ± 40 seconds, you have a significant problem. Alternatively, if you can make procedural changes or eliminate error to the point that you can reduce the variation to 1 minute $\pm$ 10 seconds, that may be a level of variability that you can work with. Frequently, observing the standard deviation of measurements taken before and after a formulation or environmental change can help to identify sources of systematic error, and can make the system safer and more reliable.

In order to maximize throughput on these kinds of experiments, it can often be desirable to employ design of experiment techniques.[14] This method involves making a 2^N table of all of the factors one thinks may be affecting their data. In the classical design, both a high and a low value are selected for each factor. Iteration of this design allows for identification of the factors and interactions that significantly influence the system under study. Data analysis is usually completed with the statistical technique known as an analysis of variance (ANOVA), which tries to determine if variability in the system is due to changes in your design parameters (factors) or just random chance. Once significant factors have been identified, there are several techniques that can be used to explore the behavior of those factors over a wide range of values. Employing this type of technique will help to minimize the amount of iteration involved in redesigning the delivery procedures of candidate gels.

3.6 Future trends

Rheology can be used, as described above, in applications involving quality control, characterization, and design of novel injection techniques and materials. For tissue engineering applications under exploration, rheology can be used to characterize the way that addition of growth factors, ligands, or environmental variables affect bulk properties of gels.

For systems injected in or near the vasculature, current issues include difficulty in obtaining clinical images during injection and dangers arising from low viscosity injections causing stroke. While past research has evaluated the incorporation of radio-opaque or x-ray visible inorganic salt additives like Tantalum[15] or Conray[13] for contrast in fluoroscopy (x-ray real time imaging). Both of these techniques suffer from the significant drawback that the visibility agent is entrapped in the gel and is not chemically attached to the precursors that form the gel. An active area of current research involves the conjugation of radio-opaque molecules, like benzyl iodine, to the precursors in order to form gels that are inherently radio-opaque. An additional area of research involves the development of higher viscosity mixtures that are still injectable. By admixing monomers of different molecular weights in defined ratios, it is possible to produce solutions that have higher initial viscosity, but still provide similar strengths and creep resistance upon gelation. Development of these kinds of mixtures for clinical applications may provide additional safety and reliability that many of these systems currently lack. By increasing the initial viscosity of the injected fluid, the goal is to reduce the risk of bolus formation if the system is injected too early. Unfortunately, this type of change is also likely to cause the solution to behave in a less Newtonian fashion, and may complicate its delivery because of this. Both of the above changes are likely to make significant alterations in the kinetics and rheological properties of the basic materials. By coupling rheology with these new chemical and formulation changes, the goal will be to produce safe, reliable systems that can be used clinically.

3.7 Sources of further information and advice

As discussed above, there are several good resources to gain a more in-depth understanding of rheological properties and rheological characterization. I have found *Understanding Rheology* (Oxford University Press), and *Colloids and Cosmetics* (Ref. 4) to be very useful in explaining the intricacies and interrelated nature of the variables measured classic rheology. These types of texts are also a good place to seek understanding as to the different types of fluids and the difference between Newtonian and non-Newtonian fluids. There is additionally a wide range of scholarly papers available through PubMed or Google Scholar describing the development of specific systems for specific applications. For specific application questions, rheology sales representatives are always a good resource, and the representatives at TA Instruments and Anton Paar have been very helpful whenever I have had a question in regards to operation of their machines. Both of these manufacturers have online rheology references available at their websites. The website for the Society of Rheology can be found at: http://www.rheology.org/sor/. The website for the Society of Biomaterials can be found at: http://www.biomaterials.org/.

3.8 References

1. Alexander Ya Malkin, Avraam I. Isayev. *Rheology – Concepts, Methods, and Applications*: ChemTec Publishing; 2006.
2. Buddy D. Ratner, Allan S. Hoffman, Frederick J. Schoen, Lemons JE. *Biomaterials Science*: Academic Press; 1996.
3. Neville J. Price, John W. Cosgrove. *Analysis of Geological Structures*: Cambridge University Press; 1990.
4. *Colloids and Cosmetics in Personal care.* Vol 4: Wiley-VCH; 2008.
5. R. Greenwood, K. Kendall, S. Ritchie, M.J. Snowden. The use of poly (N-isopropylacrylamide) microgels as a multi-functional processing aid for aqueous alumina suspensions. *Journal of the European Ceramic Society.* 2000; 20: 1707–1716.
6. Y. Hemar, D. S. Horne. Dynamic rheological properties of highly concentrated protein-stabilized emulsions. *Langmuir.* 2000; 16: 3050–3057.
7. Gavin P. Andrews, Sean P. Gorman, D.S. Jones. Rheological characterisation of primary and binary interactive bioadhesive gels composed of cellulose derivatives designed as ophthalmic viscosurgical devices. *Biomaterials.* 2005; 26: 571–580.
8. Vernon B, Martinez A. Gel strength and solution viscosity of temperature-sensitive,

in situ-gelling polymers for endovascular embolization. *J Biomater Sci Polym Ed.* 2005; 16(9): 1153–1166.

9. M.J. Bratby, E.D. Lehmann, J. Bottomley, *et al.* Endovascular embolization of visceral artery aneurysms with ethylene-vinyl alcohol (Onyx): a case series. *CardioVascular and Interventional Radiology.* 2006; 29: 1125–1128.
10. T.A. Becker, D.R. Kipke, M.C. Preul, W.D. Bichard, C.G. McDougall. *In vivo* assessment of calcium alginate gel for endovascular embolization of a cerebral arteriovenous malformation model using the Swine rete mirabile. *Neurosurgery.* 2002; 51(2): 453–459.
11. Merrill Birdno, Brent Vernon. Mechanical optimization of an arteriovenous malformation embolization material: a predictive model analysis. *Annals of Biomedical Engineering.* 2005; 33(2): 191–201.
12. Youji Soga, Mark C. Preul, Motomasa Furuse, Timothy Becker, Cameron G. McDougall. Calcium alginate provides a high degree of embolization in aneurysm models: a specific comparison to coil packing. *Neurosurgery.* 2004; 55(6): 1401–1409.
13. R. McLemore, M.C. Preul, B.L. Vernon. Controlling delivery properties of a waterborne, *in-situ*-forming material. *Journal of Biomedical Materials Research B.* 2006.
14. D.C. Montgomery. *Design and Analysis of Engineering Experiments*, 5th edn. John Wiley and Sons; 2001.
15. T.A. Becker, D.R. Kipke, M.C. Preul, W.D. Bichard, C.G. McDougall. *In vivo* assessment of calcium alginate gel for endovascular embolization of a cerebral arteriovenous malformation model using the Swine rete mirabile. *Neurosurgery.* 2002; 51(2): 453–458.

4
Improving mechanical properties of injectable polymers and composites

Y. QIU, S. K. HAMILTON and J. TEMENOFF,
Georgia Tech/Emory University, USA

Abstract: Injectable polymers and composites have been widely explored for biomedical applications due to their potential use in minimally invasive surgeries and advantages in filling irregular-shaped tissue defects. To improve overall performance and tissue integration of injectable materials, specific mechanical properties are often required. This chapter focuses on the relationship between material structure and mechanical properties, with particular emphasis on reviewing means to improve the mechanical properties of injectable polymers and composites. Potential applications of each type of injectable polymer/composite (including both hydrophilic and hydrophobic polymers) are discussed, and current challenges relating to enhancing mechanical properties of injectable biomaterials are highlighted.

Key words: injectable polymers, composites, mechanical properties, biomaterials.

4.1 Introduction

Because injectable materials can be introduced to a desired site in the body and form scaffolds *in situ*, they possess particular advantages for use in minimally invasive surgeries. At the same time, they can easily fill irregular defects, thus facilitating better integration of the implant with the native tissue. This chapter focuses on injectable polymers, which, more precisely, can be considered a class of crosslinkable precursors. They can be viscous liquids, pastes, or powders. The powder form should be soluble in water or organic diluents to allow injection into desired sites in the body, similar to the procedure utilized for liquid and paste precursors. After injection, these materials can be triggered by external cues (temperature, light, etc.) to form crosslinked network *in situ*. For various applications, different mechanical properties may be required. For example, when they are employed for hard tissues that need to support loading, the materials must be very stiff and tough with high strength. When used for replacement of blood vessels, they should exhibit toughness and a certain degree of elasticity.

This chapter will focus on the relationship between structure and mechanical properties of injectable materials and their crosslinked networks. To better understand this relationship, we will first discuss the common mechanical properties considered when characterizing injectable materials and how they are measured. We will then describe current efforts to adjust the structure of injectable materials to obtain desired mechanical properties for various expected applications. Finally, challenges and further directions in this field will also be discussed.

4.2 Mechanical properties and testing

Mechanical properties represent the responses of materials to external forces. While brittle materials break before they yield, highly elastic materials elongate to more than 1000% without breaking and recover their original shape after the force is released. Generally speaking, the responses of materials that can be easily measured are the changes of their physical shapes, including the length (l), area of the cross section (A) and angle of the sample deformation (θ). To characterize mechanical properties, well-controlled forces are imparted on a sample and responses are recorded over time using a specially designed testing machine (Nielsen and Landel, 1994; Ward and Sweeney, 2004).

Mechanical testing can be generally classified into tensile, compressive and shear testing on the basis of the mode of applied external forces (Temenoff and Mikos, 2008). In tensile testing, the force is utilized to stretch the sample. Therefore, the sample usually has a 'dog-bone' shape and a regular cross-section that is easily measured to facilitate the testing. During testing, stretch force is applied along the longitudinal axis. Two defined parameters here are stress (σ) and strain (ϵ), which can be calculated as follows:

$$\sigma = F/A_0 \qquad 4.1$$

where F is the force perpendicularly applied to the cross-section of the sample, and A_0 is the original area of cross-section before testing (Temenoff and Mikos, 2008).

$$\epsilon = (I_i - I_0)/I_0 \qquad 4.2$$

where I_0 is sample's original length and I_i is the actual length measured by the machine during the testing procedure. For further analysis, the stress is usually plotted against strain to obtain a curve, such as that seen in Fig. 4.1(a) (Schaffer, 1999). It is easy to obtain the yield stress (σ_{ys}) and ultimate tensile strength (σ_{uts}) from the curve (Fig. 4.1(a) and (b)), respectively (Schaffer, 1999). Tensile modulus can be calculated from the linear region in the area of small elongation (commonly strain < 5%). Toughness is defined as the area underneath the stress-strain curve. Generally speaking, stiff materials normally have very high tensile modulus while highly elastic materials have comparatively lower tensile modulus and can undergo large strain without breaking (e.g. 200–1000%).

Compared to tensile testing, force is applied to the sample in an opposite direction in compressive testing (Temenoff and Mikos, 2008). Moreover, the

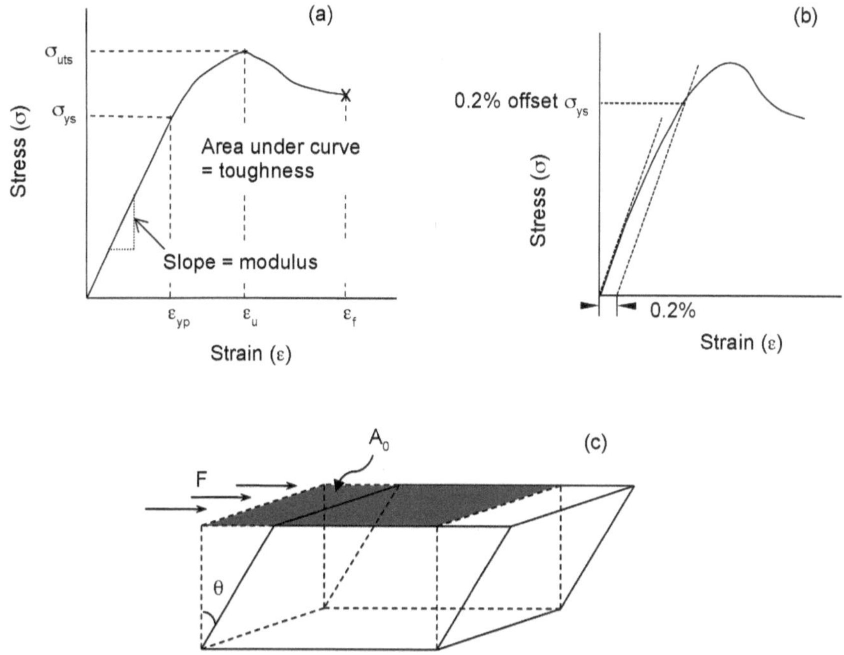

4.1 Mechanical testing parameters: (a) A representative strain–stress curve in tensile testing. Yield stress (σ_{ys}) and yield point strain (ϵ_{yp}) can be obtained by recording values at the point where the curve transitions from a linear relationship between stress and strain (elastic deformation) to a non-linear relationship (plastic deformation). Ultimate tensile strength (σ_{uts}) is the maximum stress in the curve, and the corresponding strain is called uniform strain (ϵ_u). The strain at fracture (ϵ_f) can also be obtained from the curve. (b) When the transition point between elastic and plastic deformation is difficult to identify, a 0.2% strain offset line parallel to the elastic portion is drawn to obtain the σ_{ys} or 0.2% offset σ_{ys}. (c) Schematic of the deformation that occurs when shear force is applied to a viscoelastic polymer.

specimen is usually shaped into a cylinder, and its length is normally at least twice its diameter. Compressive testing uses the same parameters (σ and ϵ) as tensile testing. However, due to the different force direction, the compressive stress and strain are calculated as negative. Therefore, the stress-strain curve in compressive testing is slightly different, but the compressive modulus can be obtained from the linear region, similar to the tensile modulus. Since compression testing does not require a dog-bone geometry and the usage of grips, it is widely applied for characterizing fragile materials such as hydrogels.

Unlike tensile or compressive testing, in shear testing, force is applied in parallel to the top and bottom surface of the sample (Fig. 4.1(c)) (Temenoff and Mikos, 2008). Shear stress (τ) is defined as:

$$\tau = F/A_0 \tag{4.3}$$

where F is the parallel force and A_0 is the original surface area. Since the shear force causes sample deformation of angle θ, shear strain (γ) is defined as

$$\gamma = \tan\theta \tag{4.4}$$

Because polymers have viscoelastic properties, rheometry is often employed to simultaneously measure both elastic and viscous parameters. To measure the viscoelastic properties using a rheometer, an oscillatory shear force/shear stress is applied to the material. Because of the viscoelasticity, the sample's deformation/shear strain exhibits a phase lag to the shear force/shear stress. When the applied shear stress is:

$$\tau = \tau_0 \sin(t\,\omega) \tag{4.5}$$

shear strain is then defined as:

$$\gamma = \gamma_0 \sin(t\,\omega + \theta) \tag{4.6}$$

where τ_0 is the maximum shear stress, t is time, ω is period of oscillation and θ is the phase lag between stress and strain. Storage modulus (G') and loss modulus (G''), which are normally used to characterize the elastic and viscous properties (respectively), can then be calculated by the following equations:

$$G' = \tau_0/\gamma_0 \cos\theta \tag{4.7}$$

$$G'' = \tau_0/\gamma_0 \sin\theta \tag{4.8}$$

4.3 Injectable hydrogels

Based on the characteristics of injectable materials, they can be divided into injectable hydrogels and non-hydrogel (hydrophobic) polymers, both of which will be reviewed in this chapter, beginning with injectable hydrogels. These types of polymers contain hydrophilic chains or segments, which makes them soluble in water. After being crosslinked, insoluble networks are formed, but their hydrophilicity encourages swelling of the material in water. Generally speaking, water molecules surrounding the polymer chains act as plasticizers, thus improving the mobility of the polymer chains and decreasing their mechanical properties. These injectable hydrogels have many applications including use in tissue engineering, drug delivery and bioadhesives. In this section, injectable hydrogels are categorized into physically, ionically and covalently crosslinked hydrogels. Mechanical properties and applications of each hydrogel type are summarized.

4.3.1 Physically crosslinked hydrogels

Mechanical properties of physically crosslinked injectable hydrogels are generally weaker than covalently crosslinked hydrogels. To improve their mechanical properties, chemically crosslinkable groups are commonly introduced into the chains of the precursors. In this section, the structures and mechanical properties of physically crosslinked injectable hydrogels are discussed. Additionally, means of improving the mechanical properties by chemical crosslinking are also presented. Two major types of physically crosslinked hydrogels include poly(N-isopropylacrylamide) (PNIPAAm) and Poloxamer (Pluronic®).

poly(N-isopropylacrylamide) (PNIPAAm)

PNIPAAm is a widely studied thermo-sensitive material. A PNIPAAm aqueous solution will undergo a sol-gel transition at its lower critical solution temperature (LCST) of about 32°C. From the molecular point of view, when the temperature is increased to the LCST, the polymer–polymer and water–water interactions become dominant compared to the hydrogen bonds between the polymer and water, which causes the PNIPAAm chains (Fig. 4.2) to quickly dehydrate and shift to a more hydrophobic structure (Schild, 1992; Ruel-Gariepy and Leroux, 2004). Through copolymerizing with more hydrophilic or hydrophobic monomers, the LCST of NIPAAm-based copolymers can be elevated or reduced, respectively (He *et al.*, 2008; Rzaev *et al.*, 2007). This sol-gel transition makes it possible to use these temperature-sensitive materials as injectable materials for blood vessel occlusion through endovascular therapy to treat arteriovenous malformations (AVMs, caused by an abnormal connection between arteries and veins) (Matsumaru *et al.*, 1996; Fleetwood and Steinberg, 2002; Hartmann *et al.*, 2007). However, the NIPAAM-based physically crosslinked gels have weak mechanical properties. Their shear storage modulus is normally less than 2 KPa (Lin and Cheng, 2001; Wu *et al.*, 2009). Moreover, the physical crosslinking of these hydrogels above their LCST is unable to stabilize them for long-term use (Cheng *et al.*, 2007). Thus, these hydrogels will creep under blood flow due to the constant and low-frequency stress.

To improve their mechanical properties, chemically crosslinkable groups, including trimethoxysilane (Ho *et al.*, 2006), cysteamine (Robb *et al.*, 2007), acrylate (Cheng *et al.*, 2007) and dimethylmaleimido (Harmon *et al.*, 2003; Kuckling *et al.*, 2002), can be introduced to the PNIPAAm chain by copolymerizing NIPAAm with functionalized monomers. After copolymerization, these crosslinkable groups exist on the polymer chains as functional groups.

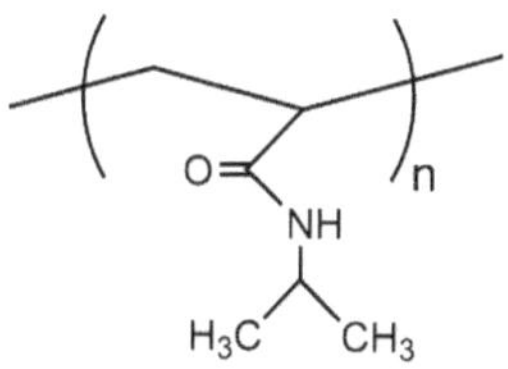

4.2 Chemical structure of PNIPAAm.

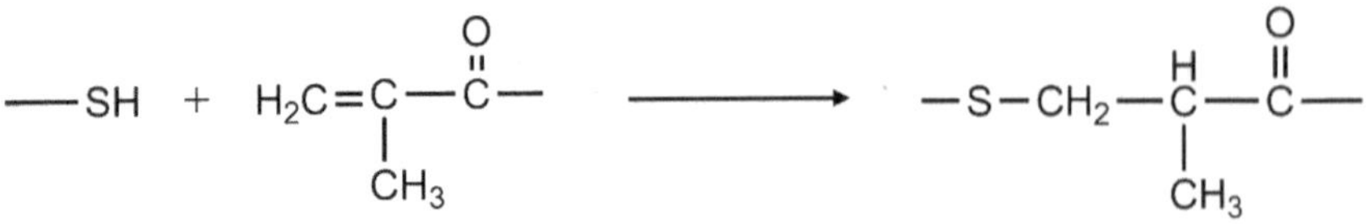

4.3 A thiol group reacts with a methacrylate group by Michael-type addition.

The functionalities can undergo chemical crosslinking as discussed below and stabilize the hydrogels after their sol-gel transition for long-term use. For example, the trimethoxysilane groups can undergo hydrolysis to create silanol groups, which crosslink by forming siloxane (Si–O–Si). A hydrogel containing 0.0005 mole ratio of trimethoxysilane monomer had a compressive modulus of ~0.6 MPa after being immersed into simulated body fluid (SBF) for five days (Ho *et al.*, 2006). Additionally, cysteamine groups can react with acrylate groups through Michael-type addition (Fig. 4.3). Therefore either cysteamines or acrylates could be introduced to the polymer chain as pendants. The modified polymer chains can be further crosslinked by addition of a crosslinker bearing the other group. The storage modulus of the hydrogels with this type of crosslinking can reach as high as ~1 MPa (Robb *et al.*, 2007). When dimethylmaleimido groups are introduced onto the polymer chains as pendants/functionalities, they can undergo dimerization upon UV exposure, thus leading to further crosslinking of the polymer chains. As the ratio of maleimido group increases, the crosslinked hydrogels will have higher chemical crosslinking density, which results in higher mechanical properties. Hydrogels with 7.2 mol% 2-(methylmaleimido)-N-ethylacrylamide had a tensile modulus of ~1.3 MPa after chemical crosslinking (Harmon *et al.*, 2003). It has been demonstrated that the increased mechanical properties of the PNIPAAm-based hydrogels through chemical crosslinking enhances their resistance to creep under the physiological conditions as well, thus making them suitable for long-term use to treat AVMs (Cheng *et al.*, 2007; Robb *et al.*, 2007).

Poloxamer (Pluronic®)

Poloxamers are another type of thermo-sensitive hydrogels with an ABA-type triblock structure (Fig. 4.4) (Kabanov *et al.*, 2002). Poloxamer 407 (Pluronic® F127, PEO_{99}-PPO_{67}-PEO_{99}) is widely employed for drug delivery because it is reported to be non-toxic and can form gels at 25°C at a concentration of 20 wt% (Dumortier *et al.*, 2006; Chiappetta and Sosnik, 2007; Nanjawade *et al.*, 2007; Bromberg, 2008). However, its applications are greatly limited by its poor mechanical properties resulting from the purely physical crosslinking. These gels are characterized by low viscosity and very high permeabilities (Sosnik *et al.*, 2003). Moreover, while they instantaneously gel upon increasing temperature above LCST in the body, they lose their structural integrity when mixed

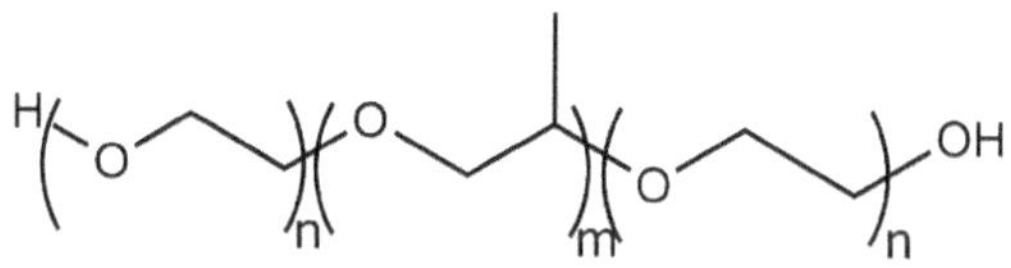

4.4 Chemical structure of PEO-PPO-PEO.

with aqueous solutions, which makes them unfit for drug delivery purposes (Sosnik *et al.*, 2003; Lee *et al.*, 2004). Like PNIPAAm polymers, much effort has been made to synthesize chemically crosslinkable poloxamers to equip them with enhanced mechanical properties. However, due to their chemical structure, reactive groups are only available at chain ends, therefore, chemically crosslinkable groups can only be used to end-cap the triblock chain. There are two main types of crosslinkable end-capping groups: methacrylate/acrylate and ethoxylsilane. Methacrylates/acrylates can be coupled to the polymer by reacting methacryloyl chloride/acryloyl chloride with the hydroxyl groups on both ends (Sosnik *et al.*, 2003; Lee *et al.*, 2004). Similarly, (3-isocyanatopropyl)triethoxysilane can be employed to react with the hydroxyl groups under catalysis of 2-ethyl-hexanoate to introduce ethoxysilane end-capping groups (Sosnik and Cohn, 2004). While the physically crosslinked gels display a compressive modulus of 142.5 ± 29.7 KPa, radically crosslinked gels using the methacrylated poloxamer and ammonium persulfate (APS) as a thermal initiator are three times stiffer, displaying a compressive modulus of 415 ± 45.7 KPa (Sosnik *et al.*, 2003). Although the exthoxysilane causes gradual chemical crosslinking (same mechanism as crosslinking of trimethoxysilane-grafted PNIPAAm-based hydrogels), their crosslinking resulted in a much higher compressive modulus: ~2600 KPa after 17 days (Sosnik and Cohn, 2004). Lysozyme has been utilized as a model protein to test the protein release profile of the diacrylated poloxamer hydrogels with higher mechanical properties. These poloxamers instantaneously formed a semi-solidified physical gel when the temperature was increased above the LCST. Then these poloxamers underwent photocrosslinking initiated by pre-mixed (4-Benzoylbenzyl)trimethylammonium chloride with UV exposure. With photocrosslinking, the gels maintained their structural integrity up to one month. While burst release of 50–70 wt% lysozyme was observed from the hydrogels in the first seven days, the remaining 30–50 wt% protein was released in a more sustained profile over a one-month period (Lee *et al.*, 2004).

4.3.2 Ionically crosslinked hydrogels

Although there are several types of ionically crosslinked hydrogels, only alginate, a polysaccharide derived from seaweed, is discussed here, because it is the only material widely used for biomedical applications. Alginate is a

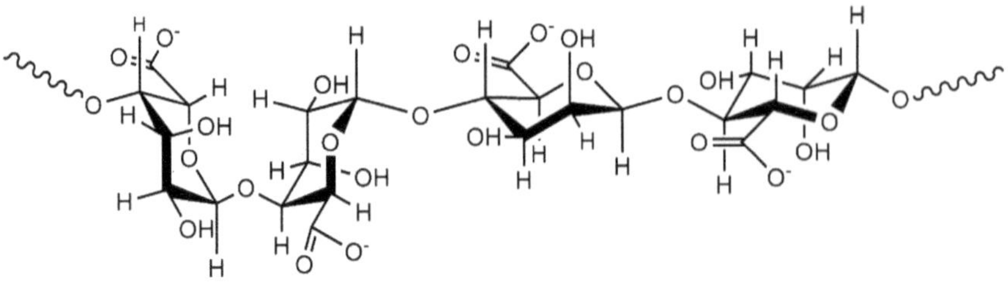

G G M M

4.5 Chemical structure of alginate.

copolymer of β-D-mannuronic acid (M) and α-L-guluronic acid (G) (Fig. 4.5). It undergoes ionic crosslinking by addition of calcium ions (Ca^{2+}) due to the reaction between Ca^{2+} and the carboxyl groups on alginate molecules (Gombotz and Wee, 1998; Augst *et al.*, 2006). For the ionically crosslinked alginate hydrogels, many factors, including alginate concentration, total calcium content, type of calcium salt crosslinker, molecular weight, and guluronic acid (G) content influence the final mechanical properties (Kuo and Ma, 2001). In general, higher concentration results in higher mechanical strength due to the increase in polymer chain density and entanglement. For example, the compressive modulus of a 1 w/v% alginate hydrogel ($M_n = 4.63 \times 10^5$) was about ~5 KPa, while it increased to ~17 KPa at a concentration of 2 w/v%. Also, when the calcium concentration is under the critical saturation concentration, higher calcium content will cause a higher degree of crosslinking, thus forming stronger gels. Different types of calcium salts will also influence the mechanical strength due to their different solubility in water. A minimally soluble calcium salt allows the gels to form at a comparatively slow rate, therefore becoming more homogenous and stronger. The use of the much slower calcium carbonate – D-glucono-δ-lactone ($CaCO_3$-GDL) system can produce structurally homogenous gels over a range of polymer concentrations with comparatively higher mechanical strength than the gels crosslinked by calcium sulfate dihydrate ($CaSO_4 \cdot 2H_2O$). 1.5 wt% hydrogel ($M_n = 3.73 \times 10^5$) crosslinked by 54 mol% $CaCO_3$-GDL (calculated from carboxyl groups) had a compressive modulus of ~80 KPa, while the compressive modulus of an alginate hydrogel crosslinked by 54 mol% $CaSO_4 \cdot 2H_2O$ at the same concentration was ~40 KPa. In addition, at lower calcium contents, alginate molecular weight plays an important role in influencing the mechanical strength because the intra-molecular covalent bonds of the polymer backbone are stronger than the inter-molecular ionic bonds formed by calcium ions. Therefore, higher molecular weight causes stronger mechanical properties. However, at higher calcium levels, the total contribution of effective ionic interactions becomes more significant than the molecular weight contribution. Since the G residues of G-blocks form an 'egg-box' structure, which controls the effective ionic crosslinking strength (Smidsrod and Skjakbraek, 1990), more G content and longer average G-block length cause higher mechanical strength.

Although the mechanical properties of alginate gels can be adjusted by the different factors discussed above and their compressive modulus can reach ~ 150 KPa, these gels are not stable for long-term use due to the uncontrollable loss of divalent cations into the surrounding environment (Malafaya *et al.*, 2007). This drawback can be overcome by chemical crosslinking. For example, methacrylate groups can be grafted onto the alginate backbone by reacting 2-aminoethyl methacrylate with the carboxyl groups of alginate using 1-ethyl-3-(3-dimethylaminopropyl)carbodiimide (EDC)/N-hydroxysuccinimide (NHS) (Jeon *et al.*, 2009). The methacrylation efficiency or the grafting ratio of methacrylate is controllable by adjusting the amount of 2-aminoethyl methacrylate during the reaction. Higher methacrylate grafting ratio results in higher crosslinking density and lower average molecular weight between crosslinks (M_C), thus producing stronger gels. The methacrylated alginate can form covalent crosslinks initiated by a photoinitiator, Irgacure 2959, with UV exposure without adding calcium ions and their mechanical properties can reach as high as that of ionically crosslinked alginate gels. For example, the alginate gels with methacrylation of 13.82% had a compressive modulus of 143.54 ± 4.84 KPa. When the methacrylation was increased to 25.23%, the gels had a compressive modulus of 174.77 ± 14.88 KPa (Jeon *et al.*, 2009).

Owing to its high cytocompatibility, alginate is usually utilized to deliver drugs (Tonnesen and Karlsen, 2002; George and Abraham, 2006; Ahmad and Khuller, 2008) or encapsulate cells for tissue engineering (Smidsrod and Skjakbraek, 1990; Rowley *et al.*, 1999; Rowley and Mooney, 2002; Augst *et al.*, 2006). For interverbral disc (IVD) regeneration, researchers have studied the effect of photocrosslinked alginate hydrogels and ionically crosslinked alginate constructs on the gene expression of encapsulated bovine nucleus pulposus (NP) cells, their ECM accumulation and distribution, and the changes of the hydrogels' mechanical properties after implantation (Chou and Nicoll, 2009). They found ionically crosslinked hydrogels exhibited inferior proteoglycan accumulation *in vitro* and lose structural integrity after implanted subcutaneously into immunocompromised 6–8 weeks old female beige mice for four weeks. On the contrary, photocrosslinked alginate gels with methacrylation of 3.5% were implanted for up to eight weeks and remained intact. The analyses further indicated the photocrosslinked alginate hydrogels resulted in both increased gene expression of type II collagen and aggrecan and enhanced production of type II collagen and sulfated glycoaminoglycans after eight weeks of implantation. Additionally, the compressive modulus increased from 1.24 ± 0.09 KPa to 4.31 ± 1.39 KPa after 8 weeks implantation, which indicated the formation of functional matrix with good mechanical properties similar to those of native NP (compressive modulus = 5–6.7 KPa).

4.3.3 Covalently crosslinked hydrogels

We have discussed the mechanical properties of physically and ionically crosslinked hydrogels and means to improve them by using chemical crosslinking in previous sections. In this section, we will focus on hydrogels that have been specifically designed to be exclusively chemically crosslinked. Covalently crosslinked hydrogels can be categorized into PEG-based and polysaccharide-based hydrogels. PEG and the polysaccharides discussed in this section do not contain crosslinkable groups in their own chemical structures. Therefore introduction of crosslinkable moieties is required for gel formation. Several factors, such as concentration of the precursors, crosslinking density and chemical structure of the polymer chains can affect the mechanical properties of covalently crosslinked hydrogels. Most of the crosslinkable moieties discussed here involve free radical polymerization in order to crosslink and form hydrogels. Therefore, initiators are usually utilized as a part of the injectable materials. The concentration of initiators is critical because it affects the toxicity of hydrogels and final mechanical properties. If the hydrogels are employed to encapsulate cells, the concentration should be below a critical value to ensure the viability of cells after encapsulation. For example, the common photoinitiator, Irgacure 2959, is normally used at concentration ≤ 0.05 wt%, which has been proved non-toxic for encapsulated cells (Williams *et al.*, 2005). In addition, when greater concentration of initiators is applied, the crosslinking will be faster, but lower double bond conversion in the same crosslinking time period will be achieved (Deng *et al.*, 2008), which will likely decrease the final mechanical properties (Ifkovits and Burdick, 2007). Therefore, appropriate initiator concentrations should be optimized for each individual polymer system since crosslinking kinetics can vary greatly depending on the chemical groups involved.

PEG-based crosslinkable hydrogels

PEG possesses hydroxyl groups on its chain ends (Fig. 4.6a). Therefore, possible routes of synthesizing crosslinkable PEG-based precursors include: 1) end-capping the PEG chain with crosslinkable groups, such as acrylate (Priola *et al.*, 1993) and methacrylate groups (Lin-Gibson *et al.*, 2005), and 2) polycondensizing with crosslinkable groups, such as fumaryl chloride, to form oligmers. Although many types of PEG-based crosslinkable hydrogels can be obtained by further reacting with other types of monomers or oligomers, only PEG-diacrylate (PEG-DA) and oligo(poly(ethylene glycol)fumarate) (OPF) are used as examples in this section to discuss the factors influencing the mechanical properties.

As shown in Figs 4.6(b) and (c), PEG-DMA and PEG-DA have methacrylate and acrylate groups at both chain ends, respectively. Both methacrylate and acrylate groups polymerize after initiation, thus forming hydrogels. For both

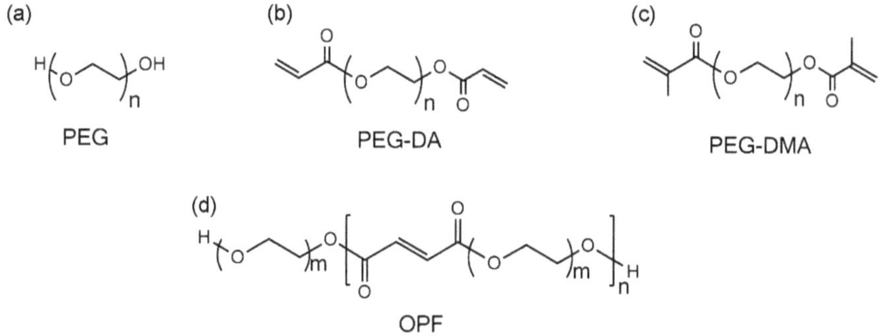

4.6 Chemical structure of PEG and PEG-based injectable materials.

types of hydrogels, the concentration of precursors and molecular weight of PEG greatly influence their mechanical properties. Similar to alginate hydrogels, higher polymer concentrations result in higher mechanical strength due to the increase in polymer chain density and entanglement (Kuo and Ma, 2001; Lin-Gibson *et al.*, 2005). Lower concentrations can cause a greater possibility of intramolecular cyclization or loop formation. The resulting loops are wasted crosslinks because they cannot contribute to the mechanical properteis of the network (Kalakkunnath *et al.*, 2006). When the molecular weight of PEG is increased, mechanical strength of the final hydrogels decreases because the M_c increases, thus decreasing the crosslinking density. For example, at concentrations of 10 wt%, 20 wt% and 30 wt%, hydrogels of PEG-DMA with a molecular weight of 2000 Da had a shear modulus of ~46 KPa, ~160 KPa and ~290 KPa, respectively. However, when the molecular weight of PEG-DMA was increased to 8000 Da, the shear modulus decreased to ~175 KPa at concentration of 30 wt% (Lin-Gibson *et al.*, 2005). Hydrogels made from PEG-DA also exhibited this trend. The shear storage modulus was ~ 1 MPa when 20 wt% PEG ($M_n = 700$) was crosslinked (Kalakkunnath *et al.*, 2006). However, when the molecular weight of PEG was increased to 6000 Da, the shear storage modulus was only ~10 KPa because of the decrease of crosslinking density (Patel *et al.*, 2005).

The crosslinking of OPF hydrogels (see Fig. 4.6d) commonly requires usage of a crosslinker, such as PEG-DA (Shin *et al.*, 2003; Temenoff *et al.*, 2002) or N-vinylpyrrolidone (NVP) (Dadsetan *et al.*, 2007) to accelerate the gelation rate because: 1) the ratio of their crosslinkable groups is comparatively lower than PEG-DA/PEG-DMA with same molecular weight of PEG and 2) the reactivity of fumarate is also comparatively lower (Busfield *et al.*, 1994). A higher ratio of crosslinker will produce stronger hydrogels because it increases the number of double bonds in the crosslinkable system. Similarly, a higher concentration of OPF results in a higher modulus. For the same reason as described for the PEG-DA system, the hydrogels made from OPF with a higher molecular weight PEG have comparatively lower tensile modulus and larger percent elongation at fracture. For example, OPF gels using PEG 3900 had a tensile modulus of 23.1 ± 12.4 KPa and percent elongation at fracture of $53.2 \pm 13.7\%$, while OPF gels with PEG 9300 had a tensile modulus of 16.5 ± 4.6 KPa and elongation of $76.0 \pm 26.4\%$. However, the PEG 860 gels had a significantly higher modulus (89.5 ± 50.7 KPa) and a significantly smaller percent elongation at fracture ($30.1 \pm 6.4\%$) (Temenoff *et al.*, 2002). PEG molecular weight did not have a significant effect on strength at fracture or toughness in these hydrogels.

PEG is becoming a very commonly used biomaterial due to advantages such as high hydrophilicity, low toxicity, low immunogenicity and high cytocompatibility (Roberts *et al.*, 2002). It is also approved by the FDA for several biomedical applications (Drury and Mooney, 2003). Moreover, it is anti-adhesive to proteins, which enables it to be not only suitable as an anti-adhesive coating (Kingshott and Griesser, 1999), but also to act as a 'blank slate' upon which to add specific biological functionalities during crosslinking (Hern and Hubbell, 1998; Burdick and Anseth, 2002; Lutolf *et al.*, 2003; Raeber *et al.*, 2005). Therefore, injectable PEG-based materials can be utilized to encapsulate cells for tissue engineering (Lutolf *et al.*, 2003; Raeber *et al.*, 2005), or to release molecules for controlled drug delivery (Greenwald *et al.*, 2003; Otsuka *et al.*, 2003). The mechanical properties of these gels are controllable to some extent by adjusting the facets discussed above, which enables PEG-based injectable gels to be employed in a wide range of regenerative medicine applications. In addition, PEG-DA is also a popular crosslinker for other types of hydrogels due to its high reactivity and wide range of molecular weights (Temenoff *et al.*, 2002; Park *et al.*, 2003; Shin *et al.*, 2003).

Hyaluronic acid-based hydrogels

Hyaluronic acid (HA) is an important component of the extracellular matrix in connective tissue (Toole, 2004). It is a polysaccharide and has a linear structure containing alternating D-glucuronic acid and N-acetyl-D-glucosamine (Fig. 4.7). Naturally occurring hyaluronic acid is easily dissolved in water due to its hydrophilic chemical structure. Chemically modified and crosslinkable HA forms hydrogels after crosslinking; it is therefore widely used for biomedical applications. The hydroxyl and carboxyl groups in the HA chain are reactive sites for introducing functional groups, such as methacrylate (Trudel and Massia, 2002; Leach *et al.*, 2003; Park *et al.*, 2003; Burdick *et al.*, 2005), to form crosslinkable HA. However, regardless of which reactive site is grafted with methacrylate groups, the mechanical properties of the resulting crosslinked hydrogels are mainly influenced by the molecular weight of HA, the concentration of HA, and the degree of substitution of crosslinkable groups on the polymer chain (Bencherif *et al.*, 2008). Lower molecular weight HA induces quicker gelation than larger molecular weight and also produces stronger hydrogels. This may be due to the higher viscosity of the larger molecular

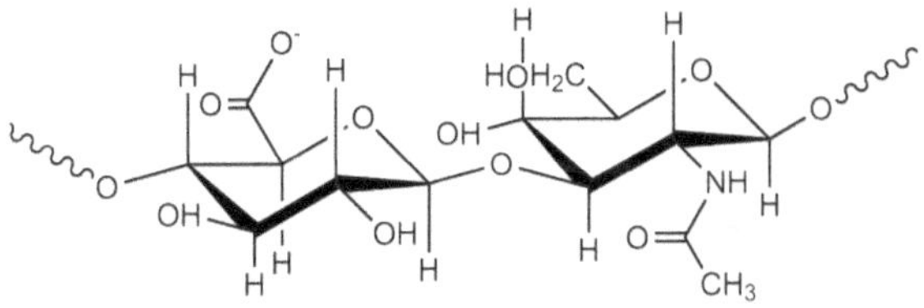

4.7 Chemical structure of hyaluronic acid.

weight HA, which limits the mobility of the chains and reduces the possibility of intermolecular reactions. Hydrogels with stronger mechanical properties can also be obtained by crosslinking higher concentrations of HA or crosslinking HA with greater degrees of substitution. The higher concentration of HA facilitates the formation of physical chain entanglements, while higher degrees of substitution result in a greater crosslinking density after crosslinking. By controlling these factors, the mechanical properties of these HA-based hydrogels can be tuned over a wide range. For example, methacrylate groups were grafted to HA with molecular weight of 50 KDa and 1100 KDa (Burdick *et al.*, 2005). Through altering the grafting ratio of methacrylate groups, the final compressive modulus of crosslinked hydrogels could be adjusted from ~2 to 100 kPa. These networks exhibited swelling ratios ranging from ~8 to 42, and degradation periods ranging from a fraction of a day up to approximately 38 days when in a solution containing 100 U/mL of hyaluronidase.

Similar to PEG-based injectable hydrogels, HA-based crosslinkable materials have many advantages, such as high cytocompatibility and low immunogenicity. Therefore, they also exhibit great potential in drug delivery and tissue engineering (Jia *et al.*, 2004; Chung *et al.*, 2006). However, one advantage of HA-based materials over PEG-based polymers is their degradability by natural enzymes. As discussed above, the mechanical properties and degradation rate of HA gels are controlled by adjusting their crosslinking density. When used for cartilage tissue engineering, the controlled degradation allows for an even distribution of glycosaminoglycan (GAG) through the whole HA network, which is similar to the GAG distribution in native tissue (Burdick *et al.*, 2005). However, the GAG is predominately constrained to the pericelluar region in a PEG-DA network because it is non-degradable. Moreover, since HA plays an important role in early development, injectable HA could also be utilized to control self-renewal and differentiation of human embryonic stem cells (hESCs) (Gerecht *et al.*, 2007).

Chondroitin sulfate-based hydrogels

Chondroitin sulfate (CS) is a sulfated polysaccharide composed of alternating N-acetylgalactoamine and glucuronic acid (Fig. 4.8) found primarily in cartilage

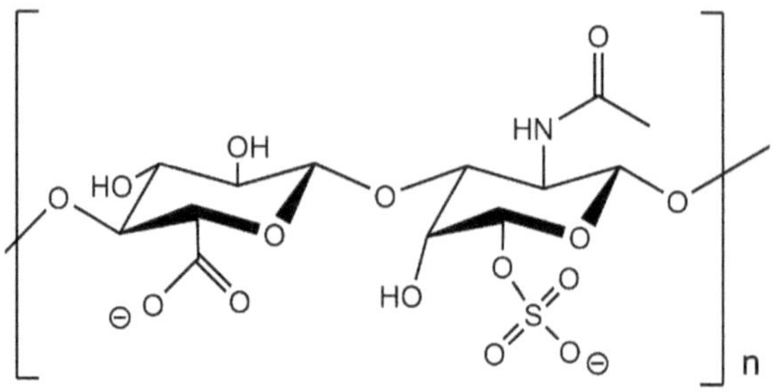

4.8 Chemical structure of chondroitin sulfate.

tissue. Therefore, much effort has been made to fabricate chondroitin sulfate-based injectable hydrogels for cartilage tissue engineering. Similar to hyaluronic acid, CS has hydroxyl and carboxyl groups on its backbone, thus allowing the introduction of methacrylate groups. Two common reagents containing methacrylate include methacrylic anhydride (Bryant *et al.*, 2004, 2005) and glycidyl methacrylate (Li *et al.*, 2004). However, the usage of different reagents results in different reaction times. While the reaction with glycidyl methacrylate was completed in 18 days (Li *et al.*, 2004), use of methacrylic anhydride decreased the reaction time to 24 hours (Bryant *et al.*, 2004). The graft ratio of methacrylate groups can be controlled by adjusting the amount of the reagents containing methacrylate. Like other covalently crosslinked hydrogels in previous sections, the graft ratio of methacrylate groups and concentration of the polymer solution greatly influence the mechanical properties. For example, when the concentration of methacrylated CS with 25 mol% of methacrylate substitution was changed from 5 wt% to 30 wt%, the compressive modulus increased from 16 ± 2 KPa to 2600 ± 400 KPa. However, the compressive modulus of methacrylated CS with < 1 mol% of methacrylate substitution at 30 wt% concentration was only 10 ± 3 KPa (Bryant *et al.*, 2004). Methacrylated CS is also utilized to crosslink other methacrylated precursors such as methacrylated poly(vinyl alcohol) (PVA) (Bryant *et al.*, 2004) and PEG-DA (Li *et al.*, 2004; Bryant *et al.*, 2005). When the total concentration of the precursors was kept constant, the ratio of methacrylated CS could be adjusted to control not only the water uptake but also the mechanical properties. For example, when 25 mol% methacrylated CS was crosslinked with 5 mol% methacrylated PVA at a total precursor concentration of 20 wt%, the compressive modulus could be adjusted from ~40 KPa to ~160 KPa by changing the ratio of two components. More interestingly, when the ratio of methacrylated CS increased, water uptake increased along with the compressive modulus due to the hydrophicility of CS, which is the opposite of many other systems that possess an inverse relationship between compressive modulus and water content (Bryant *et al.*, 2004).

When used to encapsulate chondrocytes for cartilage tissue engineering, the ratio of methacrylated CS in the hydrogel greatly influences the biological outcome. For example, no synthesis of collagen and GAGs by calf chondrocytes was detected when they were encapsulated in a 20 wt% methacrylated (methacrylation < 1 mol%) hydrogel. However, when PEG-DA ($M_n = 3400$; mole ratio of PEG-DA to methacrylated CS is 6 : 4) was incorporated into the hydrogels, calf chondrocytes had enhanced expression of collagen type II and GAGs (Bryant *et al.*, 2005).

Chitosan-based hydrogels

Chitosan is a linear polysaccharide that is composed of randomly distributed β-(1-4)-linked D-glucosamine and N-acetyl-D-glucosamine (Kumar *et al.*, 2004) (Fig. 4.9). It is commercially produced by deacetylation of chitin, which is the second abundant polysaccharide in nature and is usually found in the cell wall of fungi and exoskeletons of arthropods. Different processes produce chitosan with a deacetylation range of 60–100% (Kumar, 2000). The amino groups on chitosan allow it to react with varied types of reagents to introduce different functional groups to chitosan.

To develop an injectable bioadhesive, azide groups were introduced onto a chitosan chain to make it photocrosslinkable and enable it to bind to tissues (Ono *et al.*, 2000). Upon UV exposure, azide groups release N_2 and convert into very reactive nitrene moieties that can react rapidly with one another or with the amino groups native to the chitosan to form azo functionalties (–N=N–). Moreover, these highly reactive nitrene groups can react with amino groups on proteins, which enables modified chitosan to covalently link with tissue proteins. This strong linkage can induce firm adhesion between soft tissues and chitosan gels. Because this injectable chitosan-based hydrogel is only used as a bioadhesive, the mechanical properties we will discuss here only include binding strength and burst strength, but not tensile and compressive properties. For example, this chitosan adhesive was applied between two ham slices and tested for its binding ability. It was found that the chitosan adhesive exhibited a binding strength of about 43 g/cm^2 and the detachment of the chitosan gels from the ham surface was not observed whereas the control, fibrin glue, was easily separated from the test surfaces. In addition, the burst strength was tested on dissected pig's small intestine, aorta, and trachea. To test burst strength, one end

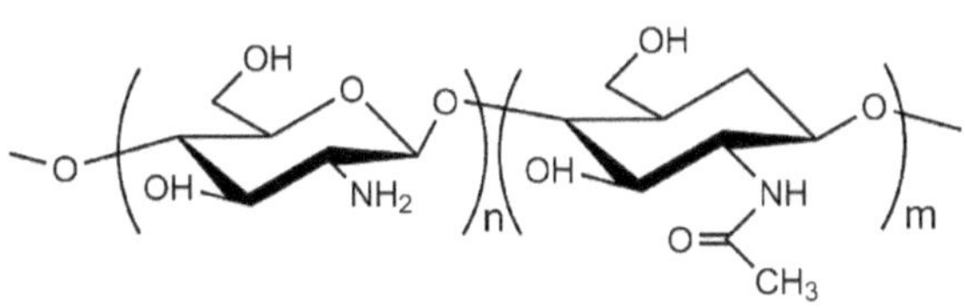

4.9 Chemical structure of chitosan.

of these tissues was tightly ligated using a suture. The other end was connected with a catheter that was attached to a syringe and an air gauge. The tissue was punctured using a needle to create a hole. Then, the bioadhesive was applied to seal the hole. The burst strength was measured by immersing the tissue in water and inflating it with the syringe until the hole burst, at which point the pressure was recorded. In these experiments, the photocrosslinked chitosan could effectively seal the pin hole and exhibited a much higher burst strength than fibrin glue. When 30 mg/ml modified chitosan was employed, a burst strength of 65 ± 5 mm Hg in the small intestine, 225 ± 25 mm Hg in the aorta and 77 ± 29 mm Hg in the trachea, respectively, was observed. Compared to the chitosan adhesive, fibrin glue demonstrated a burst strength of 48 ± 7 mm Hg in the small intestine, 65 ± 15 mm Hg in the aorta and 44 ± 16 mm Hg in the trachea (Ishihara, 2002). The photocurable chitosan was also applied *in vivo* in a New Zealand white rabbit model. Photocurable chitosan gelled faster (<1 minute) than fibrin glue (~ 3 minutes). In addition, the chitosan adhesive effectively stopped bleeding from the hole on the carotid artery and all seven rabbits survived. The rabbits were sacrificed 30 days after surgery, the histological study indicated that the chitosan adhesive allowed the hole in the artery to close completely with native tissue (Ishihara, 2002).

4.4 Non-hydrogel injectable polymers

Unlike the hydrogels reviewed in the previous section, these polymers contain mainly hydrophobic chains or segments. After being crosslinked, these polymers have compact network structures or a degree of crystallization that results in comparatively higher modulus than hydrogel materials. However, in order to obtain appropriate mobility for injection, the injectable non-hydrogel polymers should be either a viscous liquid or paste. If they are powders, they should be able to dissolve into diluents, such as NVP. In this section, three major types of injectable non-hydrogel polymers, including bone cements, trimethylene carbonate-based and polyanhydride-based materials are discussed. Mechanical properties and applications of each polymer type are summarized.

4.4.1 Bone cement

Bone cements are widely used to anchor implants, such as knee or hip replacement. They are typically viscous liquids or pastes, and able to cure with time *in situ*. Newly developed degradable cements also aim to be employed as scaffolds for bone repair and regeneration. The bone cements discussed here include an acrylic bone cement that is not degradable and a PPF-based cement that is biodegradable.

Acrylic bone cement

Although there are six commonly-used commercial formulations of acrylic bone cements in the United States, they have similar compositions (Lewis, 1997, 2003, 2006). All of these formulations contain powder and liquid monomer constituents. The powder constituents include prepolymerized poly(methyl methacrylate) (PMMA) (Fig. 4.10a), an initiator and a radiopacifier. The liquid monomer formulations contain a large amount of MMA monomer (Fig. 4.10b), small amounts of promoter or accelerator and a stabilizer. These constituents are mixed outside of the body and then injected into the appropriate site to polymerize and anchor to the artificial joint. The bone cement's main functions include amplifying the load-carrying range of the prosthesis-bone cement-bone system and/or relocating body weight and load from the prosthesis to the bone (Lewis, 1997). Therefore, mechanical properties of the cement directly influence the success of the prosthesis. Generally speaking, the cured acrylic bone cement has an ultimate tensile strength of 24–49 MPa, a tensile modulus of ~1600–4000 MPa and an elongation of ~0.86–1.62%. It also has very high compressive properties. For example, the ultimate compressive strength is ~90–115 MPa and compressive modulus is ~2623–3010 MPa. Moreover, these load-bearing materials require a long fatigue life (Lewis, 2003; Murphy and Prendergast, 2000). Fatigue life is generally measured in terms of the cycles of loading before fatigue fracture and is greatly influenced by the components and mixing process (Lewis, 1999). The usage of prepolymerized PMMA with higher molecular weight results in higher fatigue performance (Graham *et al.*, 2000), and cured cements with uniform distribution of radiopacifying agent exhibit higher fatigue strength and longer fatigue life (Lewis, 2003). Moreover, the porosity of the cured cements greatly hinders their mechanical performance. The pores in the cement may act as stress risers and induce cracks (Ishihara *et al.*, 2000; Janssen *et al.*, 2005). A number of studies indicate that higher porosity results in lower tensile modulus, compressive modulus, shear storage modulus and toughness. These pores actually arise from the mixing process and poor removal of the air bubbles. Therefore many types of mixing methods, such as centrifugation mixing (Davies *et al.*, 1987, 1988), vacuum mixing (Lidgren *et al.*, 1987; Wang

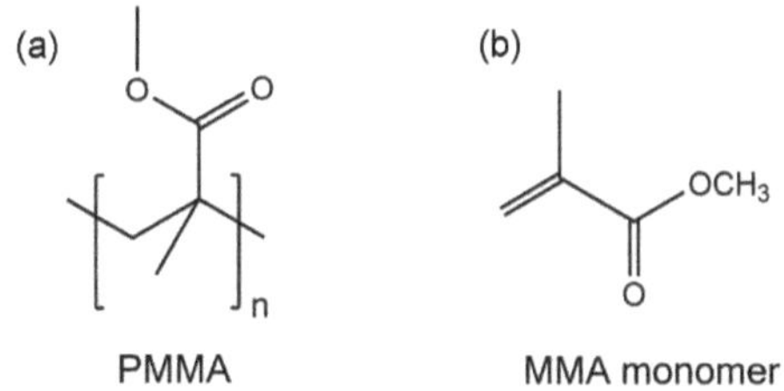

4.10 Chemical structure of PMMA powder and liquid MMA monomer used in acrylic bone cement.

et al., 1993; Geiger *et al.*, 2001; Dunne *et al.*, 2006), vibratory and shaking mixing (Linden, 1989), and sonication (Lewis, 2003), have been developed to better evacuate the air. It has been shown that the mechanical properties of these cements are significantly increased with all these methods (Lewis, 1999, 2003).

To further improve the mechanical performance of acrylic cements, many studies have incorporated particulate or fibrous toughening agents into the cement powder, such as poly(butyl methacrylate) particles, $BaSO_4$ particles, hydroxyapatite particles, titanium fibers, carbon and polyethylene terephthlate fibers (Lewis, 2003). The presence of reinforcing agents enhances the fatigue-crack propagation resistance, which, in turn, results in intensified fatigue energy dispersion and enhanced fatigue life (Lewis, 2003). For example, it was found that the fatigue life was increased 1.57 and 3.33 times when 10 wt% of 1 μm and 10 nm $BaSO_4$ particles were added, respectively (Lewis, 2003). In addition, the fatigue life of the cement was increased 55–88% when reinforcing fibers were included (Gilbert *et al.*, 1995; Topoleski *et al.*, 1995; Kim and Yasuda, 1999; Zhou *et al.*, 2009).

Poly(propylene fumarate) (PPF)-based bone cement

PPF is a linear unsaturated polyester consisting of repeat units with one unsaturated double bond that allows crosslinking of the polymer chains, and two ester groups that permit the hydrolysis of the polymer into nontoxic products (fumaric acid and propylene glycol) (He *et al.*, 2001) (Fig. 4.11). In general, crosslinked PPF has weaker mechanical properties (compressive modulus <2000 MPa) than acrylic acid-based cements due to its comparatively lower double bond ratio, slower reaction rate of fumarate groups and high molecular weight that may limit the conversion rate and crosslinking density (Busfield *et al.*, 1994; Fisher *et al.*, 2002). The biggest advantage PPF has over acrylic acid-based cements is its degradability and nontoxic degradation products (Yaszemski *et al.*, 1996). However, the degradation also results in the loss of mechanical properties, which greatly limits its application as a bone cement (Peter *et al.*, 1997, 1998; Mano *et al.*, 2004). Two possible approaches to improve the polymer's mechanical properties include: (1) increasing the double

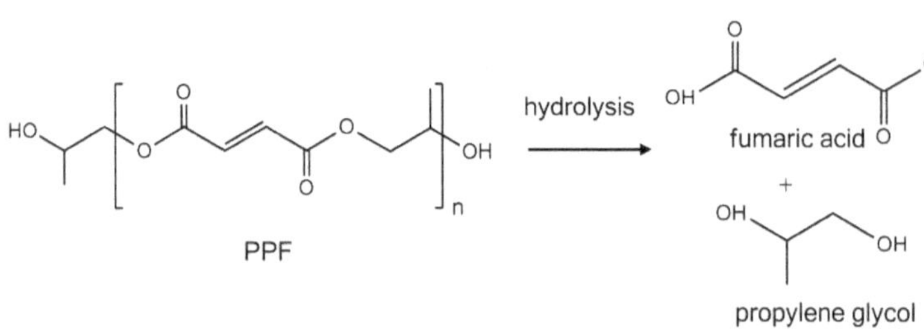

4.11 Chemical structure and degradation of PPF.

bond ratio by chemical modification or copolymerization with other polymers with higher number of double bonds per chain, and (2) fabricating composites by incorporating fillers or reinforcing agents.

Diethyl fumarate has been copolymerized with PPF to increase the double bond ratio in the system (Fisher *et al.*, 2002). The compressive properties appear to reach their maximum (compressive modulus = 195 ± 17.5 MPa, fracture strength = 68.8 ± 9.4 MPa) when 25 wt% diethyl fumarate is copolymerized with PPF. In addition, PPF can be end-capped with acrylate groups to increase the double bond ratio (He *et al.*, 2001; Hedberg *et al.*, 2002; Timmer *et al.*, 2002, 2003a). When PPF-diacrylate is incorporated with PPF, the resulting networks have a tensile modulus of 806–923 MPa and a compressive modulus of 837–1854 MPa (Timmer *et al.*, 2003b). For fabricating PPF polymer composites, many types of fillers or reinforcing agents have been utilized, which include beta-tricalcium-phosphate (Peter *et al.*, 1997, 1998, 1999), calcium sulphate (Cai *et al.*, 2009), single wall carbon nanotubes (Shi *et al.*, 2005, 2006; Sitharaman *et al.*, 2007) and alumoxane nanoparticles (Mistry *et al.*, 2007). Although these approaches increase the mechanical properties of the network to some extent, the final mechanical properties remain weaker than acrylic acid-based cements.

Due to the crosslinking properties and degradability, PPF can also be employed to fabricate porous scaffolds for bone tissue engineering. Porogens such as salt crystals are normally applied. However, the mechanical properties are significantly decreased when high porosity is created (Fisher *et al.*, 2001). For example, while a compressive modulus of 41.8 ± 15.2 MPa and yield strength of 1.84 ± 0.79 MPa were observed in scaffolds with ~60% porosity, they dropped to 0.9 ± 0.3 MPa and 0.05 ± 0.03 MPa, respectively, when the porosity increased to ~79%. Reinforcing agents, such as single wall carbon nanotubes (Shi *et al.*, 2007), have been recently explored in conjunction with PPF; however, this did not result in a significant increase in mechanical properties of the porous materials.

4.4.2 Trimethylene carbonate-based materials

To be utilized in injectable applications, polymers should be soluble in water or organic diluents, or must be viscous liquid or paste at room temperature. Most polymers become solid at room temperature when their molecular weight and/or crystallinity increase. The physical state of polymers is greatly determined by their chemical structures and molecular weight. Polymers with flexible chains have a low glass transition point (T_g). T_g describes the temperature above which the chain segments become mobile (Ward and Sweeney, 2004). In addition, polymers with asymmetric chemical structure and low molecular weight have lower crystallinity (Matsuda *et al.*, 2000). Therefore, amorphous polymer chains with comparatively low molecular weight and asymmetric chemical structure, such as the trimethylene carbonate (TMC) oligomer (see Fig. 4.12), would be a

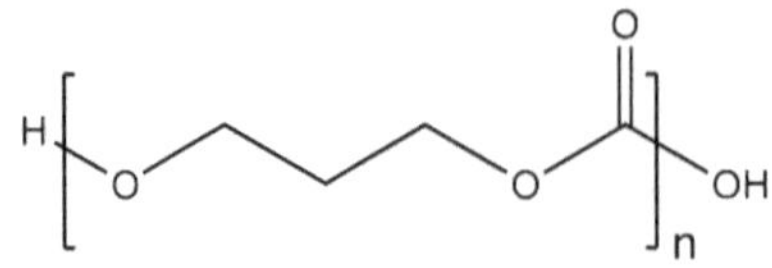

4.12 Chemical structure of poly(trimethylene carbonate) (PTMC).

likely candidate to remain as a viscous liquid or paste form at room temperature. Resulting experiments have confirmed this for both oligomers and copolymers of trimethylene carbonate (TMC). To synthesize TMC-based injectable materials, the oligomers containing hydroxyl groups as chain ends are first obtained by ring-opening of cyclic monomers using initiators that bear hydroxyl groups, such as PEG and trimethylolpropane (TMP). Then, photocurable groups, such as coumarin (Matsuda *et al.*, 2000), acrylate (Matsuda and Mizutani, 2002; Mizutani and Matsuda, 2002; Matsuda *et al.*, 2004), phenylazide (Mizutani *et al.*, 2002) and fumarate groups (Grijpma *et al.*, 2005; Hou *et al.*, 2009) are grafted on the oligomers by reacting with the hydroxyl groups. The hydrolysis and mechanical properties of the crosslinked network are strongly affected by the initiators. In particular, hydrophilicity of initiators will influence the swelling behavior and consequent mechanical properties of the resulting materials. Crosslinked networks with PEG and TMP as initiators swelled once being immersed in water and formed outmost and subsurface layers that had different mechanical strengths (Matsuda *et al.*, 2004). While the swelled network with more hydrophilic PEG-2000 resulted in a compressive modulus of ~ 10 MPa in both the outmost (E1) and subsurface (E2), the swelled network with PEG-200 demonstrated E1 of ~ 10 MPa and E2 of ~ 20–40 MPa due to the low molecular weight of the PEG. As for TMP, which has three hydroxyl groups and is less hydrophilic, its crosslinked network had E1 of ~ 15–35 MPa and E2 of ~ 100–200 MPa (Matsuda *et al.*, 2004).

For TMC-based materials, both molecular weight and molecular weight between crosslinks (M_C) can influence the mechanical properties (Hou *et al.*, 2009). While linear PTMC with a high molecular weight ($M_n = 300\,000$) has a tensile modulus of 5.21 ± 0.91 MPa, the materials resulting from fumarate-functionalizing PTMC with a lower molecular weight ($M_n = 4500$–$13\,900$) have comparatively lower tensile modulus, ranging from 1.25 ± 0.02 MPa to 2.12 ± 0.20 MPa. Unexpectedly, while a lower molecular weight crosslinkable oligomer ($M_n = 4500$) is able to result in higher crosslinking density, a higher molecular weight fumarate-functionalized PTMC ($M_n = 13\,900$) creates a network with higher tensile modulus, higher yield strength and larger elongation at yield than the lower molecular weight. This is may be explained by a greater influence of molecular weight over crosslinking density in these networks. Higher molecular weight can cause better orientation of polymer chains and close packing of chain segments upon elongation (Hou *et al.*, 2009). However, chemical crosslinking is able to increase the creep resistance of the materials. While linear PTMC with molecular weight $M_n = 300\,000$ cannot recover its original shape after stretching, the network of fumarate-functionalized PTMC ($M_n = 4500$–$13\,900$) fully recovered its shape even after 20 cycles of 50% elongation (Hou *et al.*, 2009). This elastic crosslinked network with improved creep resistance can be used as a scaffold for blood vessel tissue engineering.

The mechanical properties of the network can also be adjusted by changing the chemical composition of crosslinkable oligomers (Grijpma *et al.*, 2005). For example, D,L-lactide (DLLA) can be ring-opened with TMC in the presence of glycerol to produce star-shaped poly(TMC-co-DLLA) that can then be functionalized with fumarate groups. The incorporation of DLLA increases the T_g of the oligomers and consequently enhances the mechanical properties of the crosslinked network. While the crosslinked fumarate-functionalized network of TMC demonstated a tensile modulus of ~1.2 MPa, the network with 86% DLLA had a tensile modulus of ~5.3 MPa.

4.4.3 Polyanhydride-based materials

This category of injectable material includes low molecular weight monomers that are synthesized by reacting diacids, such as sebacic acid (SA), 1,3-bis(carboxyphenoxy) propane (CPP) and 1,6-bis(carboxyphenoxy) hexane (MCPH) with methacrylic anhydride (Burkoth and Anseth, 2000; Burkoth *et al.*, 2000) (Fig. 4.13). The end-capping methacrylate groups allow free radical polymerization using initiators to crosslink these polyanhydride-based materials. Since these monomers have comparatively low molecular weight (M_n =~ 500–1000) and crosslinking occurs only at the chain ends, their crosslinked network

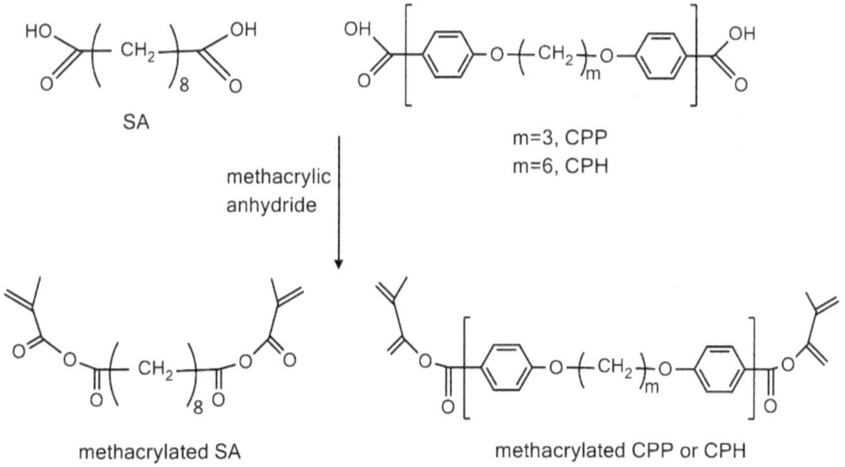

4.13 Chemical structure of polyanhydride-based injectable materials.

has higher crosslinking density and thus higher mechanical properties than most injectable materials. Methacrylated SA, once crosslinked, has a compressive strength of 40 ± 10 MPa and a tensile modulus of 1400 ± 120 MPa, while networks fabricated from methacrylated CPP have a compressive strength of 32 ± 2 MPa and a tensile modulus of 640 ± 80 MPa. The difference in moduli for these two network results from the different molecular weights of the monomers (Muggli *et al.*, 1999). Oligomerization can occur during the synthesis of the methacrylated monomer, and oligomerization occurs to a greater extent during the methacrylated CPP synthesis. Therefore, methacrylated CPP has higher molecular weight than methacrylated SA.

Compared to most biomaterials which possess bulk degradation profiles (surface and interior degrade nearly simultaneously), polyanhydrides degrade with a surface-erosion profile (degradation occurs layer by layer from the surface) due to their high hydrophobicity. This enables these materials to maintain >70% of their tensile modulus and their architectural integrity at 50% mass loss (Muggli *et al.*, 1999). Besides the superior mechanical properties discussed above, the polyanhydride-based materials are also highly osteocompatible (Anseth *et al.*, 1999; Poshusta *et al.*, 2003), which makes them suitable for orthopedic applications, particularly as load-bearing scaffolds.

4.5 Conclusion and future trends

Regardless of the classification of injectable (hydrogel or non-hydrogel polymers), these materials are designed to from crosslinked networks *in situ*. Generally speaking, the mechanical properties of these networks are greatly influenced by many factors that include the types of bonds contributing to network formation, final crosslink density, hydrophilicity of the polymer chains, and presence of any type of microporosity within the network. Moreover, toughening or reinforcing agents are often incorporated into the polymers to improve their mechanical properties. These agents are able to dissipate stress and reduce cracks. Several factors, such as the shape, size, and distribution of these agents greatly influence their efficiency.

Overall, injectable hydrogels have comparatively weaker mechanical properties than their non-hydrogel counterparts due to the water molecules that surround the polymer chains and act as plasticizers. However, because of their aqueous environment, injectable hydrogels can be used to encapsulate cells for tissue engineering. Through finely tuning the chemical and network structure of hydrogels, researchers have created hydrogels with elongation as high as ~1000–1400% and fracture strength as high as several tens of megapascals (Haraguchi and Takehisa, 2002; Haraguchi *et al.*, 2002; Gong *et al.*, 2003; Tanaka *et al.*, 2005). To fabricate highly elastic materials, N-isopropyl acrylamide was radically polymerized from the surface of clay particles to form a nanocomposite hydrogel. The clay sheets act as crosslinkers in the composite gel, which decreases the crosslinking units per volume (10 per cubic 100 nm), compared to conventionally crosslinked hydrogels (7500 per cubic 100 nm). At the same time, the polymer chains between two clay sheets are flexible and able to (cooperatively) sustain relatively high forces (Haraguchi and Takehisa, 2002; Haraguchi *et al.*, 2002). In the future, configuring such materials to allow encapsulation of cells would capitalize on this advantage of hydrophillic polymers and could therefore significantly widen the use of injectable hydrogels in mechanically active environments.

On the other hand, non-hydrogel materials have comparatively high stiffness and strength, which is due partially to their compact chain organization. Therefore, they may be more suitable for regeneration of tissues that undergo loading, such as blood vessels or orthopedic tissues. However, to enhance cell penetration and growth, porosity is usually required in these non-hydrogel materials. Unfortunately, when porosity is increased, mechanical properties of these polymers decrease dramatically. Moreover, mechanical properties usually decrease as degradation occurs. Therefore, it remains a great challenge to develop injectable polymers with high modulus, large percent porosity and well-controlled change in properties during degradation. Further exploration of composite materials holds promise to address this combination of design parameters, since it may be difficult to achieve all three of these characteristics with a homogenous material.

As discussed above, while significant progress has been made over the past ~15 years in understanding how polymer and composite structure affect mechanical properties of injectable biomaterials, additional work is required to create materials that fully match the requirements of certain high-load applications. However, many of the basic relationships elucidated to date provide direction for future efforts, particularly in the area of novel composite materials, and have highlighted the need for new materials with enhanced mechanical properties that do not sacrifice injectablity and, in many cases, biodegradability. Given the high potential impact that innovations in this field would have on improving minimally invasive surgical procedures and the concomitant decrease in recovery time for patients, the development of injectable polymers and composites remains an exciting and extremely critical area of future research for biomaterialists.

4.6 References

Ahmad, Z. & Khuller, G. K. (2008) Alginate-based sustained release drug delivery systems for tuberculosis. *Expert Opinion on Drug Delivery*, 5, 1323–1334.

Anseth, K. S., Shastri, V. R. & Langer, R. (1999) Photopolymerizable degradable polyanhydrides with osteocompatibility. *Nature Biotechnology*, 17, 156–159.

Augst, A. D., Kong, H. J. & Mooney, D. J. (2006) Alginate hydrogels as biomaterials. *Macromolecular Bioscience*, 6, 623–633.

Bencherif, S. A., Srinivasan, A., Horkay, F., Hollinger, J. O., Matyjaszewski, K. &

Washburn, N. R. (2008) Influence of the degree of methacrylation on hyaluronic acid hydrogels properties. *Biomaterials*, 29, 1739–1749.
Bromberg, L. (2008) Polymeric micelles in oral chemotherapy. *Journal of Controlled Release*, 128, 99–112.
Bryant, S. J., Davis-Arehart, K. A., Luo, N., Shoemaker, R. K., Arthur, J. A. & Anseth, K. S. (2004) Synthesis and characterization of photopolymerized multifunctional hydrogels: water-soluble poly(vinyl alcohol) and chondroitin sulfate macromers for chondrocyte encapsulation. *Macromolecules*, 37, 6726–6733.
Bryant, S. J., Arthur, J. A. & Anseth, K. S. (2005) Incorporation of tissue-specific molecules alters chondrocyte metabolism and gene expression in photocrosslinked hydrogels. *Acta Biomaterialia*, 1, 243–252.
Burdick, J. A. & Anseth, K. S. (2002) Photoencapsulation of osteoblasts in injectable RGD-modified PEG hydrogels for bone tissue engineering. *Biomaterials*, 23, 4315–4323.
Burdick, J. A., Chung, C., Jia, X. Q., Randolph, M. A. & Langer, R. (2005) Controlled degradation and mechanical behavior of photopolymerized hyaluronic acid networks. *Biomacromolecules*, 6, 386–391.
Burkoth, A. K. & Anseth, K. S. (2000) A review of photocrosslinked polyanhydrides: *in situ* forming degradable networks. *Biomaterials*, 21, 2395–2404.
Burkoth, A. K., Burdick, J. & Anseth, K. S. (2000) Surface and bulk modifications to photocrosslinked polyanhydrides to control degradation behavior. *Journal of Biomedical Materials Research*, 51, 352–359.
Busfield, W. K., Jenkins, I. D. & Heiland, K. (1994) Free-radical initiation mechanisms in the polymerization of diethyl fumarate and diethyl maleate studied by the nitroxide trapping technique. *European Polymer Journal*, 30, 1259–1267.
Cai, Z. Y., Yang, D. A., Zhang, N., Ji, C. G., Zhu, L. & Zhang, T. (2009) Poly(propylene fumarate)/(calcium sulphate/beta-tricalcium phosphate) composites: preparation, characterization and *in vitro* degradation. *Acta Biomaterialia*, 5, 628–635.
Cheng, V., Lee, B. H., Pauken, C. & Vernon, B. L. (2007) Poly(N-isopropylacrylamide-co-poly(ethylene glycol))-acrylate simultaneously physically and chemically gelling polymer systems. *Journal of Applied Polymer Science*, 106, 1201–1207.
Chiappetta, D. A. & Sosnik, A. (2007) Poly(ethylene oxide)-poly(propylene oxide) block copolymer micelles as drug delivery agents: improved hydrosolubility, stability and bioavailability of drugs. *European Journal of Pharmaceutics and Biopharmaceutics*, 66, 303–317.
Chou, A. I. & Nicoll, S. B. (2009) Characterization of photocrosslinked alginate hydrogels for nucleus pulposus cell encapsulation. *Journal of Biomedical Materials Research Part A*, 91A, 187–194.
Chung, C., Mesa, J., Miller, G. J., Randolph, M. A., Gill, T. J. & Burdick, J. A. (2006) Effects of auricular chondrocyte expansion on neocartilage formation in photocrosslinked hyaluronic acid networks. *Tissue Engineering*, 12, 2665–2673.
Dadsetan, M., Szatkowski, J. P., Yaszemski, M. J. & Lu, L. C. (2007) Characterization of photo-cross-linked oligo[poly(ethylene glycol) fumarate] hydrogels for cartilage tissue engineering. *Biomacromolecules*, 8, 1702–1709.
Davies, J. P., Burke, D. W., O'Connor, D. O. & Harris, W. H. (1987) Comparison of the fatigue characteristics of centrifuged and uncentrifuged simplex P-bone cement. *Journal of Orthopaedic Research*, 5, 366–371.
Davies, J. P., O'Connor, D. O., Burke, D. W., Jasty, M. & Harris, W. H. (1988) The effect of centrifugation on the fatigue life of bone-cement in the presence of surface irregularities. *Clinical Orthopaedics and Related Research*, 156–161.

Deng, J. P., Wu, Z. L., He, Q. X. & Yang, W. T. (2008) Photo-induced polymerization of methyl methacrylate/cyclodextrin complex in aqueous solution. *Polymers for Advanced Technologies*, 19, 1649–1655.

Drury, J. L. & Mooney, D. J. (2003) Hydrogels for tissue engineering: scaffold design variables and applications. *Biomaterials*, 24, 4337–4351.

Dumortier, G., Grossiord, J. L., Agnely, F. & Chaumeil, J. C. (2006) A review of poloxamer 407 pharmaceutical and pharmacological characteristics. *Pharmaceutical Research*, 23, 2709–2728.

Dunne, N., Xu, Y., Daly, C., Makem, J., Walker, G. & Orr, J. (2006) Development of operator independent bone cement vacuum mixing system for joint replacement surgery. *Plastics Rubber and Composites*, 35, 317–323.

Fisher, J. P., Holland, T. A., Dean, D., Engel, P. S. & Mikos, A. G. (2001) Synthesis and properties of photocross-linked poly(propylene fumarate) scaffolds. *Journal of Biomaterials Science-Polymer Edition*, 12, 673–687.

Fisher, J. P., Dean, D. & Mikos, A. G. (2002) Photocrosslinking characteristics and mechanical properties of diethyl fumarate/poly(propylene fumarate) biomaterials. *Biomaterials*, 23, 4333–4343.

Fleetwood, I. G. & Steinberg, G. K. (2002) Arteriovenous malformations. *Lancet*, 359, 863–873.

Geiger, M. H., Keating, E. M., Ritter, M. A., Ginther, J. A., Faris, P. M. & Meding, J. B. (2001) The clinical significance of vacuum mixing bone cement. *Clinical Orthopaedics and Related Research*, 258–266.

George, M. & Abraham, T. E. (2006) Polyionic hydrocolloids for the intestinal delivery of protein drugs: alginate and chitosan – a review. *Journal of Controlled Release*, 114, 1–14.

Gerecht, S., Burdick, J. A., Ferreira, L. S., Townsend, S. A., Langer, R. & Vunjak-Novakovic, G. (2007) Hyaluronic acid hydrogen for controlled self-renewal and differentiation of human embryonic stem cells. *Proceedings of the National Academy of Sciences of the United States of America*, 104, 11298–11303.

Gilbert, J. L., Ney, D. S. & Lautenschlager, E. P. (1995) Self-reinforced composite poly(methyl methacrylate) – static and fatigue properties. *Biomaterials*, 16, 1043–1055.

Gombotz, W. R. & Wee, S. F. (1998) Protein release from alginate matrices. *Advanced Drug Delivery Reviews*, 31, 267–285.

Gong, J. P., Katsuyama, Y., Kurokawa, T. & Osada, Y. (2003) Double-network hydrogels with extremely high mechanical strength. *Advanced Materials*, 15, 1155–1158.

Graham, J., Pruitt, L., Ries, M. & Gundiah, N. (2000) Fracture and fatigue properties of acrylic bone cement – the effects of mixing method, sterilization treatment, and molecular weight. *Journal of Arthroplasty*, 15, 1028–1035.

Greenwald, R. B., Choe, Y. H., McGuire, J. & Conover, C. D. (2003) Effective drug delivery by PEGylated drug conjugates. *Advanced Drug Delivery Reviews*, 55, 217–250.

Grijpma, D. W., Hou, Q. P. & Feijen, J. (2005) Preparation of biodegradable networks by photo-crosslinking lactide, epsilon-caprolactone and trimethylene carbonate-based oligomers functionalized with fumaric acid monoethyl ester. *Biomaterials*, 26, 2795–2802.

Haraguchi, K. & Takehisa, T. (2002) Nanocomposite hydrogels: a unique organic-inorganic network structure with extraordinary mechanical, optical, and swelling/de-swelling properties. *Advanced Materials*, 14, 1120–1124.

Haraguchi, K., Takehisa, T. & Fan, S. (2002) Effects of clay content on the properties of nanocomposite hydrogels composed of poly(N-isopropylacrylamide) and clay. *Macromolecules*, 35, 10162–10171.

Harmon, M. E., Kuckling, D. & Frank, C. W. (2003) Photo-cross-linkable PNIPAAm copolymers. 2. Effects of constraint on temperature and pH-responsive hydrogel layers. *Macromolecules*, 36, 162–172.

Hartmann, A., Mast, H., Choi, J. H., Stapf, C. & Mohr, J. P. (2007) Treatment of arteriovenous malformations of the brain. *Current Neurology and Neuroscience Reports*, 7, 28–34.

He, S., Timmer, M. D., Yaszemski, M. J., Yasko, A. W., Engel, P. S. & Mikos, A. G. (2001) Synthesis of biodegradable poly(propylene fumarate) networks with poly(propylene fumarate)-diacrylate macromers as crosslinking agents and characterization of their degradation products. *Polymer*, 42, 1251–1260.

He, C. L., Kim, S. W. & Lee, D. S. (2008) *In situ* gelling stimuli-sensitive block copolymer hydrogels for drug delivery. *Journal of Controlled Release*, 127, 189–207.

Hedberg, E. L., Tang, A., Crowther, R. S., Carney, D. H. & Mikos, A. G. (2002) Controlled release of an osteogenic peptide from injectable biodegradable polymeric composites. *Journal of Controlled Release*, 84, 137–150.

Hern, D. L. & Hubbell, J. A. (1998) Incorporation of adhesion peptides into nonadhesive hydrogels useful for tissue resurfacing. *Journal of Biomedical Materials Research*, 39, 266–276.

Ho, E., Lowman, A. & Marcolongo, M. (2006) Synthesis and characterization of an injectable hydrogel with tunable mechanical properties for soft tissue repair. *Biomacromolecules*, 7, 3223–3228.

Hou, Q. P., Grijpma, D. W. & Feijen, J. (2009) Creep-resistant elastomeric networks prepared by photocrosslinking fumaric acid monoethyl ester-functionalized poly(trimethylene carbonate) oligomers. *Acta Biomaterialia*, 5, 1543–1551.

Ifkovits, J. L. & Burdick, J. A. (2007) Review: Photopolymerizable and degradable biomaterials for tissue engineering applications. *Tissue Engineering*, 13, 2369–2385.

Ishihara, M. (2002) Photocrosslinkable chitosan hydrogel as a wound dressing and a biological adhesive. *Trends in Glycoscience and Glycotechnology*, 14, 331–341.

Ishihara, S., McEvily, A. J., Goshima, T., Kanekasu, K. & Nara, T. (2000) On fatigue lifetimes and fatigue crack growth behavior of bone cement. *Journal of Materials Science-Materials in Medicine*, 11, 661–666.

Janssen, D., Aquarius, R., Stolk, J. & Verdonschot, N. (2005) The contradictory effects of pores on fatigue cracking of bone cement. *Journal of Biomedical Materials Research Part B – Applied Biomaterials*, 74B, 747–753.

Jeon, O., Bouhadir, K. H., Mansour, J. M. & Alsberg, E. (2009) Photocrosslinked alginate hydrogels with tunable biodegradation rates and mechanical properties. *Biomaterials*, 30, 2724–2734.

Jia, X. Q., Burdick, J. A., Kobler, J., Clifton, R. J., Rosowski, J. J., Zeitels, S. M. & Langer, R. (2004) Synthesis and characterization of *in situ* cross-linkable hyaluronic acid-based hydrogels with potential application for vocal fold regeneration. *Macromolecules*, 37, 3239–3248.

Kabanov, A. V., Batrakova, E. V. & Alakhov, V. Y. (2002) Pluronic® block copolymers for overcoming drug resistance in cancer. *Advanced Drug Delivery Reviews*, 54, 759–779.

Kalakkunnath, S., Kalika, D. S., Lin, H. Q. & Freeman, B. D. (2006) Viscoelastic characteristics of UV polymerized poly(ethylene glycol) diacrylate networks with

varying extents of crosslinking. *Journal of Polymer Science Part B – Polymer Physics*, 44, 2058–2070.
Kim, H. Y. & Yasuda, H. K. (1999) Improvement of fatigue properties of poly(methyl methacrylate) bone cement by means of plasma surface treatment of fillers. *Journal of Biomedical Materials Research*, 48, 135–142.
Kingshott, P. & Griesser, H. J. (1999) Surfaces that resist bioadhesion. *Current Opinion in Solid State & Materials Science*, 4, 403–412.
Kuckling, D., Harmon, M. E. & Frank, C. W. (2002) Photo-cross-linkable PNIPAAm copolymers. 1. Synthesis and characterization of constrained temperature-responsive hydrogel layers. *Macromolecules*, 35, 6377–6383.
Kumar, M. N. V. R. (2000) A review of chitin and chitosan applications. *Reactive & Functional Polymers*, 46, 1–27.
Kumar, M. N. V. R., Muzzarelli, R. A. A., Muzzarelli, C., Sashiwa, H. & Domb, A. J. (2004) Chitosan chemistry and pharmaceutical perspectives. *Chemical Reviews*, 104, 6017–6084.
Kuo, C. K. & Ma, P. X. (2001) Ionically crosslinked alginate hydrogels as scaffolds for tissue engineering: Part 1. Structure, gelation rate and mechanical properties. *Biomaterials*, 22, 511–521.
Leach, J. B., Bivens, K. A., Patrick, C. W. & Schmidt, C. E. (2003) Photocrosslinked hyaluronic acid hydrogels: natural, biodegradable tissue engineering scaffolds. *Biotechnology and Bioengineering*, 82, 578–589.
Lee, J. B., Yoon, J. J., Lee, D. S. & Park, T. G. (2004) Photo-crosslinkable, thermo-sensitive and biodegradable Pluronic hydrogels for sustained release of protein. *Journal of Biomaterials Science – Polymer Edition*, 15, 1571–1583.
Lewis, G. (1997) Properties of acrylic bone cement: State of the art review. *Journal of Biomedical Materials Research*, 38, 155–182.
Lewis, G. (1999) Effect of mixing method and storage temperature of cement constituents on the fatigue and porosity of acrylic bone cement. *Journal of Biomedical Materials Research*, 48, 143–149.
Lewis, G. (2003) Fatigue testing and performance of acrylic bone-cement materials: State-of-the-art review. *Journal of Biomedical Materials Research Part B – Applied Biomaterials*, 66B, 457–486.
Lewis, G. (2006) Injectable bone cements for use in vertebroplasty and kyphoplasty: State-of-the-art review. *Journal of Biomedical Materials Research Part B – Applied Biomaterials*, 76B, 456–468.
Li, Q., Williams, C. G., Sun, D. D. N., Wang, J., Leong, K. & Elisseeff, J. H. (2004) Photocrosslinkable polysaccharides based on chondroitin sulfate. *Journal of Biomedical Materials Research Part A*, 68A, 28–33.
Lidgren, L., Bodelind, B. & Moller, J. (1987) Bone-Cement Improved by Vacuum Mixing and Chilling. *Acta Orthopaedica Scandinavica*, 58, 27–32.
Lin, H. H. & Cheng, Y. L. (2001) *In-situ* thermoreversible gelation of block and star copolymers of poly(ethylene glycol) and poly(N-isopropylacrylamide) of varying architectures. *Macromolecules*, 34, 3710–3715.
Lin-Gibson, S., Bencherif, S., Antonucci, J. M., Jones, R. L. & Horkay, F. (2005) Synthesis and characterization of poly(ethylene glycol) dimethacrylate hydrogels. *Macromolecular Symposia*, 227, 243–254.
Linden, U. (1989) Fatigue properties of bone-cement – comparison of mixing techniques. *Acta Orthopaedica Scandinavica*, 60, 431–433.
Lutolf, M. R., Weber, F. E., Schmoekel, H. G., Schense, J. C., Kohler, T., Muller, R. & Hubbell, J. A. (2003) Repair of bone defects using synthetic mimetics of

collagenous extracellular matrices. *Nature Biotechnology*, 21, 513–518.
Malafaya, P. B., Silva, G. A. & Reis, R. L. (2007) Natural-origin polymers as carriers and scaffolds for biomolecules and cell delivery in tissue engineering applications. *Advanced Drug Delivery Reviews*, 59, 207–233.
Mano, J. F., Sousa, R. A., Boesel, L. F., Neves, N. M. & Reis, R. L. (2004) Bloinert, biodegradable and injectable polymeric matrix composites for hard tissue replacement: state of the art and recent developments. *Composites Science and Technology*, 64, 789–817.
Matsuda, T. & Mizutani, M. (2002) Liquid acrylate-endcapped biodegradable poly(epsilon-caprolactone-co-trimethylene carbonate). II. Computer-aided stereolithographic microarchitectural surface photoconstructs. *Journal of Biomedical Materials Research*, 62, 395–403.
Matsuda, T., Mizutani, M. & Arnold, S. C. (2000) Molecular design of photocurable liquid biodegradable copolymers. 1. Synthesis and photocuring characteristics. *Macromolecules*, 33, 795–800.
Matsuda, T., Kwon, I. K. & Kidoaki, S. (2004) Photocurable biodegradable liquid copolymers: synthesis of acrylate-end-capped trimethylene carbonate-based prepolymers, photocuring, and hydrolysis. *Biomacromolecules*, 5, 295–305.
Matsumaru, Y., Hyodo, A., Nose, T., Ito, S., Hirano, T. & Ohashi, S. (1996) Application of thermosensitive polymers as a new embolic material for intravascular neurosurgery. *Journal of Biomaterials Science – Polymer Edition*, 7, 795–804.
Mistry, A. S., Mikos, A. G. & Jansen, J. A. (2007) Degradation and biocompatibility of a poly(propylene fumarate)-based/alumoxane nanocomposite for bone tissue engineering. *Journal of Biomedical Materials Research Part A*, 83A, 940–953.
Mizutani, M. & Matsuda, T. (2002) Liquid acrylate-endcapped biodegradable poly(epsilon-caprolactone-co-trimethylene carbonate). I. Preparation and visible light-induced photocuring characteristics. *Journal of Biomedical Materials Research*, 62, 387–394.
Mizutani, M., Arnold, S. C. & Matsuda, T. (2002) Liquid, phenylazide-end-capped copolymers of epsilon-caprolactone and trimethylene carbonate: Preparation, photocuring characteristics, and surface layering. *Biomacromolecules*, 3, 668–675.
Muggli, D. S., Burkoth, A. K. & Anseth, K. S. (1999) Crosslinked polyanhydrides for use in orthopedic applications: degradation behavior and mechanics. *Journal of Biomedical Materials Research*, 46, 271–278.
Murphy, B. P. & Prendergast, P. J. (2000) On the magnitude and variability of the fatigue strength of acrylic bone cement. *International Journal of Fatigue*, 22, 855–864.
Nanjawade, B. K., Manvi, F. V. & Manjappa, A. S. (2007) *In situ*-forming hydrogels for sustained ophthalmic drug delivery. *Journal of Controlled Release*, 122, 119–134.
Nielsen, L. E. & Landel, R. F. (1994) *Mechanical Properties of Polymers and Composites*, New York, Marcel Dekker.
Ono, K., Saito, Y., Yura, H., Ishikawa, K., Kurita, A., Akaike, T. & Ishihara, M. (2000) Photocrosslinkable chitosan as a biological adhesive. *Journal of Biomedical Materials Research*, 49, 289–295.
Otsuka, H., Nagasaki, Y. & Kataoka, K. (2003) PEGylated nanoparticles for biological and pharmaceutical applications. *Advanced Drug Delivery Reviews*, 55, 403–419.
Park, Y. D., Tirelli, N. & Hubbell, J. A. (2003) Photopolymerized hyaluronic acid-based hydrogels and interpenetrating networks. *Biomaterials*, 24, 893–900.
Patel, P. N., Smith, C. K. & Patrick, C. W. (2005) Rheological and recovery properties of poly(ethylene glycol) diacrylate hydrogels and human adipose tissue. *Journal of Biomedical Materials Research Part A*, 73A, 313–319.

Peter, S. J., Nolley, J. A., Widmer, M. S., Merwin, J. E., Yaszemski, M. J., Yasko, A. W., Engel, P. S. & Mikos, A. G. (1997) *In vitro* degradation of a poly(propylene fumarate)/beta-tricalcium phosphate composite orthopaedic scaffold. *Tissue Engineering*, 3, 207–215.

Peter, S. J., Miller, S. T., Zhu, G. M., Yasko, A. W. & Mikos, A. G. (1998) *In vivo* degradation of a poly(propylene fumarate) beta-tricalcium phosphate injectable composite scaffold. *Journal of Biomedical Materials Research*, 41, 1–7.

Peter, S. J., Kim, P., Yasko, A. W., Yaszemski, M. J. & Mikos, A. G. (1999) Crosslinking characteristics of an injectable poly(propylene fumarate)/beta-tricalcium phosphate paste and mechanical properties of the crosslinked composite for use as a biodegradable bone cement. *Journal of Biomedical Materials Research*, 44, 314–321.

Poshusta, A. K., Burdick, J. A., Mortisen, D. J., Padera, R. F., Ruehlman, D., Yaszemski, M. J. & Anseth, K. S. (2003) Histocompatibility of photocrosslinked polyanhydrides: A novel *in situ*-forming orthopaedic biomaterial. *Journal of Biomedical Materials Research Part A*, 64A, 62–69.

Priola, A., Gozzelino, G., Ferrero, F. & Malucelli, G. (1993) Properties of polymeric films obtained from UV cured poly(ethylene glycol) diacrylates. *Polymer*, 34, 3653–3657.

Raeber, G. P., Lutolf, M. P. & Hubbell, J. A. (2005) Molecularly engineered PEG hydrogels: a novel model system for proteolytically mediated cell migration. *Biophysical Journal*, 89, 1374–1388.

Robb, S. A., Lee, B. H., McLemore, R. & Vernon, B. L. (2007) Simultaneously physically and chemically gelling polymer system utilizing a poly(NIPAAm-co-cysteamine)-based copolymer. *Biomacromolecules*, 8, 2294–2300.

Roberts, M. J., Bentley, M. D. & Harris, J. M. (2002) Chemistry for peptide and protein PEGylation. *Advanced Drug Delivery Reviews*, 54, 459–476.

Rowley, J. A. & Mooney, D. J. (2002) Alginate type and RGD density control myoblast phenotype. *Journal of Biomedical Materials Research*, 60, 217–223.

Rowley, J. A., Madlambayan, G. & Mooney, D. J. (1999) Alginate hydrogels as synthetic extracellular matrix materials. *Biomaterials*, 20, 45–53.

Ruel-Gariepy, E. & Leroux, J. C. (2004) *In situ*-forming hydrogels – review of temperature-sensitive systems. *European Journal of Pharmaceutics and Biopharmaceutics*, 58, 409–426.

Rzaev, Z. M. O., Dincer, S. & Piskin, E. (2007) Functional copolymers of N-isopropylacrylamide for bioengineering applications. *Progress in Polymer Science*, 32, 534–595.

Schaffer, J. P. (1999) *The Science and Design of Engineering Materials*, Boston, WCB McGraw-Hill.

Schild, H. G. (1992) Poly (N-isopropylacrylamide) – experiment, theory and application. *Progress in Polymer Science*, 17, 163–249.

Shi, X. F., Hudson, J. L., Spicer, P. P., Tour, J. M., Krishnamoorti, R. & Mikos, A. G. (2005) Rheological behaviour and mechanical characterization of injectable poly(propylene fumarate)/single-walled carbon nanotube composites for bone tissue engineering. *Nanotechnology*, 16, S531–S538.

Shi, X. F., Hudson, J. L., Spicer, P. P., Tour, J. M., Krishnamoorti, R. & Mikos, A. G. (2006) Injectable nanocomposites of single-walled carbon nanotubes and biodegradable polymers for bone tissue engineering. *Biomacromolecules*, 7, 2237–2242.

Shi, X. F., Sitharaman, B., Pham, Q. P., Liang, F., Wu, K., Billups, W. E., Wilson, L. J. &

Mikos, A. G. (2007) Fabrication of porous ultra-short single-walled carbon nanotube nanocomposite scaffolds for bone tissue engineering. *Biomaterials*, 28, 4078–4090.

Shin, H., Temenoff, J. S. & Mikos, A. G. (2003) *In vitro* cytotoxicity of unsaturated oligo[poly(ethylene glycol) fumarate] macromers and their cross-linked hydrogels. *Biomacromolecules*, 4, 552–560.

Sitharaman, B., Shi, X. F., Tran, L. A., Spicer, P. P., Rusakova, I., Wilson, L. J. & Mikos, A. G. (2007) Injectable *in situ* cross-linkable nanocomposites of biodegradable polymers and carbon nanostructures for bone tissue engineering. *Journal of Biomaterials Science – Polymer Edition*, 18, 655–671.

Smidsrod, O. & Skjakbraek, G. (1990) Alginate as immobilization matrix for cells. *Trends in Biotechnology*, 8, 71–78.

Sosnik, A. & Cohn, D. (2004) Ethoxysilane-capped PEO-PPO-PEO triblocks: a new family of reverse thermo-responsive polymers. *Biomaterials*, 25, 2851–2858.

Sosnik, A., Cohn, D., San Roman, J. S. & Abraham, G. A. (2003) Crosslinkable PEO-PPO-PEO-based reverse thermo-responsive gels as potentially injectable materials. *Journal of Biomaterials Science – Polymer Edition*, 14, 227–239.

Tanaka, Y., Gong, J. P. & Osada, Y. (2005) Novel hydrogels with excellent mechanical performance. *Progress in Polymer Science*, 30, 1–9.

Temenoff, J. S. & Mikos, A. G. (2008) *Biomaterials: the intersection of biology and materials science*. Upper Saddle River, NJ: Pearson/Prentice Hall.

Temenoff, J. S., Athanasiou, K. A., Lebaron, R. G. & Mikos, A. G. (2002) Effect of poly(ethylene glycol) molecular weight on tensile and swelling properties of oligo(poly(ethylene glycol) fumarate) hydrogels for cartilage tissue engineering. *Journal of Biomedical Materials Research*, 59, 429–437.

Timmer, M. D., Jo, S. B., Wang, C. Y., Ambrose, C. G. & Mikos, A. G. (2002) Characterization of the cross-linked structure of fumarate-based degradable polymer networks. *Macromolecules*, 35, 4373–4379.

Timmer, M. D., Ambrose, C. G. & Mikos, A. G. (2003a) *In vitro* degradation of polymeric networks of poly(propylene fumarate) and the crosslinking macromer poly(propylene fumarate)-diacrylate. *Biomaterials*, 24, 571–577.

Timmer, M. D., Carter, C., Ambrose, C. G. & Mikos, A. G. (2003b) Fabrication of poly(propylene fumarate)-based orthopaedic implants by photo-crosslinking through transparent silicone molds. *Biomaterials*, 24, 4707–4714.

Tonnesen, H. H. & Karlsen, J. (2002) Alginate in drug delivery systems. *Drug Development and Industrial Pharmacy*, 28, 621–630.

Toole, B. P. (2004) Hyaluronan: from extracellular glue to pericellular cue. *Nature Reviews Cancer*, 4, 528–539.

Topoleski, L. D. T., Ducheyne, P. & Cuckler, J. M. (1995) The effects of centrifugation and titanium fiber reinforcement on fatigue failure mechanisms in poly(methyl methacrylate) bone-cement. *Journal of Biomedical Materials Research*, 29, 299–307.

Trudel, J. & Massia, S. P. (2002) Assessment of the cytotoxicity of photocrosslinked dextran and hyaluronan-based hydrogels to vascular smooth muscle cells. *Biomaterials*, 23, 3299–3307.

Wang, J. S., Franzen, H., Jonsson, E. & Lidgren, L. (1993) Porosity of bone-cement reduced by mixing and collecting under vacuum. *Acta Orthopaedica Scandinavica*, 64, 143–146.

Ward, I. M. & Sweeney, J. (2004) *An Introduction to the Mechanical Properties of Solid Polymers*. Chichester, Wiley.

Williams, C. G., Malik, A. N., Kim, T. K., Manson, P. N. & Elisseeff, J. H. (2005) Variable cytocompatibility of six cell lines with photoinitiators used for polymerizing hydrogels and cell encapsulation. *Biomaterials*, 26, 1211–1218.

Wu, D. Q., Qiu, F., Wang, T., Jiang, X. J., Zhang, X. Z. & Zhuo, R. X. (2009) Toward the development of partially biodegradable and injectable thermoresponsive hydrogels for potential biomedical applications. *Acs Applied Materials & Interfaces*, 1, 319–327.

Yaszemski, M. J., Payne, R. G., Hayes, W. C., Langer, R. & Mikos, A. G. (1996) *In vitro* degradation of a poly(propylene fumarate)-based composite material. *Biomaterials*, 17, 2127–2130.

Zhou, Y., Yue, W. M., Li, C. D. & Mason, J. J. (2009) Static and fatigue mechanical characterizations of variable diameter fibers reinforced bone cement. *Journal of Materials Science – Materials in Medicine*, 20, 633–641.

Part II
Clinical applications

5

Drug delivery applications of injectable biomaterials

D. J. OVERSTREET, Arizona State University, USA,
H. A. VON RECUM, Case Western Reserve University, USA
and B. L. VERNON, Arizona State University, USA

Abstract: This chapter discusses the design and applications of injectable biomaterials for the controlled delivery of drugs, proteins, and other therapeutics for the treatment of various diseases. The first half of the chapter describes *in situ* forming drug delivery systems which are injectable as a liquid, forming a solid or semi-solid depot after injection which then releases the drug. The second half of the chapter discusses particulate drug delivery systems which are often injected into the circulation. Emphasis is placed on clinical applications as well as stimuli responsive and/or targeted drug delivery. Design choices relevant to each class of injectable system are highlighted.

Key words: drug delivery, targeted cancer chemotherapy, injectable drug depot, nanoparticles.

5.1 Introduction

The goal of drug delivery is to safely and effectively provide a platform for drugs to achieve a desired therapeutic effect. Drugs and their carriers can be administered by a variety of routes, including oral, topical, transmucosal, intravenous, or as implantable devices. Drug delivery systems can be designed for carrying a drug, protecting it from unwanted metabolism, localizing the drug at the desired site of action, releasing the drug at a desired controlled rate, targeting drug release to specific tissues or cells, and minimizing unwanted side effects caused by high doses and systemic delivery. Injectable biomaterials can meet these requirements, offer improved compliance through ease of administration, and allow prolonged duration of a single treatment (Langer 1990).

For effective drug delivery, several factors must be taken into account. For example, the solubility of the drug will place specific constraints on the composition and structure of the drug delivery device. Many cancer drugs are hydrophobic, so they can be delivered with greater efficiency if contained in a hydrophobic environment. Other drugs are biomolecules themselves, including growth factors, enzymes, and nucleic acids. The desired release profile must also be considered. Often it is considered desirable to have a delivery system release the drug in a controlled manner such that the drug concentration is maintained within the therapeutic window, a range of concentration in which the drug is effective but does not cause adverse effects. Another important consideration is the safe removal of the device from the body. To achieve this, many injectable biomaterials are biodegradable. Depending on the rate of degradation, this may affect the release of drug from the device as well as the degradation of the device and its subsequent removal from the body. Further important considerations include biocompatibility, stability, patient compliance and comfort, ease of storage, and sterilization.

In this chapter, two broad classes of injectable biomaterials for drug delivery will be discussed: *in situ* forming gels and particulates. *In situ* forming drug delivery systems can be loaded with drug and injected through a needle, forming a solid or semi-solid gel depot of drug inside the body at the injection site. The drug is then released by diffusion of the drug out of the depot, which can be facilitated by further swelling, or by degradation of the depot itself, which can be triggered by water content, changes in pH, enzyme activity, or other factors. Discussion of these systems is organized according to the mechanism for gelation (solvent exchange, aqueous solubility change, *in situ* crosslinking gels).

Particulate systems can be injected either at the site of action or into the circulation. These systems are suspensions of small particles on the scale of nanometers to hundreds of microns which entrap or protect the drug and then release it due to diffusion, degradation, dissociation, or metabolism. The types of particulate drug delivery platforms discussed in this chapter are polymeric particles and spheres, liposomes and micelles, and polymer-drug conjugates. A brief overview of some advantages and disadvantages of each injectable drug delivery system is shown in Table 5.1.

Injectable *in situ* forming gels typically release drugs at a rate limited either by diffusion of the drug through the material or degradation of the material itself. However, it is desirable for a variety of applications that the material be able to release drug preferentially depending on its environment. For example, rather than degrading by hydrolysis, injectable biomaterials can be designed to degrade or swell in response to specific enzymes. These so-called bioresponsive materials have found applications in drug delivery as well as other fields. Achieving effective targeting of drugs toward particular cells and tissues is a major challenge in the development of systemically injectable drug carriers which provide a therapeutic effect while minimizing side effects, particularly for highly toxic anticancer drugs. Passive targeting occurs when drug carriers injected into the circulation preferentially accumulate in certain tissues without utilizing some functionality in the carrier. Alternatively, active targeting involves the addition of specific moieties (often antibodies or ligands) onto the drug carrier surface which causes their accumulation in a desired location. In this chapter, some drug delivery applications of stimulus-responsive drug delivery and targeting will be mentioned. For a more thorough review of how biomaterials can be designed to respond to a variety of stimuli, see Chapter 12.

Table 5.1 Summary of injectable drug delivery devices

Type of material	Advantages	Disadvantages/concerns	Selected references
Solvent exchange precipitation	Allows for injection of pre-synthesized degradable polymers	Potentially toxic solvent Burst release	Lambert and Peck (1995) Hatefi and Amsden (2002)
Aqueous solubility change	Free of organic solvent Can deliver proteins, biomolecules Can be made degradable or stimulus responsive	Syneresis (shrinking) Poor mechanical properties Non-degradability	He *et al.* (2008) Hatefi and Amsden (2002) Huang and Lowe (2005) Zentner *et al.* (2001)
In situ crosslinking or polymerizing materials	Site-specific polymerization Flexible macromer design (tunable properties) Improved mechanical properties	Burst release Heat generation Toxicity from unreacted monomers or initiator	Hoare and Kohane (2008) Hubbell *et al.* (2005) Biehl *et al.* (1974) Temenoff *et al.* (2003)
Degradable polymeric microparticles	Allows for injection of pre-synthesized degradable polymers Tunable degradability Minimal burst release Predictable release rate	Poor cellular uptake	Panyam and Labhasetwar (2003a) Soppimath *et al.* (2001) Okada (1997)
Polymeric nanoparticles	Efficient cellular uptake Injectable into the circulation Capable of passive or active targeting Flexible chemistry	Potentially toxic nanoscale interactions Nonspecific uptake Inactivation of therapeutic proteins	Nel *et al.* (2006) Soppimath *et al.* (2001) Desai *et al.* (1996)

Table 5.1 Continued

Type of material	Advantages	Disadvantages/concerns	Selected references
Micelles	Small size should help avoid nonspecific uptake Can be made stimulus responsive	Instability, dose dumping Only suitable for delivering hydrophobic drugs	Burt *et al.* (1999) Gaucher *et al.* (2005) Y. Bae *et al.* (2005)
Liposomes	Easily internalized by cells Stable in the circulation Capable of passive or active targeting Tunable size Capable of carrying hydrophilic and/or hydrophobic drugs	Chemistry limited to phospholipids Thickness of membrane is unchanged Systemic toxicity	Torchilin (2005) Lorusso *et al.* (2007) Ni *et al.* (2002) Lee and Yuk (2007)
Polymer-drug conjugates	Improves water solubility of hydrophobic drugs Prolongs half-life of drugs, proteins in the circulation Capable of passive or active targeting Wide range of chemistries Improves immunocompatibility of drug	Some drugs require multi-step or site-specific chemistries Non-degradability No currently approved conjugates with low molecular weight drugs	Greenwald *et al.* (1996) Duncan (2009) Pasut and Veronese (2007) Seymour *et al.* (2002) Khandare and Minko (2006)

5.2 Solvent exchange precipitating materials

An intuitive mechanism for the generation of *in situ* forming gels is precipitation of a polymer by solvent exchange. In this method, the polymer and drug are initially dissolved in a water-miscible organic solvent with low toxicity, such as *N*-methyl-2-pyrrolidone (NMP) or dimethyl sulfoxide (DMSO). Most solvent exchange systems involve the use of copolymers of lactic acid and glycolic acid. These materials have been demonstrated for a variety of controlled drug delivery applications due to their easily tunable mechanical properties and degradation rate via adjustment of the comonomer ratio. Upon injection of the polymer and drug solution, the organic solvent is gradually replaced by water, causing precipitation of the polymer, which forms a solid gel and entraps the drug. However, drug delivery applications of these materials have been limited due to high risks of burst release and solvent toxicity. A brief discussion of the investigation of these materials is still important because it represents some of the first work done using injectable materials to deliver drugs.

Burst release occurs from solvent exchange systems because there is a significant amount of time required for the polymer to precipitate *in situ*. Several factors are known to affect the amount of burst release, including the polymer concentration and molecular weight, solvent used, and inclusion of a surfactant (Lambert and Peck 1995; Radomsky *et al.* 1993; Chandrashekar *et al.* 2000; Shah *et al.* 1993). Higher concentrations of polymer will typically precipitate more quickly, which can reduce burst release. Lambert and Peck demonstrated this using poly(D,L-lactide-*co*-glycolide) (PLGA) in NMP and DMSO for the release of fluorescently labeled bovine serum albumin (FITC-BSA). Using a high molecular weight (75–115 kDa) polymer, the burst release was reduced from 60% to 20% when the polymer concentration was increased from 15% to 20% by weight (Lambert and Peck 1995). Using a lower molecular weight (10–15 kDa) polymer, burst release was eliminated when the concentration of polymer was elevated to 40%. After precipitation, the release rate of FITC-BSA was higher from the lower molecular weight gels at higher concentrations, with a constant release rate over about one week rather than three weeks or more for the higher molecular weight polymer.

An alternative approach was investigated by Jain *et al.*, who reported *in situ* forming microspheres using the solvent exchange mechanism for release of myoglobin and cytochrome C (Jain *et al.* 2000). The system contains droplets of PLGA and drug solution dispersed in a continuous oil phase. As the continuous phase is replaced by water, the polymer precipitates into drug-loaded microspheres. Depending on the composition of the continuous oil phase, Jain *et al.* reported a burst release between 30 and 50%, with sustained release thereafter for up to 15 days (Jain *et al.* 2000). Burst release in this case was attributed primarily to drug that was soluble in the continuous oil phase. They also showed that the structure of each protein was retained throughout the fabrication of the microspheres. This material could have been made injectable had it been preformed as microspheres and delivered as a suspension in water.

The most significant concern with solvent exchange systems is the use of organic solvents. A study by Kranz *et al.* showed the PLGA and poly(lactide) dissolved in either NMP, DMSO, or 2-pyrrolidone were all myotoxic when injected intramuscularly (Kranz *et al.* 2001). Similar studies have produced similar results for candidate solvents propylene glycol and triacetin (Chandrashekar and Udupa 1996; Singh *et al.* 1997). Another hazard for many solvents used in these systems is the risk of hemolysis (Fu *et al.* 1987; Medlicott *et al.* 2000).

5.3 Aqueous solubility change materials

Temperature responsive materials that are water-soluble at room temperature and insoluble at body temperature have been widely investigated for drug delivery applications. Most of these materials have a lower critical solution temperature (LCST), a temperature below which the material is soluble and above which the material is insoluble. Some also have an upper critical solution temperature (UCST), at which the material becomes insoluble upon cooling. At sufficient concentrations of the polymer, a hydrogel will form when the polymer is heated above its LCST. The LCST of a polymer is affected by a number of factors including polymer composition, concentration, ionic strength, and pH. For a material to be injectable, it typically must have an LCST below 37°C. These materials have many advantages over solvent exchange systems. In particular, because the materials are water-borne, they are more biocompatible and capable of safely delivering a wider range of drugs, including proteins, without use of toxic solvents. Also, these materials are usually capable of forming gels more quickly and therefore offer reduced risk of initial burst release.

5.3.1 *N*-isopropylacrylamide (NIPAAm)-based systems

Though many materials have an LCST, two families of materials have been investigated most extensively for injectable drug delivery systems. The first are polymers of *N*-isopropylacrylamide (NIPAAm). Poly(NIPAAm) is fairly unique among materials with an LCST in that it exhibits a narrow and reversible phase transition in the range of 29–33°C. However, unmodified poly(NIPAAm) has some undesirable features for drug delivery including poor mechanical stability, rapid or poorly controlled shrinkage, and non-degradability. These limitations are typically addressed by incorporating comonomers into polymers which are predominantly composed of NIPAAm and therefore retain their temperature-responsive behavior.

As a poly(NIPAAm) solution is heated above its LCST, the material becomes hydrophobic and exhibits a significant amount of syneresis (shrinkage), leading to rapid expulsion of drug solution. Though early studies proposed temperature-dependent swelling of NIPAAm-based copolymers for fast release of heparin, typically rapid non-specific release is undesirable or best obtained by injection of drug without a carrier (Gutowska *et al.* 1992). A simple strategy to control syneresis is to include a hydrophilic comonomer with NIPAAm such as acrylic acid (AAc) to increase the water content of the resulting gel. Vernon *et al.* developed poly(NIPAAm-co-AAc) gels with between 0 and 3 mol% AAc, achieving almost no shrinkage for the first 4 hours after gelation at 37°C for all the gels with at least 1% AAc, whereas homopolymer gels undergo a 60% volume reduction after 4 hours (Vernon *et al.* 2000). However, a disadvantage of this strategy is that comonomer content affects the polymer LCST. Hydrophilic comonomers such as AAc have been shown to increase the LCST, while hydrophobic comonomers decrease the LCST (Feil *et al.* 1993). Accordingly, Vernon *et al.* reported LCST values over 45°C for copolymers with 2.61% AAc (Vernon *et al.* 2000). Because NIPAAm block length has a larger impact on the polymer LCST than hydrophilic content, large hydrophilic comonomers can be used to reduce syneresis without changing the LCST (Chen and Hoffman 1995). An approach using this principle which limits syneresis without substantially affecting the LCST was developed by Pollock and Healy, in which PEG side chains were incorporated via polymerization of NIPAAm with methoxy poly(ethylene glycol) methacrylate (Pollock and Healy 2010). These high molecular weight copolymers had an LCST of about 33°C and some underwent little syneresis over 10 days. However, a significant reason that these gels were stable was due to the extremely high molecular weight of the polymer, which without degradation could cause chronic inflammation and foreign body response if the polymer remains unsolubilized, or renal toxicity if the high molecular weight polymer solubilizes in a drug delivery application. A common rule of thumb is that non-degradable molecules with molecular weights exceeding 30–50 kDa accumulate in the kidney (Yamaoka *et al.* 1993; Duncan *et al.* 2001).

Because poly(NIPAAm) chains are non-degradable, alternative strategies have been implemented in order to make copolymer gels become soluble after gelation *in situ*. Several groups have developed materials which exhibit time-dependent increases in LCST. Comonomers in these materials often contain side groups which are water-degradable. As water becomes increasingly accessible to the polymer over time, ester groups on the comonomer are hydrolyzed to carboxylic acids, increasing the comonomer hydrophilicity. For example, Neradovic *et al.* synthesized NIPAAm copolymers with ester side groups that exhibit an LCST increase upon hydrolysis, releasing lactic acid as a byproduct (Neradovic *et al.* 1999). Another approach described by Cui *et al.* uses the comonomer dimethyl-γ-butyrolactone acrylate, which was shown to have a time-dependent increase in LCST without low molecular weight byproducts (Cui *et al.* 2007). Huang and Lowe evaluated similar temperature responsive copolymers with a dextran macromer containing multiple degradable lactate units for delivery of methylene blue and bovine serum albumin (BSA) as hydrophilic model drugs (Huang and Lowe 2005). They found that drug release was controlled by the molecular size of the drug and the hydrophilicity and degradation of the hydrogel. While these materials suffered from high burst release of up to 40%, BSA was released in a sustained fashion for about 10 days thereafter. Somewhat surprisingly, many non-degradable NIPAAm-based polymers have been investigated for drug delivery since the development of their degradable counterparts. Nevertheless, it would be rather easy to convert any material already designed for a specific functionality and impart a time-dependent LCST property into it simply through the addition of a comonomer such as dimethyl-γ-butyrolactone acrylate or another ester-containing group. Some debate exists regarding the biocompatibility of polymers based on NIPAAm, but degradable formulations have been shown to exhibit no toxicity after material degradation (Henderson *et al.* 2009).

A variety of NIPAAm-based materials have been developed with crosslinks degradable by water or enzymes. Crosslinked polymers may be desirable for drug delivery due to their increased stability relative to physical gels. Assuming the material is hydrophilic enough that its equilibrium swelling is high, these materials may dissociate into insoluble polymer chains – however, the polymer will not become soluble unless the material LCST increases to above body temperature. Another disadvantage of crosslinking a NIPAAm-based polymer is that, for sufficiently high crosslink density, the material will not be injectable as a liquid. Kim and Healy developed a NIPAAm-based copolymer with a peptide crosslinker containing the MMP-13 labile sequence Pro-Gln-Gly-Leu-Ala (Kim and Healy 2003). Yoshida *et al.* used a poly(amino acid) crosslinker which was enzyme-degradable depending on the temperature (Yoshida *et al.* 2003). In some cases, syneresis is reduced in crosslinked NIPAAm-based gels by adding a high molecular weight hydrophilic molecule such as PEG or poly(acrylic acid), forming a semi-interpenetrating polymer network, or semi-IPN. In addition to reduced syneresis, Stile *et al.* reported increased complex shear modulus as an additional benefit of incorporation of 450 kDa poly(acrylic acid) into poly(NIPAAm-co-AAc) hydrogels (Stile *et al.* 2004). Alvarez-Lorenzo *et al.* developed a lightly cross-linked chitosan-poly(NIPAAm) IPN which significantly increased the loading capacity of the low molecular weight drug diclofenac compared to poly(NIPAAm) hydrogels (Alvarez-Lorenzo *et al.* 2005). Liu *et al.* have promoted IPN structures (with both hydrophobic and hydrophilic polymer networks) as suitable delivery systems for amphiphilic drugs (Liu, Fan *et al.* 2006). To this end, they developed IPNs of poly(NIPAAm-co-AAc) with poly(ethyl acrylate) which had pH-dependent swelling attributed to the carboxyl group on the acrylic acid. IPNs swelled less than poly(NIPAAm-co-AAc) hydrogels due to the hydrophobic poly(ethyl acrylate) component, which retained its properties within the IPN. Using daidezin as a model drug, hydrogels showed an initial burst release which was absent in the IPN (Liu, Shao *et al.* 2006).

Grafts of poly(NIPAAm) have also been used to impart temperature responsive behavior to natural biomaterials for drug delivery, converting them into physically crosslinking hydrogels above the LCST of the poly(NIPAAm) portions. For example, poly(NIPAAm) grafted onto hyaluronic acid formed a gel upon injection which had a 12-hour burst release of riboflavin followed by sustained release (Ha *et al.* 2006). Similarly, chitosan with grafted poly(NIPAAm) was shown to release 5-fluorouracil at a controlled rate (J.W. Bae *et al.* 2006).

Hydrogels of poly(NIPAAm-co-AAc) have been demonstrated by Na *et al.* for the delivery of multiple drugs (dexamethasone, ascorbate, and TGF β-3) to encourage chondrogenic differentiation in rabbits while also serving as a synthetic ECM (Na *et al.* 2006). An example of a targeted application of poly(NIPAAm-co-AAc) is the use of an enzyme-sensitive crosslinker 4,4′-bis(methacryloylamino)azobenzene (BMAAB) for colon-specific drug delivery investigated by Li and Liu (2008). The pH sensitivity inherent in the material causes it to collapse at low pH (when the AAc is protonated and therefore less hydrophilic) and swell at higher pH, making the azo-containing crosslink more accessible to azoreductase enzymes in the colon. Under the desired conditions for release *in vitro*, BSA was released from the hydrogels at a constant rate for 4 days (Li and Liu 2008). While this material was not injectable due to high crosslink density, a similar formulation with lighter crosslinking could be developed to be injectable and responsive to a different stimulus.

5.3.2 Temperature-responsive block copolymer systems

Temperature-responsive block copolymers are another class of materials that have been investigated for drug delivery. These materials often have a central hydrophobic block such as poly(propylene oxide) (PPO) and two hydrophilic end blocks, almost always poly(ethylene oxide) (PEO, also called PEG for poly(ethylene glycol)). One reason these materials have been studied so extensively is because their components are already FDA approved for other applications. These materials may be injectable because of either LCST or UCST behavior (in which case the material is heated to become suitable for injection and gels upon cooling), which varies greatly as a function of the length and composition of each copolymer block and the polymer concentration. Various formulations of PEG-PPO-PEG triblock copolymers are known as Pluronic® (BASF) or Poloxamer® (ICI). Concentrated aqueous solutions of these polymers undergo two reversible phase transitions based on temperature – a sol-gel transition at the LCST and a gel-to-sol transition at the UCST. The phase transition mechanisms of Pluronic solutions have been heavily investigated (Rassing and Attwood 1983; Attwood *et al.* 1985; Vadnere *et al.*

1984; Zhou and Chu 1988; Wanka *et al.* 1990; Brown *et al.* 1991; Glatter and Scherf 1994; Jorgensen *et al.* 1997; Song *et al.* 2000; Mortensen and Brown 1993). The LCST is more relevant for most drug delivery applications, and it is thought to occur based on increased hydrophobicity of the PPO segment upon heating, followed by micellar aggregation (Attwood *et al.* 1985; Vadnere *et al.* 1984). Both transition temperatures of Pluronics are much more sensitive to polymer concentration than poly(NIPAAm)-based polymers, and dilute solutions often do not undergo a phase transition at all.

Pluronics that are most desirable for drug delivery applications are in the solution state at room temperature, precipitating to form a gel at body temperature. Temperature responsive block copolymers are capable of incorporating hydrophilic or hydrophobic drugs due to an ordered micellar packing structure and intermicellar entanglements (He *et al.* 2008). While Pluronic hydrogels prolong the release of drugs, there are still several challenges in using Pluronics for effective drug delivery, including poor mechanical stability, high permeability, and non-degradability (Ruel-Gariepy and Leroux 2004). The molecular weight must also be limited in order for Pluronics to be safely cleared through the kidneys (Ruel-Gariepy and Leroux 2004).

Several degradable Pluronics have been developed for improved drug delivery. Degradability by water is introduced by the incorporation of degradable bonds (such as esters or anhydrides) into the block copolymers. This is achieved either by coupling PEG or PPO with compounds to form an ester or directly using degradable monomers, usually in place of the PPO segments. Coupling of Pluronic P85 with terephthaloyl chloride yielded biodegradable multiblock copolymers with molecular weights of 4 to 40 kDa (Ahn *et al.* 2005). Depending on the molecular weight, the dissolution time of the hydrogels could be varied *in vitro* from 8 hrs to 4 weeks. Degradable multiblock polymers have also been synthesized via coupling of PEG and PPO with carbonyl chloride or diacyl chloride, forming hydrogels with increased viscosity relative to Pluronic F127 (Sosnik and Cohn 2005). The non-degradable crosslinker hexamethylene diisocyanate (HMDI) has been used to couple Pluronics to each other for increased mechanical stability, including a degradable version with coupled oligo(ester) blocks on Pluronic F127 (Cohn *et al.* 2003; 2006). One such material was shown to slow the release of an anti-restenosis model drug from 7 days to 40 days (Cohn *et al.* 2003). Pluronics have been modified with pendant degradable polyesters and investigated for drug delivery of both procain hydrochloride (hydrophilic) and 9-(methylaminomethyl) anthracene (hydrophobic) (Xiong *et al.* 2005; 2006). Adding poly(D,L-lactide) (PDLLA) or poly(ϵ-caprolactone) (PCL) to form a pentablock copolymer did not affect the sol-gel transition temperature of F87, and no initial burst release was observed from either hydrogel.

Temperature-responsive block copolymers with degradable hydrophobic core-forming blocks of poly(L-lactide) (PLLA) were originally developed by

Jeong *et al.* (1997). Drug-loaded gels were prepared by heating aqueous polymer solutions to 45°C, then cooling to 37°C to form a gel. Sustained release of fluorescein isothiocyanate (FITC) labeled dextran (20 kDa) was achieved for up to 12 days. Burst release of dextran occurred from 23 wt% gels, but not from 35 wt% gels (Jeong *et al.* 1997). A disadvantage of this particular system is that protein drugs would have to be loaded into the device at an elevated temperature. Factors affecting the phase transition from these materials include hydrophilic/hydrophobic balance, block length, and stereoregularity of the degradable segment (i.e. PLLA vs. PDLLA) (Jeong *et al.* 1999; Choi *et al.* 1999). Jeong *et al.* also developed triblock copolymers of PEG-PLGA-PEG (Jeong *et al.* 2000). Ketoprofen, a model hydrophilic drug, was released by diffusion over two weeks with moderate burst release and a first-order release profile while spironolactone, a model hydrophobic drug, was released over eight weeks with a unique S-shaped release profile which was attributed to partitioning of the drug in the hydrophobic cores of the aggregated micelles. The release rate was reduced with increasing PLGA block length (Jeong *et al.* 2000).

Using a central hydrophilic block with pendant hydrophobic blocks (PLGA-PEG-PLGA) is another method for making temperature-responsive block copolymer hydrogels, as seen in the commercially available delivery vehicle ReGel® (1500-1000-1500 Da blocks of PLGA-PEG-PLGA). An advantage of using this system is that the synthesis is easier because it does not require a coupling procedure using HMDI. The materials also have thermoreversible sol-gel and gel-sol phase transitions with increasing temperature which can be adjusted by block length, composition, and additives (Lee *et al.* 2001; Shim *et al.* 2002). Zentner *et al.* investigated the release of several proteins and low molecular weight drugs from ReGel® (Zentner *et al.* 2001). Hydrophobic drugs paclitaxel and cyclosporin A were solubilized by the copolymers and released in a sustained manner for about 50 days, compared to release from Pluronic F127 in about one day. ReGel®/paclitaxel also showed higher anti-tumor efficacy and reduced side effects in mice with human breast tumor xenografts compared to the maximum tolerated dose of free paclitaxel (Zentner *et al.* 2001). The gel was also demonstrated for sustained release of proteins porcine growth hormone, glycosylated insulin, and recombinant hepatitis B surface antigen. Release profiles ranging from two to eight weeks were controlled by adjusting the comonomer ratio of lactide to glycolide. A later study was able to improve insulin levels with sustained release of the incretin hormone glucagons-like peptide-1 (GLP-1), a drug very useful for treatment of type 2 diabetes but unstable in the circulation. Choi *et al.* were able to obtain elevated plasma insulin concentration in rats for up to two weeks by subcutaneous injection of ReGel® for the delivery of zinc-complexed GLP-1 (Choi *et al.* 2004). Controlled release from temperature responsive PLGA-PEG-PLGA has also been demonstrated for testosterone, levonorgestrel, and interleukin-2 (Chen and Singh 2005a,b; Samlowski *et al.* 2006).

Triblock copolymers PEG-PCL-PEG and PCL-PEG-PCL have also been reported (Hwang *et al.* 2005; S.J. Bae *et al.* 2005). PCL is a degradable polyester which hydrolyzes more slowly than PLGA copolymers and is FDA approved. Aqueous solutions of both copolymers undergo a transition from sol to gel to turbid sol when heated from 10 °C to 60 °C, with the LCST dependent on polymer concentration. It was concluded that PCL-PEG-PCL is the easier of the triblock copolymers to synthesize as it forms a gel over a wider range of temperatures, and forms gels with higher modulus. A potential drawback of this system is that it spontaneously forms a solid gel within one hour at room temperature due to crystallization of the polymer, so it needs to be coupled into multiblock copolymers to have sufficient stability in solution (S.J. Bae *et al.* 2006). Some other hydrophobic polyesters used in temperature responsive degradable triblock copolymers include poly(hydroxybutyrate), poly(δ-valerolactone), poly(hexamethylene adipate), poly(ethylene adipate), and poly(ethylene succinate), and poly(propylene fumarate) (Kim *et al.* 2004; Song *et al.* 2003; Behravesh *et al.* 2002; Loh *et al.* 2007). Other non-degradable hydrophobic block materials include poly(trimethylene carbonate), poly(ethyl-2-cyanoacrylate), and temperature responsive poly(NIPAAm) (S.Y. Kim *et al.* 2007; Choi *et al.* 2007; Li, Tang *et al.* 2005; Li, Buurma *et al.* 2005).

Sensitivity of drug delivery systems to pH is relevant for delivery to sites where pH changes occur, including the stomach, intestines, lysosome, tumors, and other sites (He *et al.* 2008). Several block copolymer hydrogels have been developed toward this end by using blocks with ionizable groups (i.e. polyelectrolytes). The range of pH over which the material is most responsive is determined by the pKa of the ionizable group. In general, polyelectrolytes with pKa values between 3 and 10 are suitable for applications in medicine (Schmaljohann 2006). Acidic pH-responsive blocks often contain carboxylic acid groups, while basic pH-responsive blocks often contain tertiary amines such as poly(2-(dimethylamino) ethyl methacrylate) (PDMAEMA) and poly(2-(diethylamino) ethyl methacrylate) (PDEAEMA) (Butun *et al.* 2001). An example of pH-responsive block copolymer gels for drug delivery is based on triblock copolymers of poly(2-diisopropylamino)ethyl methacrylate) (PDPAEMA) or PDEAEMA with a central block of poly(2-methacryloyloxyethyl phosphorylcholine) (PMPC) (Ma *et al.* 2003). The pH-responsive PDPAEMA and PDEAEMA have pKa values of 6.0 and 7.3, respectively (Butun *et al.* 2001). In the pH range of 7–8, triblock polymer solutions of sufficient concentration formed gels due to hydrophobic interactions of deprotonated pH-responsive groups aiding in the formation of a micellar network (Castelletto *et al.* 2004). In pH 3 buffer, the gels dissolved. A hydrophobic model drug, dipyrimadole, was released *in vitro* from 10 to 20 wt% gels at pH 7.4, with slow release of between 2 and 4% of the payload over 3 hours, whereas the drug was released rapidly when the gel was placed in pH 3 buffer (Ma *et al.* 2003). Alternatively, PDEAEMA has been used by Determan *et al.* for end blocks of a pentablock copolymer with Pluronic F127 to make hydrogels responsive to both pH and temperature (Determan *et al.* 2007). An interesting finding of this work is that drug release rate was altered within a narrow range of pH between 7.4 and 8.0 (slow release) and 7.0 (fast release). Other pH- and temperature responsive block copolymer hydrogels have been developed using Pluronics coupled by a carboxylic acid-containing compound (Suh *et al.* 2005).

Enzyme-degradable, temperature responsive block copolymer hydrogels have recently been developed by Jeong *et al.* (2009). The materials are based on diblock copolymers of PEG with poly(alanine-co-phenylalanine), a polypeptide segment that allows for degradation by a variety of enzymes including cathepsin B, cathepsin C, and elastase. The material was developed in part to improve the shelf life of degradable block copolymer solutions because an enzyme-degradable material will remain stable in water for a long time, degrading only after injection due to various enzymes. After an initial burst release of about 15%, insulin was released at a diffusion-limited rate from a subcutaneous implant over 16 days after injection, leading to a pronounced hypoglycemic effect in rats (Jeong *et al.* 2009).

5.3.3 Chitosan-based systems

Besides poly(NIPAAm)-based materials and block copolymers, solutions of the natural biomaterial chitosan have also been investigated for injectable drug delivery systems based on solubility change in aqueous solution (Chenite *et al.* 2000; Fang *et al.* 2008; Mi *et al.* 2002; Ruel-Gariepy *et al.* 2004). Chitosan is a deacetylated version of chitin, a nitrogen-containing polysaccharide found in crustacean shells. In solutions below pH 6.2, chitosan is soluble in aqueous solutions. Neutralization causes a sol-gel phase transition. A study by Chenite *et al.* used this behavior to make the gelation of chitosan temperature dependent by adding polyol salts to chitosan solutions (Chenite *et al.* 2000). The gels were demonstrated for delivery of growth factors for promoting bone formation *in vivo* as well as for encapsulation of explanted chondrocytes for tissue engineering. Similar gels under the trade name BST-Gel™ were investigated for local delivery of paclitaxel in mice, with one hydrogel injection having reduced systemic toxicity and equal efficacy relative to four intravenous injections of unmodified drug (Ruel-Gariepy *et al.* 2004).

5.4 *In situ* crosslinking or polymerizing materials

The formation of covalent crosslinks between injectable precursor materials is a mechanism for creating solid gels after injection. These materials can crosslink or polymerize at the injection site due to various stimuli including temperature and light. Depending on the solubility of the precursors, the precursors may be injected as an aqueous solution or as an emulsion. Crosslinking generally provides increased material strength compared to physical gels, whereas polymerization after injection may be desirable if the polymer itself cannot be injected by other means. The precursors are either monomers or macromers. Monomers are small molecules which can be bonded together in long chains to form polymers. Macromers are polymers themselves which have functional groups capable of further polymerization. For example, poly(ethylene glycol) diacrylate (PEGDA) is a simple hydrophilic macromer that has unsaturated double bonds which allow for free radical or step-growth polymerization *in situ*. Macromers can be designed to control the properties of the final gel such as swelling or degradability.

In thermally activated reactions, an initiator gives rise to free radicals which react with functional groups to cause the polymerization or crosslinking reaction. The timing of the reaction must be controlled because many of the precursor materials are cytotoxic. The initiators can also be cytotoxic, particularly at high concentrations. In light activated reactions, a photoinitiator is included with the precursor materials. At the desired site, fiber-optic cables are used to create free radicals from the photoinitiator, leading to polymer formation in the desired location. Drug delivery from these systems depends on a number of factors including the photoinitiator, light intensity, and wavelength of light used. Other gelation mechanisms used for drug delivery include step-growth polymerization, ionic interactions, and biologically inspired complex formation (Salem *et al.* 2003; Sanborn *et al.* 2002). In general, the rate of drug release from *in situ* crosslinking or polymerizing materials can be controlled by a number of factors, including gelation kinetics, polymer concentration, hydrophobicity, porosity, crosslink density, and degradation rate.

5.4.1 Thermally activated systems

As an alternative strategy to solvent exchange, thermally activated crosslinking reactions were investigated by Moore *et al.* for enabling the injectability of degradable polyesters (Moore *et al.* 1995). A liquid macromer of PCL with acrylic ester groups was synthesized by reaction of polycaprolactone triol with acryloyl chloride, then mixed with drug and initiator in coupled syringes and injected subcutaneously. Initiators for this system were benzoyl peroxide or *N,N*-dimethyl-*p*-toluidine which caused formation of a crosslinked PCL gel through polymerization of the vinyl groups on each macromer. Systems loaded with flurbiprofen exhibited a burst release of about 20% within the first hour, followed by controlled release for the next seven days.

Several concerns have arisen for thermally activated systems in drug delivery applications. Burst release occurs in the time between injection and full curing of the liquid precursor materials (Hatefi and Amsden 2002). The use of free radical initiators may be undesirable for several reasons. Some of these reactions, such as in clinically used poly(methyl methacrylate) bone cement, can generate a substantial amount of heat, leading to tissue necrosis (Biehl *et al.* 1974; Sund and Rosenquist 1983). Peroxide radicals may play a role in promoting the growth of tumors (Gimenez-Conti *et al.* 1998; Slaga 1981). Another class of initiators for polymerization in aqueous media is redox initiators such as ammonium persulfate, but a tradeoff exists between the drug delivery requirements of fast gelation time and low initiator cytotoxicity (Temenoff *et al.* 2003). These factors may be controlled, though not independently, by the choice and concentration of initiator used.

5.4.2 Photoactivated systems

Photopolymerization has some select advantages over thermally activated polymerization, providing rapid polymerization rates at physiological temperatures and greater control over the shape and location of the polymer. While *in situ* forming photopolymerized gels have been mostly applied to other areas including preformed drug delivery matrices, some applications in injectable drug delivery have been investigated as well. Hubbell used degradable macromers of oligo(lactate)-PEG-oligo(lactate) diacrylate, with 2,2-dimethoxy-2-phenylacetophenone as the photoinitiator (Hubbell 1996). Several proteins with varying molecular weight were released *in vitro* from this system at a steady rate over a period of days, with higher molecular weight leading to slower release via diffusion of the protein through the gel. Above a given molecular weight threshold, protein would not release by diffusion until the gel was hydrolyzed. Another system based on PEG-oligoglycolyl-acrylate macromers with eosin as a photoinitiator was demonstrated for controlled release of water-soluble drugs and enzymes due to either visible or UV light sources (Hubbell *et al.* 2005). The light source can have a substantial effect on the properties of a photopolymerizable gel. For example, argon laser light sources improve the depth and extent of polymerization while decreasing the polymerization time. However, these polymers also exhibit higher syneresis, so the burst release from such a material may not be improved (Fleming and Maillet 1999). Recently, Sharifi *et al.* demonstrated a photopolymerizable crosslinked gel of PCL-fumarate with N-vinyl-2-pyrrolidone (NVP) as a crosslinking agent (Sharifi *et al.* 2009). NVP content was shown to reduce the swelling of the photocrosslinked gels below a critical level, at which point the NVP remained unreacted. Release of the anti-cancer agent tamoxifen citrate occurred over four days, but showed only mild cytotoxicity to reduce the viability MCF-7 breast cancer cells *in vitro*.

5.4.3 *In situ* crosslinking systems

In situ crosslinking chemistries are desirable for biomedical applications because they do not require an initiator or external activation source. The most common of these are described in a review by Hoare and Kohane: (a) reaction of an aldehyde with an amine to form a Schiff base, (b) reaction of an aldehyde with a hydrazide to form a hydrazone, (c) Michael-type addition of an acrylate and either a primary amide to form a secondary amine or a thiol to form a sulfide (Hoare and Kohane 2008). The gelation time depends on the types of precursor materials, pH, and other considerations, but is typically on the order of a few minutes (Hiemstra *et al.* 2007; Elbert *et al.* 2001; Shu *et al.* 2006; Bulpitt and Aeschlimann 1999). Hydrazone formation from an aldehyde and a hydrazide has been demonstrated for crosslinking of hyaluronic acid for controlled protein release (Ito *et al.* 2007a). Similar chemistry has been employed for other modified natural materials as well as synthetic materials (Ito *et al.* 2007b; Ossipov *et al.* 2007).

Michael-type addition is desirable for a range of injectable applications because of the minimal cytotoxicity of the precursor materials (Hoare and Kohane 2008; Vernon *et al.* 2003). Thiolated heparin and hyaluronic acid conjugated to PEG diacrylate forms a hydrogel was shown to prolong the release of fibroblast growth factor *in vivo* (Cai *et al.* 2005). To aid in the design of these systems, mathematical models have been developed for the gelation, degradation, and release kinetics of model proteins (either dissolved or covalently bound) from various PEG-based hydrogels formed by Michael-type addition (DuBose *et al.* 2005; Metters and Hubbell 2005).

In situ crosslinking has also been investigated for improving the stability of injectable gels formed by other gelation mechanisms (Robb *et al.* 2007). An example of a drug delivery application of this is the crosslinking of a poly(propylene fumarate) gel which forms by solvent exchange precipitation from NMP (Ueda *et al.* 2007). Because this system was administered into the eye, unsaturated double bonds on the chains on the polymer could crosslink either thermally or photochemically. Crosslinked gels provided *in vitro* release of fluocinolone acetonide for up to 400 days, with elevated release for 10 days after gelation. The approximately steady release thereafter was attributed to counterbalancing effects of hydrogel degradation and drug diffusion. Crosslinking of the gel was shown to increase the time with a clinically relevant release rate by approximately 140 days relative to uncrosslinked gels.

5.5 Microparticles and nanoparticles

Injecting a drug into the bloodstream is often a desirable route of administration because it avoids first-pass clearance – metabolism of a drug during its 'first pass' from the digestive system through the liver before entering the rest of the circulation. However, parenteral (non-oral) drug administration is not always sufficient in delivering a dose of drug to the desired site of action. Injected drugs can become unstable and break down or be metabolized in the circulation. They may end up being distributed randomly throughout the body or quickly cleared from the body by the kidneys. Further, many hydrophobic drugs, including cancer drugs, have limited water solubility and would require a very large volume of water to get the drug into the circulation.

Particulate drug delivery systems have the ability to address each of the above challenges to successful drug delivery following parenteral administration. They form a carrier to protect and stabilize a drug after injection. Additionally, they can provide a high-payload carrier for either hydrophobic or hydrophilic drugs, depending on their composition. Size and degradability of the carrier can also be controlled to achieve a long treatment duration while minimizing burst release. Targeting of the particles by active and passive mechanisms can improve the delivery efficiency while minimizing side effects.

Particulate carriers are often investigated for drug delivery to solid tumors because their size allows for passive targeting by the enhanced permeability and retention (EPR) effect. The high metabolic demand of tumors requires the formation of newly formed vasculature, which is unorganized relative to normal vasculature. Pores with sizes ranging from 10 to 1000 nm can be found, which enable nanoscale carriers to accumulate in the tumor tissue. Additionally, the lymphatic drainage of tumors is poor (Gaucher *et al.* 2005). To achieve effective passive tumor targeting, the plasma concentration of the drug carrier must be sustained for a significant period of time, preferably over six hours (Greish *et al.* 2003). For polymer-drug conjugates, the EPR effect can lead to drug concentrations as much as 10-fold higher in the tumor tissue than in the plasma (Pasut and Veronese 2007).

5.5.1 Nomenclature and synthesis

A common type of particulate delivery system is based on biodegradable polymers such as PLGA. Depending on the size, they are called microparticles (1–500 μm) or nanoparticles (10–300 nm). Microparticles have poorer uptake by individual cells than nanoparticles, so most applications of microparticles involve injection at the site of action, while nanoparticles are often injected intravenously (Desai *et al.* 1996). Nanoparticles are substantially smaller than a cell, which allows them to cross the epithelial lining and be taken up by cells (Vinogradov *et al.* 2002). Because nanoparticles interact with their environment on a length scale where specific physical and chemical interactions are involved, nanoparticles may have other substantially different properties, including toxicity, than microparticles with identical composition (Nel *et al.* 2006). More specific nomenclature applies based on the structure of the particle. Microspheres or nanospheres consist of a solid hydrophobic polymer matrix in which the hydrophobic drug is uniformly distributed. On the other hand, microcapsules or nanocapsules have a polymer capsule surrounding a cavity filled with aqueous drug solution.

Several methods have been demonstrated for the synthesis of microparticles and nanoparticles. The most popular among these is the solvent evaporation method. To prepare spheres, the polymer and drug are dissolved in a water-immiscible, volatile organic solvent such as dichloromethane, ethyl acetate, or chloroform. The solution is then added to an aqueous solution and emulsified, leading to an oil-in-water emulsion. Homogenization or sonication is used to reduce the particle size, and a surfactant is used to prevent aggregation. The solvent is then allowed to evaporate, and drug-loaded spheres are obtained. Capsule synthesis is similar, but it requires two emulsifying steps – a so-called double emulsion. Aqueous drug solution is emulsified in a solution of polymer in organic solvent, and then the product is emulsified again in water, leading to precipitation of the capsule's polymer shell and entrapping the aqueous drug solution. A large number of factors affect the final product of the solvent evaporation method. While a further description of nanoparticle synthesis methods exceeds the scope of this text, interested readers are encouraged to read a review by Soppimath which describes many of the other synthesis methods used (Soppimath *et al.* 2001).

Drugs can be incorporated into particulate systems either by incorporation of the drug during production or by incubating the particles in a drug solution. While incubation may be easier, lower drug loading is achieved, and accordingly more drug is wasted (Alonso *et al.* 1991; Ueda *et al.* 1998). For the adsorption method, the drug binding is dependent on the drug structure as well as the choice of polymer (Couvreur *et al.* 1979). For the direct incorporation method, Radwan found that an increase in monomer concentration increased the fraction of drug loaded into the particles and also decreased the normalized release rate of theophylline from the particles (Radwan 1995).

A wide variety of polymers have been used in nanoparticle drug delivery systems. Natural polymers such as albumin, gelatin, alginate, collagen, and chitosan typically offer a relatively short duration of drug release (Panyam and Labhasetwar 2003a). Synthetic polymers, such as PLGA and PCL offer greater flexibility in terms of drug release due to their tunable degradability. Because the degradation products lactic and glycolic acid are formed at a slow rate and removed from the body, PLA and PLGA nanoparticles have excellent biocompatibility and have been the most commonly investigated formulation for particulate drug delivery systems (Jain 2000). An important consideration for the application of long-circulating particulate systems *in vivo* is avoiding uptake by the reticuloendothelial system (RES) (Soppimath *et al.* 2001). RES uptake reduces the availability of the drug in the circulation and can potentially be toxic to the RES itself. To this end, strategies for reducing protein adsorption have been developed. Surfaces of nanoparticles coated in hydrophilic polymers such as PEG or surfactants such as poloxamine have been demonstrated for reducing protein adsorption (Peracchia *et al.* 1999; De Jaeghere *et al.* 1999; Illum and Davis 1983; 1984; Moghimi and Gray 1997).

5.5.2 Protein delivery

Drug release from PLGA particles occurs by diffusion of the drug through the polymer and by material degradation (Anderson and Shive 1997). Degradation rate is adjustable by copolymer composition and molecular weight. For example, 50/50 PLGA copolymer microspheres degrade more quickly (and release drug more quickly) than similar PLLA microspheres (Lin *et al.* 2000). Lupron® depot, a suspension of porous PLGA or PLA microspheres containing the luteinizing hormone-releasing hormone agonist leuprolide acetate for the treatment of endometriosis, was one of the first FDA approved injectable drug delivery devices (Okada 1997). Different comonomer ratios allow for either 1-month or 3-month formulations which maintain a steady concentration of drug in the circulation, providing prolonged suppression of hormone levels.

Water-soluble therapeutic proteins and peptides can be delivered using porous nanospheres or nanocapsules formed by a double emulsion solvent evaporation procedure. A concern with the delivery of proteins by nanoparticles is the loss of protein activity before its release. Desai *et al.* showed about 30% of tetanus toxoid activity was lost due after encapsulation and release from nanoparticles (Desai *et al.* 1996). Protein may be inactivated due to denaturation based on exposure to organic solvents and adsorption onto the oil-water interface during fabrication (van de Weert *et al.* 2000; Lu *et al.* 2000). A strategy for reducing adsorption of the therapeutic protein is the incorporation of human or bovine serum albumin in the aqueous phase, which restricts the access of the therapeutic protein to the phase interface (Kim and Park 1999). Another proposed cause of protein inactivation is decreased local pH experienced by the encapsulated protein due to acidic degradation byproducts. This can be addressed by including an alkaline buffer into the aqueous phase (Zhu *et al.* 2000).

5.5.3 Intracellular targeting of nanoparticles

For gene delivery as well as avoidance of multi-drug resistance proteins (MRPs) or membrane bound p-glycoprotein in tumor cells, it may be important to target specific compartments or organelles within cells (Tachibana *et al.* 1998; de Verdiere *et al.* 1997; Bart *et al.* 2000). Nanoparticles can be taken up by cells by various processes including fluid-phase pinocytosis, phagocytosis, or receptor-mediated endocytosis (Foster *et al.* 2001; Suh *et al.* 1998). Following uptake, nanoparticles enter the endo-lysosome, where the pH is acidic (Panyam and Labhasetwar 2003b). A fraction of the internalized nanoparticles are transported to the cytoplasm where they can provide sustained release. In experiments on vascular smooth muscle cells, intracellular nanoparticle amounts are maintained when the extracellular concentration is maintained, but after extracellular nanoparticles are removed, the intracellular amount in reduces by about 65% in 30 minutes (Panyam and Labhasetwar 2003a). One factor responsible for accelerating exocytosis is the amount of protein adsorption onto the nanoparticles (Panyam and Labhasetwar 2003b; Tomoda *et al.* 1989). Delivery and specific targeting to cells and organelles based on antigen recognition, receptor-ligand complexation, and other stimuli is currently a topic of substantial investigation on all forms of particulate drug delivery systems including nanoparticles.

Degradable nanoparticles have been demonstrated for gene delivery based on their ability to protect nucleic acids from lysosomal degradation (Hedley *et al.* 1998). One early study by Labhasetwar *et al.* used two marker genes in PLGA nanoparticles to induce gene expression *in vitro* in media with serum (Labhasetwar *et al.* 1999). They then demonstrated a similar result in a bone defect model, suggesting that a gene delivery strategy based on these particles could facilitate bone healing. However, this approach and others have the potential disadvantage of poor shelf life and variability in the final product, because the particles have to be used within a short time after fabrication or they can degrade. Another study showing sustained gene expression was performed by Cohen *et al.* (2000). Interestingly, polymeric nanoparticles showed poorer transfection *in vitro* but one to two orders of magnitude greater transfection *in vivo*. An explanation of this result is that there may be a large difference in efficacy between results *in vitro* and *in vivo* for some drug delivery systems due to biocompatibility and tissue toxicity issues, which are minimal in PLGA-based systems as compared to viruses or liposomes (Cohen *et al.* 2000).

5.5.4 Active targeting of nanoparticles

Farokhzad *et al.* developed aptamer-functionalized PLGA-PEG nanoparticles carrying docetaxel for preferential delivery to prostate cancer cells compared to non-functionalized nanoparticles and reduced toxicity compared to free drug (Farokhzad *et al.* 2006). Another example of an active targeting mechanism by degradable polymeric nanoparticles is based on the serum glycoprotein transferrin, which delivers iron from the circulation into cells through receptor binding and receptor-mediated endocytosis (Qian and Tang 1995). Receptor-mediated endocytosis of nanoparticles is desirable because it may avoid the p-glycoprotein-mediated drug resistance pathway by sequestration in endosomes (Wong *et al.* 2006). Also, transferrin has been investigated for targeting toward cancer cells because of the overexpression of the transferrin receptor in tumor tissues relative to healthy tissues (Qian *et al.* 2002). Sahoo and Labhasetwar used PLGA nanoparticles conjugated with transferrin to improve the duration of the anti-proliferative effect of paclitaxel *in vitro* (Sahoo and Labhasetwar 2005). They attributed the improved effect to a greater intracellular retention of the nanoparticles relative to retention of unconjugated nanoparticles.

The half-life of systemically injected particulate drug delivery systems (including but not limited to polymeric nanoparticles) within the circulation is an important consideration. Some of the factors that affect half-life include polymer composition, particle size, and surface modifications (Alexis *et al.* 2008). Targeting ligands can further influence the accumulation of the drug carrier in specific tissues. For further discussion on targeting mechanisms for degradable microspheres and nanospheres, see a recent review by Mohamed and van der Walle (2008).

5.5.5 Gold nanoparticles

Other than PLGA-based degradable nanoparticles, there are some other materials used in particulate systems used in drug delivery applications. Gold nanoparticles are interesting for drug delivery applications due to their resistance to oxidation and responsiveness to light via plasmon resonance, leading to heating of the particles (Pissuwan *et al.* 2006). Both gold nanospheres and nanorods have tunable resonance wavelengths over the near-infrared range, which is useful because the body is reasonably transparent to near-infrared light (Loo *et al.* 2004; Sershen *et al.* 2000; O'Neal *et al.* 2004). An example this approach in drug delivery is the use of gold nanoshells coated with crosslinked temperature responsive poly(NIPAAm-co-acrylic acid) (Sershen *et al.* 2000). When exposed to near-infrared irradiation, the gold nanoparticles lead to thermally induced shrinking of the polymer coating, expelling drug at an increased rate. Natural materials such as chitosan have also been investigated, mostly due to the benefit of biocompatibility and flexibility in delivery properties due to adjustable crosslink density. Many applications of chitosan microparticles relate to oral and mucosal routes of administration rather than injection due to chitosan's mucoadhesive properties and degradability only under certain conditions (Agnihotri *et al.* 2004; Lorenzo-Lamosa *et al.* 1998; Berscht *et al.* 1993). Some injectable applications have been investigated in drug and gene delivery, which is aided by formation of polyelectrolyte complexes between chitosan and DNA (Mao *et al.* 2001; Janes *et al.* 2001; Chew *et al.* 2003).

5.6 Micelles and liposomes

Self-assembling nanoscale particles have been investigated for drug delivery due to many of the same advantages as polymeric nanoparticles, including prolonged treatment duration, increased payload of hydrophobic drugs, protection from unwanted metabolism, and potential for either active or passive targeting.

5.6.1 Introduction to micelles

Micelles are formed at sufficiently high concentrations of amphiphilic or oppositely charged block copolymers. Diblock copolymers are most commonly used, but triblock copolymers and dendrimers have also been investigated. While the chemistry used for designing micelles for drug delivery is rather flexible, PEG is often used as the hydrophilic block. The minimum polymer concentration required to form micelles is called the critical micelle concentration (CMC) or critical association concentration (CAC). Above the CMC, the hydrophobic polymer segments spontaneously aggregate, forming the core of the micelles, with the hydrophilic segments forming the outer corona. Their extremely small size (10–100 nm) is desirable for avoiding uptake by the reticuloendothelial system. Micelles are used to deliver hydrophobic drugs, which are held in the core of the micelle until dissociation. However, because dissociation is concentration dependent, a major concern remains the instability of micelles upon injection into the circulation. If the local concentration falls below the CMC, drug will be released – when this happens upon injection, dose dumping occurs. Due to this concern, most of the investigation on using micelles for drug delivery applications has been pursued with the goal of increasing stability of the micelles upon injection, i.e. lowering the CMC, as well as prolonging drug retention within the micelles.

Drug is loaded into micelles by either direct dissolution or solvent removal (Allen *et al.* 1999). In direct dissolution, the copolymer and drug are dissolved in aqueous solvent. The hydrophobic drug preferentially is loaded into the hydrophobic core of the resulting micelles. Sometimes heat must be added in order to induce micellization. Solvent-removal procedures involve making a solution of copolymer and drug in an organic solvent. If the solvent is water miscible, the solvent can be exchanged by dialysis against water, causing formation of drug-loaded micelles. Alternatively, non-water miscible solvents can be used to create an oil-in-water emulsion, where micellization occurs as the hydrophobic segments enter the oil phase. Evaporation and lyophilization of some solvents have also been used for preparation of drug-loaded micelles by simply resuspending the dry copolymer-drug mixture in aqueous solution (Lavasanifar *et al.* 2002). The drug loading and composition of the final product depend on the method of preparation and depend on a number of factors which must be determined experimentally (Sant *et al.* 2004; Vangeyte *et al.* 2004).

5.6.2 Factors affecting stability

Several material design factors affect the stability of drug-loaded micelles in the circulation. In general, the rate of drug release by micellar dissociation depends on the properties of the micellar core. Longer core-forming segments tend to result in a lower CMC and reduced drug release *in vitro* (Jette *et al.* 2004; Kang and Leroux 2004). Likewise, increased hydrophobicity of the core-forming segment leads to a lower CMC and reduced drug release rate (Adams and Kwon 2003; Adams *et al.* 2003; Opanasopit *et al.* 2004). For example, Opanasopit *et al.* used diblock copolymers of PEG-poly(L-aspartate) which were modified with varying content of benzyl ester side groups in the poly(L-aspartate) block

(Opanasopit *et al.* 2004). They found that increasing benzyl ester on the polymer led to increased micelle stability and controlled release of camptothecin. Micellar stability can be improved by hydrophobic segment with a glass-transition temperature over 37°C, so that the molecular motion within the core is restricted (Allen *et al.* 1999; Yamamoto *et al.* 2002; Burt *et al.* 1999). Use of core forming micelles which form stereocomplexes (such as PEG-PDLA with PEG-PLLA) can increase the melting point and crystallinity of the core relative to either polymer independently (Slager and Domb 2003). Chemical cross-linking has also been demonstrated for decreasing or eliminating the CMC altogether (Thurmond II *et al.* 1999; Shuai *et al.* 2004; Bontha *et al.* 2006).

Interactions between the core-forming segment and the drug affect micelle stability as well. Lee *et al.* functionalized the hydrophobic block of PEG-*b*-PDLLA copolymers with carboxylic acid to obtain improved drug loading and slower release (days rather than hours) attributed to hydrogen bonding between the drug and polymer (J. Y. Lee *et al.* 2004). Drug release can also be slowed by covalent conjugation of the drug to the core-forming segment (Li and Kwon 2000).

Despite typically including PEG as a hydrophilic block for the reduction of protein adsorption, the stability of block copolymer micelles can be affected by proteins, even under well-controlled *in vitro* conditions. Toncheva *et al.* found that the stability of PEG-*b*-poly(ortho ester)-*b*-PEG micelles in presence of bovine serum albumin depended most on the length of the PEG blocks (Toncheva *et al.* 2003). A study by Liu *et al.* found that bovine serum albumin did not affect the stability of PEG-*b*-poly(5-benzyloxytrimethylene carbonate) micelles, but the drug release was accelerated in the presence of protein (Liu *et al.* 2005).

With few exceptions, poor half-life in the circulation has been a problem for micellar drug delivery vehicles. Burt *et al.* reported rapid release of paclitaxel from PEG-*b*-PDLLA micelles within minutes of administration, and the polymer was found to quickly accumulate in the kidney (Burt *et al.* 1999). This is insufficient for passive tumor targeting, which requires a drug delivery vehicle to be in the circulation for at least six hours (Greish *et al.* 2003). One approach for improving the circulation time towards the levels observed *in vitro* besides increasing the PEG block size is to functionalize the end of the PEG chains with negative surface charges. Using this approach, Yamamoto *et al.* functionalized PEG-*b*-PDLLA micelles with an anionic peptide (Yamamoto *et al.* 2001). Despite a rapid clearance of 50% of the micelles, about 25% remained in the circulation 24 hours post-injection. Another concern is that hydrophobic compounds may reduce the rate at which micelles are internalized by cells (Maysinger *et al.* 2001).

5.6.3 Selected applications of micelles

Some pH-responsive micelle formulations have been developed. A simple example is a triblock copolymer of PEG-*b*-PDMAEMA-*b*-PDEAEMA which forms micelles at neutral pH (7.1–7.3), dissociating and delivering dipyridamole at pH 3 (Tang *et al.* 2003). However, this is significantly less than most pH differences of relevance to drug delivery, including the acidic environment of tumor tissue (E. S. Lee *et al.* 2003). Bae *et al.* reported the use of an pH-sensitive hydrazone linker between the polymer and drug for increasing drug release after cellular uptake in response to the low pH environment of the endosome and lysosome (Y. Bae *et al.* 2005). Other micelles responding to pH have shown promising results for increasing the bioavailability of drugs delivered orally (Jones *et al.* 2003; Sant *et al.* 2005).

Over the last five years, some micellar drug delivery formulations have entered clinical trials in Japan, Korea, and the United States (Matsumura *et al.* 2004; D. W. Kim *et al.* 2007; K. S. Lee *et al.* 2007; Davis *et al.* 2008). A biodegradable methoxy-PEG-*b*-PDLLA micelle formulation for the delivery of paclitaxel branded under the name Genexol®-PM is approved in South Korea. As of April 2010, it is currently being investigated in three clinical trials, including two Phase III trials, in the United States for various types of cancers. Genexol®-PM shows significantly greater antitumor activity and reduced toxicity in mice compared to the currently available Taxol®, which is a solution of paclitaxel in Cremophor EL and ethanol (S. C. Kim *et al.* 2001). Other formulations using PEG-*b*-poly(aspartate) for delivery of doxorubicin have also been investigated in clinical trials (Matsumura *et al.* 2004; Hamaguchi *et al.* 2005; 2007). Despite their poor stability relative to other particulate systems, these formulations are promising for their ease of preparation, adequate stability in the circulation, and ability to sequester hydrophobic drugs.

5.6.4 Introduction to liposomes

Liposomes are nanoscale capsules with phospholipid bilayer shells, similar to a cell membrane. Phospholipids have a hydrophilic head and hydrophobic tail region, so the corresponding liposomes have both a hydrophilic cavity and a hydrophobic region inside the shell in which low molecular weight or macromolecular drugs can be placed (Lee and Yuk 2007). Based on the synthesis process, the structure can be adjusted to either make small unilamellar vesicles (100 nm), large unilamellar vesicles (200–800 nm), or large multi-lamellar vesicles (500 nm–5 μm, which contain several concentric bilayers). Another unique advantage of liposomes is that they have the potential to deliver drugs efficiently into cells by fusing with cell membranes. Uptake by the reticuloendothelial system is a concern for drug delivery due to the larger size of liposomes relative to micelles. Also, liposome chemistry (thickness of the shell, degradability) is rather inflexible since the composition is limited to phospholipids. The gold standard for avoiding unwanted uptake is coating with PEG, which forms a water shell around the liposome, limiting adhesion and recognition by opsonins (Klibanov *et al.* 1990). Several liposomal formulations of drugs are currently available or in clinical trials, and many other formulations are being researched, many of which incorporate surface moieties involved in targeting or stimulus responsiveness. While the intravenous route of administration is most common, liposomes have also been investigated for drug delivery via the lungs, mouth, and skin (Torchilin 2005).

Liposomes are prepared by dissolving phospholipids and lipid-soluble drugs (if desired) in an organic solvent, followed by evaporation or freeze drying of the solvent, leaving behind a series of lipid films, or lipid cake. As the lipids are rehydrated under agitation in aqueous solution (containing water-soluble drug if desired), the lipids self-close, forming liposomes (Szoka Jr. and Papahadjopoulos 1978). Some common phospholipids used to make liposomes include *N*-glutarylphosphatidylethanolamine (NGPE), phosphatidylethanolamine (PE), and phosphatidylcholines (Torchilin 2005).

5.6.5 Intracellular targeting of liposomes

The metabolism of liposomes at the cellular level also makes them desirable drug delivery vehicles. A liposome can either adsorb onto the cell membrane or fuse with the cell membrane, releasing its contents into the cytoplasm. Alternatively, liposomes can undergo endocytosis and be delivered to the lysosome for degradation or can itself destabilize the endosome, both of which trigger drug release within the cell. For example, pH-responsive liposomes can be made to destabilize in the endosome, releasing a hydrophobic drug contained within the lipid bilayer (Torchilin 2005). Liposomes can also be modified with viral components such as the *trans*-activating transcriptional activator (TAT) protein from HIV-1 in order to achieve efficient intracellular delivery through specific interactions with cells (Torchilin, Rammohan *et al.* 2001).

5.6.6 Long-circulating liposomes

Liposomal formulations with PEG-grafted surfaces have already been approved for some clinical applications and are considered a standard starting point for long-circulating liposome design (Torchilin 2005). Some other hydrophilic polymers investigated for resistance of protein adhesion include poly(*N*-(2-hydroxypropyl)methacrylamide), degradable peptide-based polymer-lipid conjugates, and poly(*N*-vinyl pyrrolidones) (Whiteman *et al.* 2001; Torchilin, Levchenko *et al.* 2001; Metselaar *et al.* 2003). However, the specificity of these vehicles is based solely on the EPR effect. Most of the research on liposomal drug delivery systems over the last 10 years has been directed at improving drug targeting toward cancer cells using liposomes with various targeting ligands or stimulus responsive groups in addition to long-circulating behavior. For example, Immunoglobulin G (IgG) family proteins have been investigated widely for this purpose because they can be incorporated into liposomes either through covalent or physical interactions (Torchilin 1985). However, without also including a polymer for long-circulating properties such as PEG, most of the so-called immunoliposomes will accumulate in the liver by RES uptake before effective targeting is achieved (Torchilin 2005).

5.6.7 Delivery of low molecular weight drugs

Several liposomal drug formulations are already approved and many more are under investigation, mostly for the treatment of various cancers (Gabizon 2003). DaunoXome, an approved liposomal formulation of daunorubicin, has been shown to provide a sustained concentration of drug within tumors over days due to passive targeting (Forssen *et al.* 1996). In a pharmacokinetic study comparing skin and tumor tissue, drug accumulated preferentially in tumor tissue when delivered in a liposomal formulation but not when delivered as drug alone. Amphotericin B is approved for delivery using the liposomal formulation AmBisome for the treatment or prophylaxis of fungal infections, leading to reduced toxicity and an elevated peak plasma concentration (Tollemar *et al.* 1993; Ringden *et al.* 1991; Adler-Moore 1994). The first approved PEGylated liposomal formulation of a drug to receive FDA approval was Doxil (liposomal doxorubicin). The half-life of Doxil in the circulation is on the order of 2–3 days, compared to 5 minutes for free drug (Gabizon 2003). However, despite increased uptake by tumor cells, cutaneous and mucosal toxicity remains a problem (Lorusso *et al.* 2007; Lotem *et al.* 2000; Gordon *et al.* 1995; Ellerhorst *et al.* 1999).

Newer developments in cancer treatment reported in the literature involve the use of specific ligands or reactive groups to induce uptake by specific cells or in specific regions throughout the body. For a review of the bioconjugate chemistry schemes used for liposomal modification, please see a review by Torchilin (2005). A variety of antibodies have been conjugated to liposomes for improved uptake by cancer cells. For example, Lukyanov *et al.* synthesized a modified version of Doxil conjugated with nucleosome-specific antibodies, which are capable of binding to nucleosomes on the surface of tumor cells (Lukyanov *et al.* 2004). They demonstrated increased cytotoxicity towards tumor cells relative to unmodified Doxil. Another common targeting mechanism is conjugation of folate to liposomes, due to the overexpression of folate receptors on cancer cells (Sudimack and Lee 2000). Significantly increased cytotoxicity has been reported for liposomal formulations of both daunorubicin and doxorubicin toward cancer cells (Ni *et al.* 2002; Pan *et al.* 2003). Pan *et al.* used an *in vivo* mouse model which shows increased tumor inhibition compared to both liposomes without folate and free drug. Transferrin receptor is also upregulated in a variety of cancers and has been investigated as a target using transferrin-conjugated liposomal drugs (Hatakeyama *et al.* 2004; Ishida *et al.* 2001). Liposomes have also been developed to be responsive to a number of other biological stimuli, including pH (promoting intracellular release from the endosome, for example) and enzyme action (Simoes *et al.* 2004; Davidsen *et al.* 2001; Pak *et al.* 1998). Externally applied stimuli such as magnetic field and light are particularly interesting because they enable differential release in a chosen location (Liburdy *et al.* 1986; Paasonen *et al.* 2007; Troutman *et al.* 2009).

5.6.8 Protein and gene delivery

Beyond applications in delivering low molecular weight compounds, liposomes have hydrophilic core suitable for delivery of therapeutic proteins. Gaspar *et al.* used liposomes for encapsulation of L-asparaginase which breaks down L-asparagine, an amino acid required for tumor proliferation (Gaspar *et al.* 1996). They reported reduced toxicity, reduced anaphylactic reaction and increased survival time in a xenograft tumor model relative to free enzyme. Heeremans *et al.* demonstrated a liposomal formulation of tissue-type plasminogen activator for increased thrombolytic activity in a rabbit jugular vein thrombosis model (Heeremans *et al.* 1995). Insulin has also been delivered from long-circulating liposomal formulations. In a rat diabetic model, liposomal formulations both with and without PEG were shown to suppress glucose levels for about 24 hours (Kim *et al.* 1999).

Liposomes with positively charged surfaces also can provide an alternative vector to viruses for gene delivery. For example, cationic liposomes have been developed for complexation with DNA with high loading and efficient transfection (Lasic *et al.* 1999; Matsuura *et al.* 2003). Transferrin-conjugated cationic liposomes have been investigated in a xenograft model for targeted delivery of wild type p53, a gene that often mutates in radiation-resistant cancer cells (Xu *et al.* 1999). When administered in combination with radiation, the transferrin-conjugated cationic liposomes suppressed tumor growth successfully whereas other formulations did not.

5.7 Polymer-drug conjugates

Chemical conjugation of therapeutics including low molecular weight drugs, peptides, proteins, or nucleic acids with polymers is used for injectable drug delivery applications due to several advantages. Like other injectable carriers, polymer conjugation can improve the water solubility of hydrophobic drugs while protecting the drug from unwanted or uncontrolled metabolism. Polymer-drug conjugates (particularly those using PEG) can also provide reduced immune response through steric hindrance – antibiotics, enzymes, and cells are blocked from accessing the drug by the polymer. The half-life of the drug in the circulation is additionally increased due to increased hydrodynamic radius (which slows clearance through the kidney). Depending on the activity of the conjugate, it is either an active drug itself or a prodrug (i.e. inactive precursor).

A prodrug is then converted into active drug at the site of action. As with other systems injectable into the circulation, they can be used for either passive or active targeting of particular tissues.

5.7.1 Design considerations

Drugs suitable for polymer conjugation typically have poor water solubility, instability in the body, high toxicity, and poor internalization by target cells. Correspondingly, ideal polymers for these systems should be degradable or low enough molecular weight (<50 kDa) to be safely cleared from the body, as monodisperse as possible, have a long half-life in the circulation, and the proper number of functional groups, depending on the application (Pasut and Veronese 2007). For example, polymers for protein conjugation should have one functional group to avoid crosslinking, while many functional groups for small molecular weight drug conjugation may improve the drug loading efficiency. While no polymer satisfies all of the above criteria, the most commonly investigated polymers for drug conjugation are PEG, polyglutamic acid, and *N*-(2-hydroxypropyl) methacrylamide (HPMA) copolymers. HPMA is a hydrophilic, biocompatible polymer which was chosen as a candidate soluble polymeric drug carrier as early as 1973 in work done by Kopecek and colleagues (Kopecek and Bazilova 1973; Bohdanecky *et al.* 1974). HPMA emerged as a candidate due to its hydrolytic stability, ease of synthesis, availability for copolymerization with degradable oligopeptides which could be used as drug attachment sites (Kopecek *et al.* 2000). Drugs can be conjugated to HPMA either by aminolysis of reactive polymer precursors or by copolymerization of HPMA monomer with polymerizable drug derivatives (Chytry *et al.* 1977; Solovsky *et al.* 1983; Obereigner *et al.* 1979). In order to synthesize a conjugate, both the polymer and drug need to have reactive chemical groups, such as carboxylic acids, primary amines, thiols, or alcohols (Khandare and Minko 2006). The presence of multiple identical reactive groups can make conjugation more complicated, requiring protection and deprotection during synthesis.

There are many other considerations for both conjugate features and the *in vivo* behavior of the conjugate which are more thoroughly reviewed elsewhere (Pasut and Veronese 2007). Two of the most important features are worth mentioning here – activity and linker stability. The efficient development of polymer-drug conjugates based on structure-activity relationships is an active area of research. Depending on the attachment location, the attached polymer may substantially affect the drug's function. This may be desirable for avoiding side effects. However, it is important for the drug to become active once at the site of action. In order to achieve this, degradable bonds or spacers joining the polymer and drug are often used. While it is possible to design spacers to be water-degradable (esters, anhydrides) or enzyme-degradable (peptide spacers specific to a given enzyme), the release rate can be difficult to tightly control and was too fast in early clinical trials, causing toxicity comparable to free drug (Meerum Terwogt *et al.* 2001; Schoemaker *et al.* 2002). The incorporation of a linker which releases drug at a sufficient rate is still an active area of research and represents a major challenge in the development of conjugates of low molecular weight drugs (Duncan 2009).

5.7.2 Conjugates of high molecular weight drugs

One of the most common applications of bioconjugates to date is the conjugation of PEG to therapeutic proteins, often called PEGylation. An example application is in the treatment of hepatitis C. While interferon α-2 is known to mediate the activity of chronic hepatitis C virus, it is rapidly cleared from the circulation, having a serum half-life between 4 and 16 hours (Wills 1990; Uzé *et al.* 1995). Two PEGylated versions of interferon α-2 are currently approved for use. The first, marketed under the name PEG-Intron®, is a mixture of 14 positional isomers of the protein functionalized with one 12 kDa mono-methoxyPEG chain (Wang *et al.* 2002). Each positional isomer in the blend reduces the protein activity by a different amount. The most common positional isomer in PEG-Intron (His^{34}) was shown to retain 37% of the original antiviral activity, with the overall blend retaining 28% activity. Despite the decrease in activity, PEG-Intron is effective due to its prolonged half-life in the circulation (Glue, Rouzier-Panis *et al.* 2000; Glue, Fang *et al.* 2000; Manns *et al.* 2001). An advantage of this system is that it can be administered once per week. The other approved version of PEGylated interferon-α-2 is a mixture of four positional isomers functionalized with one branched 40 kDa PEG, marketed under the name Pegasys® (Bailon *et al.* 2001). The *in vitro* activity of Pegasys® was shown to be only 7% of the original activity, likely due to increased steric hindrance caused by large branched PEG molecules, reducing the accessibility of the active site. However, the *in vivo* antitumor activity was greatly enhanced compared to free protein due to a 70-fold increase in serum half-life and a corresponding 50-fold increase in residence time in the circulation following subcutaneous injection in rats (Bailon *et al.* 2001). The results were later confirmed in humans, leading to the conjugate's approval for treatment of hepatitis C as well as investigation for other applications (Zeuzem *et al.* 2000; Motzer *et al.* 2002). Many other therapeutic proteins and enzymes have been PEGylated for improved circulation half-lives. A comprehensive review of the applications of these conjugates alone is an extensive field beyond the scope of this text, with several reviews available in the literature discussing PEGylated protein synthesis and applications (Pasut *et al.* 2004; Harris and Chess 2003; Deiters *et al.* 2004; Roberts *et al.* 2002; Chapman 2002).

The smallest drug in a currently approved conjugate is pegaptanib, an anti-VEGF aptamer (oligonucleotide strand) conjugated to 40 kDa PEG for the treatment of neovascular age-related macular degeneration which is injected intravitreously (Ng *et al.* 2006). On average, patients treated with pegaptanib for two years lost 55% of the visual acuity that similar patients lost using the standard-of-care (D'Amico *et al.* 2006; Ng and Adamis 2005). Whereas unmodified oligonucleotides have half-lives on the order of seconds to a few minutes, pegaptanib has an elimination half-life of 9.3 hours (Tucker *et al.* 1999). This allows the conjugate to have a significant anti-angiogenic effect lacking in the aptamer alone – similar studies have demonstrated this approach for other aptamers as well as other conjugated polymers (de Smidt *et al.* 1991; Griffin *et al.* 1993).

5.7.3 Conjugates of low molecular weight drugs

Conjugates of polymers to low molecular weight drugs have also been investigated and in several clinical trials since 1994, but as of yet none is in routine clinical use (Duncan and Vicent 2010). HPMA has some advantages for drug conjugation relative to PEG, including multifunctionality and formation of unimolecular micelle structures in solution which protect hydrophobic drugs within the micellar core. However, HPMA has the disadvantages of no prior regulatory approval and greater heterogeneity with respect to molecular weight and structure. The non-degradability of both HPMA and PEG remains a concern as well (Duncan and Vicent 2010). Most of the linkers are degradable intracellularly or in tumors, i.e. by acidic pH or lysosomal enzymes (Kratz *et al.* 1999; Shen and Ryser 1981; Duncan *et al.* 1983; Rejmanova *et al.* 1983). On the other hand, polyglutamic acid is itself degradable, and drug release occurs as the polymer backbone is degraded by lysosomal enzymes (Langer 2004).

Several pre-clinical and clinical studies have been performed based on conjugates of these polymers for cancer chemotherapy. An HPMA copolymer containing camptothecin underwent Phase I clinical trials for various solid cancers (Schoemaker *et al.* 2002). While the pharmacokinetics were altered significantly by conjugation to HPMA, serious bladder toxicity was observed within three days of treatment. Conjugates of paclitaxel also failed in Phase I clinical trials due to severe neurotoxicity (Meerum Terwogt *et al.* 2001). Other HPMA conjugates of anticancer drugs doxorubicin and platinates passed Phase I trials but currently have not passed Phase II (Seymour *et al.* 2009). For a thorough review of the results of several anticancer HPMA conjugates through 2009, see a review by Duncan (2009).

Development of PEG conjugates of low molecular weight anticancer drugs has also been relatively unsuccessful. Despite promising *in vitro* data demonstrating equal toxicity to Taxol®, a three times larger dose of one type of PEG-paclitaxel was shown to have less toxicity *in vivo* than a standard dose of Taxol® (Greenwald *et al.* 1996). Also, a design tradeoff exists with PEG conjugates in which a molecular weight of at least 30 kDa is required in order to prevent rapid elimination of the PEG-drug (Greenwald *et al.* 1996). As the molecular weight is increased over 30 kDa, the circulation time will increase, but renal toxicity will worsen. Another limitation is that only the end-groups of PEG are reactive, and dendrimer structures which afford improved loading may lead to a multi-step synthesis (Pasut and Veronese 2007). PEG (40 kDa)-camptothecin under the name Prothecan or Pegamotecan passed Phase I clinical trials in the treatment of several cancers (Rowinsky 2003). Despite promising Phase II results for treatment of adenocarcinoma of the stomach and gastro-esophageal junction, the conjugate is no longer being pursued (Davis *et al.* 2008; Scott *et al.* 2008).

Polyglutamic acid conjugates have been developed, and some have reached Phase III trials. In the Phase III trials of polyglutamic acid-paclitaxel (under the name Xyotax™, since changed to Opaxio™) for the treatment of non-small-cell lung cancer, no significant overall improvement in patient survival was achieved when compared to a variety of other treatments. However, the conjugates provided comparable efficacy with reduced side effects (Singer *et al.* 2005; Bonomi 2007). The reduction in side effects is attributable to the inactivation of paclitaxel when bound to the polymer through its 2′ hydroxyl group (Langer 2004).

A few conjugates based on materials other than PEG, HPMA, and polyglutamate have been investigated – most notably those based on the polysaccharide dextran. A conjugate of 70 kDa dextran with doxorubicin failed Phase I clinical trials due to toxicity from RES uptake (Danhauser-Riedl *et al.* 1993). Dextran was among the first materials investigated for conjugation to therapeutic proteins. However, multiple reactive groups present on dextran present a risk of crosslinking with proteins, which provides a heterogeneous product (Pasut and Veronese 2007).

5.7.4 Active targeting of polymer-drug conjugates

Current bench scale research on polymer-drug conjugates is largely focused on incorporating active targeting to enhance tumor targeting beyond that achieved by the EPR effect. Conjugates of heparin-folate-paclitaxel were reported by Cho *et al.* to show improved antitumor efficacy than either free drug or heparin-paclitaxel alone (Cho *et al.* 2008). Other systems are designed to target lectins, proteins that bind to specific glycans in cell membranes. Because cancer cells can express different glycans than normal cells, the lectins corresponding to cancer cells may be suitable targeting agents (Bies *et al.* 2004). Either the lectin or glycan can be conjugated to the drug, and used to target the other species (Minko 2004). The polymer-drug conjugate PK2 is an actively targeted version of HPMA-doxorubicin bound with galactosamine for targeting of the hepatic asialoglycoprotein receptor (Seymour *et al.* 2002). Gamma-camera imaging showed improved targeting toward the liver while the same formulation without galactosamine (PK1) showed no targeting (Seymour *et al.* 2002). Phase I and II clinical trials have been completed using this system for treatment of liver cancer.

5.8 Conclusion and future trends

Injectable biomaterials in the form of both solid gels and particulate systems constitute a significant fraction of the materials used for drug delivery applications. These systems have several advantages including ease of administration, high bioavailability, protection of therapeutic biomolecules, and flexibility in the rate of drug release. System-specific design factors which may include the material composition, molecular weight, hydrophilicity, and sensitivity to stimuli allow for modulation of both the drug release rate as well as spatial targeting.

Still, there is no singular cure-all or 'magic bullet'. Drug delivery is a discipline riddled with trade-offs. If drug is delivered too slowly or too rapidly, the benefit of a device could be negligible or worse. The earliest injectable drug delivery systems allowed for degradability, but introduced toxic solvents into the body. Alternatively, injectable aqueous systems still often lack either degradability, controlled swelling behavior, or sufficient mechanical properties. Particulate systems have trade-offs as well. Many systems rely solely on the EPR effect to achieve efficient targeting of cancer cells. Uptake by the reticuloendothelial system remains a concern. Micelles offer design flexibility, but often have been unsafe due to poor stability. Despite improved circulation times, conjugates of toxic anti-cancer drugs have not yet made it to market.

Future drug delivery systems will continue to address these challenges. New bioconjugation techniques now allow for reliable functionalization of injectable systems with an ever increasing range of ligands. Likewise, new polymerization chemistries have improved material homogeneity. Discoveries in related fields including biochemistry, cell biology, imaging, and materials science are constantly providing new mechanisms that can be exploited in the next generation of drug delivery devices.

For further reading on selected topics, many review articles are available in the literature covering topics ranging from polymer design to clinical applications. Review articles covering the topics presented in this chapter include those on solid gels (Hatefi and Amsden 2002; Hoare and Kohane 2008), stimuli-responsive gels (Schmaljohann 2006; He *et al.* 2008; Ulijn *et al.* 2007), protein delivery (Lee and Yuk 2007), particulate system pharmacokinetics (Alexis *et al.* 2008), polymeric microspheres and nanospheres (Chandrashekar and Udupa 1996; Soppimath *et al.* 2001; Mohamed and van der Walle 2008), micelles (Allen *et al.* 1999; Gaucher *et al.* 2005; Torchilin 2006), liposomes (Torchilin 2005), injectable materials for cancer treatment (Cho *et al.* 2008; Davis *et al.* 2008), targeting mechanisms (Bies *et al.* 2004; Qian *et al.* 2002; Sudimack and Lee 2000), PEGylation (Chapman 2002; Harris and Chess 2003;

Pasut *et al.* 2004), and polymer-drug conjugates (Pasut and Veronese 2007; Khandare and Minko 2006; Duncan 2009; Duncan *et al.* 2001).

5.9 References

Adams, M.L. and Kwon, G.S., 2003. Relative aggregation state and hemolytic activity of amphotericin B encapsulated by poly(ethylene oxide)-*block*-poly(*N*-hexyl-L-aspartamide)-acyl conjugate micelles: effects of acyl chain length. *Journal of Controlled Release*, 87, 23–32.

Adams, M.L., Andes, D.R. and Kwon, G.S., 2003. Amphotericin B encapsulated in micelles based on poly(ethylene oxide)-*block*-poly(L-amino acid) derivatives exerts reduced *in vitro* hemolysis but maintains potent *in vivo* antifungal activity. *Biomacromolecules*, 4(3), 750–757.

Adler-Moore, J., 1994. AmBisome targeting to fungal infections. *Bone Marrow Transplant.*, 14(Suppl 5), S3–7.

Agnihotri, S.A., Mallikarjuna, N.N. and Aminabhavi, T.M., 2004. Recent advances on chitosan-based micro-and nanoparticles in drug delivery. *Journal of Controlled Release*, 100(1), 5–28.

Ahn, J.S. *et al.*, 2005. Slow eroding biodegradable multiblock poloxamer copolymers. *Polymer International*, 54(5), 842–847.

Alexis, F. *et al.*, 2008. Factors affecting the clearance and biodistribution of polymeric nanoparticles. *Molecular Pharmaceutics*, 5(4), 505–515.

Allen, C., Maysinger, D. and Eisenberg, A., 1999. Nano-engineering block copolymer aggregates for drug delivery. *Colloids and Surfaces B: Biointerfaces*, 16, 3–27.

Alonso, M.J. *et al.*, 1991. Approaches to improve the association of amikacin sulphate to poly (alkylcyanoacrylate) nanoparticles. *International Journal of Pharmaceutics*, 68(1–3), 69–76.

Alvarez-Lorenzo, C. *et al.*, 2005. Temperature-sensitive chitosan-poly (N-isopropylacrylamide) interpenetrated networks with enhanced loading capacity and controlled release properties. *Journal of Controlled Release*, 102(3), 629–641.

Anderson, J.M. and Shive, M.S., 1997. Biodegradation and biocompatibility of PLA and PLGA microspheres. *Advanced Drug Delivery Reviews*, 28(1), 5–24.

Attwood, D., Collett, J.H. and Tait, C.J., 1985. The micellar properties of the poly(oxyethylene)-poly(oxypropylene) copolymer Pluronic F127 in water and electrolyte solution. *Int. J. Pharm.*, 26, 25–33.

Bae, J.W. *et al.*, 2006. Thermosensitive chitosan as an injectable carrier for local drug delivery. *Macromolecular Research*, 14(4), 461.

Bae, S.J. *et al.*, 2005. Thermogelling poly(caprolactone-*b*-ethylene glycol-*b*-caprolactone) aqueous solutions. *Macromolecules*, 38(12), 5260–5265.

Bae, S.J. *et al.*, 2006. Gelation behavior of poly(ethylene glycol) and polycaprolactone triblock and multiblock copolymer aqueous solutions. *Macromolecules*, 39(14), 4873–4879.

Bae, Y. *et al.*, 2005. Preparation and biological characterization of polymeric micelle drug carriers with intracellular pH-triggered drug release property: tumor permeability, controlled subcellular drug distribution, and enhanced *in vivo* antitumor efficacy. *Bioconjugate Chemistry*, 16(1), 122–130.

Bailon, P. *et al.*, 2001. Rational design of a potent, long-lasting form of interferon: a 40 kDa branched polyethylene glycol-conjugated interferon α-2a for the treatment of hepatitis C. *Bioconjugate Chemistry*, 12(2), 195–202.

Bart, J. *et al.*, 2000. The blood-brain barrier and oncology: new insights into function and modulation. *Cancer Treatment Reviews*, 26, 449–462.

Behravesh, E. *et al.*, 2002. Synthesis and characterization of triblock copolymers of methoxy poly(ethylene glycol) and poly(propylene fumarate). *Biomacromolecules*, 3(1), 153–158.

Berscht, P.C. *et al.*, 1993. Incorporation of basic fibroblast growth factor into methylpyrrolidone chitosan fleeces and determination of the *in vitro* release characteristics. *Biomaterials*, 15(8), 593–600.

Biehl, G., Harms, J. and Hanser, U., 1974. Experimental studies on heat development in bone during polymerization of bone cement. Intra-operative measurement of termperature in normal blood circulation and in bloodlessness. *Arch. Orthop. Unfallchir.*, 78(1), 62–69.

Bies, C., Lehr, C. and Woodley, J.F., 2004. Lectin-mediated drug targeting: history and applications. *Advanced Drug Delivery Reviews*, 56(4), 425–435.

Bohdanecky, M., Bazilova, H. and Kopecek, J., 1974. Poly[N-(2-hydroxypropyl) methacrylamide] – II: Hydrodynamic properties of dilute solutions. *European Polymer Journal*, 10(5), 405–410.

Bonomi, P., 2007. Paclitaxel poliglumex (PPX, CT-2103): macromolecular medicine for advanced non-small-cell lung cancer. *Expert Review of Anticancer Therapy*, 7(4), 415–422.

Bontha, S., Kabanov, A.V. and Bronich, T.K., 2006. Polymer micelles with cross-linked ionic cores for delivery of anticancer drugs. *Journal of Controlled Release*, 114, 163–174.

Brown, W., Schillen, K. and Almgren, M., 1991. Micelle and gel formation in a poly(ethylene oxide)/poly(propylene oxide)/poly(ethylene oxide) triblock copolymer in water solution. Dynamic and static light scattering and oscillatory shear measurements. *Journal of Physical Chemistry*, 95, 1850–1858.

Bulpitt, P. and Aeschlimann, D., 1999. New strategy for chemical modification of hyaluronic acid: preparation of functionalized derivatives and their use in the formation of novel biocompatible hydrogels. *Journal of Biomedical Materials Research Part A*, 47(2), 152–169.

Burt, H.M. *et al.*, 1999. Development of copolymers of poly(D,L-lactide) and methoxypolyethylene glycol as micellar carriers of paclitaxel. *Colloids and Surfaces B: Biointerfaces*, 16, 161–171.

Butun, V., Armes, S.P. and Billingham, N.C., 2001. Synthesis and aqueous solution properties of near-monodisperse tertiary amine methacrylate homopolymers and diblock copolymers. *Polymer*, 42, 5993–6008.

Cai, S. *et al.*, 2005. Injectable glycosaminoglycan hydrogels for controlled release of human basic fibroblast growth factor. *Biomaterials*, 26(30), 6054–6067.

Castelletto, V. *et al.*, 2004. Microstructure and physical properties of a pH-responsive gel based on a novel biocompatible ABA-type triblock copolymer. *Langmuir*, 20(10), 4306–4309.

Chandrashekar, B.L. *et al.*, 2000. Controlled release liquid delivery compositions with low initial drug burst. US Patent, 6 143 314.

Chandrashekar, G. and Udupa, N., 1996. Biodegradable injectable implant systems for long term drug delivery using poly(lactic-co-glycolic) acid copolymers. *J. Pharm. Pharmacol.*, 48(7), 669–674.

Chapman, A.P., 2002. PEGylated antibodies and antibody fragments for improved therapy: a review. *Advanced Drug Delivery Reviews*, 54(4), 531–545.

Chen, G. and Hoffman, A.S., 1995. Graft copolymers that exhibit temperature-induced phase transitions over a wide range of pH. *Nature*, 373, 49–52.

Chen, S. and Singh, J., 2005a. Controlled delivery of testosterone from smart polymer solution based systems: *in vitro* evaluation. *International Journal of Pharmaceutics*, 295(1–2), 183–190.

Chen, S. and Singh, J., 2005b. *In vitro* release of levonorgestrel from phase sensitive and thermosensitive smart polymer delivery systems. *Pharmaceutical Development and Technology*, 10(2), 319–325.

Chenite, A. *et al.*, 2000. Novel injectable neutral solutions of chitosan form biodegradable gels *in situ*. *Biomaterials*, 21(21), 2155–2161.

Chew, J.L. *et al.*, 2003. Chitosan nanoparticles containing plasmid DNA encoding house dust mite allergen, Der p 1 for oral vaccination in mice. *Vaccine*, 21, 2720–2729.

Cho, K. *et al.*, 2008. Therapeutic nanoparticles for drug delivery in cancer. *Clinical Cancer Research*, 14(5), 1310–1316.

Choi, B.G., Sohn, Y.S. and Jeong, B., 2007. Closed-loop sol-gel transition of PEG-PEC aqueous solution. *The Journal of Physical Chemistry B*, 111(27), 7715–7718.

Choi, S.W. *et al.*, 1999. Thermoreversible gelation of poly(ethylene oxide) biodegradable polyester block copolymers. II. *Journal of Polymer Science Part A: Polymer Chemistry*, 37, 2207–2218.

Choi, S., Baudys, M. and Kim, S.W., 2004. Control of blood glucose by novel GLP-1 delivery using biodegradable triblock copolymer of PLGA-PEG-PLGA in type 2 diabetic rats. *Pharmaceutical Research*, 21(5), 827–831.

Chytry, V., Vrana, A. and Kopecek, J., 1977. Synthesis and activity of a polymer which contains insulin covalently bound on a copolymer of *N*-(2-hydroxypropyl) methacrylamide and *N*-methacryloyldiglycyl *p*-nitrophenyl ester. *Macromolecular Chemistry and Physics*, 179(2), 329–336.

Cohen, H. *et al.*, 2000. Sustained delivery and expression of DNA encapsulated in polymeric nanoparticles. *Gene Therapy*, 7, 1896–1905.

Cohn, D., Sosnik, A. and Levy, A., 2003. Improved reverse thermo-responsive polymeric systems. *Biomaterials*, 24, 3707–3714.

Cohn, D. *et al.*, 2006. PEO–PPO–PEO-based poly(ether ester urethane)s as degradable reverse thermo-responsive multiblock copolymers. *Biomaterials*, 27, 1718–1727.

Couvreur, P. *et al.*, 1979. Polycyanoacrylate nanocapsules as potential lysosomotropic carriers: preparation, morphological and sorptive properties. *J. Pharm. Pharmacol.*, 31(5), 331–332.

Cui, Z., Lee, B.H. and Vernon, B.L., 2007. New hydrolysis-dependent thermosensitive polymer for an injectable degradable system. *Biomacromolecules*, 8(4), 1280–1286.

D'Amico, D.J. *et al.*, 2006. Pegaptanib sodium for neovascular age-related macular degeneration: two-year safety results of the two prospective, multicenter, controlled clinical trials. *Ophthalmology*, 113(6), 992–1001.

Danhauser-Riedl, S. *et al.*, 1993. Phase I clinical and pharmacokinetic trial of dextran conjugated doxorubicin (AD-70, DOX-OXD). *Investigational New Drugs*, 11(2), 187–195.

Davidsen, J. *et al.*, 2001. Drug delivery by phospholipase A_2 degradable liposomes. *Int. J. Pharm.*, 214, 67–69.

Davis, M.E., Chen, Z. and Shin, D.M., 2008. Nanoparticle therapeutics: an emerging treatment modality for cancer. *Nature Reviews Drug Discovery*, 7, 771–782.

De Jaeghere, F. *et al.*, 1999. Formulation and lyoprotection of poly(lactic acid-*co*-ethylene oxide) nanoparticles: influence on physical stability and *in vitro* cell uptake. *Pharmaceutical Research*, 16(6), 859–866.

Deiters, A. *et al.*, 2004. Site-specific PEGylation of proteins containing unnatural amino

acids. *Bioorganic and Medicinal Chemistry Letters*, 14(23), 5743–5745.
Desai, M.P. *et al.*, 1996. Gastrointestinal uptake of biodegradable microparticles: effect of particle size. *Pharmaceutical Research*, 13(12), 1838–1845.
Determan, M.D., Cox, J.P. and Mallapragada, S.K., 2007. Drug release from pH-responsive thermogelling pentablock copolymers. *Journal of Biomedical Materials Research Part A*, 81A(2), 326–333.
DuBose, J.W., Cutshall, C. and Metters, A.T., 2005. Controlled release of tethered molecules via engineered hydrogel degradation: model development and validation. *Journal of Biomedical Materials Research Part A*, 74A(1), 104–116.
Duncan, R., 2009. Development of HPMA copolymer-anticancer conjugates: clinical experience and lessons learnt. *Advanced Drug Delivery Reviews*, 61, 1131–1148.
Duncan, R. and Vicent, M.J., 2010. Do HPMA copolymer conjugates have a future as clinically useful nanomedicines? A critical overview of current status and future opportunities. *Advanced Drug Delivery Reviews*, 62, 272–282.
Duncan, R. *et al.*, 1983. Polymers containing enzymatically degradable bonds, 7. Design of oligopeptide side-chains in poly[N-(2-hydroxypropyl)methacrylamide] copolymers to promote efficient degradation by lysosomal enzymes. *Die Makromolekulare Chemie*, 184(10), 1997–2008.
Duncan, R. *et al.*, 2001. Polymer-drug conjugates, PDEPT and PELT: basic principles for design and transfer from the laboratory to clinic. *Journal of Controlled Release*, 74, 135–146.
Elbert, D.L. *et al.*, 2001. Protein delivery from materials formed by self-selective conjugate addition reactions. *Journal of Controlled Release*, 76(1–2), 11–25.
Ellerhorst, J.A. *et al.*, 1999. Phase II trial of doxil for patients with metastatic melanoma refractory to frontline therapy. *Oncol. Rep.*, 6(5), 1097–1099.
Fang, J.Y. *et al.*, 2008. Temperature-sensitive hydrogels composed of chitosan and hyaluronic acid as injectable carriers for drug delivery. *European Journal of Pharmaceutics and Biopharmaceutics*, 68(3), 626–636.
Farokhzad, O.C. *et al.*, 2006. Targeted nanoparticle-aptamer bioconjugates for cancer chemotherapy *in vivo*. *Proceedings of the National Academy of Sciences USA*, 103(16), 6315–6320.
Feil, H. *et al.*, 1993. Effect of comonomer hydrophilicity and ionization on the lower critical solution temperature of *N*-isopropylacrylamide copolymers. *Macromolecules*, 26(10), 2496–2500.
Fleming, M.G. and Maillet, W.A., 1999. Photopolymerization of composite resin using the argon laser. *Journal of the Canadian Dental Association*, 65, 447–452.
Forssen, E.A. *et al.*, 1996. Fluorescence imaging studies for the disposition of daunorubicin liposomes (DaunoXome) within tumor tissue. *Cancer Research*, 56, 2066–2075.
Foster, K.A., Yazdanian, M. and Audus, K.L., 2001. Microparticulate uptake mechanisms of *in-vitro* cell culture models of the respiratory epithelium. *Journal of Pharmacy and Pharmacology*, 53(1), 57–66.
Fu, R.C. *et al.*, 1987. The biocompatibility of parenteral vehicles – *in vitro*/*in vivo* screening comparison and the effect of excipients on hemolysis. *J. Parenter. Sci. Technol.*, 41(5), 164–168.
Gabizon, A., 2003. Emerging role of liposomal drug carrier systems in cancer chemotherapy. *Journal of Liposome Research*, 13(1), 17–20.
Gaspar, M.M., Perez-Soler, R. and Cruz, M.E.M., 1996. Biological characterization of L-asparaginase liposomal formulations. *Cancer Chemotherapy and Pharmacology*, 38, 373–377.

Gaucher, G. *et al.*, 2005. Block copolymer micelles: preparation, characterization and application in drug delivery. *Journal of Controlled Release*, 109(1–3F), 169–188.

Gimenez-Conti, I.B. *et al.*, 1998. Comparison of the skin tumor-promoting potential of different organic peroxides in SENCAR mice. *Toxicology and Applied Pharmacology*, 143, 73–79.

Glatter, O. and Scherf, G., 1994. Characterization of a poly(ethylene oxide)-poly(propylene oxide) triblock copolymer (EO_{27}-PO_{39}-EO_{27}) in Aqueous Solution. *Macromolecules*, 27, 6046–6054.

Glue, P., Fang, J. *et al.*, 2000. Pegylated interferon-alpha2b: pharmacokinetics, pharmacodynamics, safety, and preliminary efficacy data. Hepatitis C Intervention Therapy Group. *Clinical Pharmacology and Therapeutics*, 68(5), 556–567.

Glue, P., Rouzier-Panis, R. *et al.*, 2000. A dose-ranging study of pegylated interferon alfa-2b and ribavirin in chronic hepatitis C. *Hepatology*, 32(3), 647–653.

Gordon, K.B. *et al.*, 1995. Hand-foot syndrome associated with liposome-encapsulated doxorubicin therapy. *Cancer*, 75(8), 2169–2173.

Greenwald, R.B. *et al.*, 1996. Drug delivery systems: water soluble taxol 2-poly (ethylene glycol) ester prodrugs – design and *in vivo* effectiveness. *J. Med. Chem*, 39(2), 424–431.

Greish, K. *et al.*, 2003. Macromolecular therapeutics: advantages and prospects with special emphasis on tumour targeting. *Clinical Pharmacokinetics*, 42(13), 1089–1105.

Griffin, L.C. *et al.*, 1993. *In vivo* anticoagulant properties of a novel nucleotide-based thrombin inhibitor and demonstration of regional anticoagulation in extracorporeal circuits. *Blood*, 81(12), 3271.

Gutowska, A. *et al.*, 1992. Heparin release from thermosensitive hydrogels. *Journal of Controlled Release*, 22, 95–104.

Ha, D.I. *et al.*, 2006. Preparation of thermo-responsive and injectable hydrogels based on hyaluronic acid and poly(N-isopropyl-acrylamide) and their drug release behaviors. *Macromolecular Research*, 14(1), 87.

Hamaguchi, T. *et al.*, 2005. NK105, a paclitaxel-incorporating micellar nanoparticle formulation, can extend *in vivo* antitumour activity and reduce the neurotoxicity of paclitaxel. *British Journal of Cancer*, 92(7), 1240–1246.

Hamaguchi, T. *et al.*, 2007. A phase I and pharmacokinetic study of NK105, a paclitaxel-incorporating micellar nanoparticle formulation. *British Journal of Cancer*, 97(2), 170–176.

Harris, J.M. and Chess, R.B., 2003. Effect of pegylation on pharmaceuticals. *Nature Reviews Drug Discovery*, 2(3), 214–221.

Hatakeyama, H. *et al.*, 2004. Factors governing the *in vivo* tissue uptake of transferrin-coupled polyethylene glycol liposomes *in vivo*. *Int. J. Pharm.*, 281, 25–33.

Hatefi, A. and Amsden, B., 2002. Biodegradable injectable *in situ* forming drug delivery systems. *Journal of Controlled Release*, 80, 9–28.

He, C., Kim, S.W. and Lee, D.S., 2008. *In situ* gelling stimuli-sensitive block copolymer hydrogels for drug delivery. *Journal of Controlled Release*, 127, 189–207.

Hedley, M.L., Curley, J. and Urban, R., 1998. Microspheres containing plasmid-encoded antigens elicit cytotoxic T-cell responses. *Nature Medicine*, 4(3), 365–368.

Heeremans, J.L. *et al.*, 1995. Thrombolytic treatment with tissue-type plasminogen activator (t-PA) containing liposomes in rabbits: a comparison with free t-PA. *Thromb. Haemost.*, 73(3), 488–494.

Henderson, E. *et al.*, 2009. *In vivo* evaluation of injectable thermosensitive polymer with time-dependent LCST. *Journal of Biomedical Materials Research Part A*, 90A(4), 1186–1197.

Hiemstra, C. *et al.*, 2007. Rapidly *in situ*-forming degradable hydrogels from dextran thiols through michael addition. *Biomacromolecules*, 8(5), 1548–1556.

Hoare, T.R. and Kohane, D.S., 2008. Hydrogels in drug delivery: progress and challenges. *Polymer*, 49(8), 1993–2007.

Huang, X. and Lowe, T.L., 2005. Biodegradable thermoresponsive hydrogels for aqueous encapsulation and controlled release of hydrophilic model drugs. *Biomacromolecules*, 6(4), 2131–2139.

Hubbell, J.A., 1996. Hydrogel systems for barriers and local drug delivery in the control of wound healing. *Journal of Controlled Release*, 39, 305–313.

Hubbell, J.A. *et al.*, 2005. Photopolymerizable biodegradable hydrogels as tissue contacting materials and controlled release carriers. US Patent, 5 410 016.

Hwang, M.J. *et al.*, 2005. Caprolactonic poloxamer analog: PEG-PCL-PEG. *Biomacromolecules*, 6(2), 885–890.

Illum, L. and Davis, S.S., 1983. Effect of the nonionic surfactant poloxamer 338 on the fate and deposition of polystyrene microspheres following intravenous administration. *Journal of Pharmaceutical Sciences*, 72(9), 1086–1089.

Illum, L. and Davis, S.S., 1984. The organ uptake of intravenously administered colloidal particles can be altered using a non-ionic surfactant (Poloxamer 338). *FEBS Letters*, 167(1), 79–82.

Ishida, O. *et al.*, 2001. Liposomes bearing polyethyleneglycol-coupled transferrin with intracellular targeting property to the solid tumors *in vivo*. *Pharmaceutical Research*, 18(7), 1042–1048.

Ito, T., Yeo, Y., Highley, C.B., Bellas, E., Benitez, C.A. *et al.*, 2007a. The prevention of peritoneal adhesions by *in situ* cross-linking hydrogels of hyaluronic acid and cellulose derivatives. *Biomaterials*, 28(6), 975–983.

Ito, T., Yeo, Y., Highley, C.B., Bellas, E. and Kohane, D.S., 2007b. Dextran-based *in situ* cross-linked injectable hydrogels to prevent peritoneal adhesions. *Biomaterials*, 28(23), 3418–3426.

Jain, R.A.,, 2000. The manufacturing techniques of various drug loaded biodegradable poly(lactide-*co*-glycolide) (PLGA) devices. *Biomaterials*, 21, 2475–2490.

Jain, R.A. *et al.*, 2000. Controlled release of drugs from injectable *in situ* formed biodegradable PLGA microspheres: effect of various formulation variables. *European Journal of Pharmaceutics and Biopharmaceutics*, 50, 257–262.

Janes, K.A. *et al.*, 2001. Chitosan nanoparticles as delivery systems for doxorubicin. *Journal of Controlled Release*, 73, 255–267.

Jeong, B. *et al.*, 1997. Biodegradable block copolymers as injectable drug-delivery systems. *Nature*, 388, 860–862.

Jeong, B. *et al.*, 1999. New biodegradable polymers for injectable drug delivery systems. *Journal of Controlled Release*, 62, 109–114.

Jeong, B., Bae, Y.H. and Kim, S.W., 2000. Drug release from biodegradable injectable thermosensitive hydrogel of PEG–PLGA–PEG triblock copolymers. *Journal of Controlled Release*, 63, 155–163.

Jeong, Y. *et al.*, 2009. Enzymatically degradable temperature-sensitive polypeptide as a new *in-situ* gelling biomaterial. *Journal of Controlled Release*.

Jette, K.K. *et al.*, 2004. Preparation and drug loading of poly(ethylene glycol)-*block*-poly(epsilon-caprolactone) micelles through the evaporation of a cosolvent azeotrope. *Pharmaceutical Research*, 21(7), 1184–1191.

Jones, M.C., Ranger, M. and Leroux, J.C., 2003. pH-Sensitive unimolecular polymeric micelles: synthesis of a novel drug carrier. *Bioconjugate Chemistry*, 14(4), 774–781.

Jorgensen, E.B. *et al.*, 1997. Effects of salts on the micellization and gelation of a triblock copolymer studied by rheology and light scattering. *Macromolecules*, 30, 2355–2364.

Kang, N. and Leroux, J.C., 2004. Triblock and star-block copolymers of *N*-(2-hydroxypropyl)methacrylamide or *N*-vinyl-2-pyrrolidone and D,L-lactide: synthesis and self-assembling properties in water. *Polymer*, 45, 8967–8980.

Khandare, J. and Minko, T., 2006. Polymer-drug conjugates: progress in polymeric prodrugs. *Progress in Polymer Science*, 31(4), 359–397.

Kim, A. *et al.*, 1999. Pharmacodynamics of insulin in polyethylene glycol-coated liposomes. *Int. J. Pharm.*, 180, 75–81.

Kim, D.W. *et al.*, 2007. Multicenter phase II trial of Genexol-PM, a novel Cremophor-free, polymeric micelle formulation of paclitaxel, with cisplatin in patients with advanced non-small-cell lung cancer. *Annals of Oncology*, 18, 2009–2014.

Kim, H.K. and Park, T.G., 1999. Microencapsulation of human growth hormone within biodegradable polyester microspheres: protein aggregation stability and incomplete release mechanism. *Biotechnology and Bioengineering*, 65, 659–667.

Kim, M.S. *et al.*, 2004. Preparation of methoxy poly(ethylene glycol)/polyester diblock copolymers and examination of the gel-to-sol transition. *Journal of Polymer Science Part A: Polymer Chemistry*, 42(22), 5784–5793.

Kim, S. and Healy, K.E., 2003. Synthesis and characterization of injectable poly(*N*-isopropylacrylamide-*co*-acrylic acid) hydrogels with proteolytically degradable cross-links. *Biomacromolecules*, 4(5), 1214–1223.

Kim, S.C. *et al.*, 2001. *In vivo* evaluation of polymeric micellar paclitaxel formulation: toxicity and efficacy. *Journal of Controlled Release*, 72, 191–202.

Kim, S.Y. *et al.*, 2007. Reverse thermal gelling PEG–PTMC diblock copolymer aqueous solution. *Macromolecules*, 40(15), 5519–5525.

Klibanov, A.L. *et al.*, 1990. Amphipathic polyethyleneglycols effectively prolong the circulation time of liposomes. *FEBS Letters*, 268(1), 235–237.

Kopecek, J. and Bazilova, H., 1973. Poly[N-(2-hydroxypropyl)methacrylamide] – I. Radical polymerization and copolymerization. *European Polymer Journal*, 9(1), 7–14.

Kopecek, J. *et al.*, 2000. HPMA copolymer-anticancer drug conjugates: design, activity, and mechanism of action. *European Journal of Pharmaceutics and Biopharmaceutics*, 50(1), 61–81.

Kranz, H. *et al.*, 2001. Myotoxicity studies of injectable biodegradable *in-situ* forming drug delivery systems. *Int. J. Pharm.*, 212, 11–18.

Kratz, F., Beyer, U. and Schütte, M.T., 1999. Drug-polymer conjugates containing acid-cleavable bonds. *Critical Reviews in Therapeutic Drug Carrier Systems*, 16(3), 245–288.

Labhasetwar, V. *et al.*, 1999. Gene transfection using biodegradable nanospheres: results in tissue culture and a rat osteotomy model. *Colloids and Surfaces B: Biointerfaces*, 16, 281–290.

Lambert, W.J. and Peck, K.D., 1995. Development of an *in situ* forming biodegradable poly-lactide-co-glycolide system for the controlled release of proteins. *Journal of Controlled Release*, 33, 189–195.

Langer, C.J., 2004. CT-2103: a novel macromolecular taxane with potential advantages compared with conventional taxanes. *Clinical Lung Cancer*, 6, 85–88.

Langer, R., 1990. New methods of drug delivery. *Science*, 249(4976), 1527–1533.

Lasic, D.D., Vallner, J.J. and Working, P.K., 1999. Sterically stabilized liposomes in cancer therapy and gene delivery. *Curr. Opin. Mol. Ther.*, 1(2), 177–185.

Lavasanifar, A., Samuel, J. and Kwon, G.S., 2002. Poly(ethylene oxide)-*block*-poly(L-amino acid) micelles for drug delivery. *Advanced Drug Delivery Reviews*, 54, 169–190.

Lee, D.S. *et al.*, 2001. Novel thermoreversible gelation of biodegradable PLGA-block-PEO-block-PLGA triblock copolymers in aqueous solution. *Macromolecular Rapid Communications*, 22(8), 587–592.

Lee, E.S., Na, K. and Bae, Y.H., 2003. Polymeric micelle for tumor pH and folate-mediated targeting. *Journal of Controlled Release*, 91, 103–113.

Lee, J.Y., Cho, E.C. and Cho, K., 2004. Incorporation and release behavior of hydrophobic drug in functionalized poly(D,L-lactide)-*block*-poly(ethylene oxide) micelles. *Journal of Controlled Release*, 94, 323–335.

Lee, K.S. *et al.*, 2007. Multicenter phase II trial of Genexol-PM, a Cremophor-free, polymeric micelle formulation of paclitaxel, in patients with metastatic breast cancer. *Breast Cancer Research and Treatment*, 108(2), 241–250.

Lee, K.Y. and Yuk, S.H., 2007. Polymeric protein delivery systems. *Prog. Polym. Sci.*, 32, 669–697.

Li, C., Buurma, N.J. *et al.*, 2005. Synthesis and characterization of biocompatible, thermoresponsive ABC and ABA triblock copolymer gelators. *Langmuir*, 21(24), 11026–11033.

Li, C., Tang, Y. *et al.*, 2005. Synthesis and characterization of biocompatible thermo-responsive gelators based on ABA triblock copolymers. *Biomacromolecules*, 6(2), 994–999.

Li, S. and Liu, X., 2008. Synthesis, characterization, and evaluation of enzymatically degradable poly(N-isopropylacrylamide-co-acrylic acid) hydrogels for colon-specific drug delivery. *Polymers for Advanced Technologies*, 19, 1536–1542.

Li, Y. and Kwon, G.S., 2000. Methotrexate esters of poly(ethylene oxide)-*block*-poly(2-hydroxyethyl-L-aspartamide). Part I: Effects of the level of methotrexate conjugation on the stability of micelles and on drug release. *Pharmaceutical Research*, 17(5), 607–611.

Liburdy, R.P., Tenforde, T.S. and Magin, R.L., 1986. Magnetic field-induced drug permeability in liposome vesicles. *Radiation Research*, 108, 102–111.

Lin, S.Y. *et al.*, 2000. *In vitro* degradation and dissolution behaviours of microspheres prepared by three low molecular weight polyesters. *Journal of Microencapsulation*, 17(5), 577–586.

Liu, J., Zeng, F. and Allen, C., 2005. Influence of serum protein on polycarbonate-based copolymer micelles as a delivery system for a hydrophobic anti-cancer agent. *Journal of Controlled Release*, 103, 481–497.

Liu, Y.Y., Fan, X. *et al.*, 2006. pH-responsive amphiphilic hydrogel networks with IPN structure: a strategy for controlled drug release. *Int. J. Pharm.*, 308, 209–209.

Liu, Y.Y., Shao, Y.H. and Lu, J., 2006. Preparation, properties and controlled release behaviors of pH-induced thermosensitive amphiphilic gels. *Biomaterials*, 27(21), 4016–4024.

Loh, X.J., Goh, S.H. and Li, J., 2007. New biodegradable thermogelling copolymers having very low gelation concentrations. *Biomacromolecules*, 8(2), 585–593.

Loo, C. *et al.*, 2004. Nanoshell-enabled photonics-based imaging and therapy of cancer. *Technology in Cancer Research and Treatment*, 3(1), 33–40.

Lorenzo-Lamosa, M.L. *et al.*, 1998. Design of microencapsulated chitosan microspheres for colonic drug delivery. *Journal of Controlled Release*, 52, 109–118.

Lorusso, D. *et al.*, 2007. Pegylated liposomal doxorubicin-related palmar-plantar erythrodysesthesia ('hand-foot' syndrome). *Annals of Oncology*, 18, 1159–1164.

Lotem, M. *et al.*, 2000. Skin toxic effects of polyethylene glycol-coated liposomal doxorubicin. *Arch. Dermatol.*, 136, 1475–1480.

Lu, L., Stamatas, G.N. and Mikos, A.G., 2000. Controlled release of transforming growth factor beta-1 from biodegradable polymer microparticles. *Journal of Biomedical Materials Research*, 50, 440–451.

Lukyanov, A.N. *et al.*, 2004. Tumor-targeted liposomes: doxorubicin-loaded long-circulating liposomes modified with anti-cancer antibody. *Journal of Controlled Release*, 100, 135–144.

Ma, Y. *et al.*, 2003. Synthesis of biocompatible, stimuli-responsive, physical gels based on ABA triblock copolymers. *Biomacromolecules*, 4(4), 864–868.

Manns, M.P. *et al.*, 2001. Peginterferon alfa-2b plus ribavirin compared with interferon alfa-2b plus ribavirin for initial treatment of chronic hepatitis C: a randomised trial. *The Lancet*, 358(9286), 958–965.

Mao, H.Q. *et al.*, 2001. Chitosan-DNA nanoparticles as gene carriers: synthesis, characterization and transfection efficiency. *Journal of Controlled Release*, 70, 399–421.

Matsumura, Y. *et al.*, 2004. Phase I clinical trial and pharmacokinetic evaluation of NK911, a micelle-encapsulated doxorubicin. *British Journal of Cancer*, 91(10), 1775–1781.

Matsuura, M. *et al.*, 2003. Polycation liposome-mediated gene transfer *in vivo*. *Biochimica et Biophysica Acta*, 1612, 136–143.

Maysinger, D. *et al.*, 2001. Block copolymers modify the internalization of micelle-incorporated probes into neural cells. *Biochimica et Biophysica Acta*, 1539, 205–217.

Medlicott, N.J. *et al.*, 2000. Comparison of the effects of potential parenteral vehicles for poorly water soluble anticancer drugs (organic cosolvents and cyclodextrin solutions) on cultured endothelial cells (HUV-EC). *Journal of Pharmaceutical Sciences*, 87(9), 1138–1143.

Meerum Terwogt, J.M. *et al.*, 2001. Phase I clinical and pharmacokinetic study of PNU166945, a novel water-soluble polymer-conjugated prodrug of paclitaxel. *Anti-Cancer Drugs*, 12(4), 315.

Metselaar, J.M. *et al.*, 2003. A novel family of L-amino acid-based biodegradable polymer-lipid conjugates for the development of long-circulating liposomes with effective drug-targeting capacity. *Bioconjugate Chemistry*, 14(6), 1156–1164.

Metters, A.T. and Hubbell, J.A., 2005. Network formation and degradation behavior of hydrogels formed by michael-type addition reactions. *Biomacromolecules*, 6(1), 290–301.

Mi, F.L. *et al.*, 2002. *In vivo* biocompatibility and degradability of a novel injectable-chitosan-based implant. *Biomaterials*, 23(1), 181–191.

Minko, T., 2004. Drug targeting to the colon with lectins and neoglycoconjugates. *Advanced Drug Delivery Reviews*, 56(4), 491–509.

Moghimi, S.M. and Gray, T., 1997. Triggering macrophage clearance of long-circulating particles. *Clinical Science*, 93, 371–379.

Mohamed, F. and van der Walle, C.F., 2008. Engineering biodegradable polyester particles with specific drug targeting and drug release properties. *Journal of Pharmaceutical Sciences*, 97(1), 71–87.

Moore, L.A. *et al.*, 1995. An injectable biodegradable drug delivery system based on acrylic-terminated poly e-caprolactone. *Trans. Soc. Biomater.*, 18, 186.

Mortensen, K. and Brown, W., 1993. Poly(ethylene oxide)-poly(propylene oxide)-poly(ethylene oxide) triblock copolymers in aqueous solution. The influence of relative block size. *Macromolecules*, 26, 4128–4135.

Motzer, R.J. *et al.*, 2002. Phase II trial of branched peginterferon-α 2a (40 kDa) for patients with advanced renal cell carcinoma. *Annals of Oncology*, 13(11), 1799.

Na, K. *et al.*, 2006. Delivery of dexamethasone, ascorbate, and growth factor (TGF β-3) in thermo-reversible hydrogel constructs embedded with rabbit chondrocytes. *Biomaterials*, 27, 5951–5957.

Nel, A. *et al.*, 2006. Toxic potential of materials at the nanolevel. *Science*, 311(5761), 622–627.

Neradovic, D. *et al.*, 1999. Poly(*N*-isopropylacrylamide) with hydrolyzable lactid acid ester side groups: a new type of thermosensitive polymer. *Macromolecular Rapid Communications*, 20, 577–581.

Ng, E.W.M. and Adamis, A.P., 2005. Targeting angiogenesis, the underlying disorder in neovascular age-related macular degeneration. *Canadian Journal of Ophthalmology. Journal Canadien D'ophtalmologie*, 40(3), 352–368.

Ng, E.W.M. *et al.*, 2006. Pegaptanib, a targeted anti-VEGF aptamer for ocular vascular disease. *Nature Reviews Drug Discovery*, 5(2), 123–132.

Ni, S., Stephenson, S.M. and Lee, R.J., 2002. Folate receptor targeted delivery of liposomal daunorubicin into tumor cells. *Anticancer Research*, 22(4), 2131–2135.

Obereigner, B. *et al.*, 1979. Preparation of polymerizable derivatives of N-(4-aminobenzenesulfonyl)-n′-butylurea. *Journal of Polymer Science: Polymer Symposia*, 66(1), 41–52.

Okada, H., 1997. One- and three-month release injectable microspheres of the LH-RH superagonist leuprorelin acetate. *Advanced Drug Delivery Reviews*, 28(1), 43–70.

O'Neal, D.P. *et al.*, 2004. Photo-thermal tumor ablation in mice using near infrared-absorbing nanoparticles. *Cancer Letters*, 209(2), 171–176.

Opanasopit, P. *et al.*, 2004. Block copolymer design for camptothecin incorporation into polymeric micelles for passive tumor targeting. *Pharmaceutical Research*, 21(11), 2001–2008.

Ossipov, D.A. *et al.*, 2007. Formation of the first injectable poly(vinyl alcohol) hydrogel by mixing of functional PVA precursors. *Journal of Applied Polymer Science*, 106(1), 60–70.

Paasonen, L. *et al.*, 2007. Gold nanoparticles enable selective light-induced contents release from liposomes. *Journal of Controlled Release*, 122, 86–93.

Pak, C.C. *et al.*, 1998. Triggerable liposomal fusion by enzyme cleavage of a novel peptide-lipid conjugate. *Biochimica et Biophysica Acta*, 1372, 13–27.

Pan, X.Q., Wang, H. and Lee, R.J., 2003. Antitumor activity of folate receptor-targeted liposomal doxorubicin in a KB oral carcinoma murine xenograft model. *Pharmaceutical Research*, 20(3), 417–422.

Panyam, J. and Labhasetwar, V., 2003a. Biodegradable nanoparticles for drug and gene delivery to cells and tissue. *Advanced Drug Delivery Reviews*, 55(3), 329–347.

Panyam, J. and Labhasetwar, V., 2003b. Dynamics of endocytosis and exocytosis of poly (D,L-lactide-co-glycolide) nanoparticles in vascular smooth muscle cells. *Pharmaceutical Research*, 20(2), 212–220.

Pasut, G. and Veronese, F.M., 2007. Polymer–drug conjugation, recent achievements and general strategies. *Progress in Polymer Science*, 32(8–9), 933–961.

Pasut, G., Guiotto, A. and Veronese, F.M., 2004. Protein, peptide and non-peptide drug PEGylation for therapeutic application. *Expert Opinion on Therapeutic Patents*, 14(6), 859–894.

Peracchia, M.T. *et al.*, 1999. Stealth® PEGylated polycyanoacrylate nanoparticles for intravenous administration and splenic targeting. *Journal of Controlled Release*, 60(1), 121–128.

Pissuwan, D., Valenzuela, S.M. and Cortie, M.B., 2006. Therapeutic possibilities of plasmonically heated gold nanoparticles. *Trends in Biotechnology*, 24(2), 62–67.

Pollock, J.F. and Healy, K.E., 2010. Mechanical and swelling characterization of poly(N-isopropyl acrylamide-co-methoxy poly(ethylene glycol) methacrylate) sol–gels. *Acta Biomaterialia*, 6(4), 1307–1318.

Qian, Z.M. and Tang, P.L., 1995. Mechanisms of iron uptake by mammalian cells. *Biochimica et Biophysica Acta (BBA)-Molecular Cell Research*, 1269(3), 205–214.

Qian, Z.M. *et al.*, 2002. Targeted drug delivery via the transferrin receptor-mediated endocytosis pathway. *Pharmacological reviews*, 54(4), 561.

Radomsky, M.L. *et al.*, 1993. The controlled release of Ganirelix from the Atrigel injectable implant system. *Proc. Intern. Symp. Control. Rel. Bioact. Mater.*, 20.

Radwan, M.A., 1995. *In vitro* evaluation of polyisobutylcyanoacrylate nanoparticles as a controlled drug carrier for theophylline. *Drug Development and Industrial Pharmacy*, 21(20), 2371–2375.

Rassing, J. and Attwood, D., 1983. Ultrasonic velocity and light-scattering studies on the polyoxyethylene-polyoxypropylene copolymer Pluronic F127 in aqueous solution. *Int. J. Pharm.*, 13, 47–55.

Rejmanova, P. *et al.*, 1983. Polymers containing enzymatically degradable bonds, 8. Degradation of oligopeptide sequences in N-(2-hydroxypropyl)methacrylamide copolymers by bovine spleen cathepsin B. *Die Makromolekulare Chemie*, 184(10), 2009–2020.

Ringden, O. *et al.*, 1991. Efficacy of amphotericin B encapsulated in liposomes (Ambisome) in the treatment of invasive fungal infections in immunocompromised patients. *Journal of Antimicrobial Chemotherapy*, 28, 73–82.

Robb, S.A. *et al.*, 2007. Simultaneously physically and chemically gelling polymer system utilizing a poly(NIPAAm-*co*-cysteamine)-based copolymer. *Biomacromolecules*, 8(7), 2294–2300.

Roberts, M.J., Bentley, M.D. and Harris, J.M., 2002. Chemistry for peptide and protein PEGylation. *Advanced Drug Delivery Reviews*, 54(4), 459–476.

Rowinsky, E.K., 2003. A Phase I and pharmacokinetic study of pegylated camptothecin as a 1-hour infusion every 3 weeks in patients with advanced solid malignancies. *Journal of Clinical Oncology*, 21(1), 148–157.

Ruel-Gariepy, E. and Leroux, J.C., 2004. *In situ*-forming hydrogels – review of temperature-sensitive systems. *European Journal of Pharmaceutics and Biopharmaceutics*, 58, 409–426.

Ruel-Gariepy, E. *et al.*, 2004. A thermosensitive chitosan-based hydrogel for the local delivery of paclitaxel. *European Journal of Pharmaceutics and Biopharmaceutics*, 57, 53–63.

Sahoo, S.K. and Labhasetwar, V., 2005. Enhanced antiproliferative activity of transferrin-conjugated paclitaxel-loaded nanoparticles is mediated via sustained intracellular drug retention. *Molecular Pharmaceutics*, 2(5), 373–383.

Salem, A.K. *et al.*, 2003. Porous polymer and cell composites that self-assemble *in situ*. *Advanced Materials*, 15(3), 210–213.

Samlowski, W.E. *et al.*, 2006. ReGel® polymer-based delivery of interleukin-2 as a cancer treatment. *Journal of Immunotherapy*, 29(5), 524–535.

Sanborn, T.J., Messersmith, P.B. and Barron, A.E., 2002. *In situ* crosslinking of a biomimetic peptide-PEG hydrogel via thermally triggered activation of factor XIII. *Biomaterials*, 23, 2703–2710.

Sant, V.P., Smith, D. and Leroux, J.C., 2004. Novel pH-sensitive supramolecular assemblies for oral delivery of poorly water soluble drugs: preparation and

characterization. *Journal of Controlled Release*, 97, 301–312.
Sant, V.P., Smith, D. and Leroux, J.C., 2005. Enhancement of oral bioavailability of poorly water-soluble drugs by poly(ethylene glycol)-*block*-poly(alkyl acrylate-*co*-methacrylic acid) self-assemblies. *Journal of Controlled Release*, 104, 289–300.
Schmaljohann, D., 2006. Thermo- and pH-responsive polymers in drug delivery. *Advanced Drug Delivery Reviews*, 58, 1655–1670.
Schoemaker, N.E. *et al.*, 2002. A phase I and pharmacokinetic study of MAG-CPT, a water-soluble polymer conjugate of camptothecin. *British Journal of Cancer*, 87(41), 608–614.
Scott, L.C. *et al.*, 2008. A phase II study of pegylated-camptothecin (pegamotecan) in the treatment of locally advanced and metastatic gastric and gastro-oesophageal junction adenocarcinoma. *Cancer Chemotherapy and Pharmacology*, 63(2), 363–370.
Sershen, S.R. *et al.*, 2000. Temperature-sensitive polymer/nanoshell composites for photothermally modulated drug delivery. *J. Biomed. Mater. Res.*, 51, 293–298.
Seymour, L.W. *et al.*, 2002. Hepatic drug targeting: phase I evaluation of polymer-bound doxorubicin. *Journal of Clinical Oncology*, 20(6), 1668.
Seymour, L.W. *et al.*, 2009. Phase II studies of polymer-doxorubicin (PK1, FCE28068) in the treatment of breast, lung and colorectal cancer. *International Journal of Oncology*, 34(6), 1629–1636.
Shah, N.H. *et al.*, 1993. A biodegradable injectable implant for delivering micro and macromolecules using poly(lactic-co-glycolic) acid (PLGA) copolymers. *Journal of Controlled Release*, 27, 139–147.
Sharifi, S. *et al.*, 2009. Injectable *in situ* forming drug delivery system based on poly (ϵ-caprolactone fumarate) for tamoxifen citrate delivery: gelation characteristics, *in vitro* drug release and anti-cancer evaluation. *Acta Biomaterialia*, 5(6), 1966–1978.
Shen, W.C. and Ryser, H.J.P., 1981. *cis*-Aconityl spacer between daunomycin and macromolecular carriers: a model of pH-sensitive linkage releasing drug from a lysosomotropic conjugate. *Biochemical and Biophysical Research Communications*, 102(3), 1048–1054.
Shim, M.S. *et al.*, 2002. Poly(D,L-lactic acid-co-glycolic acid)-b-poly(ethylene glycol)-b-poly (D,L-lactic acid-co-glycolic acid) triblock copolymer and thermoreversible phase transition in water. *Journal of Biomedical Materials Research*, 61, 188–196.
Shu, X.Z. *et al.*, 2006. Synthesis and evaluation of injectable, *in situ* crosslinkable synthetic extracellular matrices for tissue engineering. *Journal of Biomedical Materials Research Part A*, 79A(4), 902–912.
Shuai, X. *et al.*, 2004. Core-cross-linked polymeric micelles as paclitaxel carriers. *Bioconjugate Chemistry*, 15(3), 441–448.
Simoes, S. *et al.*, 2004. On the formulation of pH-sensitive liposomes with long circulation times. *Advanced Drug Delivery Reviews*, 56, 947–965.
Singer, J.W. *et al.*, 2005. Paclitaxel poliglumex (XYOTAX; CT-2103): an intracellularly targeted taxane. *Anti Cancer Drugs*, 16(3), 243–254.
Singh, U.V. *et al.*, 1997. Enhanced antitumor efficacy of methotrexate poly(lactic-co-glycolic) acid injectable gel implants in mice bearing sarcoma-180. *Pharm. Sci.*, 3, 133–136.
Slaga, T.J., 1981. Skin tumor-promoting activity of benzoyl peroxide, a widely used free radical-generating compound. *Science*, 213(4511), 1023–1025.
Slager, J. and Domb, A.J., 2003. Biopolymer stereocomplexes. *Advanced Drug Delivery Reviews*, 55, 549–583.
de Smidt, P.C. *et al.*, 1991. Association of antisense oligonucleotides with lipoproteins

prolongs the plasma half-life and modifies the tissue distribution. *Nucleic Acids Research*, 19(17), 4695–4700.

Solovsky, M., Ulbrich, K. and Kopecek, J., 1983. Synthesis of N-(2-hydroxypr opyl) methacrylamide copolymers with antimicrobial activity. *Biomaterials*, 4(1), 44–48.

Song, M.J. *et al.*, 2000. Dielectric behavior during sol-gel transition of PEO-PPO-PEO triblock copolymer aqueous solution. *Polymer Bulletin*, 43, 497–504.

Song, M.J. *et al.*, 2003. Thermosensitive sol-gel transition behaviors of poly (ethylene oxide)/aliphatic polyester/poly (ethylene oxide) aqueous solutions. *Journal of Polymer Science Part A: Polymer Chemistry*, 42(3), 772–784.

Soppimath, K.S. *et al.*, 2001. Biodegradable polymeric nanoparticles as drug delivery devices. *Journal of Controlled Release*, 70(1–2), 1–20.

Sosnik, A. and Cohn, D., 2005. Reverse thermo-responsive poly(ethylene oxide) and poly(propylene oxide) multiblock copolymers. *Biomaterials*, 26, 349–357.

Stile, R.A. *et al.*, 2004. Poly (N-isopropylacrylamide)-based semi-interpenetrating polymer networks for tissue engineering applications. Effects of linear poly (acrylic acid) chains on rheology. *Journal of Biomaterials Science, Polymer Edition*, 15(7), 865–878.

Sudimack, J. and Lee, R.J., 2000. Targeted drug delivery via the folate receptor. *Advanced Drug Delivery Reviews*, 41, 147–162.

Suh, H. *et al.*, 1998. Regulation of smooth muscle cell proliferation using paclitaxel-loaded poly(ethylene oxide)-poly(lactide/glycolide) nanospheres. *Journal of Biomedical Materials Research*, 42, 331–338.

Suh, J.M., Bae, S.J. and Jeong, B., 2005. Thermogelling multiblock poloxamer aqueous solutions with closed-loop sol-gel-sol transitions upon increasing pH. *Advanced Materials*, 17(1), 118–120.

Sund, G. and Rosenquist, J., 1983. Morphological changes in bone following intramedullary implantation of methyl methacrylate. *Acta Orthop. Scand.*, 54, 148–156.

Szoka Jr., F. and Papahadjopoulos, D., 1978. Procedure for preparation of liposomes with large internal aqueous space and high capture by reverse-phase evaporation. *Proceedings of the National Academy of Sciences USA*, 75(9), 4194–4198.

Tachibana, R. *et al.*, 1998. Intracellular regulation of macromolecules using pH-sensitive liposomes and nuclear localization signal: qualitative and quantitative evaluation of intracellular trafficking. *Biochemical and Biophysical Research Communications*, 251, 538–544.

Tang, Y. *et al.*, 2003. Solubilization and controlled release of a hydrophobic drug using novel micelle-forming ABC triblock copolymers. *Biomacromolecules*, 4(6), 1636–1645.

Temenoff, J.S. *et al.*, 2003. *In vitro* cytotoxicity of redox radical initiators for cross-linking of oligo(poly(ethylene glycol) fumarate) macromers. *Biomacromolecules*, 4(6), 1605–1613.

Thurmond II, K.B. *et al.*, 1999. Shell cross-linked polymer micelles: stabilized assemblies with great versatility and potential. *Colloids and Surfaces B: Biointerfaces*, 16, 45–54.

Tollemar, J. *et al.*, 1993. Randomized double-blind study of liposomal amphotericin B (Ambisome) prophylaxis of invasive fungal infections in bone marrow transplant recipients. *Bone Marrow Transplant.*, 12(6), 577–582.

Tomoda, H., Kishimoto, Y. and Lee, Y.C., 1989. Temperature effect on endocytosis and exocytosis by rabbit alveolar macrophages. *Journal of Biological Chemistry*, 264(26), 15445–15450.

Toncheva, V. *et al.*, 2003. Use of block copolymers of poly(ortho esters) and poly(ethylene glycol) micellar carriers as potential tumour targeting systems. *Journal of Drug Targeting*, 11(6), 345–353.

Torchilin, V.P., 1985. Liposomes as targetable drug carriers. *Crit. Rev. Ther. Drug Carrier Syst.*, 2(1), 65–115.

Torchilin, V.P., 2005. Recent advances with liposomes as pharmaceutical carriers. *Nature Reviews Drug Discovery*, 4, 145–160.

Torchilin, V.P., 2006. Micellar nanocarriers: pharmaceutical perspectives. *Pharmaceutical Research*, 24(1), 1–16.

Torchilin, V.P., Levchenko, T.S. *et al.*, 2001. Amphiphilic poly-*N*-vinylpyrrolidones: synthesis, properties and liposome surface modification. *Biomaterials*, 22, 3035–3044.

Torchilin, V.P., Rammohan, R. *et al.*, 2001. TAT peptide on the surface of liposomes affords their efficient intracellular delivery even at low temperature and in the presence of metabolic inhibitors. *Proceedings of the National Academy of Sciences USA*, 98(15), 8786–8791.

Troutman, T.S., Leung, S.J. and Romanowski, M., 2009. Light-induced content release from plasmon-resonant liposomes. *Advanced Materials*, 21(22), 2334–2338.

Tucker, C.E. *et al.*, 1999. Detection and plasma pharmacokinetics of an anti-vascular endothelial growth factor oligonucleotide-aptamer (NX1838) in rhesus monkeys. *Journal of Chromatography B*, 732(1), 203–212.

Ueda, H. *et al.*, 2007. Injectable, *in situ* forming poly(propylene fumarate)-based ocular drug delivery systems. *Journal of Biomedical Materials Research Part A*, 83A(3), 656–666.

Ueda, M., Iwara, A. and Kreuter, J., 1998. Influence of the preparation methods on the drug release behaviour of loperamide-loaded nanoparticles. *Journal of Microencapsulation*, 15(3), 361–372.

Ulijn, R.V. *et al.*, 2007. Bioresponsive hydrogels. *Materials Today*, 10(4), 40–48.

Uzé, G., Lutfalla, G. and Mogensen, K.E., 1995. Alpha and beta interferons and their receptor and their friends and relations. *Journal of Interferon and Cytokine Research*, 15(1), 3–26.

Vadnere, M. *et al.*, 1984. Thermodynamic studies on the sol-gel transition of some pluronic polyols. *Int. J. Pharm.*, 22, 207–218.

Vangeyte, P., Gautier, S. and Jerome, R., 2004. About the methods of preparation of poly(ethylene oxide)-b-poly(ϵ caprolactone) nanoparticles in water: Analysis by dynamic light scattering. *Colloids and Surfaces A: Physicochemical and Engineering Aspects*, 242, 203–211.

de Verdiere, A.C. *et al.*, 1997. Reversion of multidrug resistance with polyalkylcyanoacrylate nanoparticles: towards a mechanism of action. *British Journal of Cancer*, 76(2), 198.

Vernon, B.L., Kim, S.W. and Bae, Y.H., 2000. Thermoreversible copolymer gels for extracellular matrix. *Journal of Biomedical Materials Research Part A*, 51(1), 69–79.

Vernon, B.L. *et al.*, 2003. Water-borne, *in situ* crosslinked biomaterials from phase-segregated precursors. *Journal of Biomedical Materials Research*, 64A, 447–456.

Vinogradov, S.V., Bronich, T.K. and Kabanov, A.V., 2002. Nanosized cationic hydrogels for drug delivery: preparation, properties and interactions with cells. *Advanced Drug Delivery Reviews*, 54(1), 135–147.

Wang, Y.S. *et al.*, 2002. Structural and biological characterization of pegylated recombinant interferon alpha-2b and its therapeutic implications. *Advanced Drug Delivery Reviews*, 54(4), 547–570.

Wanka, G., Hoffmann, H. and Ulbricht, W., 1990. The aggregation behavior of poly-(oxyethylene)-poly-(oxypropylene)-poly-(oxyethylene)-block-copolymers in aqueous solution. *Colloid and Polymer Science*, 268(2), 101–117.

van de Weert, M. *et al.*, 2000. The effect of a water/organic solvent interface on the structural stability of lysozyme. *Journal of Controlled Release*, 68(3), 351–359.

Whiteman, K.R. *et al.*, 2001. Poly(HPMA)-coated liposomes demonstrate prolonged circulation in mice. *Journal of Liposome Research*, 11, 153–164.

Wills, R.J., 1990. Clinical pharmacokinetics of interferons. *Clinical Pharmacokinetics*, 19(5), 390–399.

Wong, H.L. *et al.*, 2006. A mechanistic study of enhanced doxorubicin uptake and retention in multidrug resistant breast cancer cells using a polymer-lipid hybrid nanoparticle system. *Journal of Pharmacology and Experimental Therapeutics*, 317(3), 1372.

Xiong, X.Y., Tam, K.C. and Gan, L.H., 2005. Synthesis and thermal responsive properties of P(LA-*b*-EO-*b*-PO-*b*-EO-*b*-LA) block copolymers with short hydrophobic poly(lactic acid) (PLA) segments. *Polymer*, 46, 1841–1850.

Xiong, X.Y., Tam, K.C. and Gan, L.H., 2006. Synthesis and thermally responsive properties of novel Pluronic F87/polycaprolactone (PCL) block copolymers with short PCL blocks. *Journal of Applied Polymer Science*, 100(5), 4163–4172.

Xu, L. *et al.*, 1999. Transferrin-liposome-mediated systemic p53 gene therapy in combination with radiation results in regression of human head and neck cancer xenografts. *Human Gene Therapy*, 10, 2941–2952.

Yamamoto, Y. *et al.*, 2001. Long-circulating poly(ethylene glycol)-poly(D,L-lactide) block copolymer micelles with modulated surface charge. *Journal of Controlled Release*, 77, 27–38.

Yamamoto, Y. *et al.*, 2002. Temperature-related change in the properties relevant to drug delivery of poly(ethylene glycol)-poly(D,L-lactide) block copolymer micelles in aqueous milieu. *Journal of Controlled Release*, 82, 359–371.

Yamaoka, T., Tabata, Y. and Ikada, Y., 1993. Distribution and tissue uptake of poly(ethylene glycol) with different molecular weights after intravenous administration to mice. *Journal of Pharmaceutical Sciences*, 83(4), 601–606.

Yoshida, T. *et al.*, 2003. Newly designed hydrogel with both sensitive thermoresponse and biodegradability. *Journal of Polymer Science Part A: Polymer Chemistry*, 41, 779–787.

Zentner, G.M. *et al.*, 2001. Biodegradable block copolymers for delivery of proteins and water-insoluble drugs. *Journal of Controlled Release*, 72, 203–215.

Zeuzem, S. *et al.*, 2000. Peginterferon alfa-2a in patients with chronic hepatitis C. *The New England Journal of Medicine*, 343(23), 1666.

Zhou, Z. and Chu, B., 1988. Light-scattering study on the association behavior of triblock polymers of ethylene oxide and propylene oxide in aqueous solution. *Journal of Colloid and Interface Science*, 126(1), 171–180.

Zhu, G., Mallery, S.R. and Schwendeman, S.P., 2000. Stabilization of proteins encapsulated in injectable poly (lactide-co-glycolide). *Nature Biotechnology*, 18(1), 52–57.

6
Tissue engineering applications of injectable biomaterials

S. KONA, A. S. WADAJKAR and K. T. NGUYEN,
University of Texas at Arlington, USA

Abstract: Recently, injectable biomaterials have been applied extensively in the field of tissue engineering, due to their minimally invasive nature, reduced patient discomfort and complications along with a decrease in health care costs. Moreover, injectable biomaterials can form scaffolds *in situ* when they are exposed to various physiological conditions. This chapter outlines the major requirements and challenges faced in using injectable biomaterials for tissue engineering. It also summarizes the various gelation mechanisms, including both physical and chemical methods, at physiological conditions and discusses in brief selected injectable biomaterials and their composites along with their tissue engineering applications.

Key words: tissue engineering, *in situ* scaffolds, gelation mechanics, injectable composites.

6.1 Introduction

Over the last decade, tissue-engineering scaffolds made from various biomaterials have been developed to repair or replace injured and/or lost tissues. Although certain human tissues, such as the liver, exhibit an incredible ability for regeneration, other human tissues, such as skin and bones, can regenerate only if injuries are below a critical size. For injuries that are above critical size, tissue engineering scaffolds can be applied to replace lost or damaged tissue. To develop a viable biological replacement that has the ability to restore, maintain or improve tissue functions, the principles of both biological sciences and engineering are applied so that the cells seeded in scaffolds can adhere and interact with the surrounding extracellular matrix (ECM), proliferate, and perform their specific functions as shown in Fig. 6.1 (Zhang and Suggs, 2007). Thus three major factors, namely, cells, the scaffold upon which the cells are seeded, and any external stimuli (chemical factors or mechanical stimulus) are required in tissue-engineering scaffolds (Fig. 6.2). Of these factors, the scaffold or matrix assists in the regeneration of tissues by providing a three-dimensional (3D) structural support for initial cell attachment and subsequent proliferation to form new tissues. The scaffold also has the ability to load and release factors that

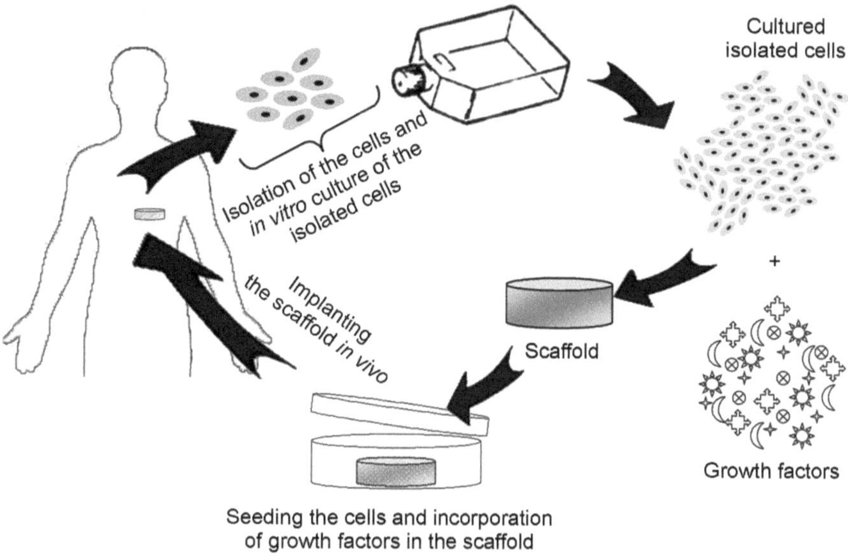

6.1 Schematic of concept of tissue engineering (inspired by online image seen at http://biomed.brown.edu/Courses/BI108/BI108_2007_Groups/group12/homepage.html).

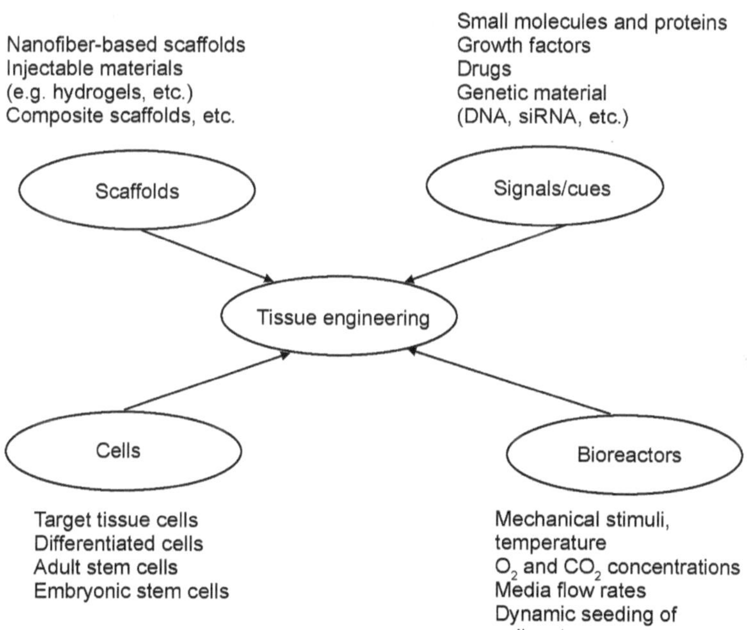

6.2 Key elements of tissue engineering (inspired by image on page 5 of the book *Nanotechnology and Tissue Engineering: The Scaffold,* Laurencin C.T. & Nair L.S., CRC Press).

facilitate proliferation of cells and maintain their differentiated functions (Hutmacher, 2001). Several materials including injectable materials have been used in the formation of scaffolds for tissue engineering. The following sections of this chapter will cover a brief discussion of the requirements of injectable biomaterials for tissue engineering applications and review of the types of injectable materials with their various tissue engineering applications.

6.2 Requirements of injectable materials for tissue engineering

There are several requirements that tissue engineering scaffolds need to satisfy for viable tissue regeneration. Along with being porous, the scaffold provides a 3D structure for cell attachment, growth, proliferation, differentiation and migration of the new cells, while allowing the cells to maintain their physiological functions. In addition, they act as space fillers to prevent unwanted cells from invading the affected area. The porous scaffold also facilitates an efficient transport of nutrients and growth factors and of waste removal (Laurencin and Nair, 2008). Moreover, scaffolds aid in vascularization, neotissue formation and tissue remodeling. Besides providing the above-listed critical functions for tissue engineering scaffolds, injectable biomaterials can also form scaffolds *in situ* and offer several benefits compared to pre-formed scaffolds. Along with being minimally invasive, injectable materials can easily fill irregular-shaped defects, overcome the difficulties of cell seeding, cell adhesion and delivery of therapeutic agents as these factors can be mixed with the material solution before being injected *in situ*. In addition, unlike the preformed scaffolds, scaffolds formed from injectable materials would have minimal amounts of toxic residual solvents and/or monomers (Gutowska *et al.*, 2001).

Therefore, all injectable materials must fulfill certain basic criteria for consideration as a suitable tissue engineering material to form functional scaffolds. These include adequate mechanical properties, biocompatibility (no adverse physiological or immune response), degradability, porosity, tissue-specific and cell–scaffold interactions, toxicity of the material itself and its degradation products, the elimination route of the degradation products and scaffold resorption rate. For instance, the mechanical properties of the material should be similar to the tissue that it is replacing. In addition, scaffolds made from these injectable materials should support attachment of cells, growth, differentiation and proliferation of the cells and should allow the cells to form their extracellular matrix. It should also degrade at a rate that is proportional to the rate of the new tissue formation and be easy to fabricate into a 3D scaffold. In addition to the above general considerations, properties of injectable biomaterials like gelation kinetics are important in tissue engineering applications. The gel kinetics, for example, is directly affected by methods of gelation. Thermal gelation is faster than gelation by pH or ionic changes, since the limiting step is heat transfer as opposed to mass transfer in case of pH or ionic gelation (Gutowska *et al.*, 2001). This in turn will also determine the cell distribution and spacing within the injected medium. Another important factor for injectable materials in tissue engineering applications is to overcome the possible interference of the gel matrix with the new tissue formation.

6.3 Injectable biomaterials: methods of gelation and tissue engineering applications

Injectable biomaterials are materials that can be handled and processed at room or ambient temperatures and subsequently be injected into the desired site where they then solidify in response to body conditions to take the shape of the defect. The advantage of these materials is that they can be prepared just before application and are easy to prepare. The injectable biomaterials are versatile in nature and in their applications. Possible areas of injectable materials in tissue engineering include bone, cartilage, cardiovascular tissues, bone cements, filling for bone defects and skin. Since, the materials will be injected into the body, the injectable formulations should ideally be prepared in a physiologically compatible solvent and should not release cytotoxic products during the transformation process or during the course of degradation (Hubbell, 1998). Depending upon their mode of fabrication and *in situ* hardening, injectable biomaterials can be classified into various categories like *in situ* crosslinking/polymerizing, precipitating systems and injectable gels (Hatefi and Amsden, 2002). Some of these materials along with the types and their applications are discussed in the next sections and summarized in Table 6.1.

6.3.1 Chemical polymerization materials

In situ polymerization of certain polymers occurs by chemically activated crosslinking reactions. In this type of polymerization, a chemical initiator forms free radicals that react with the functional groups (usually unsaturated bonds) in the monomers or macromers. This crosslinking reaction proceeds until all the monomer is crosslinked. This method of crosslinking improves the mechanical properties of the injectable scaffolds. By varying the chemical initiator concentrations and the type of crosslinkers, the density of crosslinking networks can be altered, which in turn varies the properties of the formed scaffolds (Timmer *et al.*, 2003a,b). Though this system has the benefit of being activated with change in amount or type of chemical initiators, a major limitation is the control of the gelling time so as to minimize necrosis of the surrounding tissue.

An example of this type of material is oligo(poly(ethylene glycol) fumarate (OPF). Successful formulation of cell-OPF scaffolds was achieved within 10 minutes at 37°C using a cytocompatible and water soluble thermal radical initiation system. In this system ammonium persulfate/*N*,*N*,*N*',*N*'-tetramethyl-

Table 6.1 Injectable biomaterials: methods of gelation and tissue engineering applications

Method of gelation	Materials	Tissue engineering applications	References
Chemical polymerization	OPEGF	Orthopedic	Temenoff *et al.* (2003), Park *et al.* (2007)
	HA derivatives	Cartilage	Zheng Shu *et al.* (2004), Kurisawa *et al.* (2005)
	PLAF	Bone	Jabbari and He (2008)
Thermoplastic pastes	MPEG-PCL	Bone	Kim *et al.* (2006)
	PDLLA-PEG-PDLLA, PLLA-PEO-PLLA	Soft tissue	Aamer *et al.* (2004), Zhang *et al.* (1996)
	PCL-PEG-PCL	Intraocular cavity	Reis and Romaìn (2005)
	PLGA-PEG-PLGA	Corneal wound repair	Pratoomsoot *et al.* (2008)
	MMA, AgCA, PPF, m-PEG	Tissue fillers	Zhang *et al.* (2006), Epple and Kirschnick (1997), Timmer *et al.* (2003a), Qiu and Yan (2009)
In situ photo-polymerization	PEGMA/PEGDA, PEO, PVA, DEF/PPF, PEG-RGD	Controlled release vehicles, adhesion prevention barriers	Sabnis *et al.* (2009), Nguyen and West (2002), Beck *et al.* (2007)
	Pluronics, OPEGF, HA, PPE, polyanhydrides based on sebasic acid/1,3-bis(p-caboxyphenoxy) propane/ 1,6-bis(p-carboxyphenoxy) hexane	Cell/islet encapsulation, bone	Burkoth *et al.* (2000), Burdick and Anseth (2002), Bryant and Anseth (2001), Mann *et al.* (2001), Salinas and Anseth (2008), Lin and Anseth (2009), Nguyen and West (2002), Missirlis *et al.* (2005, 2006), Park *et al.* (2003), Halstenberg *et al.* (2002), Jo *et al.* (2001a, 2001b), Zhao *et al.* (2003), Poshusta *et al.* (2003), Muggli *et al.* (1998)
In situ polymerization by ionic crosslinking	Alginate with $CaCO_3$	Cartilage	Gutowska *et al.* (2001), Park *et al.* (2009a), Paige *et al.* (1995)
		Soft tissue	Halberstadt *et al.* (2002), Loebsack *et al.* (2001)
		Vesicular reflux, urinary incontinence	Atala *et al.* (1993, 1994)

	Polysaccharide and protein-based hydrogels	Tissue repair and reconstruction	Westhaus and Messersmith (2001)
	Pentaerythritol tetrakis 3′-mercaptopropionate, PEGDA and pentaerythritol triacrylate	Hard tissue	Vernon *et al.* (2003)
pH crosslinking	Chitosan	Bone, cartilage, intervertebral disk tissue	Klokkevold *et al.* (1996), Di Martino *et al.* (2005), Chenite *et al.* (2000), Lu *et al.* (1999), Subramanian *et al.* (2005), Mwale *et al.* (2005)
Shear-thinning gels	HA, Restylane™	Soft tissue, lip augmentation Bone fracture, wound healing	Duranti *et al.* (1998), Nettles *et al.* (2004) Gutowska *et al.* (2001), Radomsky *et al.* (1998)
Self-polymerization	Tisseel®, fibrin gel, PLGA, porogens, peptide hydrogels	Adhesive sealant, dental and hard tissue	Kretlow *et al.* (2009), Krebs *et al.* (2009), Haines Butterick *et al.* (2007), Firth *et al.* (2006), Kirkham *et al.* (2007)
In situ precipitation	PCL, PLA, PLGA	Urinary incontinence	Coombes *et al.* (2004), Eliaz and Kost (2000), Oh *et al.* (2006), Shah *et al.* (1993)
Stimuli-sensitive injectable hydrogels			
Temperature-sensitive	PNIPA, PDEA, Pluronics	Biosensors, tissue fillers, bone	Kim *et al.* (2009), Hejcl *et al.* (2008), Jeong *et al.* (1997)
pH-sensitive	PAA, PDEAEM, chitosan	Bone, biosensors, permeation switches	Kim *et al.* (2009)
Electro-sensitive	Polyacrylamides	Actuators, artificial muscles	Shiga *et al.* (2003)
Light-sensitive	TPM leuco derivatives, sodium copper chlorophyllin	Photo-responsive artificial muscles, switches, memory devices	Mamada *et al.* (1990), Suzuki and Tanaka (1990)
Salt, ion, antigen, mechanical	PNIPAAm, PDADMACl, thixotrophic material	Tissue fillers, bone	Park and Hoffman (1993), Miyata *et al.* (1999), Barbucci *et al.* (2006)

ethylenediamine (APS/TEMED) was used as the chemical initiator, poly(ethylene glycol)–diacrylate (PEGDA) was the crosslinker for crosslinking of the polymer oligo(poly(ethylene glycol) fumarate) (OPF) (Temenoff *et al.*, 2003). This system was tested as an injectable carrier material for bone marrow mesenchymal stem cells (MSCs) to be used in orthopedic tissue engineering applications. Another example is the use of injectable biodegradable hydrogel OPF with encapsulated rabbit MSCs and gelatin microparticles (MPs) loaded with transforming growth factor-beta1 (TGF-β1) for cartilage tissue engineering applications. Results from this study indicate that encapsulated rabbit MSCs remained viable over the culture period, and differentiated into chondrocyte-like cells, suggesting the potential use of OPF hydrogels for localized delivery of stem cells and bioactive molecules (Park *et al.*, 2007).

In addition to OPF, hyaluronic acid (HA) derivatives are another example of chemical polymerization materials. When two thiolated HA derivatives were coupled to four alpha, beta-unsaturated ester and amide derivatives of poly (ethylene glycol) (PEG), they gelled *in situ* within 7–10 minutes (Zheng Shu *et al.*, 2004). Results of this study exhibited the potential use of this novel hydrogel as an *in situ* crosslinkable, injectable material for tissue engineering. Interestingly, an enzymatic oxidative coupling reaction that is found in one of the body's biosynthetic pathways has been used in injectable chemical crosslinking hydrogels. For instance, conjugates of hyaluronic acid–tyramine (HA-Tyr) were used in a study along with a peroxidase-catalysed oxidation reaction. This reaction is usually observed in the biosynthetic pathway of melanin formation in the body. In this study, when HA-Tyr solution, H_2O_2 (oxidant of horseradish peroxidase (HRP)) and HRP (a model catalyst that induces oxidative coupling of phenol moiety in the body) were injected, they formed hydrogels *in vivo* (Kurisawa *et al.*, 2005). From this study it was observed that this material was a potential biomaterial for tissue engineering.

Besides the above materials, unsaturated ultra low molecular weight (ULMW) poly (L-lactide) (PLA) (ULMW PLA), can also be used as an injectable *in situ* crosslinkable macromer for tissue engineering. Jabbari and He mixed ULMW PLA with fumaryl chloride to make unsaturated *in situ* crosslinkable poly (lactide fumarate) (PLAF) macromer. When this PLAF macromer was injected and crosslinked with 1-vinyl-2-pyrrolidinone (NVP) in the presence of NaCl crystals as porogen, porous scaffold was formed *in situ* (Jabbari and He, 2008). These porous scaffolds showed osteoconductive behavior and led to new bone formation when implanted in nude mice.

6.3.2 Thermoplastic pastes

Thermoplastic pastes are polymer solutions that have a low melting point, usually lower than 65°C. When these polymer solutions are injected into the targeted body site, the polymer solution cools rapidly to body temperature forming a partially crystallized structure (Hatefi and Amsden, 2002). Thermoplastic pastes usually have a low molecular weight which makes them suitable for injection (Hatefi and Amsden, 2002). In addition, these materials have a melting point close to body temperature, exhibit low melt viscosity and show a moderate degree of crystallinity so that neither cell growth within the scaffold is impeded nor release of growth factors or drugs occurs during the scaffold formation process (Amsden *et al.*, 2004). At a given temperature, the melt viscosity of thermoplastic pastes decreases with decreasing molecular weight of the polymer. Additionally, melt viscosity of the thermoplastic polymer solution is determined by the nature and relative amounts of monomers or co-monomers used (Carreau, 1997). Thus, to have a low melt viscosity, the monomer or one of the monomers must make a polymer with low glass transition temperatures (Amsden *et al.*, 2004). The stability of the gel after injection may also be altered by changing the ratios of slow to fast degrading monomers (Winternitz *et al.*, 1996). When the monomers are heated above their melting temperature to form polymers, the process is called as bulk polymerization (Wang *et al.*, 2002). Examples of thermoplastic pastes include polymers, copolymers or blends based on the biocompatible polyesters like poly (ϵ-caprolactone), poly(lactides) and poly(ethylene glycol).

A major limitation of these types of injectable materials is the requirement of high temperatures to melt or soften the polymers. This can cause pain and mild burns in patients and can also induce some amount of tissue necrosis. This is true even in polymers that exhibit very low melt temperatures (the temperature at the time of injection is 20°C to 25°C above body temperature). One way to overcome this drawback is to adjust the copolymerization or blending ratios of the constituent polymers. For example, addition of 30% of methoxy-poly(ethylene glycol) (MePEG) to PCL brought down the melting point to 50°C (Winternitz *et al.*, 1996). When such diblock copolymer solutions of methoxy poly (ethylene glycol)-poly(ϵ-caprolactone) (MPEG-PCL) were injected subcutaneously into Sprague-Dawley rats, they formed a gel at body temperature. After four weeks the gels were encased by a thin fibrous capsule and showed the presence of multipotent rat bone marrow stem cells (rBMSCs) as well as new bone formation (Kim *et al.*, 2006). In another instance, addition of 70% or more of lactide in poly(D,L-lactide)-poly(ethylene glycol)-poly(D,L-lactide) (PDLLA-PEG-PDLLA) copolymers prevented the crystallization and transformed the copolymer in a viscous liquid with melting point between 50°C and 60°C (Zhang *et al.*, 1996). A study by Aamer *et al.*, using PLLA–PEO–PLLA triblock copolymer hydrogels, showed that the elastic modulus of these triblock gels was similar to that of several soft tissues and was strongly dependent upon block length of PLLA. Hence, these materials were a suitable choice for a range of soft tissue engineering applications (Aamer *et al.*, 2004). In another study, it was possible to obtain formulations with melting temperature as low as 38°C, by adjusting the molecular weight of PCL-PEG-PCL triblock copolymers and this was found advantageous for injection into sensitive areas like the intraocular cavity (Reis and Romaìn, 2005). In a similar finding, it was seen that the triblock PLGA–PEG–PLGA polymer had suitable gelling characteristics and that this material exhibited a potential use in corneal wound repair (Pratoomsoot *et al.*, 2008). Other examples include methyl methacrylate, silver chloroacetate, poly(propylene fumarate), and methoxyl-PEG that are useful as tissue fillers and scaffolds in tissue engineering applications (Zhang *et al.*, 2006, Epple and Kirschnick, 1997, Timmer *et al.*, 2003a, Qiu and Yan, 2009).

6.3.3 *In situ* photo-polymerization materials

Photo-crosslinking materials have been investigated extensively for use in tissue engineering as a major benefit of these materials is that they can be formed *in situ* at a specific site by photo-polymerization. Photo-polymerization reactions for *in vivo* applications provide a convenient mean of polymerization with rapid polymerization rates at physiological temperatures, while allowing spatial and temporal control of the process. Since the pre-polymer materials are either liquid solutions or moldable putties, the systems can be easily placed in complex shapes and photo-polymerized *in situ* to form a scaffold. Adhesion of the *in situ* formed polymer to the surrounding tissue also improves significantly because of intimate contact of the polymer with the tissue during formation. Moreover, the invasiveness of surgical techniques can be minimized as the macromer is easily introduced at the defect and can be photo-cured with fiber optic cables, or even through tissues (Burkoth and Anseth, 2000).

Various photo-polymerizable polymers have been studied for tissue engineering applications. Examples include (di)methacrylic or (di)acrylic derivatives of poly(ethylene glycol), poly(ethylene oxide), poly(vinyl alcohol), and diethyl fumarate/poly(propylene fumarate). Of the photo-crosslinking materials, PEG-based materials are widely investigated for biomedical applications due to their advantageous properties such as biocompatibility, low immunogenicity, and ease of use. PEG functionalized with diacrylate (called PEG diacrylate or PEGDA) or dimethacrylate (PEGMA) groups crosslink to form non-degradable materials that are used in various biomedical applications like micro-encapsulation of islets, controlled release vehicles, adhesion prevention barriers and bone restorations (Sabnis *et al.*, 2009, Nguyen and West, 2002, Beck *et al.*, 2007). Moreover, photo-polymerizable PEG materials modified with arginine-glycine-aspartate (RGD) adhesive peptides have been used as cell encapsulation injectable materials (Burkoth *et al.*, 2000, Burdick and Anseth, 2002, Bryant and Anseth, 2001, Mann *et al.*, 2001, Salinas and Anseth, 2008, Lin and Anseth, 2009, Nguyen and West, 2002).

In addition to PEG-based materials, other materials such as polyphosphoester, polyanhydrides, poly(ethylene oxide)-poly(propylene oxide)-poly(ethylene oxide) (Pluronic), oligo(poly(ethylene glycol) fumarate) and hyaluronic acid have also been modified to form scaffolds for similar tissue engineering applications (Missirlis *et al.*, 2005, 2006, Park *et al.*, 2003, Halstenberg *et al.*, 2002, Jo *et al.*, 2001a,b). Polyphosphoester (PPE) (or polyphosphate when the side chain linking to the phosphorus atom is an alkoxy group) have been proposed for biomedical applications because of their ability to photo-crosslink, biodegradability, potential biocompatibility and versatility (Zhao *et al.*, 2003). Moreover, a group of polyanhydrides based on sebasic acid or its copolymers with either 1,3-bis(p-caboxyphenoxy)propane or 1,6-bis(p-carboxyphenoxy) hexane have also been developed as *in situ* photo-crosslinkable materials (Poshusta *et al.*, 2003, Burkoth *et al.*, 2000, Muggli *et al.*, 1998).

Although photo-polymerized injectable materials have been developed and applied in various tissue engineering applications, there are still some challenges. For instance, UV crosslinking to form scaffolds *in situ* can be harmful to the surrounding tissues. To overcome this limitation, photo-crosslinking can be carried out using visible light (in the blue region of the visible spectrum) (Sharifi *et al.*, 2009). Materials and methods to form polymers *in vivo* must also be considered for their biocompatibility and ease of use, respectively. The reaction conditions for *in vivo* applications are quite stringent. Other issues include a narrow range of physiologically acceptable temperatures, toxicity of monomers and of photoinitiators and/or solvents, moist and oxygen rich environments, the need for rapid processing, and clinically suitable rates of polymerization (Sabnis *et al.*, 2009, Nguyen and West, 2002, Burkoth and Anseth, 2000, Garrett *et al.*, 1999).

6.3.4 *In situ* crosslinking/polymerization materials

In this category of injectable biomaterials, the gel is formed between the liquid monomers or macromers and a suitable polymerization/crosslinker initiator in response to either ionic or pH changes. Advantages of these kinds of materials include easy placement and subsequent polymerization to fill complex shaped defects that otherwise would be difficult to fill, improved adhesion of the polymer to the surrounding tissue due to close mechanical interlocking with the micro-roughened surface of the tissue.

Polymerization by ionic crosslinking

Charged polymers that are soluble in aqueous solvents or water form gels when they react with di- or tri-valent counter ions. The process is a reversible gelation and upon removal of the cations such as Ca^{2+}, the gel becomes liquid. A well-known example of ionically crosslinked polymer gels are the alginate gels. When aqueous solutions of alginate are mixed with divalent cations like calcium carbonate, or other calcium salts, they form gels. The order of gelation varies in the order $Mg^{2+} < Ca^{2+} < Sr^{2+} < Ba^{2+}$. These gels have been studied at length for various tissue engineering applications like cartilage tissue engineering (Gutowska *et al.*, 2001, Park *et al.*, 2009a) and soft tissue reconstruction (Halberstadt *et al.*, 2002, Loebsack *et al.*, 2001). In alginates, the cations bind between the guluronic acid blocks of adjacent alginate chains, forming ionic interchain bridges (Rowley *et al.*, 1999). By controlling parameters such as alginate and calcium concentration and the molecular weight and composition of the alginate, it was possible to fabricate gels with desirable properties which supported *in vitro* cell cultures. Alginate gels have also shown promise as cell-encapsulation materials and as 3D injectable matrix for *in vivo* cell delivery and soft tissue engineering applications.

One example is the use of slowly polymerizing calcium alginate gels as injectable delivery vehicles of isolated chondrocytes for cartilage formation (Paige *et al.*, 1995). Freshly isolated articular chondrocytes from calf forelimbs were mixed with the alginate solution and injected subcutaneously in athymic mice. The formed tissue constructs were removed after six weeks and evaluated. Formation of new cartilage was seen in all cases and this was verified by histological examination. The chondrocytes also showed the ability to form hyaline cartilage as demonstrated by the immunohistochemistry results. In another instance, a rapid curing stable and uniform gel was formed using a 2% solution of alginate and $CaCl_2$. The gelation kinetics of these gels could be altered by varying the concentrations of alginate and calcium salts (Stevens *et al.*, 2004). In addition, it was seen that when cultured with chondrocytes, Ca-alginate gel was able to support periosteum-derived chondrogenesis. In another study, Ca-alginate gels formed with poorly water-soluble salts of calcium like $CaCO_3$ and $CaSO_4$ were shown to have a significant impact on the gelation rate and the mechanical properties (Kuo and Ma, 2001).

Another remarkable method of gel formation by ionic crosslinking is the use of thermal release of calcium from lipid vesicles/liposomes. This method of stimulating quick gelation of polysaccharide and protein-based hydrogels mimicked the biological approach of triggered release of Ca^{2+} from liposomal compartments of the cell. Westhaus and Messersmith formulated thermally triggerable liposomes by encapsulating $CaCl_2$ within liposomes formed from 90% dipalmitoylphosphatidylcholine and 10% dimyristoylphosphatidylcholine. These liposomes released more than 90% of entrapped Ca^{2+} when heated to 37°C. In addition, this thermally triggered Ca^{2+} release from liposomes was used to activate enzyme-catalyzed crosslinking of proteins to form hydrogels. In addition, when these Ca-loaded liposomes were mixed with fibrinogen and a Ca^{2+}-dependent transglutaminase enzyme and heated to 37°C, it formed a gel very quickly. This bioinspired material could be used for tissue repair and reconstruction (Westhaus and Messersmith, 2001).

Injectable materials formed by ionic crosslinking have been used in various tissue engineering applications. For example, in addition to being useful in cartilage tissue engineering applications, alginate gels have also been used for the treatment of vesicular reflux. Freshly isolated calf chondrocytes mixed with alginate solution were injected subcutaneously in athymic mice (Atala *et al.*, 1993, 1994). It was observed that the time taken to form the gel depended upon the calcium ions concentration and the temperature at which the chondrocytes were added to the polymer. These studies concluded that alginate could be used as a delivery system for chondrocytes and may be potentially useful in the treatment of reflux. The alginate gels could also be used for the treatment of urinary incontinence, reconstructive surgery, as well as anywhere in the human body where an injectable, biodegradable, and biocompatible material is necessary.

Another application example of injectable materials formed by ionic crosslinking is the use of water-borne biomaterials for hard tissue repair from injectable precursors (Vernon *et al.*, 2003). The phase-segregated precursors form crosslinked materials *in situ* under physiological conditions, by utilizing addition donors like pentaerythritol tetrakis 3′-mercaptopropionate (QT) and addition acceptors like poly(ethylene glycol) diacrylate (PEGDA), pentaerythritol triacrylate (TA), and poly(propylene oxide) diacrylate (PPODA). This study showed that it is possible to obtain an injectable high-modulus material with suitable mechanical properties and gelation kinetics for tissue augmentation and stabilization applications like mechanical stabilization of the intervertebral disc annulus.

Polymerization by pH crosslinking

In response to changes in pH of the solution, some of the charged water soluble polymers form pH-reversible gels. A specific example of this kind of injectable biomaterials is chitosan – a derivative of chitin. Deacetylation of chitin converts it into soluble chitosan. The degree of acetylation influences the physicochemical properties (e.g. solubility, reactivity, biodegradability) and cellular responses of chitosan (Freier *et al.*, 2005, Khor and Lim, 2003). Chitosan exhibits unique properties like biocompatibility, biodegradability, hydrophilicity, adsorption capability and high reactivity. In addition, chitosan is a cationic polysaccharide that exhibits a sol–gel transition at a pH of around 7. When the pH changes from neutral to slightly acidic, it reverts to liquid state; on the other hand, the polymer forms a gel when pH changes back to neutral ($pH = 7$). The effect of chitosan on osteoblast differentiation and *in vitro* bone formation have been studied (Klokkevold *et al.*, 1996). Results of this study indicated that chitosan promotes the differentiation of osteoprogenitor cells and may thus aid in the development of new bone. In another approach, neutral solutions of chitosan/polyol salt formulations formed monolithic gels at body temperature and physiological pH. These formulations were injected *in vivo* to form gel implants *in situ* and they successfully formed a matrix with living chondrocytes for cartilage tissue engineering applications (Chenite *et al.*, 2000).

In addition, Lu *et al.* also studied the effects of chitosan on rat knee cartilage formations (Lu *et al.*, 1999). Results of the samples after 1, 3 and 6 weeks of injecting 0.1% chitosan solution inside the rat knee articular cavity, found that chitosan decreased epiphyseal cartilage thicknesses and increased articular cartilage chondrocyte densities significantly. This suggested that chitosan, as an injectable material, could help in the tissue engineering of the articular cartilage. Chitosan has also shown some promise in tissue engineering of the intervertebral disk. A study of crosslinked chitosan hydrogels showed good results when injected into the degenerated nucleus pulposus of human cadaveric intervertebral disk, demonstrating its suitability as a scaffold for disk tissue engineering (Mwale *et al.*, 2005). Moreover, variations of chitosan have shown promise in articular cartilage, intervertebral disk and bone tissue engineering (Di Martino *et al.*, 2005).

Shear-thinning gels

A shear-thinning highly viscous polymer solution or slightly crosslinked gel is capable of forming a thick gel *in situ* when the shear force generated by injection is removed. Hyaluronic acid exhibits such a behavior and has been used for tissue engineering applications. For instance, Restylane™ (Q-Med Ltd, London, UK), a nonanimal hyaluronic acid gel was used as an injectable biomaterial for soft tissue augmentation (Duranti *et al.*, 1998). It has also been demonstrated that HA network can encapsulate articular chondrocytes *in vivo* (Nettles *et al.*, 2004). Modified hyaluronic acid had a long-lasting effect while maintaining good biocompatibility and was very suitable for lip augmentation and facial soft tissue recontouring (Beer, 2007, Bosniak *et al.*, 2004, Carruthers and Carruthers, 2005, Dastoor *et al.*, 2007, Kanchwala *et al.*, 2005, Klein, 2006, Schweiger *et al.*, 2008). Hyaluronic acid has also shown promise in bone fracture repair and wound healing (Gutowska *et al.*, 2001). In addition, single injection of sodium hyaluronate along with growth factor – basic fibroblast growth factor (bFGF) into a freshly created rabbit fibula fracture showed an increased bone and callus formation as well as an earlier restoration of mechanical strength at the fracture side. Moreover, a combined effect of sodium hyaluronate and b-FGF was also seen in this study (Radomsky *et al.*, 1998). Other studies of highly elasto-viscous solutions and gels of hyaluronan and its derivatives have also shown that these materials can be used as intercellular matrices for regeneration, viscosupplementation and developing new tissues (Balazs, 2004).

Self-polymerization

Certain materials form gels *in situ* without the aid of chemical initiators or any external factors by self-polymerization. Tisseel® (Baxter Biosciences, USA) is one of the earliest developed and clinically most successful phase separation systems. It uses a dual injection of fibrinogen and thrombin to form a fibrin clot or scaffold. Thrombin cleaves soluble fibrinogen into insoluble fibrin that then self assembles into fibrils resulting in formation of a fibrin gel. This material is widely used as an adhesive sealant to achieve hemostasis during surgical procedures (Kretlow *et al.*, 2009). Recent research showed that self-assembling peptide hydrogel that undergo shear thinning (i.e. material thins into a low viscosity gel under a shear stress), are promising candidates for injectable tissue applications (Haines-Butterick *et al.*, 2007). Self-assembling peptide amphiphiles have also shown their ability to mineralize under physiological conditions and have demonstrated some promise in dental and other hard tissue engineering applications (Firth *et al.*, 2006, Kirkham *et al.*, 2007).

6.3.5 *In situ* precipitation

In situ precipitation injectable materials are polymer solutions that precipitate when they come in contact with a non-solvent (physiological fluids) when injected into the body. Usually such polymers are hydrophobic in nature. The polymer solutions are prepared in physiologically tolerant solvents like dimethyl sulfoxide (DMSO) that are also miscible with water. Thus, when the polymer solution is injected into the body, the solvent diffuses and mixes with the physiological fluids while the polymer precipitates out to form the gel as it is not soluble in water. Major examples of this injectable material group include PCL, PLA and PLGA (poly(lactic-co-glycolic) acid) (Coombes *et al.*, 2004, Eliaz and Kost, 2000).

There are several applications of injectable materials that form scaffolds by *in situ* precipitation. For example, a copolymer of lactic and glycolic acid (PLGA) was formulated as an *in situ* precipitation system by dissolving in glycofurol, and the release of proteins was seen in this system (Eliaz and Kost, 2000). High amounts of protein (higher than 10%) generated numerous interconnected pores inside the matrix, greatly increasing the release kinetics. It was possible to control the release kinetics of the proteins from this system by increasing the polymer concentration or the molecular weight. In another study by Oh *et al.*, PLGA solution (10 wt% in tetraglycol) with PCL microparticles was used to prepare an injectable bulking agent for the effective prevention of particle migration and volume retention at the applied site (Oh *et al.*, 2006). After injection of this microparticle dispersed PLGA solution, the PLGA dissolved in tetraglycol solidified by the exchange of tetraglycol into water allowing for formation of solidified PLGA matrix. This enabled stable deposition of PCL particles in the PLGA matrix without the particle migration while the matrix is also able to maintain its initial volume, owing to the well-packed PCL microparticles. Then in the later stage, it is expected that tissue will be infiltrated into the space of the degraded PCL microparticles and thus can still maintain its volume. This PCL microparticle-dispersed PLGA solution could be used as an injectable bulking agent in treating urinary incontinence (Oh *et al.*, 2006). It should be noted that the polymer concentration determines the uniformity and stability of the gel matrix. The amount of the polymer or co-polymer ratio also controls the release (over a period of weeks to months) of the loaded therapeutics (drug or growth factors) from the gel scaffold. For example, the *in vitro* release studies of macromolecules (growth factors and proteins) showed that release occurs only via diffusion through the interconnecting channels formed by the macromolecules present in the gel matrix. In addition, the release was also influenced by the polymer concentration, the physico-chemical properties of the molecule, manner in which the molecule is incorporated as well as presence of other excipients in the formulation (Shah *et al.*, 1993).

6.3.6 Stimuli-sensitive injectable hydrogels

In addition to liquid macromonomer or prehydrogel solutions that can be polymerized *in situ*, different types of external stimuli (physical and chemical) can also be applied to induce hydrogel formation *in situ* and to provide a means for controlling 'on-off' release of the encapsulated therapeutic reagents within the scaffolds. The physical stimuli include temperature, electric fields, solvent composition, light, pressure, sound and magnetic fields; while the chemical stimuli include pH, ions and specific molecular recognition events. Further, these hydrogels can be classified based on the stimuli (Qiu and Park, 2001), as listed below.

Temperature-sensitive hydrogels

Most injectable hydrogels are temperature-dependent polymerizing hydrogels. The presence of hydrophobic groups, such as methyl, ethyl and propyl groups is the common characteristic of the temperature-sensitive polymers. Poly(*N*-isopropylacrylamide) (PNIPAAm), poly(*N,N*-diethylacrylamide) (PDEA) and Pluronics are the most widely used temperature-sensitive polymers. These materials have a lower critical solution temperature (LCST) in the range of 25–32°C. At LCST these polymers undergo a phase transition. The reverse thermal gelation phenomenon is a good strategy for the development of injectable biomedical systems (Jeong *et al.*, 1997, Qiu and Park, 2001) for the applications such as biosensors, scaffolds, tissue fillers, bone tissue engineering (Kim *et al.*, 2009) and spinal cord injury repair (Hejcl *et al.*, 2008).

pH-sensitive hydrogels

These polymer networks contain pendant acidic or basic groups that either accept or release protons in response to changes in pH. The most commonly used pH-sensitive polymers are poly(acrylic acid) (PAA), poly(*N*,*N*-diethyl-aminoethyl methacrylate) (PDEAEM) and chitosan. The presence of ionizable groups on polymer chains results in swelling of the hydrogels (Qiu and Park, 2001). Applications of pH-sensitive hydrogels include biosensors, permeation switches, and bone tissue engineering (Kim *et al.*, 2009).

Electro-sensitive hydrogels

Hydrogels sensitive to electric field or current are usually made of poly-electrolytes. They swell or shrink upon application of an electric field. Partially hydrolyzed polyacrylamide hydrogels in contact with anode and cathode electrodes undergo phase transition by a change in electric potential across the gel. The hydrated H^+ ions migrate toward the cathode resulting in loss of water at the anode side while negatively charged acrylic acid groups are electro-statically attracted towards the anode surface creating a uniaxial stress along the gel axis. This leads to shrinking of the hydrogel at anode side (Qiu and Park, 2001). Electro-sensitive hydrogels convert chemical energy to mechanical energy and therefore, can function as actuators and/or artificial muscles (Shiga *et al.*, 2003, Qiu and Park, 2001).

Light-sensitive hydrogels

Light-sensitive hydrogels are categorized into UV-sensitive and visible light-sensitive hydrogels. The UV-sensitive hydrogels contain a leuco derivative molecule, bis(4-dimethylamino) phenylmethyl leucocyanide. Upon UV irradiation, triphenylmethane leuco derivatives dissociate into ion pairs producing triphenylmethyl cations. Presence of UV irradiation swells the hydrogels due to an increase in osmotic pressure within the gel. Visible light-sensitive hydrogels contain a temperature-sensitive polymer and a light-sensitive chromophore such as trisodium salt of copper chlorophyllin. The chromophore absorbs light (e.g. 488 nm) which is then dissipated locally as heat by radiationless transitions. The temperature increase alters the swelling behavior of the polymer hydrogel (Qiu and Park, 2001). Light-sensitive hydrogels have applications in the development of photo-responsive artificial muscles, switches and memory devices (Mamada *et al.*, 1990, Qiu and Park, 2001, Suzuki and Tanaka, 1990).

Other stimuli-sensitive hydrogels

Some hydrogels are sensitive to specific ions and molecules. For instance, PNIPAAm and poly (diallyldimethylammonium chloride) hydrogels are sensitive to a critical concentration of sodium chloride in aqueous solution. The LCST of the hydrogel is lowered by increasing the chloride concentration, although the mechanism of this ion-sensitivity is unknown (Park and Hoffman, 1993).

Further, some hydrogels respond to specific antigens. These gels shrink by crosslinking interactions upon antigen–antibody binding and swell in the presence of free antigens reducing the crosslinking density (Miyata *et al.*, 1999). Another class of hydrogels show a thixotrophic property, where the thixotrophic material turns into a fluid in the presence of a mechanical stimulus and resumes its original consistency when the stimulus is removed. The possibility of injecting a preformed hydrogel avoids any problems due to *in situ* synthesis (Barbucci *et al.*, 2006).

6.4 Injectable composites and applications in tissue engineering

Recently, a combination of injectable biomaterials has been investigated for tissue engineering applications. These can be categorized as composite injectable materials that have two or more types of materials in the same injectable system. Use of these composite materials provides the advantage of versatility in tissue engineering applications. Depending upon the type of materials used, they can either be natural and natural origin composites or synthetic composite materials. A few of these composite injectable materials for tissue engineering applications are given in this section and outlined in Table 6.2.

6.4.1 Natural injectable composites

Several natural composite materials made of polysaccarides and proteins have been developed as injectable materials for tissue engineering applications. These materials include fibrin, polysaccharides – dextran, cellulose sulphate, pectin, starch, laminarin, xanthan gum, carrageenan and gellan gum. Natural materials offer the advantage of being similar to the biological macromolecules so that the host environment recognizes them and is able to metabolically use and degrade them (Mano *et al.*, 2007). In addition, they exhibit similarity with the extracellular matrix (ECM), enabling them to avoid chronic inflammation or immunological reactions, which are often observed with use of synthetic polymers. These natural materials can be extracted from plants, animal sources, algae, by fermentation of micro-organisms (Widner *et al.*, 2005) or produced *in vitro* by enzymatic processes (Chung *et al.*, 2003, Kobayashi *et al.*, 2003). Limitations of these materials include weak mechanical strength and fast degradation rate. Another important aspect to consider on the use of natural materials is that they can induce an undesirable immune response due to the presence of impurities and endotoxins, depending on the source of the material. Nevertheless, as knowledge about these natural materials increases, new approaches in control of material properties (mechanical and degradation rate) and enhancing material biocompatibility would be possible. This would enable development of better scaffolding materials to support functional tissue

Table 6.2 Injectable composites and applications in tissue engineering

Composite type	Materials	Tissue engineering applications	References
Natural composites	Fibrin with alginate, HA, chondroitin-sulfate	Cell delivery, cartilage, cardiomyoplasty treatment, myocardial infarction, skeletal muscles, skin regeneration	Perka *et al.* (2000), Park *et al.* (2005c), Chekanov *et al.* (2005), Christman *et al.* (2004), Beier *et al.* (2006), Wei *et al.* (2008), Hubbell (2003)
	Alginate with $Ca_3(PO_4)_2$, gelatin, chitosan	Wound healing, trabecular bone formation, cartilage	Luginbuehl *et al.* (2005), Balakrishnan *et al.* (2005, 2006), Balakrishnan and Jayakrishnan (2005), Park *et al.* (2005a), Li and Zhang (2005)
	Chitosan with collagen, PEG, Pluronics, PNIPA, chitin, PEO, acryloyl-PEG-RGD, anhydrides, aldehydes, glycerol phosphate, gelatin	Cartilage, corneal implants, cell delivery, vesicoureteral reflux or reflux esophagitis treatment, bladder cartilage formation, bone, periodontal surgery	Nettles *et al.* (2002), Rafat *et al.* (2008), Bhattarai *et al.* (2005a, 2005b), Chung *et al.* (2005a, 2005b), Chen and Cheng (2006), Cho *et al.* (2004), da Silva *et al.* (2008), Wang *et al.* (2009), Kuo and Ku (2008), Yeo *et al.* (2007b), Park *et al.* (2009b), Gerentes *et al.* (2002), Chenite *et al.* (2000), Hoemann *et al.* (2005a, 2005b), Shi *et al.* (2005a, 2005b), Xia *et al.* (2004)
	HA with Hylaform^{TM}, DTPH, RGD, PEGDA, gelatin, fibrin, carrageenan, chitosan, PNIPAAm, poly(NIPA-co-AAc)	Vocal fold insufficiency treatment, soft tissue, cartilage, ligament and bone formation, adipose tissue	Hallen *et al.* (1999), Shu *et al.* (2004, 2006), Zheng Shu *et al.* (2004), Pereira *et al.* (2009), Yamane *et al.* (2005), Tan *et al.* (2009a, 2009b), Chen *et al.* (2008), Na *et al.* (2007a, 2007b)

Table 6.2 Continued

Composite type	Materials	Tissue engineering applications	References
Synthetic composites	CM-chitin-HA, $Ca_3(PO_4)_2$ cement-PLGA, $\beta Ca_3(PO_4)_2$-alginate, Ca alginate-HAp-collagen, $Ca_3(PO_4)_2$-HA	Bone, osteochondral defects	Tokura and Tamura (2001, Ruhe *et al.* (2003, 2006), Matsuno *et al.* (2008), Tan *et al.* (2009b), Gao *et al.* (2002)
Bioactive composites			
Bioactive composite bone cement	Ca_3SiO_5 with $\beta Ca_3(PO_4)_2$, $Ca(H_2PO_4)_2 \cdot H_2O$	Bone	Huan and Chang (2009), Zhao *et al.* (2005)
Bioactive glass composites	Bioactive glass with chitosan-β-GP, PCL-PLA, PMMA	Orthopedic, bone fillers	Couto *et al.* (2009), Aho *et al.* (2004), Gonzalez Corchon *et al.* (2006)
Hydroxyapatite composites	HAp with agarose gel	Orthopedic, oral, maxillofacial surgery	Watanabe *et al.* (2007)
Calcium phosphate composites	$Ca_3(PO_4)_2$ with MHPC, $Ca_4(PO_4)_2$, and α-$Ca_3(PO_4)_2$	Bone, dental and craniofacial augmentation	Grimandi *et al.* (1998), Xu *et al.* (2008), Montufar *et al.* (2009)
Nanoparticles/microparticles-based composite hydrogels	PLGA NPs in HA, PNIPAAm NPs in PEGDA, PLGA MPs in PNIPAAm-chitosan, PLGA MPs in PVA, liposomes in HEC and PHEMA, gelatin MPs in PEGF hydrogels	Wound healing, contact lenses, cartilage	Yeo *et al.* (2007b), Ramanan *et al.* (2006), Sabnis *et al.* (2009), Gulsen *et al.* (2005), Park *et al.* (2005b)

regeneration. A brief discussion of natural based biomaterial composites (Fig. 6.3) of fibrin, alginate, chitin and hyaluronic acid follows.

Fibrin

Fibrin has shown promise as a cell delivery matrix in combination with other biodegradable materials, such as alginate (Perka *et al.*, 2000) or hyaluronic acid (Park *et al.*, 2005c) for cartilage tissue engineering. Fibrin glue (composite of fibrinogen and thrombin) has been demonstrated as a potential biomaterial scaffold to improve cellular cardiomyoplasty treatment and in myocardial infarction (Chekanov *et al.*, 2005, Christman *et al.*, 2004). Another tissue engineering application of this material is the use of myoblast-fibrin injection for reconstruction of skeletal muscle defects *in vivo* (Beier *et al.*, 2006). In addition, the use of fibrin-chondroitin-sulfate matrices as three-dimensional scaffolds for cartilage tissue engineering have shown promise in promoting adipose-derived adult stem cells differentiation into chondrocytes (Wei *et al.*, 2008). Thus, fibrin in combination with various growth factors, cells and polymers like PLGA, has shown promise as a biological scaffold for stem or primary cells to regenerate adipose tissue, bone, cartilage, liver, nervous tissue, ocular tissue, skin, tendons, and ligaments (Ahmed *et al.*, 2008).

Polysaccharides

Another group of natural materials that can be injected to form scaffolds *in situ* are polysaccharides. For this group of materials the physical properties, including solubility, flow behavior, gelling potential and/or surface and interfacial properties are determined by the composition of the monosaccharides, linkage types and patterns, chain shapes and their molecular weights. Some examples of polysaccharide injectable materials include alginate (alginic acid), chitin or chitosan and hyaluronic acid.

Alginate

Alginate mixed with other polymers or compounds has been used to form injectable scaffolds for tissue engineering. For instance, alginate in the presence of tricalciumphosphate and insulin-like growth factor, has been shown to promote gelation, assist bone cell attachment and provide osteoconductive conditions leading to an increase in the proliferation rate of osteoblast-like cells (Luginbuehl *et al.*, 2005). In another study, hepatocytes were successfully encapsulated in an injectable gel formed by periodate-oxidized sodium alginate crosslinked to gelatin in the presence of borax (Balakrishnan and Jayakrishnan, 2005). The cells remained viable for more than four weeks in this study. This composite also shows as a very good *in situ*-forming hydrogel wound dressing

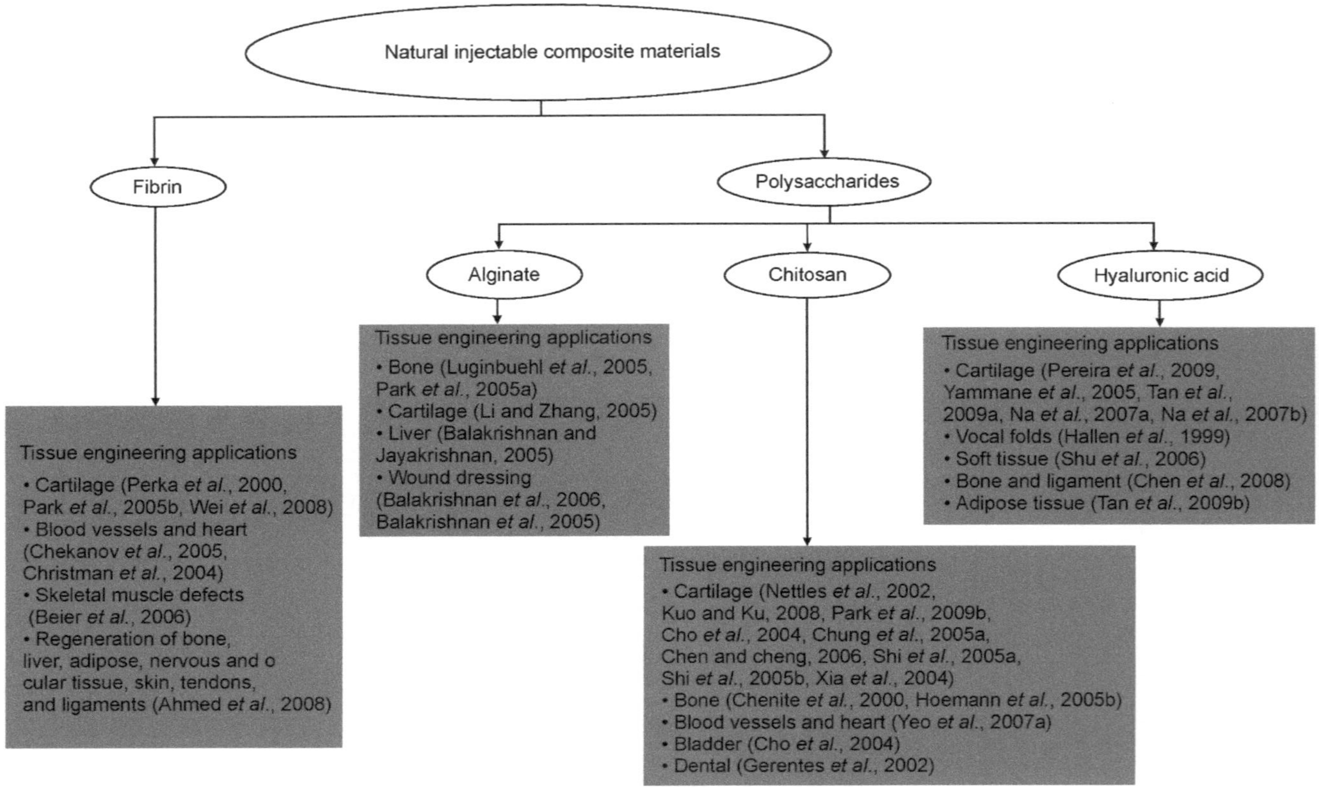

6.3 Flow chart depicting the various natural injectable materials and some of their tissue engineering applications.

material (Balakrishnan *et al.*, 2005, 2006). Sodium–alginate and chitosan solutions when combined with mesenchymal stem cells and BMP-2 (bone morphogenic protein-2) and injected subcutaneously, were able to stimulate new trabecular bone formation (Park *et al.*, 2005a). Study of alginate–chitosan scaffolds showed that these scaffolds promoted cell proliferation, enhanced phenotypic expression of HTB-94 chondrocytes and could potentially be used as an improved alternative to chitosan scaffolds for cartilage tissue engineering (Li and Zhang, 2005). However, a major drawback of alginate-based hydrogels is that the degradation occurs via a slow and unpredictable dissolution process *in vivo* (Rowley *et al.*, 1999, Boontheekul *et al.*, 2005, Bouhadir *et al.*, 2001).

Chitosan

Another injectable polysaccharide material widely used in tissue engineering applications is chitosan. Chitin-based polymers are versatile, can be processed into various forms and have been used for many tissue engineering applications in combination with other materials. Studies by Nettles *et al.* suggest that chitosan composite scaffolds may be a useful alternative to synthetic cell scaffolds for cartilage tissue engineering (Nettles *et al.*, 2002). For instance, collagen-chitosan composite hydrogels were studied for application as corneal implants and were found to have excellent optical properties, optimum mechanical properties and suturability, as well as good permeability to glucose and albumin (Rafat *et al.*, 2008). In addition, chitosan has been used in preparation of composite injectable materials by grafting synthetic temperature-sensitive polymers with low critical solution temperature (LCST) character to it. Examples include the grafting of polyethylene glycol (PEG) (Bhattarai *et al.*, 2005a,b), pluronic (Chung *et al.*, 2005a,b) and poly(*N*-isopropylacrylamide) (PNIPAAm) (Chen and Cheng, 2006, Cho *et al.*, 2004, da Silva *et al.*, 2008, Wang *et al.*, 2009) to a chitosan backbone. In PEG-chitosan grafts, hydrogen bonds between hydrophilic groups of PEG and water predominate at low temperature, while hydrophobic interactions between polymer chains prevail as temperature increases (Bhattarai *et al.*, 2005a). It was also observed that regeneration of cartilaginous components in bovine knee could be manipulated simply by controlling the composition of PEO, chitin, and chitosan in the novel PEO/chitin/chitosan hybrid scaffolds (Kuo and Ku, 2008). Furthermore, a blend of photocrosslinkable chitosan and acryloyl-poly(ethylene glycol)-RGDS (Az-chitosan/Acr-PEG-RGD) for myocyte cell culture and myocardial injection exhibited promising results (Yeo *et al.*, 2007a).

In addition to PEG-based chitosan composites, temperature-sensitive chitosan composites have also been developed for tissue engineering applications by grafting of pluronics onto chitosan. This composite material formed a thermo-sensitive hydrogel that exhibited a transition temperature of 30–35°C when the grafting percentage was altered (Chung *et al.*, 2005b). These thermosensitive chitosan-Pluronic (CP) hydrogels showed potential as injectable cell delivery carriers for cartilage tissue engineering and regeneration (Park *et al.*, 2009b). Moreover, when chitosan was grafted with PNIPAAm to form a blend of PNIPAAm-*g*-chitosan, it supported the culture of MSCs and allowed their differentiation into chondrocytes both *in vitro* and *in vivo* (Cho *et al.*, 2004, Chung *et al.*, 2005a). It was also observed that the hydrogel not only preserved the viability and phenotypic morphology of the entrapped cells (chondrocytes and meniscus cells) but also stimulated the initial cell–cell interactions (Chen and Cheng, 2006). In another study, thermo-sensitive composite gel (chitosan-g-PNIPAAm) was evaluated for its ability to differentiate mesenchymal stem cells (MSCs) into chondrocytes and form cartilage *in vivo* after injecting a thermo-sensitive gel complex. Formation of neo-cartilage suggested the use of this material in treatment of vesicoureteral reflux or reflux esophagitis by the effective mass effect as well as in cartilage formation (Cho *et al.*, 2004).

Chitosan-based thermally gelling materials can also be formed by chemical modification of chitosan with alcohol, anhydrides or aldehydes (Gerentes *et al.*, 2002) and has shown promise for use in periodontal surgery and tissue regeneration. Furthermore, when acidic chitosan (C) solutions are neutralized with glycerol phosphate (GP) they form a thermally gelling solution (C–GP) at approximately neutral pH (6.8–7.2) (Chenite *et al.*, 2000). These C–GP gels could deliver active bone protein *in vivo* leading to new cartilage and bone formation. Furthermore, Hoemann *et al.* found then when loaded with primary articular chondrocytes, the C–GP gels preserved the viability and phenotype of the chondrocytes. The gel was also present in a mobile osteochondral defect for a week and served as a scaffold to help build new tissue (Hoemann *et al.*, 2005b). Moreover, C–GP/blood implant in microfracture defects improved cartilage repair compared with microfracture alone by increasing the amount of tissue and improving its biochemical composition and cellular organization (Hoemann *et al.*, 2005a). When chitosan was blended with type II collagen, it formed a porous 3-D biomimetic matrix that supported chondrocyte growth for cartilage tissue engineering (Shi *et al.*, 2005a,b). It was also demonstrated that chitosan-gelatin scaffold exhibited successful engineering of elastic cartilages at the porcine abdomen subcutaneous tissues, using autologous auricular cartilage cells (Xia *et al.*, 2004). However, an important drawback with use of chitosan is its acute inflammatory response when injected subcutaneously (Molinaro *et al.*, 2002). The higher the degree of deacetylation, the stronger is the inflammatory response.

Hyaluronic acid

Hyaluronic acid (HA), an important component of connective tissue, synovial fluid (the fluid that lubricates joints) and the vitreous humor of the eye, exhibits clear viscoelastic properties that makes it an excellent biological absorber, lubricant and an injectable material for tissue engineering applications. Hyaluronan cross-linked with divinyl sulfone (Hylaform^{TM}) was shown to be a good candidate material for treatment of vocal fold insufficiency in humans (Hallen *et al.*, 1999). Studies also showed that attachment, spreading, and proliferation of cells was significantly enhanced on a thiol-modified HA (3,3′-dithiobis(propanoic dihydrazide) (HA-DTPH) containing the Arg-Gly-Asp (RGD) sequence crosslinked with PEGDA and that only modest accelerated *in vivo* tissue formation was seen in these composite materials (Shu *et al.*, 2004). Results with HA-DTPH-PEGDA hydrogels confirm the potential utility of this material as an *in situ* crosslinkable, injectable material for tissue engineering (Zheng Shu *et al.*, 2004). When hyaluronan (HA–DTPH), chondroitin sulfate (CS–DTPH) and gelatin (Gtn–DTPH) (three chemically modified thiolated dithiopropionylhydrazide derivatives) were crosslinked with each other, it was seen that the HA-Gtn and CS-Gtn hydrogels supported growth and proliferation of cultured murine fibroblasts *in vitro*. Moreover, subcutaneous injection of a suspension of murine fibroblasts with these hydrogels into nude mice resulted in the formation of viable and uniform soft tissue *in vivo* (Shu *et al.*, 2006). Furthermore, composites of hyaluronic acid, fibrin and carrageenan hydrogels have been demonstrated as a novel delivery system for cartilage tissue engineering (Pereira *et al.*, 2009). This material was able to regenerate and repair a lesion made in bovine articular cartilage in immunodeficient mice, as shown in this study (Pereira *et al.*, 2009).

Composites of HA with other materials such as chitosan and temperature-sensitive polymers showed great promise as cartilaginous tissue scaffolds (Yamane *et al.*, 2005). For instance, a study using N-succinyl-chitosan (S-CS) and aldehyde hyaluronic acid (A-HA) observed that the composite hydrogel supported encapsulation of bovine articular chondrocytes and the cells retained chondrocytic morphology (Tan *et al.*, 2009a). In addition, conjugation of hyaluronic acid-tethered bone morphogenetic protein-2 stimulated periosteal progenitor cells, fibrocartilagenous attachment and new bone formation in an extra-articular tendon-bone healing model, indicating that it would be effective in formation of anterior cruciate ligament (Chen *et al.*, 2008). Composites of hyaluronic acid with temperature-sensitive hydrogels demonstrate their potential use in various tissue engineering applications. For example, hyaluronic acid blended with PNIPAAm-co-AAc was found to be an efficient injectable cell vehicle and supporting matrix for the chondrogenic differentiation of chondrocytes in rabbits (Na *et al.*, 2007a). Moreover, the same thermo-reversible hydrogel composite showed significantly higher differentiation and cartilage-specific ECM production indicating neocartilage formation in the presence of HA (Na *et al.*, 2007b). In addition to cartilage tissue engineering applications, HA composite injectable materials also demonstrate their potential to replace other tissues. For instance, when human adipose-derived stem cells (ASCs) were encapsulated in the thermosensitive copolymer hydrogel, aminated hyaluronic acid-g-poly (*N*-isopropylacrylamide) (AHA-g-PNIPAAm), they preserved the viability of the entrapped cells and showed formation of adipose tissue *in vivo* suggesting that this material could be used as an injectable hydrogel for adipose tissue engineering and other tissue engineering applications (Tan *et al.*, 2009b).

Another example of an injectable bone tissue engineering material is the use of inorganic materials such as calcium phosphate, hydroxyapatite (HAp) and hydrogel materials like alginate, collagen and HA derivatives. For instance, a composite injectable material made of beta-tricalcium phosphate (beta-TCP) beads as the solid phase and alginate as the gel phase exhibited the ability to support osteogenic differentiation of mesenchymal stem cells (MSC) and new bone formation (Matsuno *et al.*, 2008). In addition, the use of an injectable and *in situ*-forming gel composite (GC) comprised of calcium alginate hydrogel and nano-hydroxyapatite/collagen (nHApC), exhibited the controllable initial and final setting time. It also demonstrated that the injectability of GC was tunable, suggesting its suitability for bone repair and bone tissue engineering (Tan *et al.*, 2009c). The composite material composed of injectable calcium phosphate (ICP) and hyaluronan (HA) derivate also showed evidence of extensive osteoclastic and osteoblastic activities in the bone tissue surrounding the defect edge and the injected composite material in young adult rabbit knee (Gao *et al.*, 2002). In addition, healing tissue of the ICP-HA material loaded with autologous bone marrow-derived progenitor cells (MPCs) showed a higher cellular density and better integration with the surrounding cartilage than ICP-HA material not loaded with MPCs, suggesting that the use of a two-phase composite graft holds promise as an injectable material in the repair of osteochondral defects (Gao *et al.*, 2002).

6.4.2 Synthetic composite materials

Similar to the materials that are natural in origin, some synthetic man-made composite materials have also shown promise as injectable materials. Some of these materials are composed of inorganic compounds (for example calcium) and gel *in situ*. When used in combination with other hydrogel materials, it is possible to control their initial and final setting time, tune their injectability and *in situ* pore formation. These materials are used mostly for bone and cartilage regeneration. The advantage of using such a synthetic composite graft is that it not only provides the mechanical support required for new bone formation but also serves as a scaffold for the repair of cartilage and bone tissue.

There are several synthetic composite materials and their applications in tissue engineering are versatile. For instance, in one study a composite of carboxymethyl-chitin (CM-chitin) with hydroxyapatite (HAp) was examined for its ability to repair bone in animals. New bone formation of CM-chitin-HAp composite was superior to that of CM-chitin, HAp, and control (Tokura and Tamura, 2001). The porous CM-chitin-HAp composite was also a functional material which could act as a scaffold for osteoblast cells as well as provide a barrier for growth of fibrous connective tissues (Tokura and Tamura, 2001). In another example, an injectable composite of calcium phosphate cement containing PLGA microparticles for sustained delivery of recombinant human bone morphogenetic protein-2 (rhBMP-2) for new bone formation was studied (Ruhe *et al.*, 2003). The ability of porous calcium phosphate (Ca-P)/poly(DL-lactic-co-glycolic acid) cement composite in reconstruction of bone defects was also studied by the same group (Ruhe *et al.*, 2006). Ca-P cements are injectable, self-setting ceramic pastes, known for their favorable bone response. In this system, the initial porosity could be induced by CO_2 foaming during setting of the cement, whereas secondary porosity could develop after hydrolysis of incorporated PLGA microparticles. Ingrowth of bone and subsequent degradation rates can be enhanced by the inclusion of macropores. Histological analysis of explanted composites revealed that bone and fibrous tissue ingrowth was facilitated by addition of PLGA microparticles with significant increase in composite density due to bone ingrowth. In addition, bone-like mineralization in subcutaneous implants suggested that the porous PLGA/Ca-P cement composites exhibit osteoinductive properties (Ruhe *et al.*, 2006).

6.4.3 Bioactive composites

Bioactive composite materials have been investigated to overcome limitations of various synthetic materials including cell and tissue integration. Some materials like certain ceramics and glasses tend to promote tissue regeneration when they come in contact with human plasma. Though ceramic-based injectable materials have been proposed for use in tissue engineering, they typically generate considerable amounts of heat during the curing of the polymer, so cells and growth factors cannot be introduced in these materials. However, the use of injectable hydrogel bioactive composite systems can overcome this limitation. Examples of these materials include bioactive composites of bone cements, bioglass, hydroxyapatite, and calcium phosphates which are discussed below in brief.

Bioactive composite bone cements

Bioactive composite bone cements can be formed by incorporation of tricalcium silicate (Ca_3SiO_5, C_3S) into a brushite bone cement composed of beta-tricalcium phosphate (beta-$Ca_3(PO_4)_2$, beta-TCP) and monocalcium phosphate monohydrate ($Ca(H_2PO_4)_2{\cdot}H_2O$, MCPM). This material exhibited higher injectability, setting time, short- and long-term mechanical strength as well as increased compressive strength with an increase in the aging time. These materials also showed significant *in vitro* bioactivity in simulated body fluid (SBF) and ability to stimulate osteoblast proliferation and promote osteoblastic differentiation of the bone marrow stromal cells. These results indicate that TCP/MCPM/C_3S cements can serve as a bioactive material for bone regeneration (Huan and Chang, 2009). In addition, tricalcium silicate (Ca_3SiO_5) also showed promise as an injectable bioactive and dissolvable material. In the *in vitro* bioactivity study it showed that it could induce hydroxyapatite (HAp) formation in SBF, suggesting its potential use as an injectable material for bone tissue repair and regeneration (Zhao *et al.*, 2005).

Bioactive glass composites

Bioactive glass materials have been incorporated with other materials including chitosan–β-glycerophosphate salt formulations to serve as temporary injectable scaffolds for orthopedic reconstructive and regenerative applications. *In vitro* bioactivity tests in SBF with this material showed the formation of bone-like apatite formation in the hydrogels, and the density of the apatite formed increased with increasing bioactive glass content and soaking time in SBF (Couto *et al.*, 2009). Furthermore, an injectable composite of particulate bioactive glass $S_{53}P_4$ (BAG) and poly(ϵ-caprolactone-co-D,L-lactide) was used as bone fillers in cancellous and cartilagineous subchondral bone defects in rabbits. Results showed that the glass granules of the composites resulted in good osteoconductivity and bone bonding at the interface between the glass and the host bone. The bone bioactivity index (BBI) indicating bone contacts between BAG and bone, as well as the bone coverage index (BCI) indicating bone ongrowth, correlated with the amount of glass in the composites. This composite material is also used in the articular surface cartilage regeneration (Aho *et al.*, 2004). In addition, injectable self-curing systems based on phosphate-free bioactive glasses and poly (methyl methacrylate) (PMMA) were investigated *in vivo* by injecting a cement dough into a defect created in the femur of rabbits and curing the cement *in situ*. In contrast to control PMMA, all bioactive formulations containing bioactive glass showed resorption of the PMMA cement. This could be attributed to the presence of the resorbable bioactive glass. Furthermore, cements formulated with bioactive glasses showed maximum neo-bone formation within two weeks and a more stable bone at the end of the eight weeks (Gonzalez Corchon *et al.*, 2006).

Hydroxyapatite composites

HAp composite materials have been used in bone tissue engineering applications. When a quick forming hydroxyapatite (HAp)/agarose gel composite was injected into the medial femoral condyle of rabbits, newly-formed bone was observed at the edge of the bone defect site two weeks postoperatively (Watanabe *et al.*, 2007). At four weeks postoperatively, excellent bone regeneration was observed and the composite gradually degraded, and disappeared at eight weeks postoperatively. These results indicated that the composite dissolved rapidly, and was replaced by newly formed bone, suggesting that the quick-forming HAp/agarose gel composites were also a good candidate as an injectable biomaterial for application in the fields of orthopedic, oral, and maxillofacial surgery (Watanabe *et al.*, 2007).

Calcium phosphate composites

Composites of calcium phosphate have shown promise in bone tissue engineering applications. For example, an injectable multiphasic bone substitute (IBS) material composed of 2% aqueous solution of methylhydroxypropylcellulose (MHPC) and biphasic calcium phosphate (BCP, 60% hydroxyapatite and 40% beta-tricalcium phosphate) in which MHPC served as the carrier for 80–200 micron of BCP granules was evaluated for percutaneous orthopedic surgery. A preliminary *in vivo* test in rabbit femoral epiphysis showed bone ingrowth into the scaffold after one week. This bone ingrowth increased regularly from the surface inward at 2, 4, and 10 weeks. At the same time, smaller BCP granules (less than 80 microns in diameter) were degraded and resorbed. Water solubility and viscosity of the polymer allowed cells to recolonize, with *in situ* bonding of the mineral phase (Grimandi *et al.*, 1998). In addition, *in situ*-hardening calcium phosphate cement (CPC) composite scaffolds were also investigated for probable application in dental and craniofacial applications (Montufar *et al.*, 2009, Xu *et al.*, 2008). Tetracalcium phosphate (TTCP: $Ca_4(PO_4)_2O$) and dicalcium phosphate (DCPA: $CaHPO_4$) were used to fabricate self-setting calcium phosphate cement. In this study, osteoblast cells were able to infiltrate into the macropores, establish cell–cell junctions, and anchor to the nano-apatite walls of the pores. Thus this material has potential dental and craniofacial uses including mandibular and maxillary ridge augmentation (Xu *et al.*, 2008). Furthermore, novel fully synthetic self-setting injectable calcium phosphate foam was developed recently, by mixing α-tricalcium phosphate (α-TCP) powder with a foamed polysorbate 80 solution. *In vitro* assessment of these foams showed their ability to sustain proliferation and differentiation of osteoblastic-like cells, indicating its ability for bone regeneration (Montufar *et al.*, 2009).

6.4.4 Nanoparticle/microparticle-based composite hydrogels

Particle-based composite hydrogels have been developed as injectable materials to provide loading and controlled release of therapeutic reagents such as growth factors for tissue engineering applications. In addition to biodegradability and *in situ* formation, the three dimensional composite networks containing chemical cues are attractive for tissue engineering. This allows delivery of drugs, growth factors and/or cells entrapped in the materials to the target tissue (Li *et al.*,

2006). Microspheres, nanoparticles and liposomes can be added to the gel solution to form composite materials. Although microspheres are easy to inject, they are difficult to formulate to have a uniform diameter and porosity. Furthermore, there is the potential problem of microsphere migration from the site of injection (Liggins *et al.*, 2000). The composite hydrogels increase the biocompatibility of these particles by hiding them within the network. They also prevent the particle migration away from the target site. The composite hydrogel networks provide multiple compartments and hence the multiple diffusion barriers for substances such as cell, growth factors and/or drugs incorporated in the network (Hoare and Kohane, 2008).

Particles entrapped in the physically crosslinked hydrogels are commonly used for tissue engineering application. For example, poly(lactic-co-glycolic acid) (PLGA) nanoparticles are embedded in a hyaluronan-based hydrogels maintaining the biocompatibility and anti-adhesion properties of the hyaluronic acid carrier (Yeo *et al.*, 2007b). PNIPAAm nanoparticles can be embedded within PEGDA hydrogels for wound healing applications (Ramanan *et al.*, 2006, Sabnis *et al.*, 2009). Few other examples include PLGA microparticles entrapped in a chitosan grafted PNIPAAm matrix and poly(vinyl alcohol) hydrogels, liposomes entrapped in hydroxyethylcellulose-based and poly(hydroxyethyl methacrylate) hydrogels for use as contact lenses (Gulsen *et al.*, 2005). Furthermore, a poly(ethylene glycol fumarate) matrix containing gelatin microparticles to deliver transforming growth factor (TGF-β1) has been developed for cartilage tissue repair (Park *et al.*, 2005b).

6.5 Conclusion and future trends

In summary injectable biomaterials can be natural or synthetic in nature. They can form gels by chemical initiation, changes in temperature and pH, by *in situ* photopolymerization, crosslinking or precipitation. In addition, these materials can be used by themselves or in combination with other materials to form composite materials. These injectable biomaterials have shown promise for various tissue engineering applications like bone, cartilage, dental, cardiovascular and soft tissue regeneration. Although these injectable materials are very versatile, permitting excellent control and ease of handling as well as being able to tailor them for a specific application, several concerns also exist with their use. These include the possible toxicity of initiators, monomers, oligomers or macromers that come in contact with the tissues before either complete polymerization or crosslinking or due to incomplete curing. Another concern with their use is the rate of polymerization. The rate of polymerization should be sufficiently quick so that the injectable material can harden in an adequate period of time. Potential harm caused by some toxic solvents used as a medium for delivery of the injectable materials is another cause for concern. Last but not the least concern is the potential injury to the surrounding tissues caused by the moderate temperature rise during the curing or gelling process. This rise in temperature is because most of the reactions for *in situ* scaffold formation are exothermic in nature. However, various alternatives such as use of block copolymers, proposed in recent years, have proven to be suitable for tissue engineering applications. Future work aimed at engineering injectable biodegradable composites with required mechanical properties and tissue-specific injectable scaffolds could provide a means for studying *in situ* scaffold–cell interactions and their effect on histogenesis. These advances in the field would not only decrease patient discomfort and costs, but would also provide an important step in the direction of minimally invasive surgery for all.

6.6 References

Aamer, K. A., Sardinha, H., Bhatia, S. R. & Tew, G. N. (2004) Rheological studies of PLLA-PEO-PLLA triblock copolymer hydrogels. *Biomaterials*, 25, 1087–93.

Ahmed, T. A., Dare, E. V. & Hincke, M. (2008) Fibrin: a versatile scaffold for tissue engineering applications. *Tissue Eng Part B Rev*, 14, 199–215.

Aho, A. J., Tirri, T., Kukkonen, J., Strandberg, N., Rich, J., Seppälä, J. & Yli-Urpo, A. (2004) Injectable bioactive glass/biodegradable polymer composite for bone and cartilage reconstruction: concept and experimental outcome with thermoplastic composites of poly(ϵ-caprolactone-co-D,L-lactide) and bioactive glass S53P4. *Journal of Materials Science: Materials in Medicine*, 15, 1165–73.

Amsden, B., Hatefi, A., Knight, D. & Bravo-Grimaldo, E. (2004) Development of biodegradable injectable thermoplastic oligomers. *Biomacromolecules*, 5, 637–42.

Atala, A., Cima, L. G., Kim, W., Paige, K. T., Vacanti, J. P., Retik, A. B. & Vacanti, C. A. (1993) Injectable alginate seeded with chondrocytes as a potential treatment for vesicoureteral reflux. *J Urol*, 150, 745–7.

Atala, A., Kim, W., Paige, K. T., Vacanti, C. A. & Retik, A. B. (1994) Endoscopic treatment of vesicoureteral reflux with a chondrocyte-alginate suspension. *J Urol*, 152, 641–3; discussion 644.

Balakrishnan, B. & Jayakrishnan, A. (2005) Self-cross-linking biopolymers as injectable *in situ*-forming biodegradable scaffolds. *Biomaterials*, 26, 3941–51.

Balakrishnan, B., Mohanty, M., Umashankar, P. R. & Jayakrishnan, A. (2005) Evaluation of an *in situ* forming hydrogel wound dressing based on oxidized alginate and gelatin. *Biomaterials*, 26, 6335–42.

Balakrishnan, B., Mohanty, M., Fernandez, A. C., Mohanan, P. V. & Jayakrishnan, A. (2006) Evaluation of the effect of incorporation of dibutyryl cyclic adenosine monophosphate in an *in situ*-forming hydrogel wound dressing based on oxidized alginate and gelatin. *Biomaterials*, 27, 1355–61.

Balazs, E. A. (2004) Viscosupplementation for treatment of osteoarthritis: from initial discovery to current status and results. *Surg Technol Int*, 12, 278–89.

Barbucci, R., Leone, G. & Lamponi, S. (2006) Thixotrophy property of hydrogels to evaluate the cell growing on the inside of the material bulk (amber effect). *J Biomed Mater Res B Appl Biomater*, 76, 33–40.

Beck, J., Angus, R., Madsen, B., Britt, D., Vernon, B. & Nguyen, K. T. (2007) Islet encapsulation: strategies to enhance islet cell functions. *Tissue Eng*, 13, 589–99.

Beer, K. R. (2007) Rejuvenation of the lip with injectables. *Skin Therapy Lett*, 12, 5–7.

Beier, J. P., Stern-Straeter, J., Foerster, V. T., Kneser, U., Stark, G. B. & Bach, A. D. (2006) Tissue engineering of injectable muscle: three-dimensional myoblast-fibrin injection in the syngeneic rat animal model. *Plast Reconstr Surg*, 118, 1113–21; discussion 1122–4.

Bhattarai, N., Matsen, F. A. & Zhang, M. (2005a) PEG-grafted chitosan as an injectable thermoreversible hydrogel. *Macromol Biosci*, 5, 107–11.

Bhattarai, N., Ramay, H. R., Gunn, J., Matsen, F. A. & Zhang, M. (2005b) PEG-grafted chitosan as an injectable thermosensitive hydrogel for sustained protein release. *J Control Release*, 103, 609–24.

Boontheekul, T., Kong, H. J. & Mooney, D. J. (2005) Controlling alginate gel degradation utilizing partial oxidation and bimodal molecular weight distribution. *Biomaterials*, 26, 2455–65.

Bosniak, S., Cantisano-Zilkha, M. & Glavas, I. P. (2004) Nonanimal stabilized hyaluronic acid for lip augmentation and facial rhytid ablation. *Arch Facial Plast Surg*, 6, 379–83.

Bouhadir, K. H., Lee, K. Y., Alsberg, E., Damm, K. L., Anderson, K. W. & Mooney, D. J. (2001) Degradation of partially oxidized alginate and its potential application for tissue engineering. *Biotechnol Prog*, 17, 945–50.

Bryant, S. J. & Anseth, K. S. (2001) The effects of scaffold thickness on tissue engineered cartilage in photocrosslinked poly(ethylene oxide) hydrogels. *Biomaterials*, 22, 619–26.

Burdick, J. A. & Anseth, K. S. (2002) Photoencapsulation of osteoblasts in injectable RGD-modified PEG hydrogels for bone tissue engineering. *Biomaterials*, 23, 4315–23.

Burkoth, A. K. & Anseth, K. S. (2000) A review of photocrosslinked polyanhydrides: *in situ*-forming degradable networks. *Biomaterials*, 21, 2395–404.

Burkoth, A. K., Burdick, J. & Anseth, K. S. (2000) Surface and bulk modifications to photocrosslinked polyanhydrides to control degradation behavior. *J Biomed Mater Res A*, 51, 352–9.

Carreau, P. J. (1997) *Rheology of Polymeric Systems: Principles and Applications*, New York, Hanser Publishers.

Carruthers, J. D. & Carruthers, A. (2005) Facial sculpting and tissue augmentation. *Dermatol Surg*, 31, 1604–12.

Chekanov, V., Kipshidze, N. & Nikolaychik, V. (2005) Cell transplantation and fibrin matrix. *J Am Coll Cardiol*, 45, 1734–5; author reply 1735–6.

Chen, C. H., Liu, H. W., Tsai, C. L., Yu, C. M., Lin, I. H. & Hsiue, G. H. (2008) Photoencapsulation of bone morphogenetic protein-2 and periosteal progenitor cells improve tendon graft healing in a bone tunnel. *Am J Sports Med*, 36, 461–73.

Chen, J. P. & Cheng, T. H. (2006) Thermo-responsive chitosan-graft-poly(*N*-isopropylacrylamide) injectable hydrogel for cultivation of chondrocytes and meniscus cells. *Macromol Biosci*, 6, 1026–39.

Chenite, A., Chaput, C., Wang, D., Combes, C., Buschmann, M. D., Hoemann, C. D., Leroux, J. C., Atkinson, B. L., Binette, F. & Selmani, A. (2000) Novel injectable neutral solutions of chitosan form biodegradable gels *in situ*. *Biomaterials*, 21, 2155–61.

Cho, J. H., Kim, S. H., Park, K. D., Jung, M. C., Yang, W. I., Han, S. W., Noh, J. Y. & Lee, J. W. (2004) Chondrogenic differentiation of human mesenchymal stem cells using a thermosensitive poly(*N*-isopropylacrylamide) and water-soluble chitosan copolymer. *Biomaterials*, 25, 5743–51.

Christman, K. L., Vardanian, A. J., Fang, Q., Sievers, R. E., Fok, H. H. & Lee, R. J.

(2004) Injectable fibrin scaffold improves cell transplant survival, reduces infarct expansion, and induces neovasculature formation in ischemic myocardium. *J Am Coll Cardiol*, 44, 654–60.
Chung, H. J., Bae, J. W., Park, H. D., Lee, J. W. & Park, K. D. (2005a) Thermosensitive chitosans as novel injectable biomaterials. *Macromol. Symp.*, 224, 275–86.
Chung, H. J., Go, D. H., Bae, J. W., Jung, I. K., Lee, J. W. & Park, K. D. (2005b) Synthesis and characterization of Pluronic® grafted chitosan copolymer as a novel injectable biomaterial. *Curr. Appl. Phys*, 5, 485–8.
Chung, J. E., Kurisawa, M., Uyama, H. & Kobayashi, S. (2003) Enzymatic synthesis and antioxidant property of gelatin-catechin conjugates. *Biotechnol Lett*, 25, 1993–7.
Coombes, A. G., Rizzi, S. C., Williamson, M., Barralet, J. E., Downes, S. & Wallace, W. A. (2004) Precipitation casting of polycaprolactone for applications in tissue engineering and drug delivery. *Biomaterials*, 25, 315–25.
Couto, D. S., Hong, Z. & Mano, J. F. (2009) Development of bioactive and biodegradable chitosan-based injectable systems containing bioactive glass nanoparticles. *Acta Biomater*, 5, 115–23.
Da Silva, R. M., Lopez-Perez, P. M., Elvira, C., Mano, J. F., Roman, J. S. & Reis, R. L. (2008) Poly(*N*-isopropylacrylamide) surface-grafted chitosan membranes as a new substrate for cell sheet engineering and manipulation. *Biotechnol Bioeng*, 101, 1321–31.
Dastoor, S. F., Misch, C. E. & Wang, H. L. (2007) Dermal fillers for facial soft tissue augmentation. *J Oral Implantol*, 33, 191–204.
Di Martino, A., Sittinger, M. & Risbud, M. V. (2005) Chitosan: a versatile biopolymer for orthopaedic tissue-engineering. *Biomaterials*, 26, 5983–90.
Duranti, F., Salti, G., Bovani, B., Calandra, M. & Rosati, M. L. (1998) Injectable hyaluronic acid gel for soft tissue augmentation. A clinical and histological study. *Dermatol Surg*, 24, 1317–25.
Eliaz, R. E. & Kost, J. (2000) Characterization of a polymeric PLGA-injectable implant delivery system for the controlled release of proteins. *J Biomed Mater Res*, 50, 388–96.
Epple, M. & Kirschnick, H. (1997) Silver chloroacetate: crystal structure and thermal polymerization mechanism. *Chem Ber./Recueil*, 130, 291–4.
Firth, A., Aggeli, A., Burke, J. L., Yang, X. & Kirkham, J. (2006) Biomimetic self-assembling peptides as injectable scaffolds for hard tissue engineering. *Nanomed*, 1, 189–99.
Freier, T., Koh, H. S., Kazazian, K. & Shoichet, M. S. (2005) Controlling cell adhesion and degradation of chitosan films by *N*-acetylation. *Biomaterials*, 26, 5872–8.
Gao, J., Dennis, J. E., Solchaga, L. A., Goldberg, V. M. & Caplan, A. I. (2002) Repair of osteochondral defect with tissue-engineered two-phase composite material of injectable calcium phosphate and hyaluronan sponge. *Tissue Eng*, 8, 827–37.
Garrett, J. S., Holland, K. M., Coonts, B. A. & Moore, L. A. (1999) *In situ*-forming biomaterials. *Providence, RI: American Mathametical Society*, 251.
Gerentes, P., Vachoud, L., Doury, J. & Domard, A. (2002) Study of a chitin-based gel as injectable material in periodontal surgery. *Biomaterials*, 23, 1295–302.
Gonzalez Corchon, M. A., Salvado, M., de la Torre, B. J., Collia, F., de Pedro, J. A., Vazquez, B. & Roman, J. S. (2006) Injectable and self-curing composites of acrylic/bioactive glass and drug systems. A histomorphometric analysis of the behaviour in rabbits. *Biomaterials*, 27, 1778–87.
Grimandi, G., Weiss, P., Millot, F. & Daculsi, G. (1998) *In vitro* evaluation of a new injectable calcium phosphate material. *J Biomed Mater Res*, 39, 660–6.

Gulsen, D., Li, C. C. & Chauhan, A. (2005) Dispersion of DMPC liposomes in contact lenses for ophthalmic drug delivery. *Curr Eye Res*, 30, 1071–80.

Gutowska, A., Jeong, B. & Jasionowski, M. (2001) Injectable gels for tissue engineering. *Anat Rec*, 263, 342–9.

Haines-Butterick, L., Rajagopal, K., Branco, M., Salick, D., Rughani, R., Pilarz, M., Lamm, M. S., Pochan, D. J. & Schneider, J. P. (2007) Controlling hydrogelation kinetics by peptide design for three-dimensional encapsulation and injectable delivery of cells. *Proc Natl Acad Sci USA*, 104, 7791–6.

Halberstadt, C., Austin, C., Rowley, J., Culberson, C., Loebsack, A., Wyatt, S., Coleman, S., Blacksten, L., Burg, K., Mooney, D. & Holder, W., Jr. (2002) A hydrogel material for plastic and reconstructive applications injected into the subcutaneous space of a sheep. *Tissue Eng*, 8, 309–19.

Hallen, L., Johansson, C. & Laurent, C. (1999) Cross-linked hyaluronan (Hylan B gel): a new injectable remedy for treatment of vocal fold insufficiency – an animal study. *Acta Otolaryngol*, 119, 107–11.

Halstenberg, S., Panitch, A., Rizzi, S., Hall, H. & Hubbell, J. A. (2002) Biologically engineered protein-graft-poly(ethylene glycol) hydrogels: a cell adhesive and plasmin-degradable biosynthetic material for tissue repair. *Biomacromolecules*, 3, 710–23.

Hatefi, A. & Amsden, B. (2002) Biodegradable injectable *in situ*-forming drug delivery systems. *J Control Release*, 80, 9–28.

Hejcl, A., Lesn, P., Prádn, M., Michálek, J., Jendelová, P., Stulík, J. & Syková, E. (2008) Biocompatible hydrogels in spinal cord injury repair. *Physiol Res*, 57, S121–32.

Hoare, T. R. & Kohane, D. S. (2008) Hydrogels in drug delivery: progress and challenges. *Polymer*, 49, 1993–2007.

Hoemann, C. D., Hurtig, M., Rossomacha, E., Sun, J., Chevrier, A., Shive, M. S. & Buschmann, M. D. (2005a) Chitosan-glycerol phosphate/blood implants improve hyaline cartilage repair in ovine microfracture defects. *J Bone Joint Surg Am*, 87, 2671–86.

Hoemann, C. D., Sun, J., Legare, A., McKee, M. D. & Buschmann, M. D. (2005b) Tissue engineering of cartilage using an injectable and adhesive chitosan-based cell-delivery vehicle. *Osteoarthritis Cartilage*, 13, 318–29.

Huan, Z. & Chang, J. (2009) Novel bioactive composite bone cements based on the beta-tricalcium phosphate-monocalcium phosphate monohydrate composite cement system. *Acta Biomater*, 5, 1253–64.

Hubbell, J. A. (1998) Synthetic biodegradable polymers for tissue engineering and drug delivery. *Current Opinion in Solid State and Materials Science*, 3, 246–51.

Hubbell, J. A. (2003) Materials as morphogenetic guides in tissue engineering. *Curr Opin Biotechnol*, 14, 551–8.

Hutmacher, D. W. (2001) Scaffold design and fabrication technologies for engineering tissues – state of the art and future perspectives. *J Biomater Sci Polym Ed*, 12, 107–24.

Jabbari, E. & He, X. (2008) Synthesis and characterization of bioresorbable *in situ* crosslinkable ultra low molecular weight poly(lactide) macromer. *J Mater Sci Mater Med*, 19, 311–18.

Jeong, B., Bae, Y. H., Lee, D. S. & Kim, S. W. (1997) Biodegradable block copolymers as injectable drug-delivery systems. *Nature*, 388, 860–2.

Jo, S., Shin, H. & Mikos, A. G. (2001a) Modification of oligo(poly(ethylene glycol) fumarate) macromer with a GRGD peptide for the preparation of functionalized polymer networks. *Biomacromolecules*, 2, 255–61.

Jo, S., Shin, H., Shung, A. K., Fisher, J. P. & Mikos, A. G. (2001b) Synthesis and characterization of oligo(poly(ethylene glycol) fumarate) macromer. *Macromolecules*, 34, 2839–44.

Kanchwala, S. K., Holloway, L. & Bucky, L. P. (2005) Reliable soft tissue augmentation: a clinical comparison of injectable soft-tissue fillers for facial-volume augmentation. *Ann Plast Surg*, 55, 30–5; discussion 35.

Khor, E. & Lim, L. Y. (2003) Implantable applications of chitin and chitosan. *Biomaterials*, 24, 2339–49.

Kim, H. K., Shim, W. S., Kim, S. E., Lee, K. H., Kang, E., Kim, J. H., Kim, K., Kwon, I. C. & Lee, D. S. (2009) Injectable *in situ*-forming pH/thermo-sensitive hydrogel for bone tissue engineering. *Tissue Eng Part A*, 15, 923–33.

Kim, M. S., Kim, S. K., Kim, S. H., Hyun, H., Khang, G. & Lee, H. B. (2006) *In vivo* osteogenic differentiation of rat bone marrow stromal cells in thermosensitive MPEG-PCL diblock copolymer gels. *Tissue Eng*, 12, 2863–73.

Kirkham, J., Firth, A., Vernals, D., Boden, N., Robinson, C., Shore, R. C., Brookes, S. J. & Aggeli, A. (2007) Self-assembling peptide scaffolds promote enamel remineralization. *J Dent Res*, 86, 426–30.

Klein, A. W. (2006) Soft tissue augmentation 2006: filler fantasy. *Dermatol Ther*, 19, 129–33.

Klokkevold, P. R., Vandemark, L., Kenney, E. B. & Bernard, G. W. (1996) Osteogenesis enhanced by chitosan (poly-*N*-acetyl glucosaminoglycan) *in vitro*. *J Periodontol*, 67, 1170–5.

Kobayashi, S., Fujikawa, S. & Ohmae, M. (2003) Enzymatic synthesis of chondroitin and its derivatives catalyzed by hyaluronidase. *J Am Chem Soc*, 125, 14357–69.

Krebs, M. D., Sutter, K. A., Lin, A. S., Guldberg, R. E. & Alsberg, E. (2009) Injectable poly(lactic-co-glycolic) acid scaffolds with *in situ* pore formation for tissue engineering. *Acta Biomater*, 5, 2847–59.

Kretlow, J. D., Young, S., Klouda, L., Wong, M. & Mikos, A. G. (2009) Injectable biomaterials for regenerating complex craniofacial tissues. *Adv Mater Deerfield*, 21, 3368–93.

Kuo, C. K. & Ma, P. X. (2001) Ionically crosslinked alginate hydrogels as scaffolds for tissue engineering: part 1. Structure, gelation rate and mechanical properties. *Biomaterials*, 22, 511–21.

Kuo, Y. C. & Ku, I. N. (2008) Cartilage regeneration by novel polyethylene oxide/chitin/chitosan scaffolds. *Biomacromolecules*, 9, 2662–9.

Kurisawa, M., Chung, J. E., Yang, Y. Y., Gao, S. J. & Uyama, H. (2005) Injectable biodegradable hydrogels composed of hyaluronic acid-tyramine conjugates for drug delivery and tissue engineering. *Chem Commun (Camb)*, 4312–14.

Laurencin, C. T. & Nair, L. S. (eds) (2008) *Nanotechnology and tissue engineering: the scaffold*, Boca Raton, FL, CRC Press.

Li, Q., Wang, J., Shahani, S., Sun, D. D., Sharma, B., Elisseeff, J. H. & Leong, K. W. (2006) Biodegradable and photocrosslinkable polyphosphoester hydrogel. *Biomaterials*, 27, 1027–34.

Li, Z. & Zhang, M. (2005) Chitosan-alginate as scaffolding material for cartilage tissue engineering. *J Biomed Mater Res A*, 75, 485–93.

Liggins, R. T., D'Amours, S., Demetrick, J. S., Machan, L. S. & Burt, H. M. (2000) Paclitaxel loaded poly(L-lactic acid) microspheres for the prevention of intraperitoneal carcinomatosis after a surgical repair and tumor cell spill. *Biomaterials*, 21, 1959–69.

Lin, C. C. & Anseth, K. S. (2009) Glucagon-like peptide-1 functionalized PEG hydrogels promote survival and function of encapsulated pancreatic beta-cells. *Biomacromolecules*, 10, 2460–7.

Loebsack, A., Greene, K., Wyatt, S., Culberson, C., Austin, C., Beiler, R., Roland, W., Eiselt, P., Rowley, J., Burg, K., Mooney, D., Holder, W. & Halberstadt, C. (2001) *In vivo* characterization of a porous hydrogel material for use as a tissue bulking agent. *J Biomed Mater Res*, 57, 575–81.

Lu, J. X., Prudhommeaux, F., Meunier, A., Sedel, L. & Guillemin, G. (1999) Effects of chitosan on rat knee cartilages. *Biomaterials*, 20, 1937–44.

Luginbuehl, V., Wenk, E., Koch, A., Gander, B., Merkle, H. P. & Meinel, L. (2005) Insulin-like growth factor I-releasing alginate-tricalciumphosphate composites for bone regeneration. *Pharm Res*, 22, 940–50.

Mamada, A., Tanaka, T., Kungwatchakun, D. & Irie, M. (1990) Photoinduced phase transition of gels. *Macromolecules*, 23, 1517–19.

Mann, B. K., Gobin, A. S., Tsai, A. T., Schmedlen, R. H. & West, J. L. (2001) Smooth muscle cell growth in photopolymerized hydrogels with cell adhesive and proteolytically degradable domains: synthetic ECM analogs for tissue engineering. *Biomaterials*, 22, 3045–51.

Mano, J. F., Silva, G. A., Azevedo, H. S., Malafaya, P. B., Sousa, R. A., Silva, S. S., Boesel, L. F., Oliveira, J. M., Santos, T. C., Marques, A. P., Neves, N. M. & Reis, R. L. (2007) Natural origin biodegradable systems in tissue engineering and regenerative medicine: present status and some moving trends. *J R Soc Interface*, 4, 999–1030.

Matsuno, T., Hashimoto, Y., Adachi, S., Omata, K., Yoshitaka, Y., Ozeki, Y., Umezu, Y., Tabata, Y., Nakamura, M. & Satoh, T. (2008) Preparation of injectable 3D-formed beta-tricalcium phosphate bead/alginate composite for bone tissue engineering. *Dent Mater J*, 27, 827–34.

Missirlis, D., Tirelli, N. & Hubbell, J. A. (2005) Amphiphilic hydrogel nanoparticles. Preparation, characterization, and preliminary assessment as new colloidal drug carriers. *Langmuir*, 21, 2605–13.

Missirlis, D., Kawamura, R., Tirelli, N. & Hubbell, J. A. (2006) Doxorubicin encapsulation and diffusional release from stable, polymeric, hydrogel nanoparticles. *Eur J Pharm Sci*, 29, 120–9.

Miyata, T., Asami, N. & Uragami, T. (1999) A reversibly antigen-responsive hydrogel. *Nature*, 399, 766–9.

Molinaro, G., Leroux, J. C., Damas, J. & Adam, A. (2002) Biocompatibility of thermosensitive chitosan-based hydrogels: an *in vivo* experimental approach to injectable biomaterials. *Biomaterials*, 23, 2717–22.

Montufar, E. B., Traykova, T., C. Gil, I. H., Almirall, A., Aguirre, A., Engel, E., Planell, J. A. & Ginebra, M. P. (2009) Foamed surfactant solution as a template for self-setting injectable hydroxyapatite scaffolds for bone regeneration. *Acta Biomaterialia*.

Muggli, D. S., Burkoth, A. K., Keyser, S. A., Lee, H. R. & Anseth, K. S. (1998) Reaction behavior of biodegradable, photo-cross-linkable polyanhydrides. *Macromolecules*, 31, 4120.

Mwale, F., Iordanova, M., Demers, C. N., Steffen, T., Roughley, P. & Antoniou, J. (2005) Biological evaluation of chitosan salts cross-linked to genipin as a cell scaffold for disk tissue engineering. *Tissue Eng*, 11, 130–40.

Na, K., Kim, S., Woo, D. G., Sun, B. K., Yang, H. N., Chung, H. M. & Park, K. H. (2007a) Combination material delivery of dexamethasone and growth factor in hydrogel blended with hyaluronic acid constructs for neocartilage formation. *J*

Biomed Mater Res A, 83, 779–86.
Na, K., Kim, S., Woo, D. G., Sun, B. K., Yang, H. N., Chung, H. M. & Park, K. H. (2007b) Synergistic effect of TGFbeta-3 on chondrogenic differentiation of rabbit chondrocytes in thermo-reversible hydrogel constructs blended with hyaluronic acid by *in vivo* test. *J Biotechnol*, 128, 412–22.
Nettles, D. L., Elder, S. H. & Gilbert, J. A. (2002) Potential use of chitosan as a cell scaffold material for cartilage tissue engineering. *Tissue Eng*, 8, 1009–16.
Nettles, D. L., Vail, T. P., Morgan, M. T., Grinstaff, M. W. & Setton, L. A. (2004) Photocrosslinkable hyaluronan as a scaffold for articular cartilage repair. *Ann Biomed Eng*, 32, 391–7.
Nguyen, K. T. & West, J. L. (2002) Photopolymerizable hydrogels for tissue engineering applications. *Biomaterials*, 23, 4307–14.
Oh, S. H., Lee, J. Y., Ghil, S. H., Lee, S. S., Yuk, S. H. & Lee, J. H. (2006) PCL microparticle-dispersed PLGA solution as a potential injectable urethral bulking agent. *Biomaterials*, 27, 1936–44.
Paige, K. T., Cima, L. G., Yaremchuk, M. J., Vacanti, J. P. & Vacanti, C. A. (1995) Injectable cartilage. *Plast Reconstr Surg*, 96, 1390–8; discussion 1399–400.
Park, D. J., Choi, B. H., Zhu, S. J., Huh, J. Y., Kim, B. Y. & Lee, S. H. (2005a) Injectable bone using chitosan-alginate gel/mesenchymal stem cells/BMP-2 composites. *J Craniomaxillofac Surg*, 33, 50–4.
Park, H., Temenoff, J. S., Holland, T. A., Tabata, Y. & Mikos, A. G. (2005b) Delivery of TGF-β1 and chondrocytes via injectable, biodegradable hydrogels for cartilage tissue engineering applications. *Biomaterials*, 26, 7095–103.
Park, H., Temenoff, J. S., Tabata, Y., Caplan, A. I. & Mikos, A. G. (2007) Injectable biodegradable hydrogel composites for rabbit marrow mesenchymal stem cell and growth factor delivery for cartilage tissue engineering. *Biomaterials*, 28, 3217–27.
Park, H., Kang, S. W., Kim, B. S., Mooney, D. J. & Lee, K. Y. (2009a) Shear-reversibly crosslinked alginate hydrogels for tissue engineering. *Macromol Biosci*, 9, 895–901.
Park, K. M., Lee, S. Y., Joung, Y. K., Na, J. S., Lee, M. C. & Park, K. D. (2009b) Thermosensitive chitosan-Pluronic hydrogel as an injectable cell delivery carrier for cartilage regeneration. *Acta Biomater*, 5, 1956–65.
Park, S. H., Park, S. R., Chung, S. I., Pai, K. S. & Min, B. H. (2005c) Tissue-engineered cartilage using fibrin/hyaluronan composite gel and its *in vivo* implantation. *Artif Organs*, 29, 838–45.
Park, T. G. & Hoffman, A. S. (1993) Sodium chloride-induced phase transition in nonionic poly(*N*-isopropylacrylamide) gel. *Macromolecules*, 26, 5045–8.
Park, Y. D., Tirelli, N. & Hubbell, J. A. (2003) Photopolymerized hyaluronic acid-based hydrogels and interpenetrating networks. *Biomaterials*, 24, 893–900.
Pereira, R. C., Scaranari, M., Castagnola, P., Grandizio, M., Azevedo, H. S., Reis, R. L., Cancedda, R. & Gentili, C. (2009) Novel injectable gel (system) as a vehicle for human articular chondrocytes in cartilage tissue regeneration. *J Tissue Eng Regen Med*, 3, 97–106.
Perka, C., Spitzer, R. S., Lindenhayn, K., Sittinger, M. & Schultz, O. (2000) Matrix-mixed culture: new methodology for chondrocyte culture and preparation of cartilage transplants. *J Biomed Mater Res*, 49, 305–11.
Poshusta, A. K., Burdick, J. A., Mortisen, D. J., Padera, R. F., Ruehlman, D., Yaszemski, M. J. & Anseth, K. S. (2003) Histocompatibility of photocrosslinked polyanhydrides: a novel in situ forming orthopaedic biomaterial. *J Biomed Mater Res A*, 64, 62–9.
Pratoomsoot, C., Tanioka, H., Hori, K., Kawasaki, S., Kinoshita, S., Tighe, P. J., Dua, H.,

Shakesheff, K. M. & Rose, F. R. (2008) A thermoreversible hydrogel as a biosynthetic bandage for corneal wound repair. *Biomaterials*, 29, 272–81.

Qiu, L. Y. & Yan, M. Q. (2009) Constructing doxorubicin-loaded polymeric micelles through amphiphilic graft polyphosphazenes containing ethyl tryptophan and PEG segments. *Acta Biomater*, 5, 2132–41.

Qiu, Y. & Park, K. (2001) Environment-sensitive hydrogels for drug delivery. *Adv Drug Deliv Rev*, 53, 321–39.

Radomsky, M. L., Thompson, A. Y., Spiro, R. C. & Poser, J. W. (1998) Potential role of fibroblast growth factor in enhancement of fracture healing. *Clin Orthop Relat Res*, S283–93.

Rafat, M., Li, F., Fagerholm, P., Lagali, N. S., Watsky, M. A., Munger, R., Matsuura, T. & Griffith, M. (2008) PEG-stabilized carbodiimide crosslinked collagen-chitosan hydrogels for corneal tissue engineering. *Biomaterials*, 29, 3960–72.

Ramanan, R. M., Chellamuthu, P., Tang, L. & Nguyen, K. T. (2006) Development of a temperature-sensitive composite hydrogel for drug delivery applications. *Biotechnol Prog*, 22, 118–25.

Reis, R. L. & Romaìn, J. S. (eds) (2005) *Biodegradable systems in tissue engineering and regenerative medicine*, Boca Raton, FL, CRC Press.

Rowley, J. A., Madlambayan, G. & Mooney, D. J. (1999) Alginate hydrogels as synthetic extracellular matrix materials. *Biomaterials*, 20, 45–53.

Ruhe, P. Q., Hedberg, E. L., Padron, N. T., Spauwen, P. H., Jansen, J. A. & Mikos, A. G. (2003) rhBMP-2 release from injectable poly(DL-lactic-co-glycolic acid)/calcium-phosphate cement composites. *J Bone Joint Surg Am*, 85-A Suppl 3, 75–81.

Ruhe, P. Q., Hedberg-Dirk, E. L., Padron, N. T., Spauwen, P. H., Jansen, J. A. & Mikos, A. G. (2006) Porous poly(DL-lactic-co-glycolic acid)/calcium phosphate cement composite for reconstruction of bone defects. *Tissue Eng*, 12, 789–800.

Sabnis, A., Wadajkar, A. S., Aswath, P. & Nguyen, K. T. (2009) Factorial analyses of photopolymerizable thermoresponsive composite hydrogels for protein delivery. *Nanomedicine*, 5, 305–15.

Salinas, C. N. & Anseth, K. S. (2008) The enhancement of chondrogenic differentiation of human mesenchymal stem cells by enzymatically regulated RGD functionalities. *Biomaterials*, 29, 2370–7.

Schweiger, E. S., Riddle, C. C., Tonkovic-Capin, V. & Aires, D. J. (2008) Successful treatment with injected hyaluronic acid in a patient with lip asymmetry after surgical correction of cleft lip. *Dermatol Surg*, 34, 717–19.

Shah, N. H., Railkar, A. S., Chen, F. C., Tarantino, R., Kumar, S., Murjani, M., Palmer, D., Infeld, M. H. & Malick, A. W. (1993) A biodegradable injectable implant for delivering micro and macromolecules using poly (lactic-co-glycolic) acid (PLGA) copolymers. *Journal of Controlled Release*, 27, 139–47.

Sharifi, S., Imani, M., Mirzadeh, H., Atai, M., Ziaee, F. & Bakhshi, R. (2009) Synthesis, characterization, and biocompatibility of novel injectable, biodegradable, and *in situ* crosslinkable polycarbonate-based macromers. *J Biomed Mater Res Part A*, 90, 830–43.

Shi, D., Cai, D. & Zhou, C. (2005a) [Fabrication and properties of a composite chitosan/type II collagen scaffold for tissue engineering cartilage]. *Zhongguo Xiu Fu Chong Jian Wai Ke Za Zhi*, 19, 278–82.

Shi, D. H., Cai, D. Z., Zhou, C. R., Rong, L. M., Wang, K. & Xu, Y. C. (2005b) Development and potential of a biomimetic chitosan/type II collagen scaffold for cartilage tissue engineering. *Chin Med J (Engl)*, 118, 1436–43.

Shiga, T., Hirose, Y., Okada, A. & Kurauchi, T. (2003) Electric field-associated

deformation of polyelectrolyte gel near a phase transition point. *J of Appl Polym Sci*, 46, 635–40.
Shu, X. Z., Ghosh, K., Liu, Y., Palumbo, F. S., Luo, Y., Clark, R. A. & Prestwich, G. D. (2004) Attachment and spreading of fibroblasts on an RGD peptide-modified injectable hyaluronan hydrogel. *J Biomed Mater Res A*, 68, 365–75.
Shu, X. Z., Ahmad, S., Liu, Y. & Prestwich, G. D. (2006) Synthesis and evaluation of injectable, *in situ* crosslinkable synthetic extracellular matrices for tissue engineering. *J Biomed Mater Res A*, 79, 902–12.
Stevens, M. M., Qanadilo, H. F., Langer, R. & Prasad Shastri, V. (2004) A rapid-curing alginate gel system: utility in periosteum-derived cartilage tissue engineering. *Biomaterials*, 25, 887–94.
Subramanian, A., Vu, D., Larsen, G. F. & Lin, H. Y. (2005) Preparation and evaluation of the electrospun chitosan/PEO fibers for potential applications in cartilage tissue engineering. *J Biomater Sci Polym Ed*, 16, 861–73.
Suzuki, A. & Tanaka, T. (1990) Phase transition in polymer gels induced by visible light. *Nature*, 346, 345–7.
Tan, H., Chu, C. R., Payne, K. A. & Marra, K. G. (2009a) Injectable *in situ*-forming biodegradable chitosan-hyaluronic acid based hydrogels for cartilage tissue engineering. *Biomaterials*, 30, 2499–506.
Tan, H., Ramirez, C. M., Miljkovic, N., Li, H., Rubin, J. P. & Marra, K. G. (2009b) Thermosensitive injectable hyaluronic acid hydrogel for adipose tissue engineering. *Biomaterials*, 30, 6844–53.
Tan, R., Niu, X., Gan, S. & Feng, Q. (2009c) Preparation and characterization of an injectable composite. *J Mater Sci Mater Med*, 20, 1245–53.
Temenoff, J. S., Shin, H., Conway, D. E., Engel, P. S. & Mikos, A. G. (2003) *In vitro* cytotoxicity of redox radical initiators for cross-linking of oligo(poly(ethylene glycol) fumarate) macromers. *Biomacromolecules*, 4, 1605–13.
Timmer, M. D., Ambrose, C. G. & Mikos, A. G. (2003a) Evaluation of thermal- and photo-crosslinked biodegradable poly(propylene fumarate)-based networks. *J Biomed Mater Res A*, 66, 811–18.
Timmer, M. D., Ambrose, C. G. & Mikos, A. G. (2003b) *In vitro* degradation of polymeric networks of poly(propylene fumarate) and the crosslinking macromer poly(propylene fumarate)-diacrylate. *Biomaterials*, 24, 571–7.
Tokura, S. & Tamura, H. (2001) O-carboxymethyl-chitin concentration in granulocytes during bone repair. *Biomacromolecules*, 2, 417–21.
Vernon, B., Tirelli, N., Bachi, T., Haldimann, D. & Hubbell, J. A. (2003) Water-borne, *in situ* crosslinked biomaterials from phase-segregated precursors. *J Biomed Mater Res A*, 64, 447–56.
Wang, J., Chen, L., Zhao, Y., Guo, G. & Zhang, R. (2009) Cell adhesion and accelerated detachment on the surface of temperature-sensitive chitosan and poly(*N*-isopropylacrylamide) hydrogels. *J Mater Sci Mater Med*, 20, 583–90.
Wang, Y., Ameer, G. A., Sheppard, B. J. & Langer, R. (2002) A tough biodegradable elastomer. *Nat Biotechnol*, 20, 602–6.
Watanabe, J., Kashii, M., Hirao, M., Oka, K., Sugamoto, K., Yoshikawa, H. & Akashi, M. (2007) Quick-forming hydroxyapatite/agarose gel composites induce bone regeneration. *J Biomed Mater Res A*, 83, 845–52.
Wei, Y., Hu, Y., Hao, W., Han, Y., Meng, G., Zhang, D., Wu, Z. & Wang, H. (2008) A novel injectable scaffold for cartilage tissue engineering using adipose-derived adult stem cells. *J Orthop Res*, 26, 27–33.
Westhaus, E. & Messersmith, P. B. (2001) Triggered release of calcium from lipid

vesicles: a bioinspired strategy for rapid gelation of polysaccharide and protein hydrogels. *Biomaterials*, 22, 453–62.
Widner, B., Behr, R., von Dollen, S., Tang, M., Heu, T., Sloma, A., Sternberg, D., DeAngelis, P. L., Weigel, P. H. & Brown, S. (2005) Hyaluronic acid production in Bacillus subtilis. *Appl Environ Microbiol*, 71, 3747–52.
Winternitz, C. I., Jackson, J. K., Oktaba, A. M. & Burt, H. M. (1996) Development of a polymeric surgical paste formulation for taxol. *Pharm Res*, 13, 368–75.
Xia, W., Liu, W., Cui, L., Liu, Y., Zhong, W., Liu, D., Wu, J., Chua, K. & Cao, Y. (2004) Tissue engineering of cartilage with the use of chitosan-gelatin complex scaffolds. *J Biomed Mater Res B Appl Biomater*, 71, 373–80.
Xu, H. H., Weir, M. D. & Simon, C. G. (2008) Injectable and strong nano-apatite scaffolds for cell/growth factor delivery and bone regeneration. *Dent Mater*, 24, 1212–22.
Yamane, S., Iwasaki, N., Majima, T., Funakoshi, T., Masuko, T., Harada, K., Minami, A., Monde, K. & Nishimura, S. (2005) Feasibility of chitosan-based hyaluronic acid hybrid biomaterial for a novel scaffold in cartilage tissue engineering. *Biomaterials*, 26, 611–19.
Yeo, Y., Geng, W., Ito, T., Kohane, D. S., Burdick, J. A. & Radisic, M. (2007a) Photocrosslinkable hydrogel for myocyte cell culture and injection. *J Biomed Mater Res B Appl Biomater*, 81, 312–22.
Yeo, Y., Ito, T., Bellas, E., Highley, C. B., Marini, R. & Kohane, D. S. (2007b) *In situ* cross-linkable hyaluronan hydrogels containing polymeric nanoparticles for preventing postsurgical adhesions. *Ann Surg*, 245, 819–24.
Zhang, G. & Suggs, L. J. (2007) Matrices and scaffolds for drug delivery in vascular tissue engineering. *Adv Drug Deliv Rev*, 59, 360–73.
Zhang, X., Jackson, J. K., Wong, W., Min, W., Cruz, T., Hunter, W. L. & Burt, H. M. (1996) Development of biodegradable polymeric paste formulations for taxol: An *in vitro* and *in vivo* study. *International Journal of Pharmaceutics*, 137, 199–208.
Zhang, Z., Zhu, X., Zhu, J. & Cheng, Z. (2006) Thermal polymerization of methyl (meth)acrylate via reversible addition-fragmentation chain transfer (RAFT) process. *Polymer*, 47, 6970–7.
Zhao, W., Wang, J., Zhai, W., Wang, Z. & Chang, J. (2005) The self-setting properties and in vitro bioactivity of tricalcium silicate. *Biomaterials*, 26, 6113–21.
Zhao, Z., Wang, J., Mao, H. Q. & Leong, K. W. (2003) Polyphosphoesters in drug and gene delivery. *Adv Drug Deliv Rev*, 55, 483–99.
Zheng Shu, X., Liu, Y., Palumbo, F. S., Luo, Y. & Prestwich, G. D. (2004) *In situ* crosslinkable hyaluronan hydrogels for tissue engineering. *Biomaterials*, 25, 1339–48.

6.7 Glossary

Biocompatibility: ability of a biomaterial to perform its desired function without eliciting any undesirable local or systemic effects in the host tissues; the material should be mechanical, chemical, pharmacological and surface compatible with surrounding tissues and host.
Biomaterial: artificial material used to replace or augment the physical and/or functional part of an organism.
Calcium phosphate: family of calcium and phosphate containing materials of natural or synthetic origin; usually used to augment or substitute bone;

prominent materials are hydroxyapatite, mono- and tri-calciumphosphate-based materials.
Composites: materials that contain two or more distinct constituent materials or phases.
Copolymer: polymers constituting two or more monomers; can be made by grafting, block, altering or random attachment of the polymer segments/chains.
Extracellular matrix (ECM): the intercellular material of a tissue or the tissue from which a structure develops.
Fibrin: elastic filamentous protein derived from fibrinogen in blood coagulation.
Gelation: process of forming a gel; formation of a gel from a sol.
Glass ceramics: glass that has been crystallized by heat treatment; exhibits ability to bond with soft and hard tissues; well-known example is bioglass.
Hydrogel: a polymer material that is capable of absorbing 30% or more of its weight in water.
Hydroxyapatite: calcium phosphate cement with composition of $Ca_{10}(PO_4)_6(OH)_2$; exhibits excellent mechanical properties and biocompatibility; major mineral constituent of the bone; also finds use as a filler to replace amputated bone and/or as a coating to promote bone ingrowth into prosthetic implants.
Initiator: a chemical used to start the addition polymerization reaction; it starts the reaction by becoming a free radical that in turn reacts with the monomer.
***In situ*:** in the original or natural place or site; in the position that it will finally occupy or stay.
Resorption: process by which a structure is remodeled; the loss and reassimilation of materials or tissue.
Scaffold: an artificial structure or surface that has the ability to support three-dimensional tissue formation.
Tissue engineering: ability to regenerate tissue with the aid of artificial materials.

6.8 List of abbreviations

AgCA	Silver chloroacetate
CM	Carboxymethyl
DEF/PPF	Diethyl fumarate/poly(propylene fumarate)
DTPH	3,3′-dithiobis(propanoic dihydrazide)
GP	Glycerophosphate
HA	Hyaluronic acid
HAp	Hydroxyapatite
HEC	Hydroxyethylcellulose
Hylaform™	Divinyl sulfone
MHPC	Methylhydroxypropylcellulose
MMA	Methyl methacrylate

M-PEG	Methoxyl-PEG
MPEG-PCL	Methoxy poly(ethylene glycol)-poly(ϵ-caprolactone)
MPs	Microparticles
NPs	Nanoparticles
OPEGF	Oligo(poly(ethylene glycol) fumarate
PAA	Poly(acrylic acid)
PDADMACl	Poly(diallyldimethylammonium chloride)
PDEA	Poly(*N,N*-diethylacrylamide)
PDEAEM	Poly(*N,N*-diethylaminoethyl methacrylate)
PEG	Poly(ethylene glycol)
PEGMA or PEGDA	Dimethacrylic or diacrylic derivatives of poly(ethylene glycol)
PEG-RGD	PEG-arginine-glycine-aspartate
PEO	Poly(ethylene oxide)
PLA	Poly (L-lactide)
PLAF	Poly(lactide fumarate)
PLGA	Poly(lactic-co-glycolic) acid
PNIPAAm	Poly(*N*-isopropylacrylamide)
PPE	Polyphosphoester
PPF	Poly(propylene fumarate)
PVA	Poly(vinyl alcohol)
TPM	Triphenylmethane

7

Vascular applications of injectable biomaterials

B. L. VERNON and C. RILEY,
Arizona State University, USA

Abstract: This chapter focuses on the vascular applications of injectable biomaterials. Two clinically relevant vascular conditions, cerebral arteriovenous malformations and intracranial aneurysm, will be discussed in terms of endovascular embolization. This chapter then outlines available embolic materials used to treat each condition, as well as highlighting new injectable biomaterials developed for embolization purposes.

Key words: endovascular embolization, arteriovenous malformations, aneurysms, embolic materials.

7.1 Introduction

The use of injectable biomaterials for the treatment of vascular conditions has become a common practice within the endovascular community. Most often, these materials are used to embolize cavernous or tortuous regions of the vascular system that are problematic, such as aneurysms and arteriovenous malformations. Injectable biomaterials are optimal for embolization therapy because they can reduce surgical invasiveness through transfemoral catheter delivery of material to the lesion site. Traditionally, embolization of such regions was done only to make surgical resection or radiation therapy easier. However, upon development of better embolic materials and techniques, embolization can now serve as a stand-alone treatment in many endovascular situations. While a variety of vascular conditions can be treated with embolization of injectable biomaterials, these conditions require specific material properties and characteristics that make some materials more suitable for use with a particular condition. Therefore, an injectable biomaterial that is used clinically to treat an aneurysm may not be suitable for embolizing an arteriovenous malformation. Injectable biomaterials for vascular embolization have taken on many forms throughout their history. From platinum coils to polymer glues, each embolic material has a unique way of accomplishing occlusion. Similarly, each material requires specialized interventional techniques in order to deliver the embolic material to the proper location. While not yet on the market, there are many new injectable biomaterials that are being investigated for embolic vascular applications. These new materials have been developed to improve upon limitations associated with traditional embolic materials.

7.2 Embolization therapy for vascular conditions

Embolization is commonly referred to as a process in which material is introduced into the circulation to purposefully occlude a vessel, abnormal structure, or an organ (Stedman, 2000). Embolization has also been used for treating hemorrhage and tumors, by limiting blood flow to the desired area. For this chapter, however, embolization of vascular conditions with injectable materials will be the focus of discussion. Two vascular conditions that will be examined in detail are cerebral arteriovenous malformations and intracranial aneurysms. Because these lesions are located in a critical area of the body, it can be more advantageous to use endovascular approaches rather than more invasive surgical procedures to treat the condition.

7.2.1 Arteriovenous malformations

Arteriovenous malformations (AVMs) have long been identified as vascular lesions capable of being embolized with injectable agents. AVMs are a specific type of vascular malformation that has an angioarchitecture construction resulting in high blood flowrates through the lesion (Legiehn and Heran, 2008). While AVMs can occur anywhere in the vasculature, cerebral AVMs are of specific interest due to the severity of potential damage upon rupture. In general, vascular malformations are a cluster of abnormally arranged blood vessels that are present at the time of birth and grow proportionally with the person. Vascular malformations are placed into different sub-categories based on the main channel containing the abnormality. Other than arteriovenous malformations, vascular malformations include venous malformations, lymphatic malformations, and capillary malformations, to name a few. Most vascular malformations are slow-flow lesions, but AVMs are fast-flow, making them at higher risk for rupture and of more urgency to treat (Legiehn and Heran, 2008).

Arteriovenous malformations are distinguished from other types of vascular malformations by the 'shunting' of blood that occurs between arteries and veins. The shunt, also called the nidus of the AVM, is made up of a hybrid artery-vein that contains mature vessel wall elements (Hashimoto *et al.*, 2007). Instead of a normal capillary network that allows the transfer of nutrients and gasses, high-flow shunts of an AVM transfer blood from the feeding arteries to the draining veins without allowing nutrient and gas transfer. The tissue surrounding an AVM may experience ischemia and hypoxia due not only to the lack of immediate nutrients, but also because blood flow from healthy vasculature nearby can be redirected into the shunt in a phenomenon called the 'local steal effect'. Changes to the angioarchitecture due to the presence of an AVM include the high flow hemodynamic profile, arterialization of the draining veins, and secondary vessel pathology upstream and downstream of the nidus, called high-flow angiopathy (Valavanis *et al.*, 2004).

Treatment of brain AVMs with injectable materials and liquid embolic agents is done in order to achieve one of three main goals: prepare the lesion for surgical resection or radiation therapy, fully embolize the lesion as a curative treatment, or reduce associated symptoms through partial embolization if the AVM cannot be fully embolized or surgically resceted (Alexander and Tolbert, 2006). There is much controversy surrounding palliative AVM embolization because some studies have shown that non-curative embolizations that are not surgically resected can lead to a higher risk of AVM rupture. In other studies, it has been shown that there is a lower risk of hemorrhage upon embolization (Valavanis *et al.*, 2004). Again, the risk of AVM rupture is related to a variety of conditions present in the AVM, so it is difficult to determine if incomplete AVM obliteration leads to an increased rupture risk.

Traditionally, embolization was used only to prepare the lesion for surgical resection. Now, embolization is being used more often as a curative therapy due to improvements in microcatheter design and embolic materials (Linfante and Wakhloo, 2007). The ability of a brain AVM to be treated in this manner depends on a variety of factors including its size, location, angioarchitectural characteristics of the nidus. AVMs can also contain local aneurysms and venous cavities, which increase the likelihood of AVM rupture and make treatment more difficult (Alexander and Tolbert, 2006). The Spetzler-Martin grade scale developed in 1986 is used predict the difficulty and morbidity of surgically resecting an AVM (Spetzler and Martin, 1986). This grade is commonly reported when performing an AVM embolization, although it has been argued that this scale is not sufficient when applied to embolization because surgical resection and embolization have different associated risk factors (Valavanis *et al.*, 2004). Even so, many considerations must be taken into account before embolizing an AVM, including the neurosurgeon's experience with a particular embolization technique and material.

Techniques for AVM embolization are specific to the material being used, but in any case the goal of curative embolization is to superselectively occlude feeding arteries as well as the nidus, while preserving local blood vessels and the venous drainage system. One of the most serious risks associated with performing an AVM embolization is the possibility of occluding the venous efflux, resulting in compromised venous outflow from the AVM and pulmonary emboli (Alexander and Tolbert, 2006). This can happen if the liquid embolic material solidifies more slowly than expected, resulting in venous occlusion. Similarly, if the material solidifies too quickly, the feeding pedicles can be occluded without ever reaching the nidus. Therefore, the surgeon's experience with embolization techniques and materials is critical in achieving a successful outcome.

AVM embolization is normally accomplished through transfemoral micro-catheter delivery of the material under fluoroscopic guidance. The microcatheter tip is placed where the feeding artery branches off from healthy vasculature and material is slowly injected under continuous fluoroscopy. This procedure is carried out for the other AVM feeding arteries until blood flow is essentially prevented from entering the nidus (Valavanis *et al.*, 2004). While the procedural explanation of AVM embolization is relatively straightforward, it is much more difficult to do in practice. For example, angiography may not show all of the feeding pedicles, requiring multiple embolization procedures to occlude all pedicles when a curative goal is desired. The injectable biomaterials used for AVM embolization differ from materials used in other embolization procedures due to the angioarchitecture of the AVM, which requires precise control over the embolic material.

7.2.2 Aneurysms

Aneurysms are another major target of embolization therapy. An aneurysm is a 'ballooning out' of an artery wall that occurs where the artery has been damaged or weakened. The hemodynamic forces of blood on the weakened artery wall can lead to aneurysm growth and eventual rupture. Most aneurysms occur within the aorta, but can happen anywhere in the arterial vasculature. An aneurysm is commonly thought of as a saccular bulge with a defined neck, but not all aneurysms have this feature. Fusiform aneurysms, for example, are characterized by bulging of an entire axial section of the artery, with no defined neck. Although these types of aneurysms can cause many physiological problems, rupture of fusiform aneurysms is relatively rare (Lohani, 2004). Of particular interest to endovascular neurosurgeons are intracranial aneurysms (ICAs), because the growth and rupture of aneurysms in the brain often leads to subarachnoid hemorrhage and stroke.

Intracranial saccular aneurysms are vascular conditions amenable to treatment through endovascular embolization. Similar to cerebral AVMs, intracranial aneurysms are often located in deep or eloquent areas of the brain, which limits the surgical options available for treatment. Endovascular embolization is therefore an attractive option, due to its minimally invasive nature and the ability to reach places in the brain that cannot be treated surgically. Aneurysm embolization has been attempted for decades, beginning in the 18th century when surgeons extravascularly introduced needles into aneurysms to induce thrombosis. Due to the inconsistent success rates of these procedures, embolization did not catch on right away as a common treatment for aneurysms. It has not been until recently, with the development of flexible catheters and better endovascular tools, that endovascular embolization has become a primary treatment option for intracranial aneurysms (Kanaan *et al.*, 2005). Microsurgical clipping was the most common treatment of intracranial aneurysms before endovascular embolization picked back up again in the early 1970s, with the advent of detachable balloons (Linfante and Wakhloo, 2007).

When detachable coils first came on the market in the early 1990s, this new endovascular technique was only used when it was considered too risky to perform microsurgical clipping (International Subarachnoid Aneurysm Trial (ISAT) Collaborative Group, 2002). Microsurgical clipping of ICAs, which involves craniotomy and physical clipping of the aneurysm neck, gained clinical acceptance in the 1960s, when the benefits were shown to outweigh the risks of the technique in a series of randomized trials by McKissock and colleagues (McKissock *et al.*, 1965). As with any surgical technique, with more clinical use, procedural experience, and better technology, the risks associated with clipping have diminished from the first reported statistics. In 2002, results from the first randomized clinical trial comparing microsurgical clipping to the new technique of endovascular coil embolization became available. The International Subarachnoid Aneurysm Trial (ISAT) involved performing one of the two techniques on patients who had ruptured ICAs that were deemed appropriate to undergo either procedure. The group analyzed patients over a year and found that coil embolization improved the chances of patient survival compared with neurosurgical clipping (International Subarachnoid Aneurysm Trial (ISAT) Collaborative Group, 2002). This groundbreaking study, while only performed on a small subset of the range of aneurysm occurrences, gave the practice of endovascular embolization significant clinical acceptance and opened the door for the development of novel embolic materials for aneurysm treatment. Owing to the attractiveness of a minimally invasive procedure to treat aneurysms, the effort to produce better embolic materials is ongoing.

7.3 Types of embolic materials

There is a wide range of materials used for endovascular embolization, from platinum coils to liquid polymerizing agents. This variety can be attributed, in part, to the many different procedural goals and types of treatment. For example, palliative treatment of a brain AVM may require a different embolization material than one that is being pre-embolized for surgical resection. For each embolic material, specific delivery techniques have been developed. While almost all of the endovascular embolic materials discussed here are introduced into the body through transfemoral catheter entry, the technique of embolization varies considerably for each material. Similarly, the conditions to be treated by endovascular embolization – cerebral AVMs and intracranial aneurysms – must be handled using different techniques. In this section, the materials used for endovascular embolization will be divided first by the type of condition they are used to treat. Then, the properties of the material will be discussed, along with the special considerations of the material related to its delivery technique.

7.3.1 Embolic materials for cerebral arteriovenous malformations

Polyvinyl alcohol particles

Polyvinyl alcohol (PVA) particles were identified for use as embolic agents in 1971, but were used clinically for other purposes since the early 1950s (Davidson and Terbrugge, 1995). One advantage of PVA particles is their ability to be produced in various, distinct sizes, allowing embolization treatment with PVA particles to be specifically tailored to the AVM being treated. PVA particles can be administered non-surgically through transfemoral guidewire-directed catheters. The mode of action that PVA particles employ to occlude an AVM has been debated. Davidson and Terbrugge (1995) explained that PVA particles act by adhering to the vessel wall and slowing blood flow, rather than actually plugging the AVM with secondary thrombosis. However, it has also been thought that the particles themselves are thrombogenic when injected into small vessels (Linfante and Wakhloo, 2007).

A variety of studies have been carried out to determine the safety and effectiveness of PVA particles used in AVM embolization. One common finding when examining PVA particle embolization is the high rate of recanalization associated with this technique (Linfante and Wakhloo, 2007). Another drawback is the relatively long amount of time it takes to occlude the AVM lumen when compared to other embolic materials. Since thrombus formation and occlusion takes minutes rather than seconds, there is a pressure increase within the AVM lumen as smaller channels are embolized. The added pressure has been shown to increase the chances of rupture and hemorrhage during embolization (Wallace *et al.*, 1995). Due to such findings, cerebral AVM embolization with PVA particles is generally reserved as a pre-surgical treatment in order to slow blood flow in the region before surgical resection.

N-butyl cyanoacrylate

N-butyl cyanoacrylate (n-BCA) is a liquid adhesive injectable material that polymerizes almost instantaneously when it comes into contact with an anionic environment such as blood (Debrun, 1997). This material, used under the trade name Histoacryl® (B. Braun), is marketed as a tissue adhesive to be used in place of sutures or stapling. Its properties of quick polymerization and slow degradation make n-BCA an optimal material for AVM embolization. Slow polymerization would result in material escaping into the vein, while material degradation would subject the lesion to recanalization. Owing to its adhesive nature, one commonly reported problem with using n-BCA during endovascular embolization is 'gluing' the catheter tip to the vessel wall. A surgeon's inability to withdraw a catheter without substantial damage to the vessel is an obvious issue that must be avoided.

This material is a colorless liquid, so introduction of the material into an AVM requires mixing it with a liquid contrast agent. In order to keep the material from reacting with the contrast agent, the agent must be very hydrophobic. Ethiodol and Lipiodol have both been used as the radio-opaque agent included prior to embolization with n-BCA (Yu *et al.*, 2004). Addition of a hydrophobic contrast agent can also slow the reaction time *in vivo* when the material contacts blood. The rate of polymerization can be adjusted to the desired speed by changing the ratio of n-BCA to contrast material. Debrun (1997) describes clinical AVM embolization procedures using a formulation of 1 mL Histoacryl and 3 mL Ethiodol.

N-butyl cyanoacrylate is commonly delivered transfemorally through a flow-directed microcatheter system. A larger guidewire (6F–8F) is used to direct the microcatheter (1.8F–1.2F) close to the base of the cranium, where the flexible microcatheter tip allows further advancement through tortuous angioarchitecture of the cerebral AVM (Goto *et al.*, 1998). Before injecting the n-BCA mixture, the surgeon must place the microcatheter tip at the entrance of or within the AVM nidus. Until the advent of flexible microcatheter tips, this task was almost impossible. Accurate tip positioning is assessed by a pre-injection of contrast agent into the nidus. If there is no proximal reflux of contrast, the embolization can proceed. If contrast does reflux, the microcatheter tip is re-positioned and the contrast pre-injection is done again (Debrun, 1997). Along with microcatheter tip placement, sometimes flow control techniques are used in order to reduce delivery complications that may arise in the high flow environment of an AVM. For example, Goto *et al.* (1998) explain that a variety of extravascular and endovascular techniques to reduce flow to the AVM nidus, such as systemic hypotension, direct carotid artery compression, temporary balloon occlusion, and adjustment of the n-BCA-contrast agent ratio. Once the tip is positioned correctly and the regional flow is controlled, the injection of n-BCA also requires specific techniques and skills. Injection of the material is done slowly and in conjunction with some type of digital subtraction angiography or biplane roadmapping in order to visualize the progression of n-BCA within the nidus. The injection is continued until a drop of glue is seen to enter the draining vein. At this point, the injection is paused, and then continued until a drop of glue is seen to enter the draining vein again. The sequence of injecting and pausing is repeated until the progression of n-BCA into the nidus is no longer observed, or the material is seen to reflux proximally (Debrun, 1997). Removal of the microcatheter and guidewire must be done carefully so the microcatheter tip does not become glued to the vessel on the way out.

N-butyl cyanoacrylate is the most commonly used cerebral AVM embolic material, and is considered by some to be the most effective (Linfante and Wakhloo, 2007). While its drawbacks include tissue adhesiveness and optimization of polymerization time, the main advantage of this material is its permanency. The curative capability of n-BCA, seen both after initial embolization and long-term follow-up, make this material a desirable choice for AVM obliteration (Yu *et al.*, 2004).

Onyx

Onyx Liquid Embolic System, manufactured by ev3, is a non-adhesive precipitating embolic material formulated from ethylene-vinyl alcohol copolymer dissolved in the organic solvent dimethylsulfoxide (DMSO). The copolymer is formed with ethylene, which is a hydrophobic subunit, and vinyl alcohol, which is hydrophilic. This mixture is dissolved in DMSO and micronized tantalum particles are added for radio-opacity. Once the solution is injected, DMSO rapidly diffuses away into the blood and the copolymer precipitates to create a spongy solid (He *et al.*, 2005). Figure 7.1 depicts a similar ethylene and vinyl alcohol copolymer as it solidifies when coming into contact with saline (Murayama *et al.*, 1998).

Owing to its non-adhesive nature and slower solidification characteristics, it has been suggested that this material can be delivered in a more sustained, controllable fashion with more nidal penetration and less chance of tissue adherence to the catheter (Velat *et al.*, 2008). However, despite less tissue adhesion, there have been reported cases of the catheter tip becoming trapped in the delivered material during Onyx delivery (Weber *et al.*, 2007). Also, it has been argued that with greater nidal penetration, there is a potential for increased complication rates due to subsequent increased venous occlusion.

Delivering Onyx to a cerebral AVM requires some special considerations given the material's chemical and physical characteristics. Inclusion of DMSO within the delivery material requires that Onyx be injected very slowly. High speeds and large volumes of DMSO injection have been shown to cause vessel necrosis (Murayama *et al.*, 1998). Also, Onyx requires the use of DMSO-

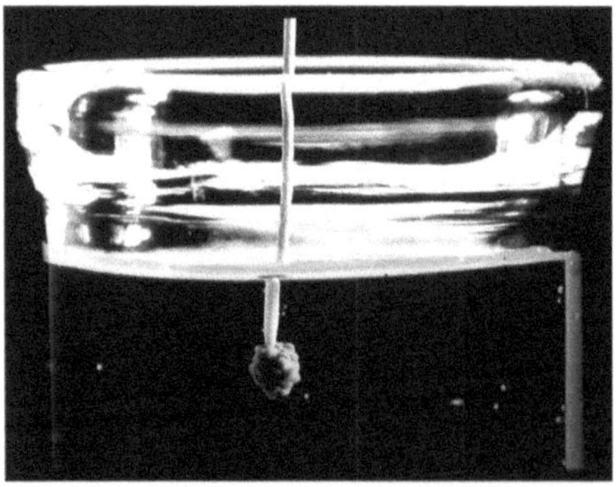

7.1 Photograph depicting the solidification of an ethylene-vinyl alcohol copolymer in contact with saline. Reproduced with permission from Murayama (1998). Copyright (1998) Lippincott, Williams & Wilkins.

compatible microcatheters, which are typically not designed with the flexible flow-directed tips, which are used for administration of n-BCA. As a result, this can cause difficulty in optimal microcatheter tip placement and greater proximal reflux of Onyx during injection, which must be taken into account prior to embolization (Velat *et al.*, 2008).

A number of delivery techniques for Onyx embolization have been described by endovascular neurosurgeons. Weber *et al.* (2007) describe the 'plug and push' technique, where a dense cast of Onyx is created around the micocatheter tip to establish vascular occlusion, and then this 'plug' is pushed further into the nidus by injecting many small volumes of Onyx. This process is repeated until the material fills the nidus, resulting in a spongy polymer mass (Weber *et al.*, 2007). He *et al.* (2005) use a technique similar to that of n-BCA administration, in which the material is injected until it is seen to proximally reflux. The injection is paused for a few minutes after observation of the reflux, and the material is injected again.

The use of Onyx for AVM embolization has become more common in the United States since it was approved by the FDA in 2005, while it has been used clinically in Europe since 1999. As neurosurgeons are gaining experience delivering the material, more information is becoming available regarding the overall safety and effectiveness of embolizing AVMs with Onyx. Velat *et al.* (2008) retroactively compared AVM embolization with n-BCA and Onyx in terms of procedure and fluoroscopy times associated with each technique. While this study did not specifically analyze factors such as recanalizaiton rates or morbidity/mortality statistics, complication rates with each embolic material were reported, and were similar. Comparing fluoroscopy and procedure time with each embolic agent does provide a measure of clinical advantage that needs to be taken into consideration. Overall, Velat *et al.* (2008) found that AVM embolization with Onyx requires significantly more fluoroscopy time than n-BCA procedures, but that the operator performing the embolization also proved to be a significant factor in total fluoroscopy time.

Despite this somewhat negative aspect of Onyx embolization, many neurosurgeons prefer Onyx because of its increased controllability over n-BCA, and its potential to provide deeper penetration into the AVM nidus and occlude more feeding pedicles. However, it should be noted that both embolic materials provide different benefits and limitations when considering an endovascular approach to AVM treatment. Instead of comparing these materials with a 'better-worse' characterization, it is more advantageous to view each material as having its place in endovascular embolization. For example, when embolizing an AVM under circumstances where material reflux is unacceptable, nBCA may be the embolic agent of choice, since Onyx has been associated with higher reflux events. Similarly, the controllability properties of Onyx may make it a better candidate for embolization of a large volume AVMs with only one feeding pedicle (Velat *et al.*, 2008). Overall, the material is not the only consideration when embolizing an AVM – many other factors, including the AVM size and location, play a large part in deciding which embolic agent to use.

7.3.2 Embolic materials for intracranial aneurysm

Endovascular coils

Endovascular coiling is now the standard practice used for intracranial aneurysm embolization. Since the advent of this technique, there has been much research and development geared towards producing better embolic coils. While platinum coils are the standard material used for aneurysm embolization, they do not come without drawbacks. One common occurrence with platinum coil embolization is aneurysm recanalization (Lanzino *et al.*, 2005). Also, as reported in the ISAT 2002 study of ruptured ICAs, coil embolization had a higher rate of rebleeding than was found with microsurgical clipping (International Subarachnoid Aneurysm Trial (ISAT) Collaborative Group, 2002). The relatively low fill percentages achieved with coil embolization are thought to be related to higher rates of recanalization and rebleeding. Coil packing percentages in intracranial aneurysms tend to be less than 30–40%, due in part to the nature of the coils, their tendencies to tangle, and resistance within an aneurysm once the first coil has been introduced (Tamatani *et al.*, 2002). Lower coil packing densities have been linked to coil compaction in a variety of studies. In particular, Kawanabe *et al.* (2001) retrospectively analyzed 33 patients who had ICAs embolized from 1994 to 1998. All of the patients who experienced coil compaction had initial coil packing densities below ~20%, while all patients who did not experience coil compaction had initial coil packing densities greater than 20% (Kawanabe *et al.*, 2001).

A number of modifications to platinum coils have been developed in recent years in order to combat aneurysm recanalization and rebleeding, such as the introduction of HydroCoil and Matrix detachable coils. HydroCoils (MicroVention, Aliso Viejo, CA) consist of platinum coils coated with an expandable hydrogel that swells when in contact with blood. In this way, the HydroCoil can potentially fill more of the aneurysm and achieve a greater occlusion volume than bare platinum coils alone. Figure 7.2 shows the profiles of a bare platinum coil placed next to a hydrogel-coated coil in both its dehydrated and hydrated forms. From observation alone, the expansion of the hydrogel around the carrier coil allows for higher initial fill percentages (Cloft and Kallmes, 2004).

In a study by Fanning *et al.* (2007) 100 intracranial aneurysms were embolized with HydroCoils in conjunction with bare platinum coils, where a 'basket' of bare platinum coils were positioned in the aneurysm, followed by the introduction of HydroCoils. The treatment group showed a 20% increase in the mean packing density when the same number of coils was used in the control

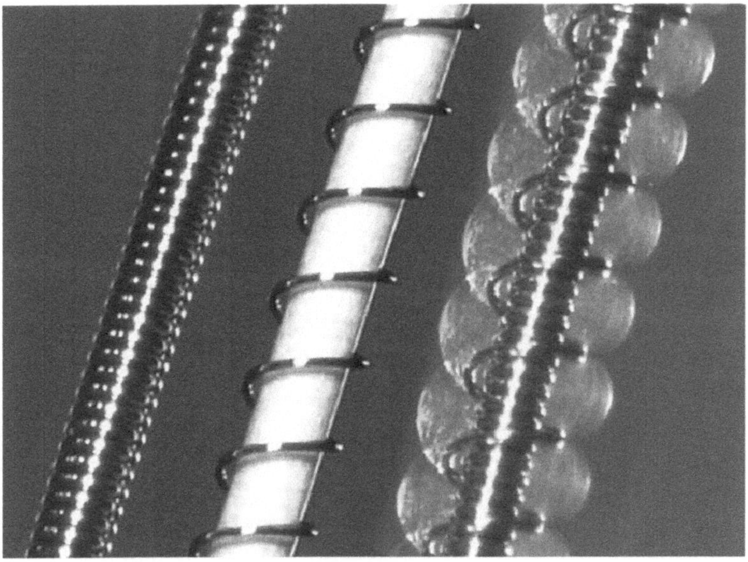

7.2 Comparison of bare platinum coil with a hydrogel-coated coil device. Left: bare platinum coil. Middle: pre-hydrated coil image. Right: post-hydration coil image, showing the expanded transcucent hydrogel. Reproduced with permission from Cloft and Kallames (2004). Copyright (2004) American Society of Neuroradiology.

group (bare platinum coils alone). Furthermore, initial angiographic results showed significantly better occlusions in the treatment group (Fanning *et al.*, 2007). While the initial post-embolization angiographic results of this method are promising, HydroCoils have yet to been investigated for long term outcomes.

Matrix detachable coils (Boston Scientific Neurovascular) are another example of modified endovascular coils, employing a stainless steel delivery wire coated with a bioabsorbable copolymer of 90% polyglycolide and 10% polylactide. In a study by Murayama *et al.* (2003), matrix detachable coils were shown to accelerate the rate of aneurysm healing in swine aneurysm models, specifically by promoting the formation of a thick neointimal layer at the aneurysm neck more quickly bare platinum coils (Murayama *et al.*, 2003). Taschner *et al.* (2005) evaluated the use of Matrix detachable coils in 25 patients with intracranial aneurysms. Again, stable embolized aneurysms were achieved over a six-month period, but only when Matrix coils were used in conjunction with bare platinum coils (Taschner *et al.*, 2005).

Another disadvantage to endovascular coiling is that the procedure is generally successful for aneurysms with well-defined necks only, excluding fusiform and giant aneurysms. Treatment of fusiform aneurysms with endovascular coils has been attempted, usually resulting in coil migration into the parent vessel. Recently, using stent-assisted coil embolization and balloon remodeling to treat fusiform aneurysms has been done with more success (Wells-Roth *et al.*, 2005).

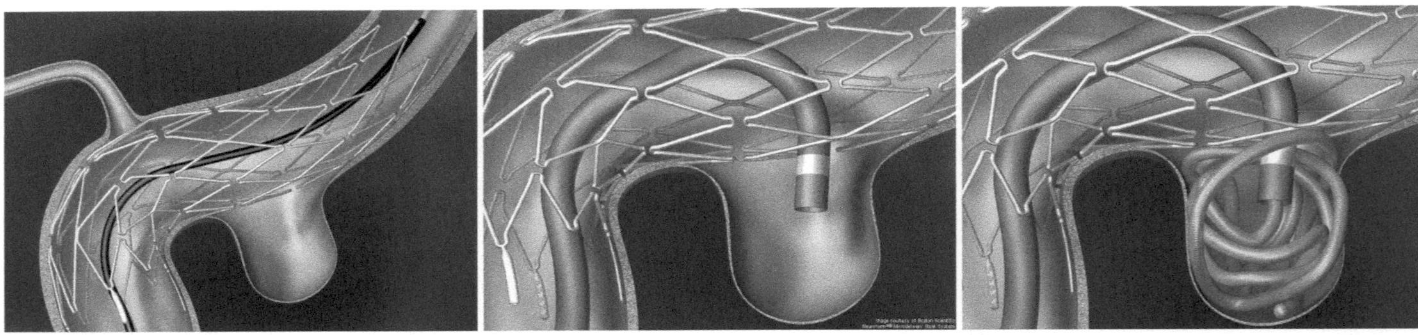

(a) (b) (c)

7.3 Schematic drawings showing stent-assisted embolization with the Neuroform stent (Boston Scientific/Target), which helps prevent coil migration into the parent vessel. (a) Stent is positioned in the parent artery over the aneurysm. (b) The microcatheter is placed through the stent mesh. (c) Coils are delivered to the aneurysm through the microcatheter. Reproduced with permission from Lanzino (2005). Copyright (2005) Lippincott, Williams & Wilkins.

Figure 7.3 is a schematic showing how stent-assisted embolization can be performed during aneurysm embolization (Lanzino *et al.*, 2005).

Onyx

While already extensively used for the treatment of AVMs, Onyx has recently been examined for occlusion of intracranial aneurysms as well. The characteristics that make this material optimal for AVM embolization, including ease of deliverability and controllability, also apply to embolization of intracranial aneurysms. In 2002, the Cerebral Aneurysm Multicenter European Onyx (CAMEO) trial investigated the clinical and angiographic outcomes of intracranial aneurysm Onyx embolization using a population of ICAs that are historically difficult to treat with coil embolization (Molyneux *et al.*, 2004). While the authors found that introduction of Onyx to the aneurysm generally required the aid of either balloon reconstruction or stent-assisted delivery, the clinical and angiographic outcomes at 3 and 12 months were surprisingly good. In fact, the angiographic occlusion rates were superior to those commonly reported for coil embolization (Molyneux *et al.*, 2004).

The procedure for Onyx administration in an aneurysm is similar to the 'plug and push' technique described for AVM embolization, but with the additional consideration of inflation and deflation of the balloon during the procedure such that blood flow in the parent artery is not restricted for an extended period of time. Overall, this may tend to increase procedure times when embolizing aneurysms with Onyx as opposed to coil embolization.

Since Onyx has shown much potential in its ability to occlude aneurysms, there has been more interest towards developing and investigating other injectable polymeric systems that may provide even more benefits than those currently on the market for embolization therapy.

7.4 Future trends

Embolic materials for both intracranial AVMs and aneurysms have come a long way since the first endovascular embolization procedure was carried out. Much advancement to this branch of neurosurgery came about because of an emphasis on development of equipment that was better suited to endovascular techniques. Some of these inventions include flow-directed microcatheters, endovascular balloons, and re-designed stents. Owing to a greater capacity to perform endovascular techniques with suitable equipment, the development of better embolic materials has followed. Now, there are a variety of techniques and materials that endovascular neurosurgeons have at their disposal, all of which provide a variety of benefits, yet have considerable drawbacks. Efforts are always being made to improve current materials and techniques, as well as to find new materials that may be better suited for embolization. A few of these developmental embolic materials are discussed here.

7.4.1 Calcium alginate gel system

Becker *et al.* (2005) have described an injectable gelling system composed of a crosslinked natural copolymer, calcium alginate. Alginate is a naturally occurring copolymer with mannuronic and guluronic acids blocks. When active guluronic acid sites associate with a divalent cation, such as calcium, polymer chains crosslink to form a gel matrix (Becker *et al.*, 2005). In order to deliver this material to a lesion site, a double-lumen microcatheter has been used to bring both sodium alginate and the calcium chloride ($CaCl_2$) initiator to the desired site without reacting. Once the materials mix in the lesion site, the Ca^{2+} replaces a Na^{+} ion on the alginate, resulting in rapid crosslinking. The byproduct of this system is NaCl, and the formed gel is nonadhesive as well as stable and biocompatible after 6 month *in vivo* studies in an AVM animal model (Becker *et al.*, 2002). The advantages of this system include the absence of organic solvents, low toxicity, and the formation of a nonadhesive tissue-like gel. Figure 7.4 depicts an *in vitro* aneurysm model that has been cut to expose the calcium alginate embolic material, showing the tissue-like nature of the solidified material (Soga *et al.*, 2004). Furthermore, the delivery properties are optimal for microcatheter delivery due to the shear-thinning properties of alginate (Becker and Kipke, 2001). While further optimization of the calcium alginate system must be done before it is used clinically, this material holds much promise as a future embolic material.

7.4.2 Michael-type addition polymer systems

Other *in situ* gelling polymeric systems under investigation for endovascular embolization include multi-functional Michael-type addition monomers that

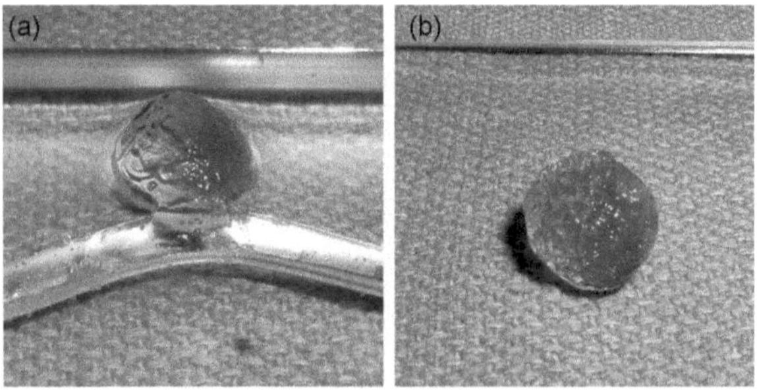

7.4 (a) An opened *in vitro* aneurysm model filled with calcium alginate in strand form. (b) Calcium alginate removed from the aneurysm model post-embolization. Reproduced with permission from Soga (2004). Copyright (2004) Lippincott, Williams & Wilkins.

undergo a thiol-acrylate reaction during polymerization. The thiol-containing monomer is deprotonated by a free hydroxide group, which is provided by incorporation of a water phase. The deprotonated thiol group then attacks an acrylate group located on the other reacting monomer in a Michael-type addition reaction. Owing to the multi-functionality of the monomers, the material crosslinks, forms a network, and becomes a solid gel. These materials are advantageous because the thiol-acrylate reaction is very rapid and very specific, leaving few unreacted monomers and allowing the gel to reach high storage modulus values. Because this system uses a water-based initiation, organic solvents are not needed, making them safer for endovascular procedures (Vernon *et al.*, 2003). This polymer system gels in a time-dependent manner based on a variety of factors. The process of mixing the water-based portion into the monomer phase, both the rate of mixing and the length of mixing, can affect the kinetics of the reaction. The pH of the water phase is also an important factor, where higher pH results in faster reaction kinetics and gel formation (McLemore *et al.*, 2006). The minor adjustments that can be made to the kinetics through alteration of the mixing process and pH of the water phase make this polymer system extremely flexible in terms of tailoring the reaction time to fit individual endovascular procedures.

7.4.3 Shape memory polymers

Shape memory polymers make up another class of injectable biomaterials for vascular applications, yet are relatively new in the field of endovascular embolization. Shape memory polymers are chemically structured so that they are able to reversibly take on a different physical shape in response to some stimuli (Small *et al.*, 2007). Usually these different shapes include a compact form and an expanded form of the polymer. In the case of endovascular embolization, the expanded polymer can be pre-formed to fit specific contours of an individual aneurysm (Ortega *et al.*, 2007). Upon interacting with some type of stimuli, such as heat or cold, the material is compacted into a shape that can be delivered through a microcatheter. The process of using shape memory polymers to embolize an aneurysm is shown in Fig. 7.5, along with samples of expanded SMPs (Ortega *et al.*, 2007).

These materials have an obvious application to fusiform aneurysms, which are difficult to treat using coils or liquid embolics due to migration into the parent vessel. Shape memory polymers can potentially remove this limitation since the device is pre-formed to the aneurysm topography. Metcalf *et al.* (2003) investigated a porous polyurethane shape memory polymer as an embolic device for fusiform aneurysms in an animal model. In this study, thick neointimal formation was found over aneurysm necks after a 12-week period. The porous nature of this material may have encouraged cell infiltration and neointimal growth to seal off the aneurysm from the rest of the vasculature (Metcalfe *et al.*,

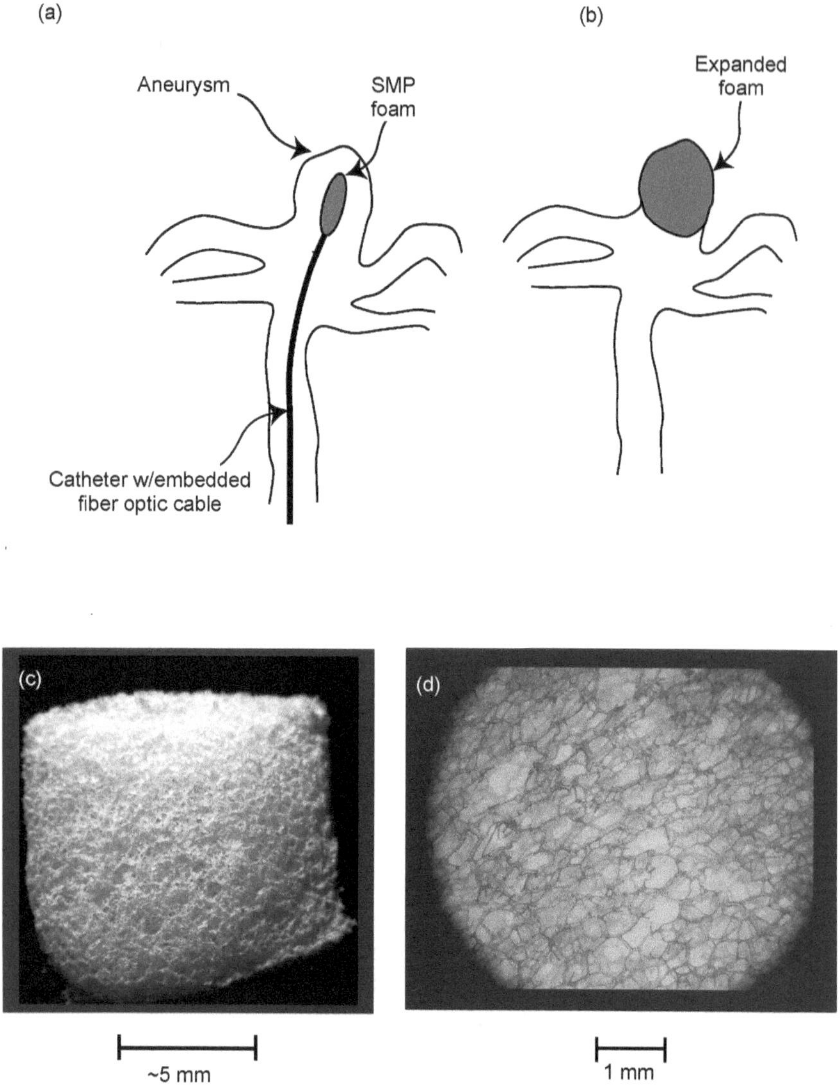

7.5 Treatment of an intracranial aneurysm with SMP foam. (a) Catheter delivery of a compressed piece of SMP foam to the aneurysm. (b) Fully expanded SMP foam within the post-treatment aneurysm. (c) Sample of SMP foam in a primary, expanded shape. (d) Close-up of the SMP foam. Reproduced with permission from Ortega (2007). Copyright (2007) Springer.

2003). Shape memory polymers, as well as the other developmental embolic materials discussed here, represent insight into future procedures that may revolutionize the practice of endovascular embolization in order to better treat critical vascular conditions.

7.5 Sources of further information and advice

For further information about intracranial aneurysms, arteriovenous malformations, endovascular embolization techniques, and interventional neuroradiology, see the books listed below.

Golzarian, J., Sun, S. & Sharafuddin, M. J. (2006) *Vascular embolotherapy: a comprehensive approach, Volume 1: General principles, chest, abdomen, and great vessels*. Berlin, Springer-Verlag.

Golzarian, J., Sun, S. & Sharafuddin, M. J. (2006) *Vascular embolotherapy: a comprehensive approach, Volume 2: Oncology, trauma, gene therapy, vascular malformations, and neck*. Berlin, Springer-Verlag.

Knaut, M. (2006) *Intracranial vascular malformations and aneurysms: from diagnostic work-up to endovascular therapy*. Springer.

Morris, P. (2001) *Interventional and endovascular therapy of the nervous system: a practical guide*. New York, Springer-Verlag.

Thompson, M., Morgan, R., Matsumura, J.S., Sapoval, M., & Loftus, I.M. (2007) *Endovascular intervention for vascular disease: principles and practice*. New York, Informa Healthcare.

7.6 References

Alexander, M. J. & Tolbert, M. E. (2006) Targeting cerebral arteriovenous malformations for minimally invasive therapy. *Neurosurgery*, 59, 178–183.

Becker, T. A. & Kipke, D. R. (2001) Flow properties of liquid calcium alginate polymer injected through medical microcatheters for endovascular embolization. *Journal of Biomedical Materials Research*, 61, 533–540.

Becker, T. A., Kipke, D. R., Preul, M. C., Bichard, W. D. & McDougall, C. G. (2002) Endovascular embolization of a cerebral arteriovenous malformation model using the swine rete mirabile. *Neurosurgery*, 51, 453–459.

Becker, T. A., Preul, M. C., Bichard, W. D., Kipke, D. R. & McDougall, C. G. (2005) Material for endovascular arteriovenous malformation embolization: six-month results in an animal model. *Neurosurgery*.

Cloft, H. J. & Kallmes, D. F. (2004) Aneurysm packing with HydroCoil embolic system versus platinum coils: initial clinical experience. *American Journal of Neuroradiology*, 25, 60–62.

Davidson, G. S. & Terbrugge, K. G. (1995) Histologic long-term follow-up after embolization with polyvinyl-alcohol particles. *American Journal of Neuroradiology*, 16, 843–846.

Debrun (1997) Embolization of the nidus of brain arteriovenous malformations with n-butyl cyanoacrylate. *Neurosurgery*, 40, 112–121.

Fanning, N. F., Berentei, Z., Brennan, P. R. & Thornton, J. (2007) HydroCoil as an adjuvant to bare platinum coil treatment of 100 cerebral aneurysms. *Neuroradiology*, 49, 139–148.

Goto, K., Uda, K. & Ogata, N. (1998) Embolization of cerebral arteriovenous malformations (AVMs): Material selection, improved technique, and tactics in the initial therapy of cerebral AVMs. *Neurologia Medicu-Chirurgica Suppl*, 38, 193–199.

Hashimoto, N., Nozaki, K., Takagi, Y., Kikuta, K.-I. & Mikuni, N. (2007) Surgery of cerebral arteriovenous malformations. *Neurosurgery*, 61, SHC375–SHC389.

He, H.-W., Jiang, C.-H., Liu, H.-B., Li, Y.-X., Zhang, J.-B. & Wu, Z.-X. (2005) Endovascular treatment of cerebral arteriovenous malformations with Onyx embolization. *Chinese Medical Journal*, 118, 2041–2045.

International Subarachnoid Aneurysm Trial (ISAT) Collaborative Group. (2002) International Subarachnoid Aneurysm Trial (ISAT) of neurosurgical clipping versus endovascular coiling in 2143 patients with ruptured intracranial aneurysms: a randomised trial. *The Lancet*, 360, 1267–1274.

Kanaan, Y., Kaneshiro, D., Fraser, K., Wang, D. & Lanzino, G. (2005) Evolution of endovascular therapy for aneurysm treatment. *Neurosurgical Focus*, 18, E2.

Kawanabe, Y., Sadato, A., Taki, W. & Hashimoto, N. (2001) Endovascular occlusion of intracranial aneurysms with Guglielmi detachable coils: correlation between coil packing density and coil compaction. *Acta Neurochirurgica*, 143, 451–455.

Lanzino, G., Kanaan, Y., Perrini, P., Dayoub, H. & Fraser, K. (2005) Emerging concepts in the treatment of intracranial aneurysms: stents, coated coils, and liquid embolic agents. *Neurosurgery*, 57, 449–459.

Legiehn, G. M. & Heran, M. K. S. (2008) Venous malformations: classification, development, diagnosis, and interventional radiologic management. *Radiologic Clinics of North America*, 46, 545–597.

Linfante, I. & Wakhloo, A. K. (2007) Brain aneurysms and arteriovenous malformations: advancements and emerging treatments in endovascular embolization. *Stroke*, 38, 1411–1417.

Lohani, B. (2004) Fusiform middle cerebral artery aneurysm. *Journal of Neuroscience*, 1, 50–52.

McKissock, W., Richardson, A. & Walsh, L. (1965) Anterior communicating aneurysms: a trial of conservative and surgical treatment. *Lancet*, 1, 873–876.

McLemore, R., Preul, M. C. & Vernon, B. (2006) Controlling delivery properties of a waterborne, *in-situ*-forming biomaterial. *Journal of Biomedical Materials Research Part B: Applied Biomaterials*, 79B, 398–410.

Metcalfe, A., Desfaits, A.-C., Salazkin, I., Yahia, L. H., Sokolowski, W. M. & Raymond, J. (2003) Cold hibernated elastic memory foams for endovascular interventions. *Biomaterials*, 24, 491–497.

Molyneux, A. J., Cekirge, S., Saatci, I. & Gal, G. (2004) Cerebral aneurysm multicenter European Onyx (CAMEO) trial: results of a prospective observational study in 20 European centers. *American Journal of Neuroradiology*, 25, 39–51.

Murayama, Y., Vinuela, F., Ulhoa, A., Akiba, Y., Duckwiler, G. R., Gobin, Y. P., Vinters, H. V. & Greff, R. J. (1998) Nonadhesive liquid embolic agent for cerebral arteriovenous malformations: preliminary histopathological studies in swine rete mirabile. *Neurosurgery*, 43, 1164–1172.

Murayama, Y., Tateshima, S., Gonzalez, N. & Vinuela, F. (2003) Matrix and bioabsorbable polymeric coils accelerate healing of intracranial aneurysms: long-term experimental study. *Stroke*, 34, 2031–2037.

Ortega, J., Maitland, D., Wilson, T., Tsai, W., Savas, O. & Saloner, D. (2007) Vascular dynamics of a shape memory polymer foam aneurysm treatment technique. *Annals of Biomedical Engineering*, 35, 1870–1884.

Small, W., Buckley, P. R., Wilson, T., Benett, W. J., Hartman, J., Saloner, D. & Maitland, D. (2007) Shape memory polymer stent with expandable foam: a new concept for endovascular embolization of fusiform aneurysms. *IEEE Transactions on Biomedical Engineering*, 54, 1157–1160.

Soga, Y., Preul, M. C., Furuse, M., Becker, T. A. & McDougall, C. G. (2004) Calcium alginate provides a high degree of embolization in aneurysm models: a specific comparison to coil packing. *Neurosurgery*, 55, 1401–1409.

Spetzler, R. F. & Martin, N. A. (1986) A proposed grading system for arteriovenous malformations. *Journal of Neurosurgery*, 65, 476–483.

Stedman, T. (2000) *Stedman's Medical Dictionary 27th ed.*, Lippincott Williams & Wilkins.

Tamatani, S., Ito, Y., Abe, T., Koike, T., Takeuchi, S. & Tanaka, R. (2002) Evaluation of the stability of aneurysms after embolization using detachable coils: correlation between stability of aneurysms and embolized volume of aneurysms. *American Journal of Neuroradiology*, 23, 762–767.

Taschner, C. A., Leclerc, X., Rachdi, H., Barros, A. M. & Pruvo, J.-P. (2005) Matrix detachable coils for the endovascular treatment of intracranial aneurysms: analysis of early angiographic and clinical outcomes. *Stroke*, 36, 2176–2180.

Valavanis, A., Pangalu, A. & Tanaka, M. (2004) Endovascular treatment of cerebral arteriovenous malformations with emphasis on the curative role of embolisation. *Swiss Archives of Neurology and Psychiatry*, 155, 341–347.

Velat, G. J., Reavey-Cantwell, J. F., Sistrom, C., Smullen, D., Fautheree, G. L., Whiting, J., Lewis, S. B., Mericle, R. A., Firment, C. S. & Hoh, B. L. (2008) Comparison of n-butyl cyanoacrylate and ONYX for the embolization of intracranial arteriovenous malformations: analysis of fluoroscopy and procedure times. *Neurosurgery*, 63, ONS75–ONS82.

Vernon, B., Tirelli, N., Bachi, T., Haldimann, D. & Hubbell, J. A. (2003) Water-borne, *in situ* crosslinked biomaterials from phase-segregated precursors. *Journal of Biomedical Materials Research*, 64A, 447–456.

Wallace, R. C., Flom, R. A., Khayata, M. H., Dean, B. L., McKenzie, J., Rand, J. C., Obuchowski, N. A., Zepp, R. C., Zabramski, J. M. & Spetzler, R. F. (1995) The safety and effectiveness of brain arteriovenous malformation embolization using acrylic and particles: the experiences of a single institution. *Neurosurgery*, 37, 606–618.

Weber, W., Kis, B., Siekmann, R., Jans, P., Laumer, R. & Kuhne, D. (2007) Preoperative embolization of intracranial arteriovenous malformations with Onyx. *Neurosurgery*, 61, 244–254.

Wells-Roth, D., Biondi, A., Janardhan, V., Chapple, K., Gobin, Y. P. & Riina, H. A. (2005) Endovascular procedures for treating wide-necked aneurysms. *Neurosurgical Focus*, 18, E7.

Yu, S. C. H., Chan, M. S. Y., Lam, J. M. K., Tam, P. H. T. & Poon, W. S. (2004) Complete obliteration of intracranial arteriovenous malformation with endovascular cyanoacrylate embolization: initial success and rate of permanent cure. *American Journal of Neuroradiology*, 25, 1139–1143.

8
Orthopaedic applications of injectable biomaterials

A. C. McLAREN and C. S. ESTES,
Banner Good Samaritan Medical Center, USA

Abstract: This chapter begins by outlining the progression in orthopaedic surgery towards biological interventions, limited exposures and closed or arthroscopic procedures. This leads to the need for materials and implants that can be introduced to the target site remotely, either percutaneously or from a distant entry portal. It then proposes a classification for injectable biomaterials from an orthopaedic perspective and proceeds to discuss specific clinical applications including implant fixation, fracture healing, bone, cartilage and intervertebral disc regeneration, viscosupplementation, drug delivery and enzymatic fasciotomy. Many of the materials discussed in the chapter are in developmental stages or under clinical investigation with long-term outcomes pending.

Key words: orthopaedic, implant fixation, fracture healing, viscosupplementation, bone morphogenic protein.

8.1 Introduction

Orthopaedics has become increasingly focused on the biology of underlying conditions and on wound healing, requiring materials and implants that are more biologically oriented rather than simply structural. Procedures have become less extensive requiring implants to be introduced to target sites through narrower exposures. Injectable biomaterials are integral to this progress.

Orthopaedia is the term that was first used to describe prevention and correction of deformity in children in 1741 [84]. Surgical intervention followed for disorders that were unresponsive to corrective splints and braces. Initially surgery was limited to soft tissue releases as might be needed for a tight Achilles tendon but progressed to larger open soft tissue releases and corrective bone realignment. The profession expanded to adults, encompassing the full spectrum of musculoskeletal disorders including fracture management, joint reconstruction, musculoskeletal tumors and sports-related conditions. Understanding the injury caused by surgical dissection itself has led orthopaedists to minimize dissection, successfully leading to less morbidity while requiring more sophisticated technology and materials. It is through understanding the fundamentals of normal biology and the pathophysiology of underlying conditions that biology can be exploited for the benefit of the patient. Prevention and regeneration, rather than mechanical reconstruction for established deformity is clearly the current direction in orthopaedics. The biology of wound healing is the central process. Angiogenesis and fibrocyte proliferation coupled with myofibroblast contraction close tissue disruptions. Cellular proliferation and differentiation into specialized tissues (cartilage, bone, ligament, tendon) regenerate lost tissue. Differentiated tissues, multi-potential cells, signaling peptides and molecular/elemental building blocks are important biologically oriented materials in contemporary orthopaedics. Metals, ceramics and polymers remain important materials to provide the structural needs for a biologically favorable environment. Less-invasive and minimally invasive approaches, 'closed' and remote procedures, and arthroscopy have created the need for biomaterials to be injectable.

Injectable biomaterials are now used in a multitude of orthopaedic procedures, notably, bone void filling, fracture healing, fracture fixation, articular cartilage regeneration, tendinosis healing, and drug delivery. Although the term injectable medically presumes percutaneous, the target site of some orthopaedic materials is inaccessible by means other that injection even when the procedure is performed through wide exposure. For this discussion, introduction of a material forced through a narrow tube is considered injection even when performed through a surgical incision.

Increasing sophistication in materials has increased the co-dependency between bioengineering and orthopaedic surgery. Bioengineers rely upon orthopaedic surgeons to guide their efforts toward clinical relevance; orthopaedic surgeons rely upon bioengineers to deliver technically sound designs. Patient safety is greatly compromised when either profession works independently. Along with the advances in surgical procedures and implantable materials comes the need to address unintended effects and adverse responses. The Federal Drug Administration (FDA) is the agency in the United States that is responsible for protection of patients from harm caused by implants and drugs. Many of the materials used in orthopaedics are used as medical devices rather than drugs, which follows a less rigorous and less costly process for FDA approval. This places the onus on everyone involved in the development and use of orthopaedic biomaterials to scrutinize the technology and clinical response, interacting closely in the process. Product development and clinical application cannot progress in isolation. Patient welfare must come ahead of commercial dominance or professional notoriety.

8.2 Classification

A clinically functional approach based on why a material is being used is a common way orthopaedists think about biomaterials: biological activity, mechanical function or both.

Materials in the biological group are related to wound healing, tissue regeneration, or maintenance of normal tissue biology. Materials in the mechanical group provide a surface, fill a void or bear load. Biologically active materials may depend upon mechanical materials to provide a favorable environment to allow their activity to occur and mechanical materials may be dependent on biological repair to share or replace their mechanical role. For this reason materials are frequently used in combination. Availability, immunogenicity and toxicity, critical factors that determine clinical applicability, are often related to the source, therefore natural and synthetic subcategories are often considered next. Over the long term, if a material does not degrade and resorb, it remains as an implant with the all the implant associated risks including mechanical failure, adverse host response, and surface colonization by bacteria. Biologically active materials are rapidly deactivated and degraded so the resorbable and non-resorbable categories generally apply to materials in the mechanical group. Further categorization by material, allows consideration of material properties and interactions with tissue or other materials.

Injectable orthopaedic biomaterials can be classified similarly:

Function → source → resorbability → material

Bioactive (wound healing)

- a. Tissues
  - i. bone:
    - 1. autograft, allograft, xenograft
    - 2. cortical or cancellous
  - ii. hyaline cartilage:
    - 1. autograft or allograft osteochondral segments
    - 2. allograft particles (juvenile)
- b. Cells
  - i. autologous bone marrow
  - ii. cultured autologous condrocytes
  - iii. mesenchymal stem cells
  - iv. multipotential stem cells
- c. signaling molecules
  - i. bone marrow (autologous)
  - ii. PRP (autologous or allogeneic)
  - iii. BMP, PDGF, ILGF, IL, TGFα (allogeneic or recombinant)
- d. enzymes:
  - i. Botulinum toxin
  - ii. Clostridial collagenase
- e. polymers
  - i. Hyaluronic acid (xenograft)

Mechanical/structural

- ii. Natural/purified
  - 1. Non-resorbable: long term

            a. bone: auto/allo/xeno graft
            b. ceramic: hydroxylapitate (HA), bioglass
        2. Resorbable: short term
            a. protein: collagen
            b. glycosaminoglycan: hyaluronic acid
            c. ceramic: CASO4
    iii. Synthetic/processed
        1. Non-resorbable: long term
            a. PMMA
            b. HA (degradable but over >10 yrs)
            c. composites
                i. cortical bone – PMMA
        2. Resorbable: short term
            a. degradable polymers
                i. PLA, PGA
            b. βTCP, CPC

8.3 Clinical applications 1: fixation

8.3.1 Implant fixation

Poly(methyl methacrylate) (PMMA) is one of the most frequently injected biomaterials in orthopaedic surgery. First described by Edward Haboush in 1953, fixation with PMMA was a key factor employed by Sir John Charnley in the 1960s to achieve success in low friction arthroplasty of the hip [114]. Entrapped air, blood and debris in the interface, and poor penetration into cancellous interstices, all associated with the finger packing technique used initially to fill intramedullary canals, were addressed by injecting the cement into the canal using a device similar to a caulking gun. Pressurizing cement in the medullary canal achieves penetration into the interstices of the endosteal and metaphyseal cancellous bone. Current cement technique for intramedullary stems uses a cement gun to retrograde fill a plugged, clean intramedullary canal with cement prepared under vacuum to minimize air bubbles. The stem is then pushed into the cement-filled canal achieving a uniform mantel 2–4 mm thick. However, many contemporary stemmed implants are fixed biologically through bone apposition or bone in-growth not using cement. Secure non-cemented fixation requires correct fit and immediate stability. When initial stability is not possible, PMMA remains the best fixation option. Non-stemmed implants are cemented by pressurizing the PMMA into the broad surfaces of epiphyseal/metaphyseal cancellous bone rather than injection into the intramedullary canal. Pressurization involves injection of the cement into the exposed cancellous bone surfaces with the nozzle of a cement gun and by capturing cement under the implant as it is impacted into place.

PMMA is also injected into vertebral bodies for fixation of fragility fractures of the spine, injected into screw holes to augment internal fixation in osteopenic bone, and injected into structural voids following resection of benign tumors to control dead space and support the surrounding bone. In many of these applications antimicrobial powder can be added to the PMMA for drug delivery when local delivery of antimicrobials is needed.

Other materials used to achieve implant fixation such as porous metal and calcium ceramics are commercially bonded to implant surfaces, not injected. With better understanding of bioactive peptides, the future may bring the use of signaling molecules to augment biologic implant fixation. Bioactive peptides could be commercially bonded to the substrate surface or injected in liquid or gel form at the time of implantation.

8.3.2 Tissue glue

Materials used to glue tissues are generally introduced by injection due to the need for accurate placement in difficult target sites. Octyl-cyanoacrylate cyanoacrylate, N-asetil 2 butyl sistein and fibrin are the most commonly used materials [5, 55]. The orthopaedic uses include meniscal repairs and repairs of the annularus fibrosis [55, 104]. Both of these applications require more strength than can be achieved by tissue glue alone but in combination with sutures tissue glue improves the contact between the apposed edges and for limited posterior horn applications might be sufficient without sutures [5, 64, 87]. Fibrin glue appears to be adequate to contain cell (chondrocyte) implantations.

8.4 Clinical applications 2: bone healing

8.4.1 Fracture healing

The role of bone graft and bone graft substitutes in fracture healing is well established. Increasingly limited exposures require preparations that can be introduced to the target site by injection. Bone graft and bone graft substitutes can function biologically, mechanically or both. They can provide a mechanical scaffold for bone growth across gaps or voids (osteoconductive), biologically stimulate local cells to form bone (osteoinductive) or deliver living bone forming cells to an atrophic site to independently form bone (osteogenic). For injection, particulate bone is made into a slurry using an inert carrier (glycerin), a biologically active carrier (platelet rich plasma (PRP), bone marrow), or blood. This slurry can be injected into a fracture site or a non-union site by closed means through the intramedullary canal from a remote entry portal using a large bore conduit such as a chest tube, prior to inserting the fixation rod. The difficulty with this technique is controlling where the graft goes. For non-unions, the potential space needed to accept the graft needs to be developed in dense scar tissue, and acute injuries can have extended wound spaces that fail to contain the graft material in the target fracture site.

Autograft can be obtained by reaming the intramedullary canal with a Reamer/Irrigator/Aspirator (Synthes USA, West Chester PA). Small acetabular reamers or burrs can be used on iliac crest donor sites to harvest particulate autograft. Allograft, demineralized allograft and ceramic (hydroxylapitate or beta tricalcium phosphate) bone graft substitutes can be ground into powder, <0.5 mm particle size, suspended and injected using a large bore needle.

Structural load-bearing applications of bone grafts cannot be performed by injection but *in situ* setting bone graft substitutes can be injected to provide structural support or fixation for metaphyseal and epiphyseal fractures.

8.4.2 Bone graft substitutes

Any material that is used to provide the bone healing role of bone graft but is not autograft bone is known as bone graft substitute, or, if mixed with autograft bone to increase the graft volume, it is known as bone graft extender. This includes bone, cells, bioactive factors, Ca/P ceramics and polymers in various combinations [66]. The choice between autograft bone and a substitute takes several factors into account. Autograft is associated with higher healing rates than individual substitute materials. It is osteoconductive, osteoinductive and osteogenic but requires a second surgical site, frequently the iliac crest, to harvest the graft. Major downside concerns are donor site pain and a limited amount of available bone.

Allograft bone has an unlimited supply, often at significant expense, and is osteoinductive, especially when BMPs in the matrix are exposed through demineralization, but, it carries the risk of transmitting disease (1:1 500 000 for human immunodeficiency virus (HIV), 1:100 000 for hepatitis B, and 1:60 000 for hepatitis C) [66]. If allograft bone is not completely cleared of cellular components, there is the potential for an immunological response, a clinical problem mostly for composite tissue transplants.

Demineralized allograft bone

Marshal Urist first described the potential of demineralized bone matrix to induce bone formation in 1965 [108]. Growth factors first termed bone morphogenic proteins (BMP) are contained in the extra cellular matrix (ECM) of bone. Cortical bone has the most BMP but the BMP is entrapped by hydroxyapitate. Acid extraction of the Ca/P mineral component exposes BMP thereby increasing the level of osteoinductive activity. The demineralization process has the added benefit of removing exposed donor cellular components, reducing antigenicity and it kills viral and bacterial microbes, sterilizing the graft [67]. Release of BMP is dependent on the exposed surface area which can be increased by using layers of thin cortical struts for structural applications. For non-structural applications demineralized cortical powder increases the exposed surface area dramatically. Suspended in a delivery vehicle such as glycerin or bone marrow aspirate, demineralized cortical powder can be introduces to target sites by injection.

Cellular bone graft substitute

Living cells with the potential to form bone are required for osteogenic activity. They are found in bone marrow and have been injected into non-union sites to induce bone healing [24, 38]. It is technically difficult to inject sufficient volume of bone marrow aspirate into non-compliant dense scar at a non-union site. In spite of positive reports, the technique has had limited use since its initial description; however, the biological basis remains valid. Bone marrow can be mixed with allograft, ceramic, or polymer scaffolds; all of which have limited anecdotal clinical experience. With more precise knowledge and improved technology, mesenchymal stem cell injections hold the potential to induce bone formation and fracture healing [24]. Selection of the stem cell fraction in bone marrow has been attempted by centrifugation [79]. This decreases the volume considerably. Clinical trials are not available. Platelet rich plasma (PRP), a source of concentrated growth factors, is not truly a cellular graft substitute as platelets lack nuclei. PRP is osteoinductive not osteogenic.

Bioactive factors

Growth factors are bioactive signaling proteins that regulate cell activity through cell surface receptors. These factors cause osteoinduction, acting through osteoblasts and osteoclasts to control and couple production and resorption of bone. The source of these factors is from bone and platelets. Growth factors found in the extracellular matrix of bone include insulin-like growth factor (IGF), transforming growth factor beta (TGF-β), platelet-derived growth factor (PDGF), fibroblast growth factor (FGF), and bone morphogenic proteins (BMP).

Growth factors important for bone regulation found in alpha granules of platelets include BMP, PDGF, TGF, vascular endothelial growth factor (VEGF), epithelial growth factor (EGF), and Vitronectin. Platelets deliver these factors to injury sites in the platelet clot that forms secondary to vascular endothelial disruption [93]. Clinically, concentrated growth factors can be injected into an injury site in the form of PRP, the platelet-rich fraction obtained from centrifuged venous blood. PRP can be obtained from autogenous or allogeneic blood and injected directly into an injury site to enhance bone or soft tissue healing. However, when injected as a liquid there is no control over where it goes. In acute injuries the PRP can disperse widely in the tissues torn by the injury and is exposed to rapid degradation. In chronic wounds, noncompliant scaring can prevent the fluid from infiltrating the tissue at the targeted site. To counter this, a potential space can be developed surgically and the bioactive factors can be delivered in a structural vehicle of protein (collagen), polymer (PLA, PGA), ceramic or bone (autograft or allograft, demineralized allograft) [93]. Clinical reports on platelet rich plasma injections are small pilot studies for acute and chronic tendon injuries, plantar fasciitis, chronic wounds, fracture healing, and spinal fusion [11, 12, 93]. Larger clinical trials are needed to better determine the efficacy of PRP for these applications.

In spite of obvious potential use, experience with injection of signaling molecules is anecdotal with insufficient data to establish efficacy or safety. FDA approved indications for use are very limited and extreme cost makes off-label use a challenge. Clinical trials, as have been done for BMP 2 and BMP 7, are required to establish indications.

Bone morphogenic proteins (BMP)

Bone morphogenic proteins (BMP) are pleiotropic regulators of bone volume, skeletal organogenesis, and fracture healing [111]. Several of the 21 currently identified BMPs have the ability to stimulate osteogenic cellular differentiation, proliferation, and matrix formation, including BMP-2, BMP-4, BMP-6, and BMP-7 [76, 111]. They are released from platelets and osteoprogenitor cells and naturally exist within the extracellular matrix of bone [111].

Human BMP is therapeutically active in milligram doses but is present in cortical bone in the concentration of only 1–2 μg/kg, making it impractical to extract sufficient quantities for clinical use. Therefore, therapeutic quantities are produced commercially through molecular biology techniques (recombinant BMP – rhBMP). Two are currently available for clinical use: rhBMP-2 (Infuse; Medtronic Sofamor Danek, Memphis, Tennessee) and rhBMP-7 (OP-1; Stryker, Kalamazoo, Michigan).

In 2001, the FDA approved rhBMP-7 for use in the treatment of recalcitrant long bone non-unions, but not acute fractures. In 2004 rhBMP-2 received FDA approval for the treatment of open (exposed to the air through a skin laceration) tibial shaft fractures, but not non-unions. The approved use requires an open procedure with delivery of the rhBMP in a collagen sponge, a collagen paste, or collagen/carboxymethycellulose sodium putty. Several small studies have investigated the efficacy and safety of BMP for off-label use to stimulate bone healing in other fracture types, typically implanting the rhBMP in a delivery vehicle such as an absorbable collagen sponge or calcium phosphate cement [111]. Injectable delivery vehicles are being developed for minimally invasive surgery and percutaneous techniques (calcium phosphate with rhBMP-impregnated microspheres) [43, 99]. Due to high cost, averaging $5000 or more per treatment and limited level one outcomes studies, the cost effectiveness of rhBMP remains controversial. If improved healing can prevent the cost of prolonged and failed treatment, this expense may be justifiable [3, 26].

rhBMP-2 was approved in 2002 for spinal fusion surgery using non-injectable methods. Numerous prospective human studies have demonstrated improved posterolateral lumbar fusion rates in patients treated with rhBMP-2 versus groups treated with iliac crest bone graft (ICBG) [29, 37]. Similar results have been reported for other lumbar fusion techniques without the pain and morbidity from a bone graft donor site [77, 111].

Off-label use is a natural consequence of surgical techniques developing faster than regulatory approval can respond. Currently more BMP2 is being used for non-approved procedures than the approved procedure. Serious complications associated with the use of BMP in anterior cervical spine fusion without improved fusion rates illustrate the need for controlled clinical trials before successful treatment for one condition can be extended to a similar condition [110].

Ceramic bone graft substitutes

Ceramics (hydroxyapitate (HA), beta tricalcium phosphate (βTCP), anhydrous calcium sulfate ($CaSO_4$), calcium phosphate cement (CPC)) are the most commonly injected bone graft substitutes. Through minimally invasive techniques, they are used to fill irregular defects and/or provide immediate mechanical stability. Essential physical properties include a fluid state, liquid or gelatinous prior to and during injection, and setting or hardening in an aqueous environment at body temperature (37°C) [61]. The material must also be biocompatible and biodegradable at the rate of bone healing/formation. If the graft substitute resorbs too quickly, loss of stability will occur before the fracture heals or the defect will be filled with fibrous tissue. If the graft substitute resorbs too slowly, blocking bone formation, it will not gain load sharing from regenerate bone, exposing it to the risk of fatigue failure from cyclic loading.

Contained bone defects that limit extravasations prior to setting are best suited for injections with liquid ceramic. Ceramics such as HA, βTCP and $CaSO_4$ have varying porosity to conduct healing bone and no osteoinductive or osteogenic properties. When used in combination with bioactive peptides, healing rates can equal or exceed fresh autograft [54].

Injectable ceramics have been used to manage osteoporotic fractures that have residual defects from compacted bone. Cancellous defects are often caused by impaction of subchondral cancellous bone. After the articular fragment is elevated there is a residual void in the cancellous bone. Although anatomic reduction and stable fixation usually requires an open procedure, percutaneous injection of calcium phosphate cement (CPC) following closed reduction and percutaneous pinning has been shown to improve early rehabilitation for distal radius fractures [20]. As an adjunct to fixation for plate and screw fixation of osteopenic fractures, *in situ* setting ceramics can provide structural stability for the fracture fragments and a scaffold for bone regeneration.

Calcium phosphate cement

Calcium phosphate cements, as an example of *in situ* setting ceramics, are made from a powder containing anhydrous calcium phosphate and an aqueous phosphate solution. Once mixed, calcium phosphate precipitates in an entanglement of crystals that form a paste [91].

Ultimately, the cement hardens to form dahllite, a carbonated apatite similar to that found in the mineral phase of bone [27, 47]. The cement has a microporous structure with pores smaller than 1 μm [86]. Calcium phosphate cement is available from multiple manufactures, as an example Norian Skeletal Repair System (SRS, Synthes West Chester, PA) consists of a liquid sodium phosphate solution and powder monocalcium phosphate monohydrate, tricalcium phosphate, and calcium carbonate. After mixing, the cement has a working time of approximately five minutes and hardens in approximately ten minutes. The material has a compressive strength of approximately 10 MPa at 10 minutes and maximum compressive strength of approximately 50 MPa within 24 hours.

The compressive strength of calcium phosphate cement is 4–10 times greater than cancellous bone and has the highest mechanical strength of any osteoconductive bone graft substitute [27, 47].

In vivo, calcium phosphate is mainly broken down through a cell-mediated process. Small particles of ceramic undergo phagocytosis by giant cells and macrophages, while larger volumes of material are broken down by osteoclasts at the bone–cement interface. Animal studies show remodeling similar to that of native bone remodeling with absorption by osteoclasts, blood vessels formation and development of haversian lamellae [31]. CPC is replaced by host bone at a faster rate than hydroxyapatite, which can persist 10 years or longer after implantation but slower than calcium sulfate, which resorbs in approximately 4–8 weeks [47, 118]. The resorption characteristics and compressive strength of CPC allow its use in load-bearing areas of the skeleton. The structural support provided by this material is particularly advantageous in osteoporotic patients who may be unable to comply with weight-bearing restrictions [47].

Osteoporosis predisposes fracture fixation to failure. To improve screw purchase, calcium phosphate cement can be injected into the porotic bone where the screw will be placed and into voids that screws pass through.

Osteoporosis also leads to insufficiency fractures of the spine in elderly patients. When the strength of the vertebral bodies is insufficient to withstand normal physiologic loads, spontaneous collapse occurs, often leading to progressive kyphosis, (humpback deformity) pain and disability. The loss of structural integrity renders surgical fixation ineffective. These fractures have been treated by vertebroplasty; percutaneous injection with PMMA or calcium-phosphate cement to stabilize the fracture and permit healing either around the PMMA or incorporating the ceramic. A significant risk of vertebroplasty is extrusion of the injected material into an area where it will impinge on nerve roots or the spinal cord. Unfortunately early reports of clinical success have not been confirmed by recent controlled clinical trials perhaps due to lack of consensus for the clinical indications [18, 59, 81].

CPC has been used successfully for the treatment of osteoporosis fractures including distal radius, tibial plateau, calcaneus fractures, and thoracolumbar compression fractures [20, 22, 51, 60, 66, 71, 72, 94, 96, 118]. The majority of these studies report improved early function, earlier return to weight bearing, and improved maintenance of fracture reduction. A meta-analysis of randomized trials for fracture stabilization in the distal radius, femoral neck, intertrochanteric femur, tibial plateau, and calcaneus concluded the use of CPC is associated with less pain and a lower risk of losing fracture reduction when compared with autogenous bone graft, particularly in the case of tibial plateau fractures [7]. Further studies are required to determine long-term outcomes. Not all of these studies injected the material percutaneously; in the open procedures the material was injected into the fracture site or bone void through the incision.

Canine studies show replacement of the CPC by bone through normal osteoclast–osteoblast coupling at a slower pace than allograft bone remodeling although mechanical integrity was preserved throughout the remodeling process [31].

One concern about injectable ceramics is inadequate porosity. Osteoconductive materials should have a three-dimensional interconnecting porosity that allows osteointegration through migration of osteogenic cells and neovascularization. Pore sizes of 150–500 μm have been reported ideal for bone ingrowth (minimum of 100 μm) [36, 65]. Insufficient porosity requires osteoclastic removal of the material slowing bone ingrowth.

Research is currently focused on the development of porous CPC. Loading the cement with particles that degrade faster and the cement, and introducing bubbles during the mixing phase have been examined as methods to create porosity [86]. Degradable microspheres of poly(lactic-co-glycolic) acid (PLGA), poly(trimethylene carbonate) (PTMC), or gelatin have been used to leave pores after degradation to enhance the osteoconductivity of the graft material [45, 46, 82]. Some of the obstacles to the development of porous CPC continue to be compromised compressive strength, poor injectability, and poragen degradation that occurs either too quickly or too slowly.

Microspheres in CPC are also being investigated for local drug delivery of growth factors and antimicrobials [43, 98]. PLGA/gentamicin sulfate microspheres in CPC releases increasing amounts of gentamicin with increased loading up to 20% (w/w) [98]. Antimicrobials have been directly mixed into CPC to control osteomyelitis in an animal model [58]. No clinical trials have been reported using CPC for local antimicrobial delivery; however, there has been at least one case report [80]. $CaSO_4$ has been more extensively studied as a local antimicrobial delivery vehicle. CPC mixed with PLGA/rhBMP-2 microparticles bridge rat cranial defects faster than controls but a substantial amount of the rhBMP-2 is trapped in the cement due to incomplete degradation [13].

Polymers

Type I collagen is a naturally occurring mammalian protein made up from repeating aminoacid subunits consisting of Glycine, X Y (¼ of x = Proline and ¼ of y = Hydroxyproline). Collagen is the most commonly used polymeric bone graft substitute. Although collagen does not independently lead to bone formation it is a very effective carrier for growth factors and mesenchymal stem cells which do lead to bone formation. Harvesting and processing autogenous collagen is impractical. Allogenic and xenogenic (bovine, porcine) collagen are potentially immunogenic; however, clinical performance has not been limited by immunologically incited inflammation. Antibodies to Type I bovine collagen do not have clinically detectable cross-reactivity to human collagen, do not cause hypersensitivity reactions, and do not affect the clinical performance of the bovine collagen [22]. Particulate microfibrilar collagen can be mixed with bone marrow aspirate for injection. Other collagen preparations in the form of sheets used for soft tissue repair are not injectable. Other injectable polymeric materials used as bone graft substitutes include hyaluronic acid (scaffold for cells), chitosan (increased fracture gap healing in dogs), polyanhydrides (surface degradation maintains strength for fracture fixation vs. bulk degrading polymers), polypropylene fumarate (vertebraplasty), polycaprolactones (scaffold for cell culture of cartilage), polyphosphazenes and polylactide-co-glycolide (water soluble hydrolysable for drug delivery), and polyurethanes (glue, cell scaffold) [14, 28, 44, 62, 70].

8.5 Clinical applications 3: prevention and regeneration

8.5.1 Viscosupplementation

Osteoarthritis (OA) is the most common joint disease affecting humans potentially affecting any joint with the neck, low back, fingers, knee and hip dominating [63]. Osteoarthritis of the knee affects more than 20 million Americans, 12% of Americans over 60 years of age. Synovial fluid is responsible for articular cartilage nutrition and lubrication in synovial joints. The high viscosity and thixotropic behavior of synovial fluid comes from the hyaluronic acid component. As OA develops, a decrease in the molecular weight of glucosaminoglycans, including hyaluronic acid, in the articular cartilage ECM occurs, decreasing the hydrophobic negative charge, increasing water content, decreasing cartilage resilience and load bearing properties. The subchondral bone experiences increased peak loads stimulating a bone response, increasing its stiffness, further degrading the joint's ability to distribute loads. The highly organized surface layer of collagen is disrupted, leading to progressive deterioration of the smooth, near frictionless gliding between joint surfaces. In response, more synovial fluid is produced. This increased volume of synovial fluid has lower viscosity with lower hyaluronic acid concentration and molecular weight. To mitigate these effects viscosupplementation with injections of hyaluronic acid has been explored as a symptomatic treatment that does not address the underlying pathophysiology.

First studied in the 1960s as a medical device, hyaluronic acid is a non-sulfated glycosaminoglycan made by fibroblasts and type B synoviocytes [32]. Five commercially available hyaluronic acid formulations of differing MW and crosslinking are in use clinically. They are purified from rooster combs or produced by bacterial fermentation. It is injected either in the form of sodium hyaluronate or covalently crosslinked hyaluronic acid molecules [56]. The treatment regimen is formulation dependent, administered by 1, 3, or 5 intra-articular weekly injections.

The exact mechanism(s) leading to symptomatic relief from viscosupplementation with hyaluronic acid is unknown; however, it is likely not related to rheological changes from the material injected. Injected Hylan A has a half-life of 8.8 hours and Hylan B 1.2 hours; shorter than the lag time between injection and onset of relief (4–6 wks) or maximum relief (8–12 wks). The symptomatic relief provided by hyaluronic acid (26 wks) is generally longer than the viscosupplement remains in the joint. The half-life of [^{3}H]acetyl-labeled hyaluronic acid has been shown to be 21 hours in normal joints and 12 hours in acutely inflamed joints using a sheep model [33]. Traces of Hylan A and B persist within the knee for up to 28 and 56 days, respectively in a goat model [56].

It is more likely that hyaluronic acid viscosupplementation produces its effects through down-regulation of aggrecanse-2, tumor necrosis factor alpha (TNF alpha), interleukin-8 (IL-8), inducible nitric oxide synthase (iNOS), and matrix metalloproteinases leading to anti-inflammatory, anabolic and analgesic effects, or through an interaction between hyaluronic acid and cell receptor CD44 [83, 95, 105, 113].

Viscosupplementation via intra-articular hyaluronic acid injections is a conservative treatment modality to be used in conjunction with other conservative management modalities including activity modification, physical therapy, analgesics, nonsteroidal anti-inflammatories (NSAIDS), and intra-articular corticosteroid injections. It is only approved by the FDA for treating osteoarthritis of the knee. Off-label use has been reported for treatment of osteoarthritis affecting the carpometacarpal joints of the thumb, apophyseal joints of the lumbar spine, hip, ankle, and foot [1, 34, 40, 92, 101].

Clinically, viscosupplementation has been shown to perform better than placebo but comparisons to intra-articular steroid injection are inconsistent [10]. It has a low complication rate but may incite an inflammatory response in some patients [23, 39, 57]. An independently funded, randomized, controlled trial has shown no statistically significant difference between viscosupplementation and intra-articular steroid injection on multiple functional outcome measures and on a visual analog pain scale [69]. A recent Cochrane Database Review reported highly variable results across products with only 5 to 13 weeks duration of 28 to 54% improvement in pain and 9 to 43% improvement in function; a marginal response for the cost ($853 to $1,844, about one-third the cost of a total knee prosthesis, plus physician and facility fees) [10, 112]. In the Clincal Practice Guidelines for non-arthroplasty treatment for OA of the knee recently issued by the American Academy of Orthopaedic Surgeons, viscosupplementation is recognized as a modality with low level support in the literature. Further level 1 studies are needed to determine its appropriate use.

8.5.2 Tissue regeneration

Bone

Bone voids are generally created by destructive lesions (giant cell tumor, aneurismal bone cyst, unicameral bone cyst) and trauma. Percutaneous techniques can be utilized to fill bone voids [90, 118]. Regenerating bone to fill the void entails all the considerations discussed above for fracture healing, bone grafts, bone graft substitutes and bone graft extenders although in specific circumstances for some benign tumors the void may be filled with PMMA. One advantage of using PMMA in the setting of a giant cell tumor is that tumor recurrence is more easily visualized on radiographs due to the contrast of the radiodense PMMA at its interface with a radiolucent active bone lesion. When a bone void or defect compromises the structural integrity of the bone, the regenerate bone needs to meet the structural needs of the bone. Temporarily the loads can be bridged by fixation devices or by structural graft.

Cartilage

Attempts at regeneration of articular cartilage produce fibrocartilage without Type II cartilage unless live chondrocytes from hyaline cartilage are implanted. Osteochondral Auto/Allograft Transplant System (OATS procedure) transplants intact articular cartilage segments from a non-weight bearing area of the joint or a donor joint, to replace a degenerative weight bearing area. These osteochondral segments are not injectable but the procedure is can be done arthroscopically using a trephine for small areas. Other techniques using injectable chondrocytes are currently being used. Autolologous Chondrocyte Implantation (ACI Procedure) uses the patient's own chodrocytes propagated in cell culture ($10,000.00; more than double the price of a total knee prosthesis) [21]. The ACI procedure involves injection of autologous chondrocytes into an articular cartilage defect contained under harvested periostium sealed with fibrin glue injected along the interface. Another technique currently being studied uses living juvenile (<12 yrs) chondrocytes in morcelized unaltered hyaline cartilage allograft (http://clinicaltrials.gov/ct2/show/NCT00791245). Surgical application does not require cell propagation in culture and it uses only fibrin glue without periostium to contain the graft [117]. Until hyaline cartilage with Type II collagen can be generated from multipotential cells and bioactive signaling molecules, articular cartilage regeneration requires living chondrocytes [88].

Nucleus pulposus regeneration

The intervertebral disc is composed of a central, gelatinous nucleus pulposus contained peripherally by the collagenous annulus fibrosus, superiorly by the cartilaginous endplate of the upper vertebral body and inferiorly by the cartilaginous endplate of the lower vertebral body. Degenerative disc disease causes weakening of the annulus fibrosus leading to annulus rupture and nucleus herniation. Desiccation of the nucleus can also occur with loss of disc height leading to overriding apophyseal joints, secondary osteoarthritis and progressive pain and functional limitation. Disc replacement is an experimental treatment used to correct loss of disc height and maintain segmental motion. Disc replacement can be done in one of two ways: prosthetic implant replacement of the entire disc or by replacement of the nucleus pulposus only using an elastomeric material [42, 68]. Experiments involving injection of silicone into degenerated discs began in the mid 1970s [97]. Currently, nucleus replacement is accomplished by inserting a dehydrated elastomeric implant that expands upon rehydration *in situ* or by injection of a self-curing polymer [68]. All injectable nucleus pulposus replacement materials are considered investigational. The curing process is typically induced through changes in temperature or pH, or by the addition of a curing agent. The nucleus replacement, once formed *in situ*, acts as a scaffold for native cells which produce extracellular matrix and then share in mechanical load bearing. A recognized complication is extrusion of the replacement material through the surgical portal in the annulus fibrosus used to inject the elastomer/polymer. The extruded material can impinge neurovascular structures causing pain and neurological deficit. In order to reduce the incidence of extrusion, a combination of annulus closure techniques has been studied. A combination of sutures and cryanoacrylate glue was found to be the most durable, but still inadequate to withstand the physical demands place on the repair [50]. Another approach entails injection into a balloon to contain the material while it cures [68].

A recombinant protein copolymer consisting of amino acid sequences derived from silk and elastin synthesized in E. coli is in clinical trials as an investigational device for nucleus pulposus regeneration (NuCore, Spine Wave, Inc. Shelton, CT) [17]. One of the elastin blocks has been modified to provide for chemical cross-linking. It has a 90-second working time once the cross-linking agent has been added before it becomes a viscous gel. The material cures within five minutes and achieves final mechanical strength at thirty minutes. Numerous other polymers are also being investigated for this purpose [48, 78, 88, 115, 116].

The endplates of the vertebral bodies, which contain the nucleus pulposus, have also become a focus of attention in nucleus pulposus replacement. There is concern that hyaline cartilage macromolecules and subchondral bone sclerosis inhibit cytokines, mesenchymal stem cell migration, and neovascularization from the adjacent vertebral bodies into the replacement material. Research is currently directed at preparation of the endplates by injecting enzymes to remove minerals and proteoglycans prior to replacement of the disc. Stem cell transplant, cytokines, and gene therapy are being investigated for future use in nucleus pulposus replacement/regeneration.

8.6 Clinical applications 4: miscellaneous

8.6.1 Drug delivery

Local drug delivery is utilized in orthopaedics for delivery of antimicrobials or osteoinductive agents such as BMP [9, 49, 106]. PMMA is the most common carrier and is often introduced to the target site by injection during polymerization, especially in conjunction with implant or fracture fixation as discussed above. Bone and bone graft substitutes, and resorbable materials including polymers (hyaluronic acid/methycellulose, collagen, PLA/PGA), ceramics (CPC, $CaSO_4$) and various combinations of these materials are also used as the carrier, many of which are or can be introduced to the target site by injection [41, 75]. Modifying these materials to control drug release through controlled resorption rates or increased permeability, and to maximize mechanical integrity are the target of extensive investigation.

8.6.2 Spasticity management: botulinum toxin

Intractable muscle spasm is a component of some orthopaedically relevant neuromuscular disorders including cerebral palsy (CP), cervical dystonia and stroke. Control of the spasm decreases pain and permits functional use of the muscles that are not affected by the spastic process. Botulinum toxin is a heptvalent neurotoxin produced by *Clostridium botulinum* that causes paralysis of skeletal muscle by preventing the release of acetylcholine at the neuromuscular junction. Purified toxins A and B are available for clinical use. Each cleaves a different protein in the SNARE complex, preventing release of acetylcholine from vesicles in the nerve end thus blocking neuromuscular transmission by different mechanisms [4]. They do not have cross antigenicity. Botox purified Type A neurotoxin (Allergan, Inc., Irvine, CA) is a low protein formulation that has less antigenicity, often used in cosmetic dermatology to relax wrinkles. Rimabotulinumtoxin B (Myobloc®, Solstice Neurosciences Inc, San Francisco, CA) is primarily used for intramuscular injection including orthopaedic conditions such as CP. About three to five months of paralysis occurs following injection into a muscle [30]. Patients with spastic CP benefit with improved function (gate, hand), posture and decreased pain. The effect can spread beyond the injected muscle and has been reported to progress to systemic botulism and death [109].

8.6.3 Enzymatic fasciotomy

Dupuytren's disease is characterized by progressive contractures in the palm of the hand and fingers secondary to the formation of contracting bands or 'cords' of collagen laid down by myofibroblasts. It occurs predominately in 40-year-old white men of Northern European decent. The pathogenic tissue is composed of collagen [3].

Historically, treatment has been surgical, including percutaneous fasciotomy or open fasciectomy [103]. Surgical complications occur in about 18% of cases (nerve injury 2.3%, arterial injury 0.4%, digital hematoma 2%, wound infection 9.5%, skin slough 2.4%, and sympathetic dystrophy 2.4%) [19]. Recurrence ranges from 27% to 80% [73, 74, 89, 107]. Numerous non-surgical modalities have been tried with limited success [52].

Enzymatic fasciotomy for the treatment of Dupuytren's disease was first attempted by Bassot in 1969, using trypsin, α-chymotrypsin, thiomcase, and hyaluronidase. Collagenase was used in the early 1970s for the debridement of severe burns and leg ulcers [16, 52]. In 1995 Starkweather *et al.* studied the effects of purified clostridial collagenase on the tensile strength of Dupuytren's cords *in vitro* and found a 93% decrease in the modulus of elasticity compared to controls [100]. The use of collagenase (Xiaflex; collagenase clostridium histoliticum, Auxilium Pharmaceuticals Malvern, PA) for the treatment of Dupuytren's disease has since progressed. In a randomized, double-blind, placebo-controlled trial 87% of 62 joints improved range of motion. Contracture recurrences were seen in five joints by 24 months follow-up. There were no serious treatment-related side effects [6]. Excellent results continue with the same authors reporting on patients in 308 cases with >40° improvement in joint range of motion and only three complications; two tendon ruptures and one complex regional pain syndrome [53].

The use of collagenase injections to correct a deforming disease, drastically reducing complications encountered from surgical intervention, is an inspiring example of enlisting biology for therapeutic effects. Additional long-term studies are needed to verify the effectiveness and determine long-term recurrence rates.

8.6.4 Sclerotherapy and embolization

Controlling blood loss during orthopaedic procedures and from musculoskeletal trauma can be achieved by pre-emptively embolizing the arterial inflow before resection of highly vascular primary bone tumors, and metastases, especially renal cell carcinoma or by therapeutically embolizing bleeding vessels for pelvic trauma [2, 8, 15, 85, 102]. Embolization is performed with 150–1000 μm Polyvinyl Alcohol Particles (TRUFILL™, Cordis Endovascular Systems, Miami, FL), collagen granules or coils. Sclerosing agents including polidocanol and ethanol can be used to therapeutically reduce vascular malformations [25, 35]. These are considered interventional radiology procedures but are intimately related to orthopaedic management of these musculoskeletal disorders.

8.7 Conclusion

Injectable biomaterials are integral to the contemporary management of musculoskeletal disorders. The capability of introducing these materials by injection is driven by the need to place them in their target sites through increasingly limited exposures and to control the distribution of delivery. With advances in biologic knowledge and refinements in technology these materials are becoming increasingly sophisticated. Many of the injectable biomaterials that are being used or investigated have been discussed, by no means exhaustively however, as new materials, new applications of known materials and new combinations of materials are evolving rapidly.

8.8 References

1. Abate, M., Pelotti, P., De Amicis D., Di Iorio A., Galletti S., Salini, V. 2008. Viscosupplementation with hyaluronic acid in hip osteoarthritis (a review). *Ups. J. Med. Sci.* 113(3), 261–277.
2. Agolini, S.F., Shah, K., Jaffe, J., Newcomb, J., Rhodes, M., Reed, J.F. 1997. Arterial embolization is a rapid and effective technique for controlling pelvic fracture hemorrhage. *J Trauma* 43, 395–399.
3. Alt, V., Heissel, A. 2006. Economic considerations for the use of recombinant human bone morphogenetic protein-2 in open tibial fractures in Europe: the German model. *Curr Med Res Opin* 22 Suppl 1, S19–22.
4. Arezzo, J.C. 2009. Basic and Therapeutic Aspects of Botulinum and Tetanus Toxins, NeuroBloc®/Myobloc®: Unique features and findings, *Toxicon* 54(5), 690–696.
5. Ayan, I., Colak, M., Comelekoglu, U., Milcan, A., Ogenler O., Oztuna, V., Kuyurtar, F. 2007. Histoacryl glue in meniscal repairs (a biomechanical study), *International Orthopaedics* 31(2), 241–246.
6. Badalamente, M.A., Hurst, L.C. 2007. Efficacy and safety of injectable mixed collagenase subtypes in the treatment of Dupuytren's contracture. *J Hand Surg Am* 32(6), 767–774.
7. Bajammal, S.S., Zlowodzki, M., Lelwica, A., Tornetta, P., Einhorn, T.A., Buckley,

R., Leighton, R., Russell, T.A., Larsson, S., Bhandari, M. 2008. The use of calcium phosphate bone cement in fracture treatment. A meta-analysis of randomized trials. *The Journal of Bone and Joint Surgery* 90(6), 1186–1196.

8. Barton, P.P., Waneck, R.E., Karnel, F.J., Ritschl, P., Kramer, J., Lechner, G.L. 1996. Embolization of Bone Metastases. *Journal of Vascular and Interventional Radiology* 7(1), 81–88.
9. Beardmore, A.A., Brooks, D.E., Wenke, J.C., Thomas, D.B. 2005. Effectiveness of local antibiotic delivery with an osteoinductive and osteoconductive bone-graft substitute. *J Bone Joint Surg Am* 87(1), 107–112.
10. Bellamy, N., Campbell, J., Robinson, V., Gee, T., Bourne, R., Wells, G. 2006. Viscosupplementation for the treatment of osteoarthritis of the knee (review). Cochrane Database of Systematic Reviews 2006, Issue 2. Art. No.: CD005321. DOI: 10.1002/14651858.CD005321.pub2.
11. Bielecki, T., Gazdzik, T.S., Szczepanski, T. 2008. Benefit of percutaneous injection of autologous platelet-leukocyte-rich gel in patients with delayed union and nonunion. *European Surgical Research* 40(3), 289–296.
12. Bielecki, T.M., Gazdzik, T.S. 2006. Percutaneous injection of autogenous growth factors in patient with nonunion of the humerus. A case report. *J Orthopaedics* 3(3), e15.
13. Bodde, E.W.H., Boerman, O.C., Russel, F.G.M., Mikos, A.G., Spauwen, P.H.M., Jansen, J.A. 2008. The kinetic and biological activity of different loaded rhBMP-2 calcium phosphate cement implants in rats. *J Biomed Mater Res A.* 87(3), 780–791.
14. Bonzania, I.C., Adhikarib, R., Houshyarb, S., Mayadunneb, R., Gunatillakeb, P., Stevensa M.M., 2007. Synthesis of two-component injectable polyurethanes for bone tissue engineering, *Biomaterials* 28(3), 423–433.
15. Börüban, S. 2007. Embolization of benign and malignant bone and soft tissue tumors of the extremities, *Diagn Interv Radio*, 13, 164–171.
16. Boxer, A.M., Gottesman, N., Bernstein, H., Mandl, I. 1969. Debridement of dermal ulcers and decubiti with collagenase. *Geriatrics* 24(7), 75–86.
17. Boyd, L.M., Carter, A.J. 2006. Injectable biomaterials and vertebral endplate treatment for repair and regeneration of the intervertebral disc. *Eur Spine J.* 15(S3), 414–421.
18. Buchbinder, R., Osborne, R. H., Ebeling, P.R., Wark, J. D., Mitchell, P., Wriedt, C., Graves, S., Staples, M.P., Murphy, B. 2009. A randomized trial of vertebroplasty for painful osteoporotic vertebral fractures. *NEJM* 361(6), 558–568.
19. Bulstrode, N.W., Jemec, B., Smith, P.J. 2005. The complications of Dupuytren's contracture surgery. *J Hand Surg Am* 30(5), 1021–1025.
20. Cassidy, C., Jupiter, J.B., Cohen, M., Delli-Santi, M., Fennell, C., Leinberry, C., Husband, J., Ladd, A., Seitz, W.R., Constanz, B. 2003. Norian SRS cement compared with conventional fixation in distal radial fractures. A randomized study. *J Bone Joint Surg Am.*85-A(11), 2127–2137.
21. The Center for Orthopaedics & Sports Medicine. 2003. *ACI: General information.* Available at: http://www.arthroscopy.com/sp08024.htm (accessed April 2, 2010).
22. Chapman, M.W., Bucholz, R., Cornell, C. 1997. Treatment of acute fractures with a collagen-calcium phosphate graft material. A randomized clinical trial. *J Bone Joint Surg Am* 79(4), 495–502.
23. Chen, A.L., Desai, P., Adler, E.M., Di Cesare, P.E. 2002. Granulomatous inflammation after Hylan GF 20 viscosupplementation of the knee, a report of six cases. *J Bone Joint Surg Am* 84, 1142–1147.
24. Connolly, J. F., 1991. *Tibial Nonunion: Diagnosis and Treatment*, AAOS Press.

25. Crawford, E.A., Slotcavage, R.L., King, J.J., Lackman, R.D. Ogilvie, C.M. 2009. Ethanol sclerotherapy reduces pain in symptomatic musculoskeletal hemangiomas. *Clin Orthop Relat Res* 467, 2955–2961.
26. Dahabreh, Z., Calori, G., Kanakaris, N., Nikolaou, V., Giannoudis, P. 2008. A cost analysis of treatment of tibial fracture nonunion by bone grafting or bone morphogenetic protein-7. *Int Orthop.* Available at: http://www.ncbi.nlm.nih.gov/pubmed/19052743 (accessed September 26, 2009).
27. De Long, W.G., Einhorn, T.A., Koval, K., McKee, M., Smith, W., Sanders, R., Watson, T. 2007. Bone grafts and bone graft substitutes in orthopaedic trauma surgery. A critical analysis. *J Bone Joint Surg Am* 89(3), 649–658.
28. Dhanan, G., Rao, J., Balasubramanian, N.N., Prathaban, S., Justin, B., Tamilnadu, W. 2009. Clinical evaluation of chitin and chitosan in the management of fractures. *J. Veterinary & Animal Sciences* 5(1), 1–3.
29. Dimar, J.R., Glassman, S.D., Burkus, K.J., Carreon, L.Y. 2006. Clinical outcomes and fusion success at 2 years of single-level instrumented posterolateral fusions with recombinant human bone morphogenetic protein-2/compression resistant matrix versus iliac crest bone graft. *Spine* 31(22), 2534–2539, discussion, 2540.
30. Dressler, D., Eleopra, R. 2006. Clinical use of non-A botulinum toxins: botulinum toxin type B, *Journal Neurotoxicity Research* 9(2–3), 121–125.
31. Frankenburg, E.P., Goldstein, S.A., Bauer, T.W., Harris, S.A., Poser, R.D. 1998. Biomechanical and histological evaluation of a calcium phosphate cement. *J Bone Joint Surg Am* 80(8), 1112–1124.
32. Fraser, J.R., Clarris, B.J., Baxter, E. 1979. Patterns of induced variation in the morphology, hyaluronic acid secretion, and lysosomal enzyme activity of cultured human synovial cells. *Ann Rheum Dis* 38(3), 287–294.
33. Fraser, J.R., Kimpton, W.G., Pierscionek, B.K., Cahill, R.N. 1993. The kinetics of hyaluronan in normal and acutely inflamed synovial joints: observations with experimental arthritis in sheep. *Semin. Arthritis Rheum* 22(6 Suppl 1), 9–17.
34. Fuchs, S., Erbe, T., Fischer, H., Tibesku, C.O. 2005. Intraarticular hyaluronic acid versus glucocorticoid injections for nonradicular pain in the lumbar spine. *J Vasc Interv Radiol* 16(11), 1493–1498.
35. Gabal, A.M. 2002. Percutaneous technique for sclerotherapy of vertebral hemangioma compressing spinal cord. *Cardiovascular and Interventional Radiology* 25(6), 494–500.
36. Gazdag, Lane, Glaser, Forster. 1995. Alternatives to autogenous bone graft: efficacy and indications. *J Am Acad Orthop Surg* 3(1), 1–8.
37. Glassman, S.D., Dimarm, J.R., Carreon, L.Y., Campbell, M.J., Puno, R.M., Johnson, J.R. 2005. Initial fusion rates with recombinant human bone morphogenetic protein-2/compression resistant matrix and a hydroxyapatite and tricalcium phosphate/collagen carrier in posterolateral spinal fusion. *Spine* 30(15), 1694–1698.
38. Goel, A., Sangwan, S., Siwach, R., Ali, A. 2005. Percutaneous bone marrow grafting for the treatment of tibial non-union. *Injury* 36(1), 203–206.
39. Goldberg, V.M., Coutts, R.D. 2004. Pseudoseptic reactions to Hylan viscosupplementation: diagnosis and treatment. *Clin Orthop Rel Res* 419, 130–137.
40. Grogan, K.A., Chang, T.J., Salk, R.S. 2009. Update on viscosupplementation in the treatment of osteoarthritis of the foot and ankle. *Clin Podiatr Med Surg* 26(2), 199–204.
41. Gupta, D., Tator, C.H., Shoichet, M.S. 2006. Fast-gelling injectable blend of hyaluronan and methylcellulose for intrathecal, localized delivery to the injured

spinal cord. *Biomaterials* 27(11), 2370–2379.
42. Guyer, R.D., Ohnmeiss, D.D. 2003. Treatment for degenerative disc disease: Intervertebral disc prostheses. *Spine* 28(15S), S15–S23.
43. Habraken, W.J.E.M., Boerman, O.C., Wolke, J.G.C., Mikos, A.G., Jansen, J.A. 2008. *In vitro* growth factor release from injectable calcium phosphate cements containing gelatin microspheres. *J Biomed Mater Res A* Available at: http://www.ncbi.nlm.nih.gov/pubmed/18985784 (accessed September 12, 2009).
44. Habraken, W.J., Wolke, J.G., Mikos, A.G., Jansen, J.A. 2006. Injectable PLGA microsphere/calcium phosphate cements: Physical properties and degradation characteristics. *J Biomater Sci Polym Ed* 17(9), 1057–1074.
45. Habraken, W.J.E.M., Wolke, J.G.C., Mikos, A.G., Jansen, J.A. 2009. Porcine gelatin microsphere/calcium phosphate cement composites: An *in vitro* degradation study. *J. Biomed. Mater. Res. Part B Appl. Biomater* Available at: http://www.ncbi.nlm.nih.gov/pubmed/19582834 (accessed September 11, 2009).
46. Habraken, W.J.E.M., Zhang, Z., Wolke, J.G.C., Grijpma, D.W., Mikos, A.G., Feijen, J., Jansen, J.A. 2008. Introduction of enzymatically degradable poly(trimethylene carbonate) microspheres into an injectable calcium phosphate cement. *Biomaterials* 29(16), 2464–2476.
47. Hak, D.J. 2007, The use of osteoconductive bone graft substitutes in orthopaedic trauma. *Journal of the American Academy of Orthopaedic Surgeons* 15(9), 525.
48. Halloran, D.O., Grad, S., Stoddart, M., Dockery, P., Alini, M., Pandit, A.S. 2008. An injectable cross-linked scaffold for nucleus pulposus regeneration. *Biomaterials* 29(4), 438–447.
49. Hanssen, A.D. 2005. Local antibiotic delivery vehicles in the treatment of musculoskeletal infection. *Clin Orthop Relat Res* 437, 91–96.
50. Heuer, F., Ulrich, S., Claes, L., Wilke, H. 2008. Biomechanical evaluation of conventional anulus fibrosus closure methods required for nucleus replacement. Laboratory investigation. *J Neurosurg Spine* 9(3), 307–313.
51. Horstmann, W.G., Verheyen, C.C.P.M., Leemans, R. 2003. An injectable calcium phosphate cement as a bone-graft substitute in the treatment of displaced lateral tibial plateau fractures. *Injury* 34(2), 141–144.
52. Hurst, L.C., Badalamente, M.A. 1999. Nonoperative treatment of Dupuytren's disease. *Hand Clinics* 15(1), 97–107.
53. Hurst, L.C., Badalamente, M.A., Hentz, V.R., Hotchkiss, R.N., Kaplan, F.T.D., Meals, R.A., Smith, T.M., Rodzvilla, J., for the CORD I Study Group. 2009. Injectable collagenase clostridium histolyticum for Dupuytren's contracture. *N Engl J Med* 361, 2578–2580.
54. Intini, G., Andreana, S., Intini, F.E., Buhite, R.J., Bobek, L.A. 2007. Calcium sulfate and platelet-rich plasma make a novel osteoinductive biomaterial for bone regeneration. *Journal of Translational Medicine* 5(1), 13.
55. Ishimura, M., Tamai, S., Fujisawa, Y. 1991. Arthroscopic meniscal repair with fibrin glue. *Arthroscopy* 7(2), 177–181
56. Jackson, D.W., Simon, T.M. 2006. Intra-articular distribution and residence time of Hylan A and B: a study in the goat knee. *Osteoarthr. Cartil* 14(12), 1248–1257.
57. Jones, K.B. 2005. Viscosupplementation pseudotumor. A case report. *The Journal of Bone and Joint Surgery* 87(5), 1113–1119.
58. Joosten, U., Joist, A., Frebel, T., Brandt, B., Diederichs, S., von Eiff, C. 2004. Evaluation of an *in situ* setting injectable calcium phosphate as a new carrier material for gentamicin in the treatment of chronic osteomyelitis: studies *in vitro* and *in vivo*. *Biomaterials* 25(18), 4287–4295.

59. Kallmes, D.F., Comstock, B.A., Heagerty, P.J., Turner, J.A., Wilson, D.J., Diamond T.H., Edwards, R., Gray, L.A., Stout, L., Owen, S., Hollingworth, W., Ghdoke, B., Annesley-Williams, D.J., Ralston, S.H., Jarvik, J.G. 2009. A Randomized trial of vertebroplasty for osteoporotic spinal fractures. *NEJM* 361(6), 569–579.
60. Keating, J.F., Hajducka, C.L., Harper, J. 2003. Minimal internal fixation and calcium-phosphate cement in the treatment of fractures of the tibial plateau. A pilot study. *J Bone Joint Surg Br* 85(1), 68–73.
61. Khan, Y., Yaszemski, M.J., Mikos, A.G., Laurencin, C.T. 2008. Tissue engineering of bone: material and matrix considerations. *J Bone Joint Surg Am* 90 Suppl 1, 36–42.
62. Kim, C., Mahar, A., Perry, A., Massie, J., Lu, L., Currier, B., Yaszemski, M.J. 2007. Biomechanical evaluation of an injectable radiopaque polypropylene fumarate cement for kyphoplasty in a cadaveric osteoporotic vertebral compression fracture model. *J Spinal Disord Tech* 20(8), 604–609.
63. Klippel, J.H., Stone, J.H., Crofford, L.E.J., White, P.H. 2008. *Primer on the Rheumatic Diseases*, 13th edn, Springer.
64. Koukoubis, T.D., Glisson, R.R., Feagin, J.A., Seaber, A.V., Vail, T.P, 1995. Augmentation of meniscal repairs with cyanoacrylate glue decreases separation of sutured menisci but not strong enough alone. *Journal of Biomedical Materials Research* 29, 715–720.
65. Kühne, J.H., Bartl, R., Frisch, B., Hammer, C., Jansson, V., Zimmer, M. 1994. Bone formation in coralline hydroxyapatite. Effects of pore size studied in rabbits. *Acta Orthop Scand* 65(3), 246–252.
66. Laurencin, C., Khan, Y., El-Amin, S.F. 2006. Bone graft substitutes. *Expert Rev Med Devices* 3(1), 49–57.
67. Laurencin, C.T., Khan, Y. 2009. Bone graft substitute materials: *eMedicine Orthopedic Surgery*. Available at: http://emedicine.medscape.com/article/1230616-overview (accessed September 7, 2009).
68. Leckie, S., Kang, J. 2009. Recent advances in nucleus pulposus replacement technology, *Current Orthopaedic Practice* 20(3), 222–226.
69. Leopold, S.S., Redd, B.B., Warme, W.J., Wehrle, P.A., Pettis, P.D., Shott, S. 2003. Corticosteroid compared with hyaluronic acid injections for the treatment of osteoarthritis of the knee: A prospective, randomized trial. *J Bone Joint Surg Am* 85A(7), 1197–1203.
70. Lim, S.M., Lee, H.J, Oh, S.H., Kim, J.M., Lee, J.H. 2009. Novel fabrication of PCL porous beads for use as an injectable cell carrier system. *J Biomed Mater Res B Appl Biomater* 90(2), 521–530.
71. Lobenhoffer, P., Gerich, T., Witte, F. Tscherne, H. 2002. Use of an injectable calcium phosphate bone cement in the treatment of tibial plateau fractures: a prospective study of twenty-six cases with twenty-month mean follow-up. *J Orthop Trauma* 16(3), 143–149.
72. Marco, R.A.W., Kushwaha, V.P. 2009. Thoracolumbar burst fractures treated with posterior decompression and pedicle screw instrumentation supplemented with balloon-assisted vertebroplasty and calcium phosphate reconstruction. *J Bone Joint Surg Am* 91(1), 20–28.
73. Mäkelä, E.A., Jaroma, H., Harju, A., Anttila, S., Vainio, J. 1991. Dupuytren's contracture: the long-term results after day surgery. *J Hand Surg Br* 16(3), 272–274.
74. McFarlane, R., McGrouther, D., Flint, M. 1990. *Dupuytren's disease: Biology and treatment*. Edinburgh: Churchill Livingstone.
75. McLaren A.C. 2004. Alternative materials to acrylic bone cement for delivery of

depot antibiotics in orthopaedic infections. *Clin Orthop and Related Research* 427, 101–106.
76. Mont, M.A., Ragland, P.S., Biggins, B., Friedlaender, G., Patel, T., Cook, S., Etienne, G., Shimmin, A., Kildey, R., Rueger, D.C., Einhorn, T.A. 2004. Use of bone morphogenetic proteins for musculoskeletal applications. An overview. *J Bone Joint Surg Am* 86-A Suppl 2, 41–55.
77. Mummaneni, P.V., Pan, J., Haid, R.W., Rodts, G.E. 2004. Contribution of recombinant human bone morphogenetic protein-2 to the rapid creation of interbody fusion when used in transforaminal lumbar interbody fusion: a preliminary report. Invited submission from the Joint Section Meeting on Disorders of the Spine and Peripheral Nerves, March 2004. *J Neurosurg Spine* 1(1), 19–23.
78. Nagae, M., Ikeda, T., Mikami, Y., Hase, H., Ozawa, H., Matsuda, K., Sakamoto, H., Tabata, Y., Kawat,a M., Kubo, T. 2007. Intervertebral disc regeneration using platelet-rich plasma and biodegradable gelatin hydrogel microspheres. *Tissue Eng* 13(1), 147–158.
79. Neiman, R. *Treatment of tibial nonunion and delayed union by percutaneous injection of concentrated autologous stem cells: An alternative to open surgical repair – A case report.* Available at: http://www.harvesttech.com/pdf/Orthopedic/Trauma/Neiman.pdf (accessed April 2, 2010).
80. Niikura, T., Tsujimoto, K., Yoshiya, S., Tadokoro, K., Kurosaka, M., Shiba, R. 2007. Vancomycin-impregnated calcium phosphate cement for methicillin-resistant *Staphylococcus aureus* femoral osteomyelitis. *Orthopedics* 30, 320–321.
81. Prather, H., Van Dillen, L., Metzler, J. P., Riew, K. D., Gilula, L. A. 2006. Prospective measurement of function and pain in patients with non-neoplastic compression fractures treated with vertebroplasty. *J Bone Joint Surg Am* 88, 334–341.
82. Qi, X., Ye, J., Wang, Y. 2008. Improved injectability and *in vitro* degradation of a calcium phosphate cement containing poly(lactide-co-glycolide) microspheres. *Acta Biomater* 4(6), 1837–1845.
83. Qiu, B., Liu, S., Peng, H., Wang, H. 2005. The effects of sodium hyaluronate on mRNA expressions of matrix metalloproteinase-1, -3 and tissue inhibitor of metalloproteinase-1 in cartilage and synovium of traumatic osteoarthritis model. *Chin. J. Traumatol* 8(1), 8–12.
84. Raney, R. B. 1949. Andry and the orthopaedia. *J Bone Joint Surg Am* 31, 675–682.
85. Rastogi, S., Varshney, M.K., Trikha, V., Khan, S.A., Choudhury, B., Safaya, R. 2006. Treatment of aneurysmal bone cysts with percutaneous sclerotherapy using polidocanol: A review of 72 cases with long-term follow-up. *J Bone Joint Surg Br* 88-B(90), 1212–1216.
86. del Real, R.P., Wolke, J.G.C., Vallet-Regí, M., Jansen, J.A. 2002. A new method to produce macropores in calcium phosphate cements. *Biomaterials* 23(17), 3673–3680.
87. Reckers, L.J., Fagundes, D.J., Cohen, M. 2009. The ineffectiveness of fibrin glue and cyanoacrylate on fixation of meniscus transplants in rabbits. *Knee* 16(4), 290–294.
88. Richardson, S.M., Curran, J.M., Chen, R., Vaughan-Thomas, A., Hunt, J.A., Freemont, A.J., Hoyland, J.A. 2006. The differentiation of bone marrow mesenchymal stem cells into chondrocyte-like cells on poly-L-lactic acid (PLLA) scaffolds. *Biomaterials* 27(22), 4069–4078.
89. Rodrigo, J.J., Niebauer, J.J., Brown, R.L., Doyle, J.R. 1976. Treatment of Dupuytren's contracture. Long-term results after fasciotomy and fascial excision.

J Bone Joint Surg Am 58(3), 380–387.
90. Rougraff, B.T. 2006. Percutaneous bone grafting of benign bone tumors. *Current Opinion in Orthopaedics* 17(6), 563–567
91. Ruhé, P.Q., Hedberg, E.L., Padron, N.T., Spauwen, P.H.M., Jansen, J.A., Mikos, A.G. 2005. Biocompatibility and degradation of poly(DL-lactic-co-glycolic acid)/ calcium phosphate cement composites. *J Biomed Mater Res A* 74(4), 533–544.
92. Salini, V., De Amicis, D., Abate, M., Natale, M.A., Di Iorio, A. 2009. Ultrasound-guided hyaluronic acid injection in carpometacarpal osteoarthritis: short-term results. *Int J Immunopathol Pharmacol* 22(2), 455–460.
93. Sampson, S., Gerhardt, M., Mandelbaum, B. 2008. Platelet rich plasma injection grafts for musculoskeletal injuries: a review. *Curr Rev Musculoskelet Med* 1(3–4), 165–174.
94. Sanchez-Sotelo, J., Munuera, L., Madero, R. 2000. Treatment of fractures of the distal radius with a remodellable bone cement: a prospective, randomised study using Norian SRS. *J Bone Joint Surg Br* 82(6), 856–863.
95. Sasaki, A., Sasaki, K., Konttinen, Y.T., Santavirta, S., Takahara, M., Takei, H., Ogino, T., Takagi, M. 2004. Hyaluronate inhibits the interleukin-1beta-induced expression of matrix metalloproteinase (MMP)-1 and MMP-3 in human synovial cells. *Tohoku J. Exp. Med* 204(2), 99–107.
96. Schildhauer, T.A., Bauer, T.W., Josten, C., Muhr,G. 2000. Open reduction and augmentation of internal fixation with an injectable skeletal cement for the treatment of complex calcaneal fractures. *J Orthop Trauma* 14(5), 309–317.
97. Schneider, P.G., Oyen, R. 1974. Surgical replacement of the intervertebral disc. First communication: replacement of lumbar discs with silicon-rubber. Theoretical and experimental investigations. *Z Orthop Ihre Grenzgeb* 112(5), 1078–1086.
98. Schnieders, J., Gbureck, U., Thull, R., Kissel, T. 2006. Controlled release of gentamicin from calcium phosphate-poly(lactic acid-co-glycolic acid) composite bone cement. *Biomaterials* 27(23), 4239–4249.
99. Seeherman, H., Li, R., Li, X.J., Wozney, J. 2003. Injectable rhBMP-2/CPM paste for closed fracture and minimally invasive orthopaedic repairs. *Journal Of Musculoskeletal and Neuronal Interactions* 3(4), 317–319.
100. Starkweather, K.D., Lattuga, S., Hurst, L.C., Badalamente, M.A., Guilak, F., Sampson, S.P., Dowd, A., Wisch, D. 1996. Collagenase in the treatment of Dupuytren's disease: an *in vitro* study. *J Hand Surg Am* 21(3), 490–495.
101. Sun, S., Chou, Y., Hsu, C., Chen, W. 2009. Hyaluronic acid as a treatment for ankle osteoarthritis. *Curr Rev Musculoskelet Med* 2(2), 78–82.
102. Sun, S., Lang, E.V. 1998. Bone metastases from renal cell carcinoma: Preoperative embolization. *Journal of Vascular and Interventional Radiology* 9(2), 263–269.
103. Swartz, W.M., Lalonde, D.H. 2008. Dupuytren's disease. *Plast. Reconstr. Surg* 121(4 Suppl), 1–10.
104. Szomor, Z.L., Murrell, G.A.C., Appleyard, R.C., Tyler, M.J. 2009. Meniscal repair with a new biological glue: An *ex vivo* study, *Techniques in Knee Surgery* 7, 261–265.
105. Takahashi, K., Goomer, R.S., Harwood, F., Kubo, T., Hirasawa, Y., Amiel, D. 1999. The effects of hyaluronan on matrix metalloproteinase-3 (MMP-3), interleukin-1beta(IL-1beta), and tissue inhibitor of metalloproteinase-1 (TIMP-1) gene expression during the development of osteoarthritis. *Osteoarthr. Cartil* 7(2), 182–190.
106. Thomas, D.B., Brooks, D.E., Bice, T.G., DeJong, E.S., Lonergan, K.T., Wenke, J.C. 2005. Tobramycin-impregnated calcium sulfate prevents infection in contaminated

wounds. *Clin. Orthop. Relat. Res* 441, 366–371.

107. Tonkin, M.A., Burke, F.D., Varian, J.P. 1985. The proximal interphalangeal joint in Dupuytren's disease. *J Hand Surg Br* 10(3), 358–364.
108. Urist, M.R. 1965. Bone: formation by autoinduction. *Science* 150(12), 893–899.
109. US Food and Drug Administration. 2009. *Update of safety review of OnabotulinumtoxinA (marketed as Botox/Botox Cosmetic), AbobotulinumtoxinA (marketed as Dysport) and RimabotulinumtoxinB (marketed as Myobloc).* Available at: http://www.fda.gov/Drugs/DrugSafety/PostmarketDrugSafetyInformationforPatientsandProviders/DrugSafetyInformationforHeathcareProfessionals/ucm174959.htm (accessed April 2, 2010).
110. Vaidya, R., Carp, J., Sethi, A., Bartol, S., Craig, J., Les, C.M. 2007. Complications of anterior cervical discectomy and fusion using recombinant human bone morphogenetic protein-2. *Eur Spine J* 16(8), 1257–1265.
111. Valdes, M., Thakur, N., Namdari, S., Ciombor, D., Palumbo, M. 2009. Recombinant bone morphogenic protein-2 in orthopaedic surgery: a review. *Arch Orthop Trauma Surg* Available at: http://www.ncbi.nlm.nih.gov/pubmed/19280204 (accessed September 25, 2009).
112. Waddell, D.D. 2007. Viscosupplementation with hyaluronans for osteoarthritis of the knee: clinical efficacy and economic implications. *Drugs Aging* 24(8), 629–642.
113. Wang, C., Lin, Y., Chiang, B., Lin, Y., Hou, S. 2006. High molecular weight hyaluronic acid down-regulates the gene expression of osteoarthritis-associated cytokines and enzymes in fibroblast-like synoviocytes from patients with early osteoarthritis. *Osteoarthritis and Cartilage* 14(12), 1237–1247.
114. Webb, J.C.J., Spencer, R.F. 2007. The role of polymethylmethacrylate bone cement in modern orthopaedic surgery. *J Bone Joint Surg Br* 89(7), 851–857.
115. Yang, S., Chen, P., Chen, Y., Lin, F. 2005. Gelatin/chondroitin-6-sulfate copolymer scaffold for culturing human nucleus pulposus cells *in vitro* with production of extracellular matrix. *J. Biomed. Mater. Res. Part B Appl. Biomater* 74(1), 488–494.
116. Yang, S., Chen, P., Chen, Y., Lin, F. 2005. An *in-vitro* study on regeneration of human nucleus pulposus by using gelatin/chondroitin-6-sulfate/hyaluronan tri-copolymer scaffold. *Artif Organs* 29(10), 806–814.
117. Zimmer Corp. 2010. *DeNovo NT Natural Tissue Graft.* [Online] (Updated 8 January 2010). Available at: http://www.zimmer.com/z/ctl/op/global/action/1/id/10497/template/MP (accessed April 2, 2010).
118. Zimmermann, R., Gabl, M., Lutz, M., Angermann, P., Gschwentner, M., Pechlaner, S. 2003. Injectable calcium phosphate bone cement Norian SRS for the treatment of intra-articular compression fractures of the distal radius in osteoporotic women. *Arch Orthop Trauma Surg* 123(1), 22–27.

9

Dental applications of injectable biomaterials

R. W. HASEL, Stanford University School of Medicine, USA
and E. COMBE, University of Minnesota School of Dentistry, USA

Abstract: This chapter focuses on dental biomaterials designed for permanent placement in the mouth. The development of flowable polymer–ceramic composites is traced and their rheological properties, such as pseudoplasticity and thixotropy, discussed. Also considered are some materials that are being developed for root canal therapy, including calcium phosphate cements. There is vast scope for research into materials development, clinical applications and fundamental mechanisms.

Key words: dental biomaterials, resin composites, flowable composites, endodontic materials, calcium phosphate cements.

9.1 Introduction

According to the *Oxford English Dictionary*, to inject is to 'to drive or force (a fluid, etc.) into a passage or cavity, as by means of a syringe, or by some impulsive power; said especially of the introduction of medicines or other preparations into the cavities or tissues of the body.'

There are a number of well-known instances where injection techniques are used in dentistry – for example, for delivering anesthetics and for the purposes of irrigation. Also, one stage of prosthodontic treatment involves the recording of an impression. Such impression materials (for example, silicones) are syringed into place. This is a particularly useful technique when a gingival retraction cord (with or without medicaments) is used to displace the gingival tissue to enable placement of the impression material (Kumbuloglu *et al.*, 2007) (Fig. 9.1).

However, this chapter focuses on dental biomaterials intended for permanent placement. Three areas of research and development are considered and critiqued:

1. directly placed tooth-colored restorative dental materials
2. materials for the obturation of root canals
3. calcium phosphate cements for endodontic treatment.

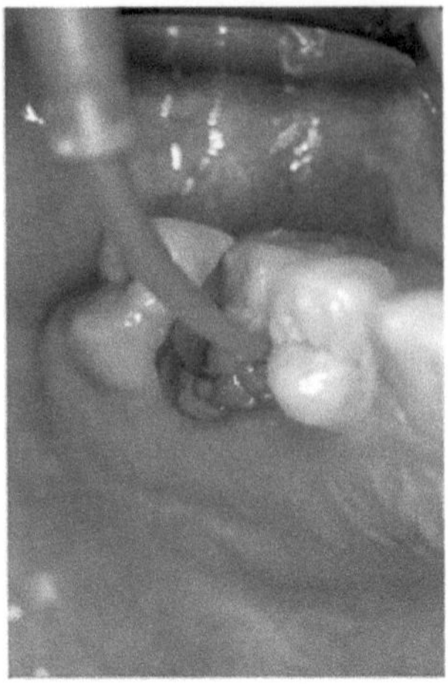

9.1 Injectable dental impression material.

9.2 Challenges in the application of biomaterials to dentistry

When a synthetic material is placed in the mouth, there are many concerns. Obviously the material must be biocompatible, with an appropriate host response (Wataha, 2001). Further, the material may be subjected to mechanical stresses (shock, fatigue and abrasion), and chemical and enzymatic degradation. Thus it is important that the material is manipulated in such a way as to obtain its optimum properties to withstand the long-term rigors imposed by the oral environment. In that regard, it is advantageous to have materials that are easier to manipulate, which in turn can promote a superior outcome. This is now being achieved in some cases by the development of injectable materials.

9.3 Directly placed tooth-colored materials

9.3.1 Composites

Until the 1970s, the only materials for permanently restoring teeth were amalgam and silicate cement. This latter material had poor durability, discolored easily and was believed to be responsible for pulpal damage to teeth. The search for a replacement led to the development of ceramic filled polymers – resin composites – following the pioneering work of Bowen (1962). These materials consist of dimethacrylate monomers filled with particulate inorganic fillers, such as silica, barium glass and zirconia/silica.

Early composite materials were supplied as two pastes (Fig. 9.2), both containing mixtures of monomers and fillers, and one paste with a polymerization initiator (typically a peroxide), and the other with an activator

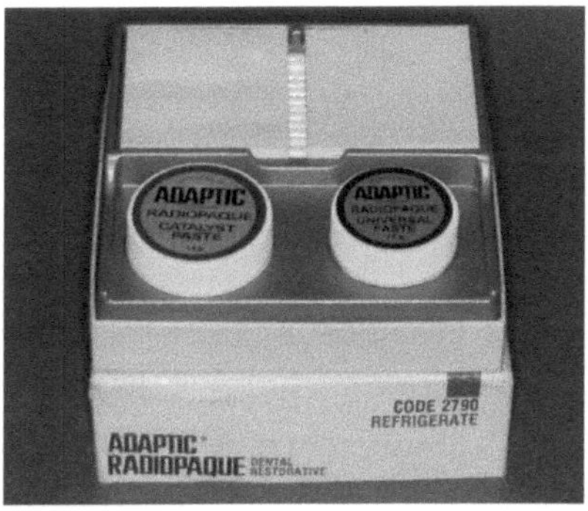

9.2 Two-part, chemical cure paste composite filling material by 3M.

(such as a tertiary amine). On mixing the two pastes together, a redox reaction generates free radicals to initiate polymerization.

For these materials, rheological considerations were always a concern, both for the manufacturer and the dental professional. The principal monomer used is usually 2,2-bis-[4-(methacryloxy-2-hydroxy-propoxy)-phenyl]-propane, known as bis-GMA or Bowen's resin, or a urethane dimethacrylate (Fig. 9.3). Despite the considerable merits of these monomers – including fast hardening by a free radical mechanism and good mechanical properties when polymerized – they have one significant drawback. Bowen's resin is very viscous, (viscosity $\eta = 719$ Pa s at 23°C) so incorporation of inorganic filler is not feasible. Thus a diluent monomer, such as triethylene glycol dimethacrylate (TEGDMA, $\eta = 0.008$ Pa s at 23°C) is required. A 70/30 w/w mix of Bis-GMA and TEGDMA has a viscosity of 2.29 Pa s at the same temperature (Beun *et al.*,

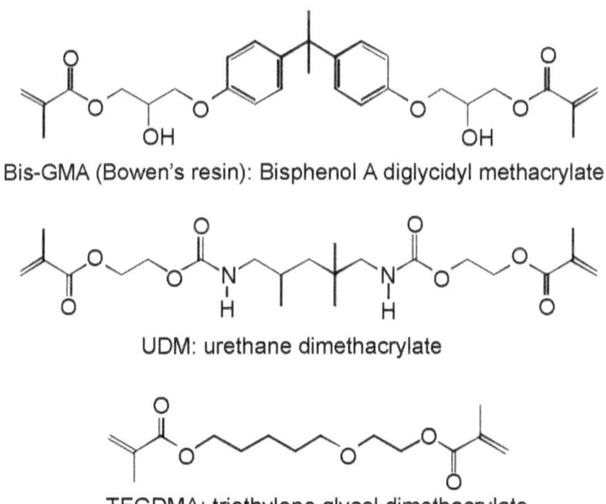

9.3 Dimethacrylate monomers employed in dental resin composites.

2009). The use of a diluent monomer gives problems, however. Polymerization shrinkage is increased leading to problems of bonding at the adhesive interface with tooth dentin (Puckett *et al.*, 2007).

With added fillers – typically 70 wt% for early materials – the dimethacrylate monomers form very viscous pseudoplastic pastes (Watts *et al.*, 1980). The manipulation of these materials was very technique-sensitive. Thorough mixing of the two pastes was essential, yet this was difficult to ensure, given that both pastes were of the same color.

Furthermore, mixing introduced air bubbles into material, resulting in poorer surfaces thus affecting and compromising the surface and marginal integrity. The situation was complicated by the fact that free radical polymerization was occurring even from the start of mixing, resulting in an increasing viscosity of the material and the development of an elastic modulus, thus compromising the ability of the material to be adapted to a tooth cavity (Jacobsen, 1976).

9.3.2 Flowable composites

Two significant developments led to the development of composites capable of being syringed. The first of these was the development of visible light cure (VLC) activation systems (Bassiouny and Grant, 1978; Watts *et al.*, 1984). These unpolymerized pastes contain chemicals (typically an α-diketone such as camphor quinone and a tertiary amine) that will generate initiating free radicals on exposure to light of wavelength 470–480 nm (Douglas *et al.*, 1979).

Supplied as a single paste, these materials involve no mixing, and will not significantly polymerize when being placed in a tooth cavity under normal ambient light conditions. Because of their greater ease of use, the VLC materials have largely displaced the two-paste systems.

In research to further facilitate the manipulation of these materials, attempts were made to develop syringes to deliver the unpolymerized paste (e.g. Galler, 1986; Mühlbauer, 1990).

An alternative approach was taken by Hasel (1999, 2001), who developed materials capable of being placed through a hypodermic syringe, from 25 to 16 gauge needles (0.260 to 1.194 mm internal diameter) (Fig. 9.4). Retaining the monomer system used with conventional materials, these new systems initially contained less filler content. This filler also included colloidal silica of particle size 0.04 μm. These are termed 'flowable composites', and are now widely available (Clinical Research Associates, 2002). Recent generations of flowable composites have been introduced that are at or above conventional paste filler rates (e.g. up to 80 wt%). This advance may open up the use and applications of flowables to any situation where conventional paste composites have been used.

In terms of rheological behavior, these materials have some significant features, which facilitate their ability to be syringed without requiring excessive

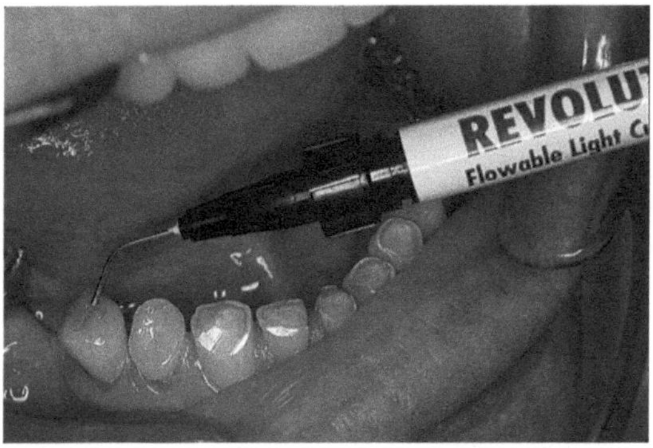

9.4 'Revolution' flowable composite filling material.

finger pressure, thus allowing precise placement in the prepared tooth cavity in controlled amounts.

- Their viscosity is lower than conventional materials because of the lower filler content and/or because of novel resin matrix formulations.
- In common with many other pastes, they are pseudoplastic (Watts *et al.*, 1980); that is, they show shear thinning, which is advantageous. (The monomers themselves are essentially Newtonian.)
- Additionally, they are thixotropic owing to the presence of colloidal silica. On shearing, hydrogen bonds are broken, which facilitates flow of the material. When the material has been syringed, the bonds re-form, and the material stays where placed, until it is adapted to shape. This important property allows the operator to easily place precise amounts in very controlled environments and to optimize polymerization and minimize the shrinkage associated with polymerization.

The thixotropy is illustrated for one material in Fig. 9.5 (Owen and Combe, unpublished results). Using a Rheometrics Dynamic Stress Rheometer, materials

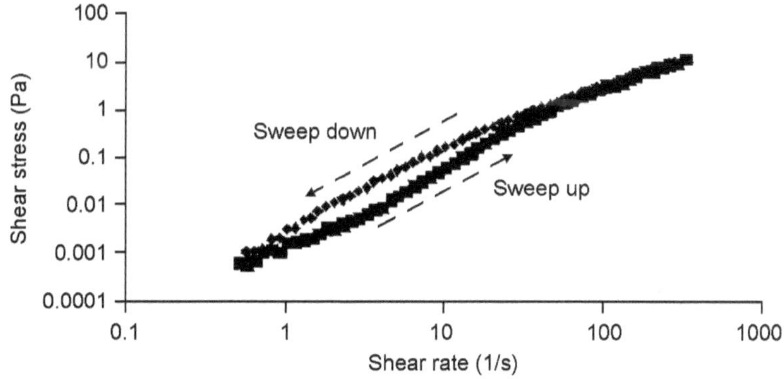

9.5 Illustration of the thixotropic behavior of a flowable composite (Aria^{TM}).

(at 25°C and protected from ambient light) were sheared between 25 mm aluminum parallel plates, separated by 1.00 mm. Steady stress sweep tests were performed, starting at high shear stress, to be more relevant to the dental situation, since composites are highly stresses as they are forced through a narrow gauge needle. The fact that a loop diagram was obtained is indicative of thixotropy.

Today, flowable materials are used not only for most classes of restoring teeth, but also as fissure sealants. Current products differ considerably in formulation and filler content (Beun *et al.*, 2008). Fissure sealants contain less than 25% inorganic filler, while conventional flowable filling materials have about 50–70% filler. Consequently there are considerable differences in properties between commercially available products. Beun *et al.* (2008) have studied the effect of these variations on rheological properties including storage modulus, and classified the products into three groups, based on their solid-like behavior.

9.3.3 Other tooth-colored materials

Since the development of resin composites, other types of directly placed tooth-colored restorative materials have been developed, some of which are formulated to be capable of being syringed. These include:

- Glass-ionomer cements, which harden not by polymerization, but by the acid-base reaction between an aqueous polyelectrolyte (poly(acrylic acid) or related co-polymers) and a basic fluoro-aluminosilicate (FAS) glass. These materials are not as tough as resin composites, but they chemically adhere to tooth tissue and are capable of releasing fluoride ions.
- Resin-modified glass-ionomers – these are similar to the above, but hardening also takes place by a free radical addition polymerization reaction, in addition to the acid-base reaction.
- Polyacid-modified resin composites (commonly known as 'compomers') – these are composites to which some of the glass-ionomer constituents have been added.

9.4 Injectable materials in root canal therapy

9.4.1 Limitations of traditional materials and techniques

In endodontic treatment, the aim is to completely seal the root canal. Traditionally this has been carried out with cones of gutta percha, also containing added zinc oxide, barium sulfate, plasticizers and coloring agents (Friedman *et al.*, 1975), packed into the canal with a 'sealer' – usually a cement containing zinc oxide and eugenol. A concern with this material system is that there is no adhesion between gutta percha and the sealer, or between the sealer and the tooth dentin. Further, complete adaptation of the material to completely obturate the root canal is not always achieved.

9.4.2 Injectable thermoplasticized gutta percha

Injectable thermoplasticized gutta percha systems have been developed in attempts to achieve good obturation – currently available systems have been reviewed by Glickman *et al.* (2000, 2001). These systems can be successful, but do not eliminate the need for careful shaping and cleaning of the root canal prior to filling.

However, it is surprising and disappointing that there appears to be no rheological data on these materials in the literature. It would be of value to know the temperature dependence of rheological properties on temperature and shear rate, and if thixotropy occurs. It would also be desirable to know if the material had any viscoelastic properties.

9.4.3 Alternative polymer systems

Alternative polymer systems have been developed for root canal obturation. These include a degradable polymer (polycaprolactone) and a bioactive glass (Elzubair *et al.*, 2006). Similar to gutta percha, these materials are thermoplastic and can be heated and injected into the root canal. As before, however, there appears to be no rheological information about them in the literature.

9.5 Injectable calcium phosphate cements

An alternative suggested approach to endodontic treatment is to use injectable bone substitute and calcium phosphate materials, which have been described as 'promising' in terms of biocompatibility, bioactivity and rheological properties (Enkel *et al.*, 2008).

9.6 Conclusion

It is evident that there is vast scope for research in injectable dental biomaterials, in terms of chemical development, establishment of new and improved clinical treatment techniques and in fundamental understanding of basic rheological mechanisms.

9.7 References

Bassiouny M A, Grant A A (1978) 'A visible light-cured composite restorative. Clinical open assessment.' *Brit Dent J*, 145, 327–330.

Beun S, Bailly C, Devaux J, Leloup G (2008) 'Rheological properties of flowable resin composites and pit and fissure sealants.' *Dent Mater*, 24, 548–555.

Beun S, Bailly C, Dabin A, Vreven J, Devaux J, Leloup G (2009) 'Rheological properties of experimental Bis-GMA/TEGDMA flowable resin composites with various macrofiller/microfiller ratio.' *Dent Mater*, 25, 198–205.

Bowen R L (1962) US Patent 3,066,112.
Clinical Research Associates (2002) 'Flowable resins, Comparison of 33 brands.' *CRA Newsletter*, 26, 3–4.
Douglas W H, Craig R G, Chen C J (1979) 'A new composite restorative based on a hydrophobic matrix.' *J Dent Res*, 58, 1981–1986.
Elzubair A, Elias C N, Suarez J C M, Lopes, H P, Vieira M V (2006) 'The physical characterization of a thermoplastic polymer for endodontic obturation.' *J Dent*, 34, 784–789.
Enkel B, Dupas C, Armengol V, Akpe A J, Bosco J, Daculsi G, Jean A, Laboux O, LeGeros R Z, Weiss P (2008) 'Bioactive materials in endodontics.' *Expert Rev Med Devices*, 5(4), 475–494.
Friedman C M, Sandrik J L, Heuer M A, Rapp, G W (1975) 'Composition and mechanical properties of gutta-percha endodontic points.' *J Dent Res*, 54, 921–925.
Galler J (1986) US Patent 4,601,662.
Glickman G N, Koch K A (2000) '21st-century endodontics.' *J Amer Dent Assoc*, 131 Suppl 39S–46S.
Glickman G N (2001) 'Injectable thermoplasticized gutta-percha systems.' *Practical Procedures & Aesthetic Dentistry*, 13, 477–482.
Hasel R W (1999) US Patent 5,944,527.
Hasel R W (2001) US Patent 6,315,567.
Jacobsen P H (1976) 'Working time of polymeric restorative materials.' *J Dent Res*, 55, 244–251.
Kumbuloglu O, User A, Toksavul S, Boyacioglu H (2007) 'Clinical evaluation of different gingival retraction cords.' *Quint Int*, 38, e92–e98.
Mühlbauer E (1990) US Patent 4,952,209.
Puckett A D, Fitchie J G, Kirk P C, Gamblin J (2007) 'Direct composite restorative materials.' *Dent Clin N Amer*, 51, 659–675.
Wataha J C (2001) 'Principles of biocompatibility for dental practitioners.' *J Prosthet Dent*, 86, 203–209.
Watts D C, Combe E C, Greener E H (1980) 'Capillary rheology of two composite resin systems.' *J Oral Rehab*, 7, 475–480.
Watts D C, Amer O, Combe E C (1984) 'Characteristics of visible-light-activated composite systems.' *Brit Dent J*, 156, 209–215.

10
Injectable polymeric carriers for gene delivery systems

R. B. AROTE, D. JERE, H.-L. JIANG, Y.-K. KIM, Y.-J. CHOI, M.-H. CHO and C.-S. CHO,
Seoul National University, Korea

Abstract: Cationic polymers that have shown significant promise as gene delivery agents are more effective than the state-of-the art, commercially available non-viral systems. Gene delivery *in vivo* involves interactions with the biophase (the effect site of drug) prior to reaching the target cells which complicates efforts to understand the mechanism of the delivery process. The ability to incorporate genetic materials such as DNA, RNA and siRNAs into functionalized nanoparticles demonstrates a new era. In this chapter, we highlight the basic overview of injectable polymeric gene carriers that have been reported as safe and successful vectors, their formulations and *in vivo* success thereof. In addition, we outline various strategies for designing polymeric carriers to overcome various biological barriers as successful gene delivery vectors.

Key words: polymers, biodegradable, poly(ester amine)s, transfection efficiency, gene expression.

10.1 Introduction

Gene therapy has gained many applications for the treatment of various diseases. The recent emergence of small interfering RNA (siRNA) to trigger RNA interference has initiated efforts to identify siRNA sequences capable of silencing a vast number of genes in human genome.[1] However, the bottleneck of this therapy remains cellular delivery. Synthetic vectors are ideally suited for this purpose as they are capable of complexing and delivering large loads of nucleic acids of virtually any size and are generally regarded as being safer than viral vectors. Moreover, various studies reported that the biocompatibility and utility of synthetic vectors can be improved by incorporation of various hydrophilic polymers and targeting ligands.[2,3] Non-viral carriers show considerable advantages over viral counterparts owing to greater control of their molecular composition for simplified manufacturing and analysis, flexibility in the size of the transgene (a gene from one species introduced into the genome of another by transgenesis) to be delivered and relatively lower immunity. Non-viral delivery systems, which are able to deliver therapeutic genes specifically to target tissues in *in vivo*, would be practically attractive for the development of therapeutics, e.g. in areas of high medical needs such as oncology, cardiovascular diseases, diseases of central nervous system (CNS). For successful gene transfer, gene carrier has to fulfil a series of delivery functions in order to overcome extra- and intracellular barriers. After the effective DNA condensation into the particles like viruses, polymers should protect DNA from degradation and undesired interactions with the biological environment during extracellular transport followed by cell binding and internalization, and ideally should have target specificity.[4,5]

For efficient transfection, the delivery vector must mediate a sequential process that comprises DNA condensation, uptake into cell, release from the endosomal compartment, migration through the cytoplasm, uptake into nucleus and finally decondensation of DNA for transcription.[6] Furthermore, for *in vivo* application, polyplexes have to face additional barriers until DNA reaches the target cells, including anatomical size constraints, non-specific interactions with biological fluids, the polyplexes must be small enough to enable blood circulation, extravasations and diffusion through tissues.[7] Recently, strategies have been developed for target-specific gene delivery *in vivo*. Specific recognition and internalization into the target cells aim to avoid undesired delivery to non-target tissues and to diminish toxic side-effects.[7] Mechanistically these non-viral carriers have been designed to combine the mechanism of DNA compaction, cellular uptake, endosomal release and to some extent nuclear uptake. Various polycations such as dendrimer, polyethylenimine (PEI), polylysine possess these mechanism that have been broadly used for gene transfer *in vitro* as well as *in vivo*.[8–10] These polymeric gene carriers are increasingly being proposed as alternatives to viral vectors for *in vivo* gene transfer because of their potential advantages in addressing the pharmaceutical issues of applying genes as drugs. Cationic polymers are increasingly being proposed as potential vectors because of the versatility in fine tuning the physicochemical properties of the carrier. Various important parameters of the cationic polymers, such as rigidity, hydrophobicity/hydrophilicity, charge density, biodegradability and molecular weight of the polymer chains, can in principle be adjusted to effect an optimal complexation with DNA. Admittedly, the desirable features of optimal complexation, other than efficient condensation into small particle size, are unclear. It is likely that, for different cells and tissues or different routes of administration *in vivo*, the desirable characteristics of polyplexes would differ. Cationic polyplexes with their multiple degrees of freedom, for optimization are nevertheless well positioned to meet the increasing challenges. In the last two to three decades various reports have provided the proof of concept of the polymeric approach along with their routes of administration.[11]

Polymeric carriers can be divided into three groups according to the administration routes: site specific, local and systemic carriers. Following the application of polycation/DNA complexes *in vivo*, additional barriers have to be overcome. For locally applied complexes, the target site, route of access and chosen therapy will determine the strategy for gene delivery. When the target site is easily accessible, local administration such as intradermal, intramuscular (IM), intratracheal, intraperitoneal (IP) or intratumoral applications can be used.[12] In the same way, surgery or catheters can deliver the polyplexes directly to the target site. Cutaneous applications via micropumps,[13] aerosol delivery,[14] or jet nebulization[15] are other physical methods used to increase polyplex gene delivery locally.

The aim of this chapter is to give an overview of the injectable polymeric gene carriers that have been reported as safer and successful vectors, their various formulations and *in vivo* success thereof. The chapter is divided into four major parts to focus on barriers to gene delivery using synthetic vectors, various overviews of injectable carriers in various formulations and *in vivo* success thereof. For instance, we describe various formulations of polymeric gene carriers such as nanoparticles, microspheres and hydrogels. In addition, we discuss various strategies for designing polymeric carriers to overcome various barriers to be successful gene carriers. Furthermore we highlight in detail hydrogels, their classification and characteristics as injectable gene carriers.

10.2 Biological barriers

Polyplexes face various extracellular as well as intracellular barriers. Most of the extracellular barriers are the factors that influence biodistribution of the administered polyplexes from the point of delivery to the site of interest and they will vary profoundly between routes of delivery.

10.2.1 Extracellular barriers

The success of gene delivery mainly depends on the targeting of vectors to specific tissues. For instance, ligand specific delivery systems have been developed for tissue specific targeting. Various ligands such as asialoglycoprotein conjugated DNA-poly-lysine complex[16], transferring,[17] have been used for receptor-mediated delivery of nucleic acid owing to the presence of asialoglycoprotein receptors on hepatocytes and high levels of transferrin receptors on cancer cells, respectively. These polyplexes with target-specific ligand showed significant results *in vitro* but failed to retain *in vivo*. Most of the synthetic vectors systems have diameters more than 50 nm, allowing them to target either components of blood stream or parenchymal cells and sinusoidal organs such as liver and spleen. However, the permeability of polyplexes can be changed, which was shown by the Chamberlain[18] group. It was found that systemic application of VEGF dramatically augmented the ability of adeno-associated virus (AAV) to gain access to muscle cells following intravenous

(IV) delivery.[18] Disorganized and leaky microvasculature of tumors was first time reported by Maeda and co-workers which is known as 'enhanced permeation and retention' effect (EPR). EPR effect constitutes the poor lymphatic drainage of tumors, which leads to inadequate interstitial fluid convection, leading to hypoxia, which in turn increases the permeability of tumor vasculature.[19,20]

Several groups reported the possibility of delivering genes via target associated receptors. Fischer *et al.* reported one strategy that combined the principles of steric and lateral stabilization with receptor-mediated targeting, resulting in receptor-mediated uptake and targeting of polymer-stabilized polyplexes using a series of targeting ligands.[21] Another barrier to gene transfer is the penetration and distribution of vectors in tissues. Vectors must penetrate endothelial cells to extravasate from blood vessels to target tissues and cells. Several viral vectors including adenovirus and adeno-associated vectors cannot penetrate endothelial cells when administered systemically.[22] Cationic liposomes, when injected into the mouse tail vein, showed that the lung was the organ where gene expression was detected primarily.[23] However, cationic liposomes cannot penetrate past the endothelial cells when injected into the vasculature.[24]

10.2.2 Intracellular barriers

Synthetic vectors need to facilitate a number of distinct steps as mentioned earlier including cell-specific binding, internalization (e.g. endocytosis), escape from endocytic vesicles, transport through the cytoplasm, translocation across the nuclear membrane and release of DNA for transcription.[11] Viral vectors have already evolved the mechanisms to overcome each of these barriers. However, these functionalities need to be incorporated into the design of synthetic vectors. Additionally the lack of techniques for the study of intracellular trafficking of polyplexes limits the progressive passage of polyplexes and this in turn limits transfection efficiency. To date, researchers have relied on quantitation of gene expression as a measure of polymer efficacy. However, the rational design of synthetic vectors will ultimately require a better understanding of the interaction of vectors with the cells at each of the intracellular barriers.[11]

Endocytosis comprises those cellular events that lead to internalization of specialized regions of plasma membrane as well as small volumes of extracellular fluid.[25] Polyethylenimine (PEI) is one of the best known and most widely studied cationic polymers which is regarded as 'gold standard' due to its ability to mediate high levels of transfection efficiency in a range of cell types.[26] Being highly cationic in nature, PEI has the ability to have strong buffering capacity and thereby a proton sponge effect. Another common strategy to overcome the endocytic barrier is to conjugate endosomolytic peptides to the synthetic vectors that are known to form pores in the lipid membrane. Melittin, a small amphiphatic protein from bee venom, was conjugated to PEI in order to enhance cytoplasmic delivery. This protein has been shown to integrate into natural or synthetic membranes and to disrupt a variety of cells and liposomes at micromolar concentration which is partly due to its detergent-like sequence.[27]

In another report, histidine-rich molecules have also been shown to exhibit membrane destabilization features in an acidic medium, resulting in enhanced nucleic acid delivery in cytosol.[28] It was found that protonation of the imidazole functionality within the histidine structure was responsible for the enhanced transfection. The pKa of imidazle group in histidine is ~6.0, in which under slightly acidic conditions, the nitrogen heterocyclic rings are protonated. Thus the imidazole group possesses a buffering capacity in the endosomal pH range which is responsible for the escape of polyplexes from endocytic vesicles.[29,30] For efficient transportation of nucleic acids into the nucleus, after endocytosis and to achieve higher gene expression, various factors are responsible for the nuclear transport such as stability of genes to nucleases in the cytoplasm, decondensation of vectors to release nucleic acids and the rate of movement of polyplexes across the cytoplasm to nucleus. Use of low molecular weight condensing peptides, which easily dissociate from DNA, is a potential strategy to facilitate intracellular delivery. Also, linear reducible cations and histidine-rich reducible polycations showed effective vector unpacking so as to release the nucleic acid for further processing.[11]

10.3 Nanoparticles

The effectiveness of a non-viral gene delivery system critically depends on providing an optimal local concentration of plasmid DNA in the target tissue and overcoming a number of barriers, including rapid degradation by extra- and intracellular endonucleases and restricted nuclear entry in non-dividing cells.[31] Some polycations have demonstrated the ability to electrostatically bind DNA and condense it into nanoparticles sufficient for cellular uptake. Biodegradable nanoparticles have been extensively investigated as carriers for various therapeutic agents including macromolecules such as proteins and peptides.[32] The main advantage of nanoparticles is their polymeric nature, which makes the system devoid of the toxicity and immunogenic concerns that are associated with viral vectors. Moreover, controlled release of encapsulated DNA from nanoparticles is expected to provide sustained gene expression.[33] Nanoparticles are submicron in size and have been demonstrated to have significantly higher cellular and tissue uptake as compared to microparticles. Various strategies and polymer systems have been investigated for the formulation of nanoparticles; however, their intracellular uptake and trafficking has been relatively less studied aspect. In order to know the mechanism of nanoparticle-mediated gene delivery, it is essential to understand how nanoparticles deliver DNA into cells. Panyam *et al.* showed that efficient internalization of nanoparticles into cells largely depends on concentration and time-dependent endocytic processes.[34] It was found that the efficiency of intracellular nanoparticle uptake was reduced at higher doses and with incubation time, suggesting that the uptake pathway is saturated or reaches an equilibrium uptake. The same group revealed that nanoparticle uptake reached a plateau within 2 h of incubation in most cell lines, suggesting a rapid process of nanoparticle uptake.[35]

The route of administration determines to some extent whether biodegradable or non-biodegradable materials can be used for preparation of the nanoparticles. For parenteral administration, the particles need to be biodegradable[36] to avoid the risk of polymer accumulation in the body and to ensure complete elimination. Biodegradable nanoparticles can also be used intravenously for sustained and constant systemic DNA release. For such applications, the surface of the nanoparticles has to be suitably modified to avoid the uptake by mononuclear phagocyte systems. Such nanoparticles, after injection, circulate in the body acting as drug/gene carriers and slow release of the drugs from the nanoparticles, leading to constant drug blood levels.[37] Followed by cellular uptake, nanoparticles are transported to primary endosomes and then to sorting endosomes where they escape to endo-lysosomes and enter the cytosolic compartment within 10 min following the incubation of cells with nanoparticles. Panyam *et al.* hypothesized that cationization of nanoparticles resulted in their interaction with vesicular membranes, leading to transient and localized destabilization of membranes and escape of nanoparticles into the cytoplasmic compartment.[34]

Highly cationic PEI was shown to escape the endo-lysosomal compartment through a 'proton sponge effect' where swelling was developed owing to osmotic pressure inside the endosome thereby causing rupture of endosomal membrane and escape of the polyplex.[38] This mechanism in turn revealed the need of highly cationic polymers for successful gene transfer. Keeping in mind the above hypothesis, our group synthesized various biodegradable poly(ester amine)s (PEAs) using several acrylate monomers such as polycaprolactone-diacrylate (PCLDA),[38] poly(ethylene glycol) diacrylate (PEGDA),[39] glycerol dimethacrylate (GDM),[40] glycerol triacrylate (GTA)[41] and poloxamer diacrylate[42] crosslinked with low molecular weight PEI. The simple synthesis of these PEAs was carried out by the Michael addition reaction. The polyplexes prepared from these PEAs have suitable physiochemical parameters showing a particle size below 200 nm and appropriate surface charge. All above PEAs were biodegradable and have shown remarkable cell viability. These PEAs have demonstrated the prompt release from endosomal compartment by proton sponge effect owing to buffering capacity of the PEI moieties. Higher luciferase and GFP gene expression shown by these PEAs further demonstrated their ability to transfer genes, which is undoubtedly the synergistic evidence of lower cytotoxicity owing to biodegradable ester linkage on one hand and proton sponge effect due to PEI moieties on the other hand, as shown in Fig. 10.1.[38–42]

Various factors which affect the intracellular uptake of nanoparticles are particle size and surface characteristics such as hydrophobicity and zeta potential. Prabha *et al.* investigated the correlation between particle size and gene transfer ability. In their study, nanoparticles prepared using PLG-PLA by the emulsion solvent evaporation method were fractionated into greater than 100 nm and smaller than 100 nm, which showed different gene transfection levels. It was found that the smaller size fraction of nanoparticles demonstrated 27-fold higher transfection efficiency in COS-7 cells than the larger particle

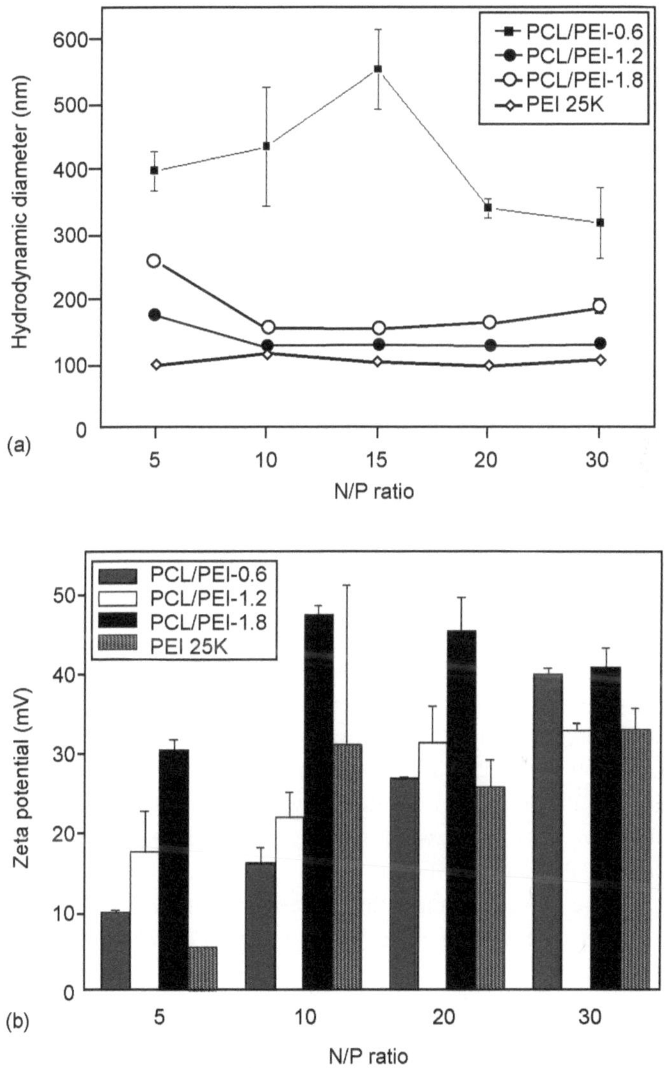

10.1 (a) Particle sizes of PCL/PEI-1.2/DNA complexes at various N/P ratios, (b) zeta potential measurement and (c) atomic force microscopy images of PCL/PEI-1.2/DNA complexes at N/P ratio 10 (error bars represent standard deviation) (cited from Ref. 38).

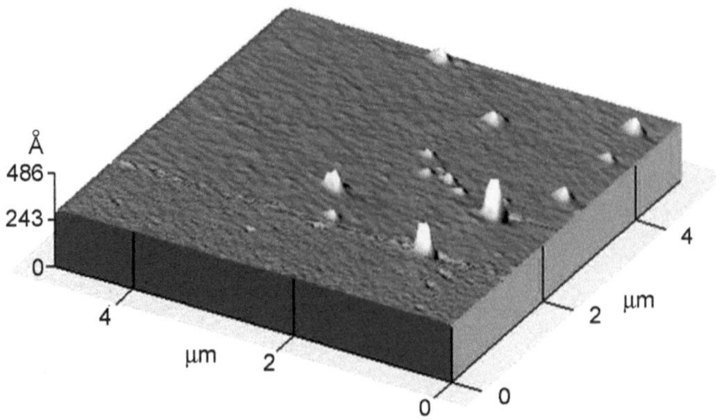

10.1 Continued.

fraction. However, higher gene transfection with the smaller size fraction was not associated with its higher cellular uptake on weight basis or DNA release rate compared to the larger size fraction.[43] PEAs synthesized by our group showed suitable particle size (below 200 nm) for intracellular delivery with comparable surface charges.[38–42]

In another interesting finding by our group, two PEAs, which were synthesized using GDM and GTA monomer with LMW-PEI, showed remarkable cellular uptake results owing to the presence of hydrophilic glycerol moieties in their backbone.[40,41] It was found that the hyperosmolarity of these glycerol-based PEAs was responsible for the increased cellular uptake of the polyplexes prepared from them, thereby increasing gene delivery ability. The superiority of these carriers (in terms of gene delivery ability) over the other PEAs prepared by us was the presence of hyperosmotic effect owing to glycerol moieties in the ester backbone synergistically with the 'proton sponge effect' owing to the presence of PEI moieties as shown in Fig. 10.2. These PEAs also revealed superior GFP expression after aerosol administration. Introduction of biodegradable ester linkages from hydrophobic/hydrophilic acrylate monomers and highly cationic PEI along with better physicochemical parameters tended to increase *in vivo* gene expression in lungs. Polyplexes prepared from biodegradable PCL/PEI and pEGFP-N2 at charge ratio of 30 were aspirated to 13-week-old female BALB/c mice. In agreement with *in vitro* results, PEAs depicted increased level of GFP expression than PEI 25K as a control (Fig. 10.3), indicating that the alveolar cells of lungs were more compatible with PEAs than cytotoxic PEI 25K owing to the introduction of biodegradable ester linkage.[38]

Hyperosmotic biodegradable GDM/PEI and GTA/PEI also revealed superior gene expression in lungs, after aerosol administration. The increased reporter gene expression shown by the glycerol-based PEAs over the other PEAs is due to the hyperosmotic effect that it exerts because of the presence of glycerol

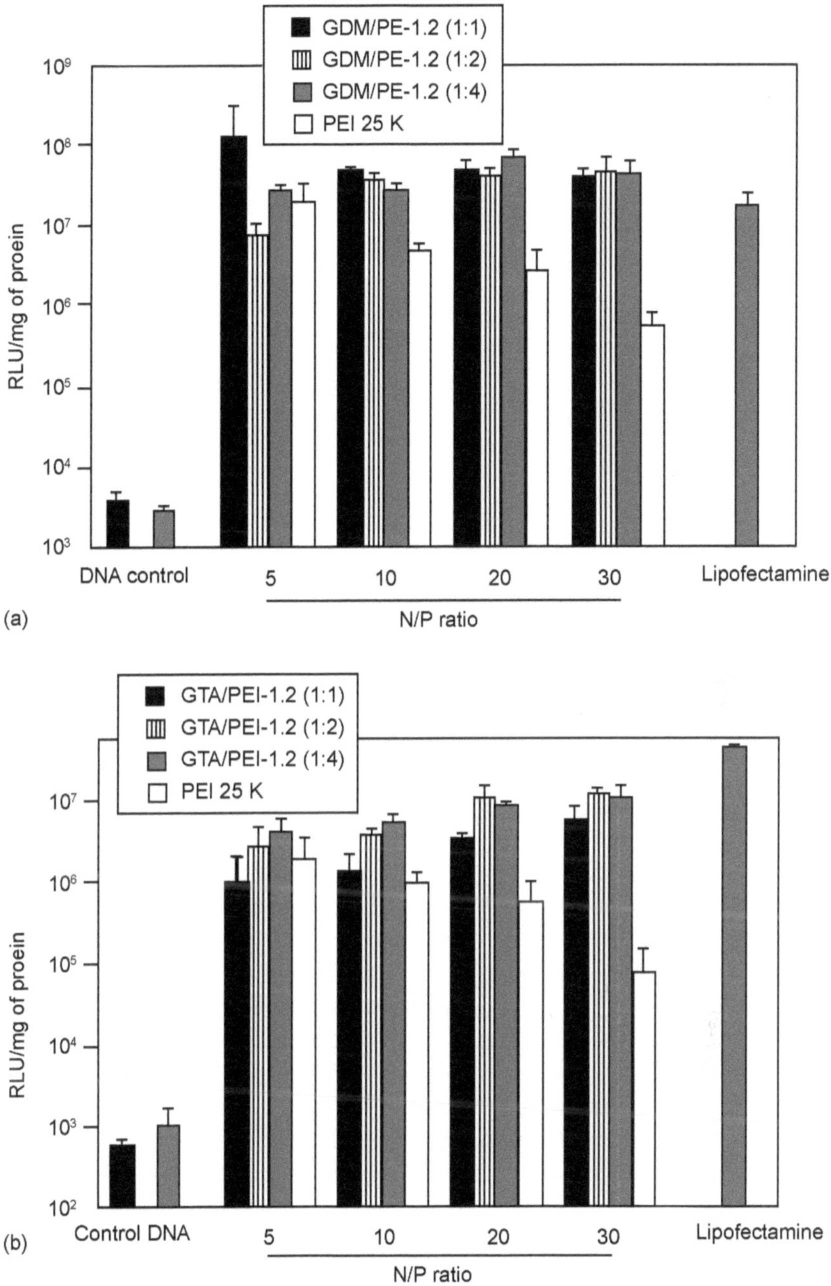

10.2 In vitro transfection efficiency of: (a) GDM/PEI-1.2 copolymers and (b) GTA/PEI-1.2 copolymers/pDNA (pGL3-control) complexes by luciferase assay on 293T cell lines at various N/P ratios (error bars represent standard deviation) (cited from Ref. 40).

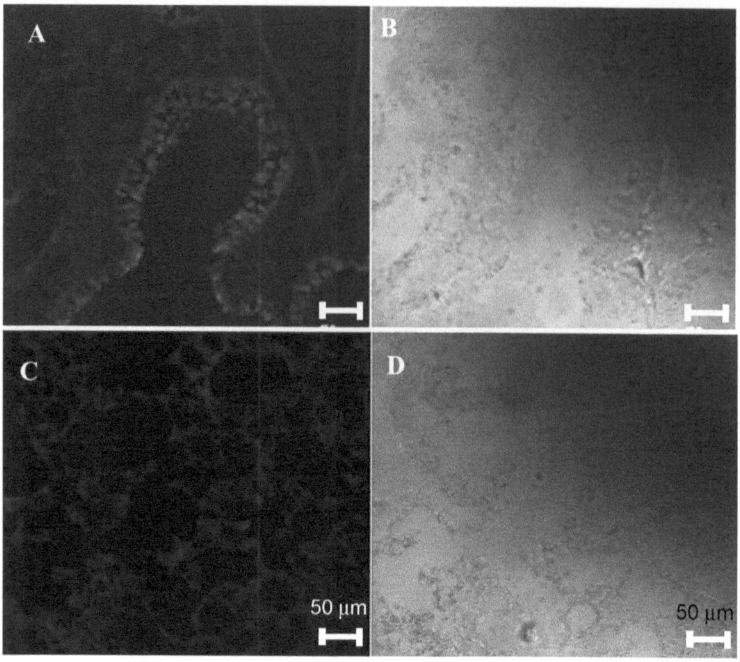

10.3 In vivo GFP expression analysis after aerosol administration to lung (bar = 50 μm). (a) Fluorescent microscopic image of PCL/PEI-1.2, (b) phage contrast image of PCL/PEI-1.2, (c) fluorescent microscopic image of PEI 25K, (d) phage contrast image of PEI 25K (cited from Ref. 38).

backbone. This exerted osmotic pressure is supposedly responsible for the subsequent cellular uptake of polyplexes and thereby increased transfection efficiency. Park *et al.* reported that after 24 h (IV) or 48 h (aerosol administration) of polyplexes containing PEG-alt-PEI, the quantity of luciferase was determined in lung, liver, spleen, kidney and heart. It was found that luciferase expression using 400 μl injection volume increased 8-fold over 100 μl injection. Luciferase expression was primarily found in lungs in agreement with previous results owing to the fact that lung is the first organ encountered by polyplexes after tail vein injection and thus positively charged polyplexes may electrostatically interact with negatively charged membrane of the endothelial cells of lungs.[44] A higher gene expression through aerosol administration was obtained than that through the IV route with any organs of mice and the gene expression in lung and liver after aerosol administration were maintained for 7 days.

In another interesting report, Jiang *et al.* showed the successful liver transfection after IP administration of galactosylated chitosan-graft-PEI (GC-g-PEI). Significant GFP expression was observed after IP administration of the polyplexes prepared from GC-g-PEI which was in agreement with the results of the successful *in vivo* biodistribution using ^{99m}Tc-GC-g-PEI by the same route of administration.[45] Apart from successful DNA delivery by injectable carriers, siRNA were also prominently delivered by biodegradable carriers developed by our group. Jere *et al.* showed the prominent results of si/shRNA delivery using biodegradable PEA based on PEGDA and LMW-PEI. It was found that 1.5 times superior and safer EGFP silencing was observed with PEAs than PEI 25K. Additionally, PEA-mediated AktshRNA delivery efficiently silenced oncoprotein Akt1 and reduced cell survival in Akt1 knock-down specific manner. In apoptosis and necrosis assays, PEI 25K-delivered shAKTsmainly caused undesirable cell necrosis while PEAs-mediated delivery primarily induced apoptosis providing superior delivery efficiency and low cytotoxicity.[46] Jere *et al.* also reported the Akt1 silencing efficiencies in lung cancer cells by sh/si/ssiRNA transfection using a reductable polyspermine carrier. Reductable polyspermine (RPS) carrier was synthesized successfully using multiple spermine units with disulfide linkages for gene expression and silencing studies. EGFP expression was found to be almost 4-fold higher and 20-fold safer with RPS carrier than with PEI25K. Also, systemic administration of RPS exhibited significantly higher EGFP expression in mice lungs. Similarly in gene silencing studies, EGFP silencing achieved was nearly 1.5 times superior with RPS carrier than PEI25K. This RPS also delivered Akt1 shRNA (shAkt), siRNA (siAkt) and ssiRNA (ssiAkt) efficiently and silenced oncoprotein Akt1 thereby decreased A549 cell survival.[47]

Generally nanoparticles escaping from the vesicles into cytoplasm intact can diffuse to the nuclear membrane. The property of polymer that would accelerate this active and passive diffusion process is currently unknown. Microinjected pDNA is rapidly degraded in cytoplasm with an apparent half-life of 50–90 min.[48] There is evidence that intact nanoparticles can be present in the nucleus of even non-dividing cells. It is generally believed that it is the unpacked DNA that translocates into the nucleus for ultimate gene expression. Also, the inclusion of viral nuclear localization signals (NLS) has been demonstrated to be effective strategy to facilitate nuclear transport.[49]

10.4 Microspheres

Several groups reported that microspheres formulated from biodegradable polymers have many inherent properties that are advantageous for gene delivery applications. Various properties such as ease of lyophillization for long-term storage and off the shelf use, protection of DNA from enzymatic attack, controlled delivery of pDNA over longer durations are promising successful gene delivery.[50] This extended release of DNA from microshperes could alleviate the disadvantage of transient expression inherent in all non-viral vectors.[12] Moreover, in case of gene delivery using biodegradable microspheres, no surgical implantation or retrieval is necessary. These microspheres can be administered locally into the tissues by bolus injection or IV administration for systemic application.[12] The rate of polymeric degradation and then the rate of DNA release is dependent on the composition and formulation of the microspheres.

Researchers reported that microspheres fabricated from hydrolytically degradable polymers such as poly(lactide-co-glycolic acid) (PLGA) have been widely used to sustain the release of encapsulated therapeutic compounds. Lynn *et al.* reported the fabrication of pH-responsive microspheres using poly(β-amino ester)s (PBAE).[51] They showed that PBAE was suitable for the fabrication of polymer microspheres ranging from 5 to 30 microns in a diameter using a double emulsion technique. Poteinei *et al.* also reported the fabrication of pH-responsive nanoparticles from the same polymer ranging from 100 to 150 nm in diameter using solvent displacement technique.[52] They successfully delivered rhodamine-123 or paclitaxel to human breast cancer cells by modifying PBAE nanoparticles with poly(ethylene oxide).

Results from various reports suggest that *in vivo* uptake of particles containing pDNA results in expression of exogeneous DNA. Gene expression was also detected following the *in vivo* administration of PLG microparticles formulated with DNA. Intramuscular injection of microparticles coated with pDNA resulted in gene expression at the site of injection up to 14 days post administration,[53] which was in contrast to the findings made after IM injection in rats with encapsulated DNA, where in some cases lower levels of protein expression were observed in comparison to naked DNA.[33] As injection of microparticle-associated DNA differs from that of naked DNA, in terms of localization of gene expression, more sophisticated experiments were carried out. A single IM injection of 30 μg encapsulated DNA resulted in transgene expression in liver, lymph node, spleen and muscles at 15 days after injection as detected by RT-PCR, whereas three IM injections of 100 μg of the same naked DNA led to expressions that were restricted to liver and muscle tissues.[54]

Intraperitoneal injection of PLG microparticles promoted uptake by CD14+ macrophages, whereas intradermal injections resulted in uptake by CD86+ dendritic cells.[55] Parenteral delivery of encapsulated DNA or DNA-coated PLG microspheres was effective at stimulating systemic β-cells and T-cell responses. Cytotoxic T-cell responses specific to encoded epitopes were generated by mice immunized with minigens encoding individual T-cell epitopes followed by either IM, subcutaneous or IP routes.[12] McKeever *et al.* showed that as little as 2 μg of encapsulated DNA was as active as 200 μg of naked DNA in eliciting T-cell responses. Administration of encapsulated DNA formulations encoding reporter antigens by IM or IV routes was shown to promote antibody responses, T-cell proliferation and T-cell mediated- release of γ-interferons.[56]

Yun *et al.* reported the *in vivo* efficacy of hyaluronan (HA)-DNA microspheres with rat hind limb model. To determine if the pDNA delivered from HA microspheres is being transcribed, the RNA extracted from the muscles 3 weeks after injection, has been purified (DNA digested) and analyzed with RT-PCR.[57] RT-PCR analysis showed positive signals for the rat hind limb muscles injected with HA-DNA and PLGA-DNA microspheres. It was also found from RT-PCR that, hind limb muscles injected with HA-DNA microspheres were transcribing a mRNA for β-gal which is foreign to the rat's genome. This confirms that skeletal tissues have been transfected by DNA released from HA or PLGA microspheres since the muscles injected with saline were negative. Furthermore, the detection of mRNA after 3-weeks injection could confirm the controlled release characteristics exhibited by HA-DNA microspheres *in vivo*.[57]

10.5 Hydrogels

Hydrogels are hydrophilic polymer networks capable of absorbing large amounts of water.[58] The hydrogels have been of great interest in a broad range of biomedical application because of their hydrophilic and biocompatible character. Most recently such hydrogels have become attractive to the new fields of tissue engineering and gene delivery.[59] Hydrogels have been employed to locally deliver non-viral vectors, and to provide a sustained release and maintain elevated concentrations.[60] Also, gene delivery using hydrogels is versatile, with the potential to target any cellular process, and gene expression can persist for a long time, which is advantageous for proteins for half-lives.[60] Crosslinking of the polymer chains can be obtained by various physical, chemical and genetic methods. Recently, research interest has focused on injectable formulations that form a macroscopic gel at the site of injection due to several advantages such as patient comfort and cost reductions.[61] In this section, various methods to create *in situ* gelling systems for gene delivery are outlined.

10.5.1 Physical hydrogels

Alginate is widely used due to its low toxicity, easy chemical modification and mild microcapsule formation with a multivalent ion.[62] These microcapsules can be used to load plasmid DNA. Aggarwal *et al.*[63] encapsulated DNA containing the bacterial β-galactosidase (LacZ) gene. The results indicated that mice inoculated orally with microcapsules containing plasmid DNA expressed LacZ in the intestine, spleen and liver. When polyelectrolytes of opposite charges are mixed, or proton-donating polymers and proton-accepting polymers are mixed, they may form a complex gel. Ismail *et al.*[64] prepared two *in situ* gel systems with plasmid DNA and salmon sperm DNA. One is polymethacrylic acid (PMA)/poly(ethylene glycol)(PEG) mixture system and the other is a hydroxypropylmethylcellulose/Carbopol mixture one. The results indicated that both gel composition and medium pH influenced the release of plasmid DNA from *in situ* gel formulations. Also, DNA was released without degradation, although they did not perform *in vivo*.

Agarose is a linear polysaccharide consisting of repeating units of agarobiose that forms double helices during cooling, which associate into a three-dimensional network with gelling.[65] The easy-gelling behavior and thermo-reversibility of the agarose have resulted in many applications in drug delivery systems.[65] Meilander *et al.*[66] used agarose hydrogel for sustained release of DNA after compaction with a polylysine-PEG conjugate *in vitro*. The results indicated that the agarose hydrogel provided the sustained release of compacted, functional DNA for over 50 days *in vitro*, although at lower levels than freshly compacted DNA. The same group studied agarose hydrogel for prolonged gene expression in skin.[67] The results indicated that the sustained release of DNA complexed with polylysine in the agarose hydrogel prolonged gene expression for 35 days after injection intradermally in rodents, whereas injections of DNA in solution produced gene expression for only 5–7 days, suggesting that it can be used to promote the local production of a therapeutic protein. Toussaint *et al.*[68] compared sustained release of DNA vaccines between osmotic pumps and agarose hydrogel implants in cattle for the bovine herpesvirus 1-specific immune response. The results showed that intradermal injection with agarose hydrogel implants induced a more efficient immune response in a single manipulation of the animals than osmotic pumps with repeated intradermal administrations.

Biodegradable triblock copolymers [PEG-poly(L-lactic acid)(PLA)-PEG] can undergo sol-gel transition with increasing temperature.[69] Huang and his co-workers used PEG-poly(D,L-lactic acid-co-glycolic acid)(PLGA)-PEG hydrogel for controlled gene delivery *in vitro* and *in vivo*.[70] The results indicated that the release of pDNA from the polymer followed the zero-order kinectics up to 12 days and maximal gene expression of luciferase was obtained at 24 h in the skin wound of CD-1 mice, although the expression dropped by nearly 94% at 72 h. They also used the thermosensitive hydrogel for controlled delivery of TGF-β1 gene to accelerate diabetic wound healing.[71] The results showed that accelerated re-epithelialization, increased cell proliferation, and organized collagen were obtained in the wound bed treated with the hydrogel containing plasmid TGF-β1 whereas the hydrogel alone was slightly beneficial for re-epithelialization at early stage of healing. Pearton *et al.*[72] used a combination of microfabricated microneedles and PLGA-PEG-PLGA hydrogel for gene delivery to the epidermal cells of human skin explants because non-viral gene expression in skin is generally inefficient and transient. The results indicated that pDNA hydrogels were shown to harbor and gradually release pDNA and microneedle-assisted delivery of pDNA hydrogels to human skin expression of the pCMVβ reporter gene was shown in the viable epidermis proximal to microchannels.

Biodegradable hydrogels based on starch were produced by free-radical polymerization with acrylic acid and applied for drug delivery carriers or bone cements.[73] Bannai *et al.*[74] used starch-grafted-polyacrylate as a carrier for a discrete deposit of antisense oligodeoxy-nucleotides (ODN) in the central nervous system of mouse. The results indicated that antisense ODNs were distributed to within 800 μm from the edge of the area where the gel is located and then gradually disappear from this area within days, but remain within 300 μm distance 7 days later and suppressed the synthesis of the target protein.

The same group used the same hydrogel for injection of antisense of ODN of glutamic acid decarboxylase (GAD) isozymes into rat ventromedical hypothalamus on food intake and locomotor activity.[75] The results showed that an injection combining both antisense ODNs significantly decreased food intake only on day 1, but body weight remained significantly lower than the control for 5 days whereas control ODN did not affect food intake, body weight and locomotor activity. Semba *et al.*[76] used starch-grafted-polyacrylate for the slow delivery of c-fos antisense ODN in the brain of mouse. It was observed that unilateral injection with c-fos antisense ODN into the rat striatum caused robust ipsilateral rotations after methamphetamine challenge 4 days post injection, suggesting that the biological effect of antisense ODN in the hydrogel can be maintained for several days even after a single injection into the brain.

Block copolymers of PEG and poly(propylene oxide)(PPG), well known as poloxamer, lead to the formation of hydrophobic domains and eventually transition of an aqueous transition to a hydrogel network as temperature increases.[77] The poloxamers have been widely used in medical, pharmaceutical, and cosmetic applications. Liaw *et al.*[78] used poloxamer as a carrier for eye-drop gene delivery of plasmid DNA with lacZ gene in mice and rabbits. It was found that reporter expression was detected around the iris, sclera, conjunctiva, and lateral rectus muscle of rabbit eyes and also in the intraocular tissues of nude mice upon *in vivo* topical application or 48 h with a DNA/poloxamer formulation. Pitard *et al.*[79] used another poloxamer [PEO(13)-PPO(30)-PEO(13)] as a carrier for gene delivery of beta-galactosidase reporter gene to skeletal and cardiac muscles of rats. The results indicated that the poloxamer permitted long-term gene expression compared with naked DNA, although poloxamer/DNA formulations were inefficient *in vitro*. They also found that intramuscular injection of plasmid DNA formulated with poloxamer provided an efficient and simple method for secretion and production of erythropoietin.[80] Agarwal *et al.*[81] synthesized cationic pentablock copolymers with poly(diethyl-amino ethyl methacrylate) blocks covalently attached to poloxamer for sustained release of DNA because these copolymers electrostatically condense DNA and further self-assemble above critical concentration to form gels at physiological temperature. The results indicated that the hydrogels had better mechanical strength than poloxamer itself and hydrogels of nanoplexes released nanoplexes up to 5 days *in vitro*, compared to rapid release of up to 90% entrapped naked DNA from poloxamer gels by day 1, although they did not perform *in vivo* study.

10.5.2 Chemical hydrogels

PEG has been widely used for the preparation of hydrogels due to safety and FDA approval for internal use.[82] Quick *et al.*[83] prepared photocrosslinked PEG hydrogels for sustained DNA delivery. The results showed that plasmid DNA was released primarily in the relaxed and supercoiled forms for periods of 6–100 days with either nearly linear or delayed burst release profiles, although chemical and physical protective agents were added to preserve the supercoiled form of the plasmid DNA during photoencapsulation.

Chun *et al.*[84] photocrosslinked Pluronic F127 for sustained delivery of plasmid DNA. The results indicated that release of DNA was dependent on the UV irradiation time and vinyl group-modified hyaluronic acid (HA) amounts, and the released DNA from the HA/Pluronic hydrogels exhibited considerable transfection efficiency without degradation of DNA by the UV irradiation.

Gelatin has been widely used for biomedical applications because its biosafety has been proved and gelatin can easily be chemically modified.[85] Tabata and his coworkers[86] synthesized cationized gelatin hydrogels through introduction of ethylenediamine and crosslinking with glutaraldehyde for controlled release of DNA. The results showed that DNA release and consequent gene expression in the hydrogels were affected by the water content of hydrogels and intramuscular implantation of DNA-incorporated hydrogels into the mice enhanced significantly expression of the DNA around the implanted site. They also reported that the gene expression by the cationized gelatin hydrogels incorporating lacZ plasmid DNA depended on the aminized percentage of gelatin[87] and, enhanced and prolonged gene expression in the femoral muscle of mice was accompanied with the *in vivo* degradation of the cationized gelatin hydrogel.[88]

Kasper *et al.*[89] prepared injectable oligo(poly(ethylene glycol)) fumarate (OPF) hydrogels crosslinked by N,N-methylenebisacrylamide for the *in vitro* release of DNA. It was found that DNA was released in a sustained, linear fashion over the course of 45–62 days and the release kinetics was dependent on the molecular weight of the PEG in the OPF.

10.5.3 Peptide-based hydrogels

There is a growing interest in peptide-based hydrogels for drug delivery systems because synthetic polymers are combined with protein domains that self-assemble through hydrophobic coiled-coil interactions and the self-assembly occurs in response to temperature and pH.[90]

Recently, progress in recombinant DNA technology has provided the synthesis of recombinant protein-based polymers with precisely defined molecular weights, compositions, sequences and stereochemistries.[91] It enables construction of new tailor-made injectable polymers for gene delivery. Ghandehari and his co-workers[92,93] synthesized genetically engineered silk-elastinlike polymer (SELP) hydrogels as a carrier for the controlled release of plasmid DNA. It was found that DNA was released from the SELP hydrogels through an ion-exchange mechanism and the release rate was affected by buffer ionic strength, SELP concentration, and SELP cure time. They also reported that the release of DNA was influenced by the SELP hydrogel geometry, DNA molecular weight, and DNA conformation, and delivery of pRL-CMV from the hydrogel resulted in increased transfection in a murine model of human breast cancer *in vivo*.[94] Furthermore, they used SELP hydrogel in controlling the release rate of adenoviruses *in vitro* and *in vivo*.[95,96] The results indicated that the SELP hydrogels released viruses over a period of 4 weeks *in vitro* while preserving their bioactivity, and a prolonged and localized expression of adenoviruses was observed after intratumoral injection into xenograft tumor models of breast and head and neck cancer in mice.

Fibrin hydrogels are formed from fibrinogen which exists as a dimer comprising two D domains and a central E domain. Fibrinogen is converted into insoluble fibrin through thrombin-mediated fibrinopeptide release, protofibril formation, and crosslinking in presence of factor XIII to yield a stabilized 3D network of fibrils known as the fibrin clot.[97] The fibrin hydrogel has been widely used as an in cell delivery because it is amenable to *in situ* delivery by simple injection at the site of interest, where it quickly polymerizes within seconds and it is a biodegradable polymer.[98] Andree *et al.*[99] used fibrin for controlled release of plasmid DNA to human keratinocytes *in vitro* and *in vivo*. The results indicated that the transfection efficiency in the human keratinocytes increased up to a 100-fold compared to control containing no EGF expression plasmid and a 180-fold increase in EGF concentration was obtained compared to control after transplantation to full thickness wounds on athymic mice. Trentin *et al.*[100] studied peptide-matrix-mediated gene transfer of an oxygen-insensitive hypoxia-inducible factor-1α from a fibrin for induction of proangiogeneic proteins, including vascular endothelial growth factor (VEGF) in a dermal wound of mouse. It was found that angiogenesis was increased comparably strongly to that induced by VEGF-A165 protein when the peptide-DNA complexes were entrapped in fibrin matrices, suggesting a powerful approach in tissue engineering and therapeutic angiogenesis. Saul *et al.*[101] used sphere-templated fibrin scaffolds for sustained transgene expression in NIH-3T3 fibroblasts. The results indicated that different transgene expression were obtained according to the spatial distribution of polyplexes within the scaffold and surface-coated polyplexes showed one order of magnitude greater expression than polyplexes embedded within the scaffold. Rieux *et al.*[102] used fibrin hydrogels for maximizing gene transfer for *in vitro* models of tissue growth after entrapping of cells and DNA in the hydrogels. The results showed that all cells had intracellular plasmid and transgene expression persisted for at least 10 days. Kulkarni *et al.*[103] also reported that the fibrin-lipoplex system showed higher transfection efficiency for two reporter genes at day 7 after topical administration in a rabbit ear ulcer model after topical when compared to lipoplexes alone. Breen *et al.*[104,105] used fibrin scaffold for delivery of the viral vector to a wound site because gene therapy using viral vectors in tissue regeneration is hindered by a short duration of transgene expression. It was found that the fibrin aided in the delivery of a low-dose viral vector, thereby avoiding a chronic inflammatory response, and allowing superior transfection than viral vector alone. Lei *et al.*[106] used fibrin hydrogels for cell-controlled and spatially arrayed gene delivery. The results indicated that cell transfection depended strongly on the local cell-pDNA microenvironments as defined by the 2D vs. 3D context, target cell type and density, as well as fibrinogen and pDNA concentrations.

10.5.4 Nanohydrogel

Nanohydrogels have gained considerable attention in recent years as a drug delivery system, because they have combined properties of hydrogels and nanosize at the same time. Therefore, they can benefit from hydrophilicity, flexibility, versatility and biocompatibility, and advantages of nanosize, mainly long life span in circulation and the possibility of being actively or passively targeted to the desired organs,[107] although only a few researches for gene delivery have been reported so far. Vinogradov *et al.*[108] synthesized crosslinked PEO and polyethylenimine (PEI) nanohydrogel for delivery of antisense oligonucleotides. It was found that interaction of oligonucleotides with PEO-cl-PEI resulted in formation of nanocomposite materials in which the hydrophobic regions form polyion-complexes that were jointed by the hydrophilic PEO chains. Also, efficient cellular uptake and intercellular release of oligonucleotides immobilized in PEO-cl-PEI nanohydrogel were obtained after modification with polypeptide ligands. Furthermore, this delivery system showed enhanced delivery of oligonucleotides across gastrointestinal epithelium and brain microvessel endothelial cells *in vitro*. Recently, Lee *et al.*[109] prepared photo-crosslinkable chitosan/Pluronicnanohydrogels for controlled release of plasmid DNA. The results indicated that release rates of plasmid DNA in the hydrogel were influenced by chitosan content and photo-irradiation time and released fractions from chitosan/Pluronic hydrogels showed better transfection efficiency in HEK 293 cells than those from Pluronic hydrogels.

10.6 Small interfering RNA (siRNA)

Recently, the discovery of RNA interference (RNAi)-mediated gene silencing strategy has gained promising interest for gene therapy because the RNAi is highly target specific and it has wide therapeutic potential including in viral infections, cancer and neurodegenerative disorders although reported research using injectable carriers is very limited at this moment. Blackburn *et al.*[110] synthesized core/shell nanohydrogels consisting of poly(N-isopropylacrylamide-co-acrylic acid) as the core and poly(N-isopropylacrylamide-co-amino propyl methacrylamide) as the shell with surface-localized peptides that specifically target ovarian carcinoma cell lines having high expression levels of the erythropoietin-producing hepatocellular (Eph) A2 receptor for targeted siRNA delivery. The results indicated that these nanohydrogels showed high effectiveness in the noncovalent encapsulation of siRNA and nanohydrogel-mediated delivery of siRNA targeted to the EGF receptor resulted in knockdown of that receptor without cytotoxicity owing to the excellent production of siRNA during endosomal uptake and endosomal escape of the nanohydrogels. Hu *et al.*[111] synthesized another pH-sensitive core/shell nanohydrogel consisting of poly(2-diethyl-amino ethyl methacrylate) as the core and poly(2-aminoethyl methacrylate) (PAEMA) as the shell or poly(methyl methacrylate) as the core and PAEMA as the shell for cytosolic delivery of siRNA into the epithelial cells. It was found that pH-sensitive core/shell nanohydrogels enabled cytosolic siRNA delivery and gene knockdown in the epithelial cells.

10.7 Conclusion

Gene therapy is a very promising approach to treat or to prevent diseases. However, progress in this field is hindered by lack of suitable vectors. Biodegradable injectable carriers offer a nontoxic and nonimmunogenic gene delivery system which is capable of delivering genes of interest at a controlled rate, resulting in sustained gene delivery. Many factors such as DNA loading, release from carriers, their cellular uptake and release from endosome could influence nano-, micro- and hydrogel-mediated gene transfections. The current review clearly outlined the design, synthesis and characterization of injectable polymeric carriers and their evaluation as a safe and potential gene carrier. These injectable polymeric carriers conjugated to specific targeting ligands will further enhance the potential of this system as a targeted gene delivery vector.

10.8 Acknowledgements

This work was supported by the Korea Science and Engineering Foundation (KOSEF) NRL Program grant funded by the Korea government (MEST) (No. ROA-2008-000-20024-0). We also acknowledge Ji-He Seo for typewriting this chapter.

10.9 References

1. Dorsett Y, Tuschl T. siRNAs: applications in functional genomics and potential as therapeutics. *Nat Rev Drug Discov*, 2004, 3(4), 318–29.
2. Cotten M, Längle-Rouault F, Kirlappos H, Wagner E, Mechtler K, Zenke M, Beug H, Birnstiel ML. Transferrin-polycation-mediated introduction of DNA into human leukemic cells: stimulation by agents that affect the survival of transfected DNA or modulate transferrin receptor levels. *Proc Natl Acad Sci USA*, 1990, 87(11), 4033–7.
3. Dash PR, Read ML, Fisher KD, Howard KA, Wolfert M, Oupicky D, Subr V, Strohalm J, Ulbrich K, Seymour LW. Decreased binding to proteins and cells of polymeric gene delivery vectors surface modified with a multivalent hydrophilic

polymer and retargeting through attachment of transferrin. *J Biol Chem*, 2000, 275(6), 3793–802.

4. Plank C, Tang MX, Wolfe AR, Szoka FC Jr. Branched cationic peptides for gene delivery: role of type and number of cationic residues in formation and *in vitro* activity of DNA polyplexes. *Hum Gene Ther*, 1999, 10(2), 319–32.
5. Wagner E. Application of membrane-active peptides for nonviral gene delivery. *Adv Drug Deliv Rev*, 1999, 38(3), 279–89.
6. Behr JP. Gene transfer with synthetic cationic amphiphiles: prospects for gene therapy. *Bioconjug Chem*, 1994, 5(5), 382–9.
7. Kircheis R, Wightman L, Wagner E. Design and gene delivery activity of modified polyethylenimines. *Adv Drug Deliv Rev*, 2001, 53(3), 341–58.
8. Huang CH, Hung MC and Wagner E. *Non-viral Vectors for Gene Therapy*, Academic Press, San Diego, 1999.
9. Haensler J, Szoka FC Jr. Polyamidoamine cascade polymers mediate efficient transfection of cells in culture. *Bioconjug Chem*, 1993, 4(5), 372–9.
10. Boussif O, Lezoualc'h F, Zanta MA, Mergny MD, Scherman D, Demeneix B, Behr JP. A versatile vector for gene and oligonucleotide transfer into cells in culture and *in vivo*: polyethylenimine. *Proc Natl Acad Sci USA*, 1995, 92(16), 7297–301.
11. Hwang L, Hung MC and Wagner E. Non-viral vectors for gene therapy, Academic Press, 1999, 267–87.
12. Amiji MM, *Polymeric Gene Delivery: Principles and Applications*, CRC Press, 2005.
13. Coll JL, Chollet P, Brambilla E, Desplanques D, Behr JP, Favrot M. *In vivo* delivery to tumors of DNA complexed with linear polyethylenimine. *Hum Gene Ther*, 1999, 10(10), 1659–66.
14. Gautam A, Densmore CL, Golunski E, Xu B, Waldrep JC. Transgene expression in mouse airway epithelium by aerosol gene therapy with PEI-DNA complexes. *Mol Ther*, 2001, 3(4), 551–6.
15. Rudolph C, Müller RH, Rosenecker J. Jet nebulization of PEI/DNA polyplexes: physical stability and *in vitro* gene delivery efficiency. *J Gene Med*, 2002, 4(1), 66–74.
16. Wu GY and Wu CH. Receptor-mediated gene delivery and expression *in vivo*. *J Biol Chem*, 1988, 263(29), 14621–4.
17. Wagner E, Zatloukal K, Cotten M, Kirlappos H, Mechtler K, Curiel DT, Birnstiel ML. Coupling of adenovirus to transferrin-polylysine/DNA complexes greatly enhances receptor-mediated gene delivery and expression of transfected genes. *Proc Natl Acad Sci USA*, 1992, 89(13), 6099–103.
18. Gregorevic P, Blankinship MJ, Allen JM, Crawford RW, Meuse L, Miller DG, Russell DW, Chamberlain JS. Systemic delivery of genes to striated muscles using adeno-associated viral vectors. *Nat Med*, 2004, 10(8), 828–34.
19. Matsumura Y, Maeda H. A new concept for macromolecular therapeutics in cancer chemotherapy: mechanism of tumoritropic accumulation of proteins and the antitumor agent smancs. *Cancer Res*, 1986, 46(12 Pt 1), 6387–92.
20. Maeda H, Seymour LW, Miyamoto Y. Conjugates of anticancer agents and polymers: advantages of macromolecular therapeutics *in vivo*. *Bioconjug Chem*, 1992, 3(5), 351–62.
21. Fisher KD, Ulbrich K, Subr V, Ward CM, Mautner V, Blakey D, Seymour LW. A versatile system for receptor-mediated gene delivery permits increased entry of DNA into target cells, enhanced delivery to the nucleus and elevated rates of transgene expression. *Gene Ther*, 2000, 7(15), 1337–43.

22. Eslami MH, Gangadharan SP, Sui X, Rhynhart KK, Snyder RO, Conte MS. Gene delivery to *in situ* veins: differential effects of adenovirus and adeno-associated viral vectors. *J Vasc Surg*, 2000, 31(6), 1149–59.
23. Wheeler CJ, Felgner PL, Tsai YJ, Marshall J, Sukhu L, Doh SG, Hartikka J, Nietupski J, Manthorpe M, Nichols M, Plewe M, Liang X, Norman J, Smith A, Cheng SH. A novel cationic lipid greatly enhances plasmid DNA delivery and expression in mouse lung. *Proc Natl Acad Sci USA*, 1996, 93(21), 11454–9.
24. Sawa Y, Suzuki K, Bai HZ, Shirakura R, Morishita R, Kaneda Y, Matsuda H. Efficiency of *in vivo* gene transfection into transplanted rat heart by coronary infusion of HVJ liposome. *Circulation*, 1995, 92(9 Suppl), II479–82.
25. Mukherjee S, Ghosh RN, Maxfield FR. Endocytosis. *Physiol Rev*, 1997, 77(3), 759–803.
26. Boussif O, Lezoualc'h F, Zanta MA, Mergny MD, Scherman D, Demeneix B, Behr JP. A versatile vector for gene and oligonucleotide transfer into cells in culture and *in vivo*: polyethylenimine. *Proc Natl Acad Sci USA*, 1995, 92(16), 7297–301.
27. Bettinger T, Read ML. Recent developments in RNA-based strategies for cancer gene therapy. *Curr Opin Mol Ther*, 2001, 3(2), 116–24.
28. Pichon C, Gonçalves C, Midoux P. Histidine-rich peptides and polymers for nucleic acids delivery. *Adv Drug Deliv Rev*, 2001, 53(1), 75–94.
29. Uster PS, Deamer DW. pH-dependent fusion of liposomes using titratablepolycations. *Biochemistry*, 1985, 24(1), 1–8.
30. Wang CY, Huang L. Polyhistidine mediates an acid-dependent fusion of negatively charged liposomes. *Biochemistry*, 1984, 23(19), 4409–16.
31. Chorny M, Polyak B, Alferiev IS, Walsh K, Friedman G, Levy RJ. Magnetically driven plasmid DNA delivery with biodegradable polymeric nanoparticles. *FASEB J*, 2007, 21(10), 2510–19.
32. Panyam J, Labhasetwar V. Biodegradable nanoparticles for drug and gene delivery to cells and tissue. *Adv Drug Deliv Rev*, 2003, 55(3), 329–47.
33. Cohen H, Levy RJ, Gao J, Fishbein I, Kousaev V, Sosnowski S, Slomkowski S, Golomb G. Sustained delivery and expression of DNA encapsulated in polymeric nanoparticles. *Gene Ther*, 2000, 7(22), 1896–905.
34. Panyam J, Zhou WZ, Prabha S, Sahoo SK, Labhasetwar V. Rapid endo-lysosomal escape of poly(DL-lactide-co-glycolide) nanoparticles: implications for drug and gene delivery. *FASEB J*, 2002, 16(10), 1217–26.
35. Davda J, Labhasetwar V. Characterization of nanoparticle uptake by endothelial cells. *Int J Pharm*, 2002, 233(1–2), 51–9.
36. Arote RB, Jere D, Cho CS, 2009 Biodegradable polyester derivatives as gene carrier. *Curr Trends Polym Sci*, 2008, 12, 1–17.
37. Jere D, Arote R, Cho MH, Cho CS, Biodegradable poly (β-amino ester) derivatives for gene and siRNA delivery. In Gustafasson WB (ed.), *New Gene Therapy and Cancer Research*, Nova Science Publishers Inc., pp. 249–278.
38. Arote R, Kim TH, Kim YK, Hwang SK, Jiang HL, Song HH, Nah JW, Cho MH, Cho CS. A biodegradable poly(ester amine) based on polycaprolactone and polyethylenimine as a gene carrier. *Biomaterials*, 2007, 28(4), 735–44.
39. Park MR, Han KO, Cho MH, Nah JW, Choi YJ and Cho C S. Degradable polyethylenimine-*alt*-poly(ethylene glycol) copolymers as novel gene carriers. *J Control Release*, 2005, 105, 367–80.
40. Arote RB, Hwang SK, Yoo MK, Jere D, Jiang HL, Kim YK, Choi YJ, Nah JW, Cho MH, Cho CS. Biodegradable poly(ester amine) based on glycerol dimethacrylate and polyethylenimine as a gene carrier. *J Gene Med*, 2008, 10(11), 1223–35.

41. Arote RB, Lee ES, Jiang HL, Kim YK, Choi YJ, Cho MH, Cho CS. Efficient gene delivery with osmotically active, hyperbranched poly(ester amine)s. *Bioconjug Chem*, 2009, 20(12), 2231–41.
42. Kim TH, Cook SE, Arote RB, Cho MH, Nah JW, Choi YJ, Cho CS. A degradable hyperbranched poly(ester amine) based on poloxamerdiacrylate and polyethylenimine as a gene carrier. *Macromol Biosci*, 2007, 7(5), 611–19.
43. Prabha S, Zhou WZ, Panyam J, Labhasetwar V. Size-dependency of nanoparticle-mediated gene transfection: studies with fractionated nanoparticles. *Int J Pharm*, 2002, 244(1–2), 105–15.
44. Park MR, Kim HW, Hwang CS, Han KO, Choi YJ, Song SC, Cho MH, Cho CS. Highly efficient gene transfer with degradable poly(ester amine) based on poly(ethylene glycol) diacrylate and polyethylenimine *in vitro* and *in vivo*. *J Gene Med*, 2008, 10(2), 198–207.
45. Jiang HL, Kwon JT, Kim YK, Kim EM, Arote R, Jeong HJ, Nah JW, Choi YJ, Akaike T, Cho MH, Cho CS. Galactosylated chitosan-graft-polyethylenimine as a gene carrier for hepatocyte targeting. *Gene Ther*, 2007, 14(19), 1389–98.
46. Jere D, Xu CX, Arote R, Yun CH, Cho MH, Cho CS. Poly(beta-amino ester) as a carrier for si/shRNA delivery in lung cancer cells. *Biomaterials*, 2008, 29(16), 2535–47.
47. Jere D, Kim JE, Arote R, Jiang HL, Kim YK, Choi YJ, Yun CH, Cho MH, Cho CS. Akt1 silencing efficiencies in lung cancer cells by sh/si/ssiRNA transfection using a reductablepolyspermine carrier. *Biomaterials*, 2009, 30(8), 1635–47.
48. Lechardeur D, Sohn KJ, Haardt M, Joshi PB, Monck M, Graham RW, Beatty B, Squire J, O'Brodovich H, Lukacs GL. Metabolic instability of plasmid DNA in the cytosol: a potential barrier to gene transfer. *Gene Ther*, 1999, 6(4), 482–97.
49. Brandén LJ, Mohamed AJ, Smith CI. A peptide nucleic acid-nuclear localization signal fusion that mediates nuclear transport of DNA. *Nat Biotechnol*, 1999, 17(8), 784–7.
50. Langer R, Cleland JL, Hanes J. New advances in microsphere-based single-dose vaccines. *Adv Drug Deliv Rev*, 1997, 28(1), 97–119.
51. Lynn DM, Amiji MM, Langer R. pH-Responsive Polymer Microspheres: Rapid Release of Encapsulated Material within the Range of Intracellular pH. *Angew Chem Int Ed Engl*, 2001, 40(9), 1707–10.
52. Potineni A, Lynn DM, Langer R, Amiji MM. Poly(ethylene oxide)-modified poly(beta-amino ester) nanoparticles as a pH-sensitive biodegradable system for paclitaxel delivery. *J Control Release*, 2003, 86(2–3), 223–34.
53. Singh M, Vajdy M, Gardner J, Briones M, O'Hagan D. Mucosal immunization with HIV-1 gag DNA on cationic microparticles prolongs gene expression and enhances local and systemic immunity. *Vaccine*, 2001, 20(3–4), 594–602.
54. Lima KM, Santos SA, Lima VM, Coelho-Castelo AA, Rodrigues JM Jr, Silva CL. Single dose of a vaccine based on DNA encoding mycobacterial hsp65 protein plus TDM-loaded PLGA microspheres protects mice against a virulent strain of Mycobacterium tuberculosis. *Gene Ther*, 2003, 10(8), 678–85.
55. Newman KD, Elamanchili P, Kwon GS, Samuel J. Uptake of poly(D,L-lactic-co-glycolic acid) microspheres by antigen-presenting cells *in vivo*. *J Biomed Mater Res*, 2002, 60(3), 480–6.
56. McKeever U, Barman S, Hao T, Chambers P, Song S, Lunsford L, Hsu YY, Roy K, Hedley ML. Protective immune responses elicited in mice by immunization with formulations of poly(lactide-co-glycolide) microparticles. *Vaccine*, 2002, 20(11–12), 1524–31.

57. Yun YH, Goetz DJ, Yellen P, Chen W. Hyaluronan microspheres for sustained gene delivery and site-specific targeting. *Biomaterials*, 2004, 25(1), 147–57.
58. Peppas NA, Bures P, Leobandung W, Ichikawa H, Hydrogels in pharmaceutical formulations. *Eur J Pharm Biopharm*, 2000, 50, 27–46.
59. Hoffman AS, Hydrogels for biomedical applications. *Adv Drug Deliv Rev*, 2002, 43, 3–12.
60. des Rieux A, Shikanov A, Shea LD, Fibrin hydrogels for non-viral vector delivery *in vitro*. *J Control Release*, 2009, 136, 148–54.
61. Hatefi A, Amsden B, Biodegradable injectable *in situ* forming drug delivery systems. *J Control Release*, 2002, 80, 9–28.
62. Drury JL, Mooney DJ, Hydrogels for tissue engineering: Scaffold design variables and applications. *Biomaterials*, 2003, 24, 4337–51.
63. Aggarwal N, Hogenesch H, Guo P, North A, Suckow M, Mittal SK, Biodegradable alginate microspheres as a delivery system for naked DNA. *Can J Vet Res*, 1999, 63, 148–52.
64. Ismail FA, Napaporn J, Hughes JA, Brazeau GA, *In situ* gel formulations for gene delivery: release and myotoxicity studies. *Pharm Dev Technol*, 2000, 5, 391–7.
65. Lead JR, Starchev K, Wilkinson KJ, Diffusion coefficients of humic substances in agarose gel and in water. *Environ Sci Technol*, 2003, 482–7.
66. Meilander NJ, Pasumarthy MK, Kowalezyk TH, Cooper MJ, Bellamkonda RV, Sustained release of plasmid DNA using lipid microtubules and agarose hydrogel. *J Control Release*, 2003, 88, 321–31.
67. Meilander NJ, Cheung PJ, Wilson DL, Bellamkonda RV, Sustained *in vivo* gene delivery from agarose hydrogel prolongs nonviral gene expression in skin. *Tissue Eng*, 2005, 11, 546–55.
68. Toussaint JF, Dubois A, Dispas M, Paquet D, Letellier C, Kerkhofs P, Delivery of DNA vaccines by agarose hydrogel implants facilitates genetic immunization in cattle. *Vaccine*, 2007, 25, 1167–74.
69. Jeong B, Bae YH, Lee DS, Kim SW, Biodegradable block copolymers as injectable drug-delivery systems. *Nature*, 1997, 388, 860–2.
70. Li Z, Ning W, Wang J, Choi A, Lee P, Tyagi P, Huang L, Controlled gene delivery system based on thermosensitive biodegradable hydrogel. *Pharm Res*, 2003, 20, 884–8.
71. Li P, Li Z, Huang L, Thermosensitive hydrogel as a TGF-β1 gene delivery vehicle enhances diabetic wound healing. *Pharm Res*, 2003, 20, 1995–2000.
72. Pearton M, Allender C, Brain K, Anstey A, Gateley C, Wilke N, Morrissey A, Birchall J, Gene delivery to the epidermal cells of human skin explants using microfabricated micro needles and hydrogel formulations. *Pharm Res*, 2007, 25, 407–16.
73. Pereira CS, Cunha AM, Reis RL, New starch-based thermoplastic hydrogels for use as bone cements or drug-delivery carriers. *J Mater Sci Mater Med*, 1998, 9, 825–33.
74. Bannai M, Ichikawa M, Nishimura F, Nishihara M, Takahashi M, Water-absorbent polymer as a carrier for a discrete deposit of antisense oligodeoxynucleotides in the central nervous system. *Brain Res Protoc*, 1998, 3, 83–7.
75. Bannai M, Ichikawa M, Nishihara M, Takahashi M, Effect of injection of antisense oligodeoxynucleotides of GAD isozymes into rat ventromedial hypothalamus on food intake and locomotor activity. *Brain Res*, 1998, 784, 305–15.
76. Semba J, Wakuta M, Suhara T, Long-term suppression of methamphetamine-induced c-Fos expression in rat striatum by the injection of c-Fos antisense oligodeoxynucleotides absorbed in water-absorbent polymer. *Psychiatry Clin*

Neurosci, 2004, 58, 531–5.
77. Van Tomme SR, Storm G, Hennink WE, *In situ* gelling hydrogels for pharmaceutical and biomedical applications. *I J Pharm*, 2008, 355, 1–18.
78. Liaw J, Chang SF, Hsiao FC, *In vivo* gene delivery into ocular tissues by eye drops of poly(ethylene oxide)-poly(propyleneoxide)-poly(ethylene oxide) (PEO-PPO-PEO) polymeric micelles. *Gene Ther*, 2001, 8, 999–1004.
79. Pitard B, Pollard H, Agbulut O, Lambert O, Vilguin JT, Cherel Y, Abadie J, Samuel JL, Rigaud JL, Menoret S, Anegon I, Escande D, A nonionic amphiphile agent promotes gene delivery *in vivo* to skeletal and cardiac muscles. *Hum Gene Ther*, 2002, 13, 1767–75.
80. Richard P, Pollard H, Lanctin C, Bello-Roufai M, Desigaus L, Escande D, Pitard B, Inducible production of erythropoietin using intramuscular injection of block copolymer/DNA formulation. *J Gene Med*, 2005, 7, 80–6.
81. Agarwal A, Unfer RC, Mallapragada SK, Dual-role self-assembling nanoplexes for efficient gene transfection and sustained gene delivery. *Biomaterials*, 2008, 29, 607–17.
82. Bailey FE, Koleske JV, *Poly(ethylene oxide)*, Academic Press, New York, 1976.
83. Quick DJ, Anseth KS, DNA delivery from photocrosslinked PEG hydrogels: in capsulation efficiency, release profiles, and DNA quality. *J Control Release*, 2004, 96, 341–51.
84. Chun KW, Lee JB, Kim SH, Park TG, Controlled release of plasmid DNA from photo-cross-linked pluronic hydrogels. *Biomaterials*, 2005, 26, 3319–26.
85. Veis A, The physical chemistry of gelatin. *Int Rev Connect Tissue Res*, 1965, 3, 113–200.
86. Fukunaka Y, Iwanaga K, Morimoto K, Kakemi M, Tabata Y, Controlled release of plasmid DNA from cationized gelatin hydrogels based on hydrogel degradation. *J Control Release*, 2002, 80, 333–43.
87. Kushibiki T, Tomoshige R, Fukunaka Y, Kakemi M, Tabata Y, *In vivo* release and gene expression of plasmid DNA by hydrogels of gelatin with different cationization extents. *J Control Release*, 2003, 90, 207–16.
88. Kushibiki T, Tomoshige R, Iwanaga K, Kakemi M, Tabata Y, Controlled release of plasmid DNA from hydrogels prepared from gelatin cationized by different amine compounds. *J Control Release*, 2006, 249–56.
89. Kasper FK, Seidlits SK, Tang A, Crowther RS, Carney DH, Barry MA, Mikos AG, *In vitro* release of plasmid DNA from oligo(poly(ethylene glycol) fumarate hydrogels. *J Control Release*, 2005, 104, 521–39.
90. Kopecek J, Yang J, Hydrogel biomaterials: a smart future? *Biomaterials*, 2007, 28, 5185–92.
91. Meyer DE, Chilkoti A, Genetically encoded synthesis of protein-based polymers with precisely specified molecular weight and sequence by recursive directional ligation: examples from the elastin-like polypeptide system. *Biomacromolecules*, 2002, 3, 357–67.
92. Megeed Z, Cappello J, Ghandehari H, Controlled release of plasmid DNA from a genetically engineered silk-elastinlike hydrogel. *Pharm Res*, 2002, 954–59.
93. Hwang D, Moolcharndani V, Dandu R, Haider M, Cappello J, Ghandehari H, Influence of polymer structure and biodegradation on DNA release from silk-elastinlike protein polymer hydrogels. *I J Pharm*, 2009, 368, 215–19.
94. Megeed Z, Haider M, Li D, O'Malley Jr. BW, Cappello J, Ghandehari H, *In vitro* and *in vivo* evaluation of recombinant silk-elastinlike hydrogels for cancer gene therapy. *J Control Release*, 2004, 94, 433–45.

95. Hatefi A, Cappello J, Ghandehari H, Adenoviral gene delivery to solid tumors by recombinant silk-elastinlike protein polymers. *Pharm Res*, 2007, 24, 773–9.
96. von Wald Cresce A, Dandu R, Burger A, Cappello J, Ghandehari H, Characterization and real-time imaging of gene expression of adnovirus embedded silk-elastinlike protein polymer hydrogels. *Mol Pharm*, 2008, 5, 891–7.
97. Ho W, Tawil B, Dunn JC, Wu BM, The behavior of human mesenchymal stem cells in 3D fibrin clots: dependence on fibrinogen concentration and clot structure. *Tissue Eng*, 2006, 12, 1587–95.
98. Isenberg BC, Williams C, Tranquillo RT, Small-diameter artificial arteries engineered *in vitro*. *Circ Res*, 2006, 98, 25–35.
99. Andree C, Voigh M, Wenger A, Erichshen T, Bittner K, Schaefer D, Walgenbach K, Borges J, Horch RE, Eriksson E, Stark B, Plasmid gene delivery to human keratinocytes through a fibrin-mediated transfection system. *Tissue Eng*, 2001, 7, 757–66.
100. Trentin D, Hall H, Wechsler S, Hubbell JA, Peptide-matrix-mediated gene transfer of an oxygen-insensitive hypoxia-inducible factor-1α variant for local induction of angiogenesis. *Proc Natl Acad Sci USA*, 2006, 103, 2506–11.
101. Saul JM, Linnes MP, Ratner BD, Giachelli CM, Pun SH, Delivery of non-viral gene carriers from sphere-templated fibrin scaffolds for sustained transgene expression. *Biomaterials*, 2007, 28, 4705–16.
102. des Rieux A, Shikanov A, Shea LD, Fibrin hydrogels for non-viral vector delivery *in vitro*. *J Control Release*, 2009, 136, 148–54.
103. Kulkarni M, Breen A, Greiser U, O'Brien T, Pandit A, Fibrin-lipoplex system for controlled topical delivery of multiple genes. *Biomacromolecules*, 2009, 10(6), 1650–4.
104. Breen AM, Dockery P, O'Brien T, Pandit AS, The use of therapeutic gene eNOS delivered via a fibrin scaffold enhances wound healing in a compromised wound model. *Biomaterials*, 2008, 29, 3143–51.
105. Breen A, Dockery P, O'Brien T, Pandit A, Fibrin scaffold promotes adenoviral gene transfer and controlled vector delivery. *J Biomed Mater Res A*, 2009, 89, 876–84.
106. Lei P, Padmashali RM, Andreadis ST, Cell-controlled and spatially arrayed gene delivery from fibrin hydrogels. *Biomaterials*, 2009, 30, 3790–9.
107. Hamidi M, Azadi A, Rafiei P, Hydrogel nanoparticles in drug delivery. *Adv Drug Deliv Rev*, 2008, 60, 1638–49.
108. Vinogradov S, Batrakova E, Kabanov A, Poly(ethylene glycol)-polyethyleniminenanogel particles: novel drug delivery systems for antisense oligonucleotides. *Colloids Surf B*, 1999, 16, 291–304.
109. Lee JI, Kim HS, Yoo HS, DNA nanogels composed of chitosan and pluronic with thermo-sensitive and photo-crosslinking properties. *I J Pharm*, 2009, 373, 93–9.
110. Blackburn WH, Dickerson EB, Smith MH, McDonald JF, Lyon LA, Peptide-functionalized nanogels for targeted siRNA delivery. *Bioconjugate Chem*, 2009, 20, 960–8.
111. Hu Y, Atukorale PU, Lu JJ, Moon JJ, Um SH, Cho EC, Wang Y, Chem J, Irvine DJ, Cytosolic delivery mediated via electrostatic surface binding of protein, virus, or siRNA cargos to pH-responsive core-shell gel particles. *Biomacromolecules*, 2009, 10, 756–65.

Part III

Technologies and developments

11

Environmentally responsive injectable materials

H. H. BEARAT and B. L. VERNON,
Arizona State University, USA

Abstract: This chapter highlights the various environmental stimuli which can be utilized as a trigger for *in situ* formation of injectable hydrogel systems, specifically to provide a more efficient and localized method for controlled delivery of drugs and molecules. These components include temperature, electric field, pH, light, magnetic field, pressure and ionic strength, as well as biomolecular stimuli such as antigens, enzymes, thrombin, and glucose. The properties of each stimulus are described as well as their particular uses in biomedical applications.

Key words: hydrogel, temperature, poly(N-isopropyl acrylamide), pH, electric field, magnetic field, pressure, light, ionic strength, enzyme, antigen, thrombin, glucose.

11.1 Introduction

Smart materials have been under immense investigation in all fields of science and in all corners of the world over the past decades. Smart materials consist of materials which respond to changes in their environment, thus rendering them stimuli-responsive. This work focuses on use of environmentally responsive hydrogels, essentially polymer networks which are capable of retaining large amounts of water without altering their structure. Many hydrogels possess the ability to undergo reversible changes in phase transition, from a solution-to-gel or gel-to-solution, depending on their chemical properties as well as the type of stimulus they are subjected to. The array of stimuli observed to trigger such changes includes temperature, electric field, pH, light, pressure, magnetic field, and ionic strength. Additionally, other hydrogels have been shown to be responsive to biomolecules including antigens, glucose, enzymes and thrombin.

There is demand for more effective, localized, and need-based systems, which can be used in a plethora of biomedical applications, such as cancer targeting, controlled drug delivery, tissue engineering or biosensors. By developing injectable hydrogels which can respond to variations in their environment and which can achieve the desired outcome (releasing a drug or biological molecule, targeting cancerous cells, or cell differentiation in scaffolds), better medical techniques can be attained.

11.2 Temperature-sensitive polymers

11.2.1 Properties

Thermosensitive materials have received much attention in recent years due to their unique characteristics when exposed to various temperatures, particularly at physiological conditions. Since temperature acts as the stimulus, these materials undergo gelation upon increase or decrease in temperature, such as a change from room to body temperature. The event of a transformation from solution to gel in an aqueous environment is known as a sol-gel transition (Klouda and Mikos 2008). This transition is marked by a critical temperature which can either be a lower critical solution temperature (LCST) or a higher critical solution temperature (HCST) (Ougizawa *et al.* 1985; Moelbert and De Los Rios 2003). Below the LCST, the polymer is hydrophilic and soluble, and can thus be found in a solution state. However, as temperature is increased to above the LCST, the polymer becomes more hydrophobic and insoluble, thus causing a collapse into a gel form (Liu and Zhu 1999; Klouda and Mikos 2008; Henderson *et al.* 2008). In the case of a UCST, a phase separation occurs at a low temperatures and the polymer solution converts into a gel as cooling occurs (Ougizawa *et al.* 1985; Moelbert and De Los Rios 2003). The phase transition temperature can be altered by varying the composition of comonomers in the polymer structure. With addition of hydrophobic comonomers, the LCST can be decreased while incorporation of hydrophilic comonomers results in an increase in LCST (Cui *et al.* 2007). It has been demonstrated that the addition of acrylic acid to poly(N-isopropyl acrylamide) leads to an increase in its LCST (Lee and Vernon 2005; Vernon *et al.* 2000), while incorporation of hydroxyethyl methacrylate-acrylate lowers its LCST (Lee *et al.* 2006). It has also been shown that increasing the molecular weight of a polymer may increase its UCST and decrease its LCST (Bae *et al.* 1991).

Although complete understanding of the phase transition of such systems has not yet been attained, various hypotheses are present. One proposition is that a LCST exists due to a local structural transition, which involves the presence of water molecules around specific portions of the polymer in solution (Solis *et al.* 2005). At low temperatures, the water molecules tend to be frozen in place, forming a sort of clathrate structure around segments of the polymer. When at lower temperatures, the water molecules do not possess sufficient energy to alter the bonding pattern and thus maintain their location within the lattice structure (Plummer and Chen 1983). This structure causes the polymer to remain water soluble and in solution form. With an increase in temperature, the water molecules gain energy, resulting in an increase of librational motion of the bonds which in turn causes hydrogen bonding disruption (Plummer and Chen 1983). The disruption of hydrogen bonds of the water molecules within the clathrate structure allows for associations to be formed between newly exposed monomers. Exposure of monomers leads to more chances of entanglement, and thus, formation of a gel.

The behavior of polymers in solution and their phase transition at different temperatures can also be described thermodynamically. Three types of interactions can occur once a polymer is dissolved in water: water–polymer, water–water, and polymer–polymer (Klouda and Mikos 2008; Solis *et al.* 2005), and they can be analyzed using the free Gibbs energy equation given below:

$$\Delta G = \Delta H - T\Delta S \qquad 11.1$$

where ΔG is the change in free energy of the system, ΔH is the change in the enthalpy of the system, T is the absolute temperature and ΔS is the change in entropy of the system. As can be seen from the equation, as temperature is increased, the entropy term ($T\Delta S$) becomes more negative compared to the enthalpy term (ΔH), leading to a negative free energy term (ΔG). What this translates to for polymers with an LCST is that as temperature is increased, a decrease in the free energy of the system occurs, which results in unfavorable conditions for polymer–water interaction and more favorable conditions for water–water and polymer–polymer interactions (Klouda and Mikos 2008). Frank and Evans in 1945 studied this phenomenon and noted that when a non-polar molecule dissolves in water at room temperature, the water molecules tend to orient themselves in a manner to produce greatest 'crystallinity' (Frank and Evans 1945). What they describe as the 'freezing' of the water molecules, as in a clathrate-like structure, was coined as the 'iceberg' theory. In this manner, the water molecules would rather form hydrogen bonds with other adjacent water molecules to construct a cage around the non-polar molecule. The greater the non-polar molecule, the greater the iceberg or cage formed. From a thermodynamic point, at low temperatures, processes tend to lower their enthalpies whereas at high temperatures, these processes reach higher entropy levels (Southall *et al.* 2002). Thus, as temperature is increased, the water molecules in this cage will gain entropy by rearranging themselves to widen their distribution; however, as they do so, the bonds between the water molecules will break, resulting in an increase in enthalpy (Southall *et al.* 2002). Different polymers behave differently at their phase transition temperature. The following sections discuss various thermo-sensitive polymers as well as their respective properties and applications.

11.2.2 N-isopropyl acrylamide

Temperature-sensitive polymers are most likely the most investigated environmental stimuli-responsive materials (Qiu and Park 2001), especially for biomedical purposes. One of the well-known thermosensitive polymers is poly(N-isopropylacrylamide), abbreviated as poly(NIPAAm) (Fig. 11.1). This particular polymer has an LCST around 32°C. Below its LCST, NIPAAm is hydrophilic and soluble in aqueous solutions. As temperature is increased above 32°C, the polymer becomes hydrophobic and insoluble, resulting in its collapse into a gel.

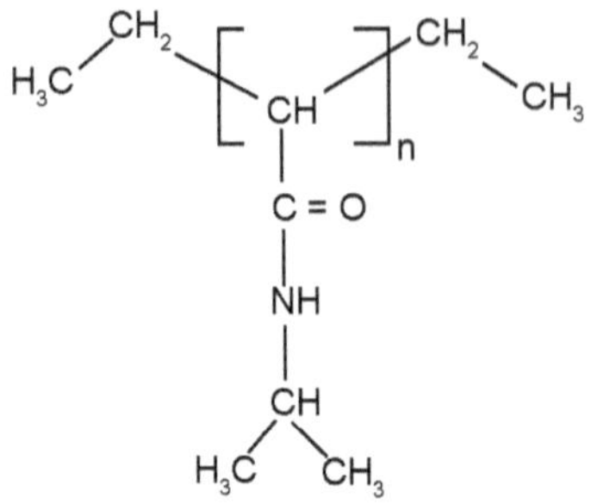

11.1 Chemical structure of thermo-sensitive polymer poly(N-isopropyl acrylamide), known as NIPAAm.

The behavior of NIPAAm around its phase transition temperature has not been fully uncovered. A possibility is, as explained earlier, that as the temperature is increased, the water molecules which formed a clathrate structure around the hydrophobic methyl groups, will unfreeze. This in turn allows the polymer chains to entangle, crosslink, and form a gel, as seen in Fig. 11.2.

NIPAAm possesses great potential for medical use due to an LCST close to body temperature. It is also important to note that the LCST of NIPAAm can be altered by copolymerization of other monomers to the poly(NIPAAm) backbone. The addition of a hydrophobic monomer leads to a decrease in the LCST, whereas the addition of a hydrophilic monomer results in an increase in LCST. An example of copolymerization of a hydrophobic monomer to poly(NIPAAm) has been done by Lee *et al.* (2006). Through free radical polymerization, the group has added

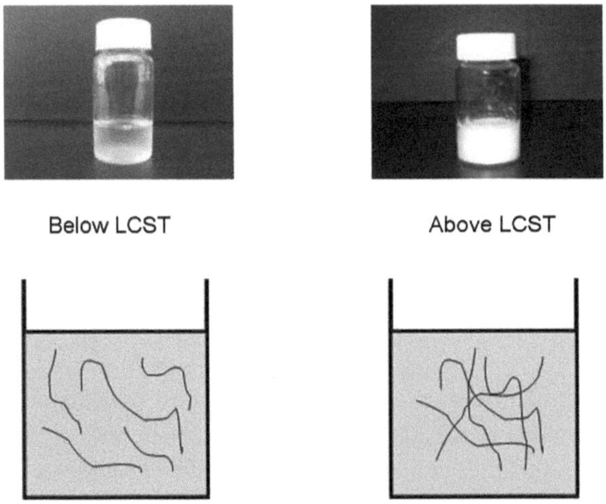

11.2 Demonstration of a thermo-sensitive polymer below and above its LCST. Below LCST, the polymer is hydrophilic and remains in solution form. As temperature is increased to above its LCST, the polymer becomes insoluble and collapses to form a gel.

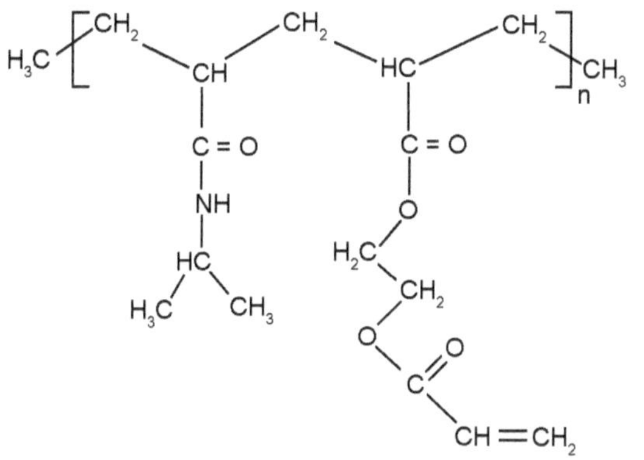

11.3 Chemical structure of thermo-sensitive polymer poly(N-isopropyl acrylamide-co-hydroxyethyl methacrylate acrylate), or poly(NIPAAm-co-HEMA-acrylate). By the copolymerization of HEMA-acrylate, a hydrophobic monomer, the LCST of the polymer decreases.

hydroxyethylmethacrylate-acrylate (HEMA-acrylate) to the backbone (Fig. 11.3). The hydrophobicity of the HEMA-acrylate monomer caused the LCST of the copolymer to decrease to 23°C (Lee *et al.* 2006). Contrarily, by the copolymerization of acrylic acid to poly(NIPAAm) (Fig. 11.4), Vernon and Martinez (2005) witnessed that as the content of acrylic acid (AAc) in the polymer is increased, an increase in LCST is simultaneously observed. They recorded that at 0 mol% AAc in THF, the LCST was 32.87°C, with 1.33 mol% AAc the LCST increased to 38.17C, whereas with 1.99 mol% AAc, the LCST reached 39.1°C (Vernon and Martinez 2005). Feil *et al.* (1993) have also investigated the addition of different comonomers to poly(NIPAAm-co-butyl methacrylate-X) where X is a hydrophobic, hydrophilic, cationic, or anionic comonomer. Their study showed that the addition of hydrophilic or charged comonomers had no direct effect on the water structure around the hydrophobic groups of the polymer, but rather caused an increase in the LCST due to the influence on the overall hydrophilicity of the polymer (Feil *et al.* 1993).

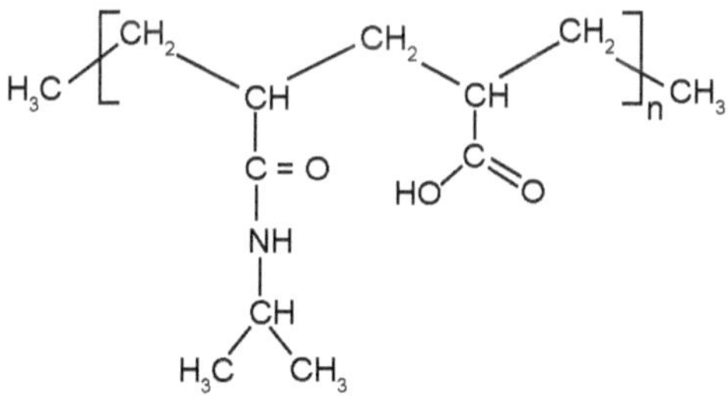

11.4 Chemical structure of thermo-sensitive polymer poly(N-isopropyl acrylamide-co-acrylic acid), or poly(NIPAAm-co-AAc). Since acrylic acid is a hydrophilic moiety, its conjugation increases the original LCST.

Poly(NIPAAm) being one of the most studied thermosensitive polymers has thus found itself used in various biomedical applications. Lee *et al.* (2006) and Robb *et al.* (2007) have taken advantage of the thermal characteristics of poly(NIPAAm) and combined it with the Michael-type addition reaction which occurs between thiols on one NIPAAm copolymer with the olefins on the second NIPAAm copolymer to form an *in situ* gel used for potential endovascular embolization of aneurysms and arteriovenous malformations (Lee *et al.* 2006, Robb *et al.* 2007). Cui *et al.* (2007) synthesized poly(NIPAAm) with dimethyl-γ-butyrolactone acrylate to form a hydrolysis-dependent thermo-sensitive gelling system, rendering the copolymer biodegradable, for injectable drug delivery (Cui *et al.* 2007). By conjugating poly(NIPAAm) with acrylic acid (AAc) and HEMA-poly(trimethylene carbonate), a biodegradable and thermo-sensitive copolymer was achieved for injection into the ventricular wall to prevent progressive remodeling of the left ventricle after myocardial infarction (Fujimoto *et al.* 2009). NIPAAm and AAc combination was also used as a carrier of chondrocytes and transforming growth factor β3 to cartilage tissue (Yun and Moon 2008). After 8 weeks of implantation in cartilage of mice, Yun and Moon observed normal histological and biochemical characteristics, and concluded this hydrogel can be used for neocartilage formation. Grafting of NIPAAm on collagen/chitosan-immobilized polypropylene nonwoven fabric has shown improved healing as well as better remodeling of the veins, epidermis and dermis of the skin injury, when compared to the non-NIPAAm grafted fabric (Wang *et al.* 2008). Kim and Lee (2009) obtained a thermosensitive gel with an LCST around 34.5°C by preparing NIPAAm with vinyl phosphonic acid. The hydrogel was then biomineralized with urea-mediation and was loaded with bovine serum albumin for a drug release model. They determined that drug release was affected by drug loading, water content and biomineralization. Through protein delivery and biomineralization, this hydrogel has potential for bone regeneration (Kim and Lee 2009). By forming branched copolymers of NIPAAm and poly(ethylene glycol) (PEG), a highly elastic and stiff material was achieved to be used for replacement of the nucleus pulposus of the intervertebral discs (Vernengo *et al.* 2008).

11.2.3 Natural thermo-sensitive polymers

Natural polymers have also been used as thermo-sensitive hydrogels, either on their own or in combination with other synthetic polymers. Popular natural polymers include chitosan, cellulose derivatives, dextran, xyloglucan and gelatin (Klouda and Mikos 2008). Chitosan is a polysaccharide derived from the shells of crustaceans and is produced by deacetylation of chitin, basically through the removal of the acetyl group using a concentrated NaOH solution (Fig. 11.5). The main advantage of chitosan for medical and pharmaceutical applications is its biocompatibility and inertness when in contact with human cells (Kumar *et al.*

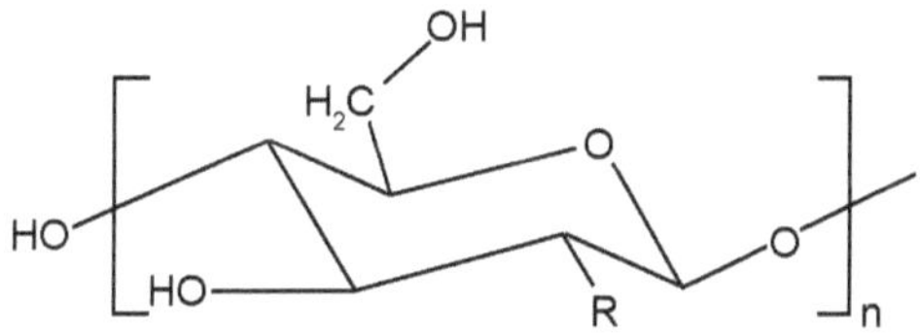

11.5 Chemical structure of chitosan, a natural thermo-sensitive polymer.

2004). It is also quite unique in that it can be degraded in the human body by enzymatic action, but can also be recognized by tumor cells and thus be used for drug delivery applications. An extensive review written on the chemistry and applications of chitosan is highly recommended for further reading (Kumar *et al.* 2004). The Leroux group has also elaborately investigated use of chitosan in drug delivery applications. Chitosan is soluble up to a slightly acidic pH of 6.2 at 85% degree of deacetylation. Once the pH is brought above this value, a gel is formed. They have determined that by using a polyol counterionic monohead salt to neutralize the pH, the chitosan solution was found to remain in liquid form for an extended period of time at or below room temperature. This discovery is important in that it allows chitosan solutions to possess pH values closer to the physiological pH of 7.4 and also results in dependence on temperature to determine the liquid or gel phase, with gel formation occurring at higher temperatures (Chenite *et al.* 2000). Chenite *et al.* (2000) used the chitosan/polyol salt solution for delivery of biologically active growth factors *in vivo* and also utilized it for tissue engineering techniques as an encapsulating matrix for living chondrocytes. Ruel-Gariépy *et al.* (2000), from the same group, looked into using chitosan with glycerophosphate (GP). They found that gelation rate depended on temperature and degree of deacetylation of chitosan (Ruel-Gariépy *et al.* 2000). When tested *in vitro*, the release profile of the chitosan/GP solution with different modeled compounds was related to GP present in the solution, molecular weight and lysozyme presence in the release media. Studies have been done which use chitosan for delivery of bovine serum albumin and anti-tumor necrosis factor agents (Shamji *et al.* 2008), for local sustained release of paclitaxel against tumor growth (Ruel-Gariépy *et al.* 2004), for nasal drug delivery by combination with poly(ethylene glycol) (Wu *et al.* 2007) or thiolated chitosan microparticles for nasal peptide delivery (Krauland *et al.* 2006), ocular delivery of liposome-chitosan nanoparticles (Diebold *et al.* 2007) and fluorescently-labeled chitosan nanoparticles (De Salamanca *et al.* 2006), as well as microspheres for a sustained and controlled drug carrier to the systemic circulation (Denkbas and Ottenbrite 2006).

Cellulose is a polysaccharide commonly found in nature which is insoluble in water. Its insolubility can be altered by substituting the hydroxyl groups on its chiral structure to hydrophobic groups, such as methyl or hydroxypropyl groups (Klouda and Mikos 2008). Methylcellulose and hydroxypropyl methylcellulose

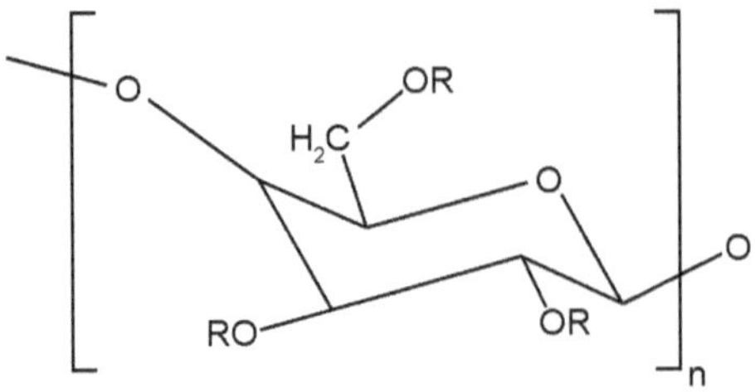

11.6 Chemical structure of methylcellulose, a derivative of the naturally occurring temperature-responsive cellulose.

undergo similar gel formation as poly(NIPAAm), in that at low temperature (and low concentrations of 1–10 wt%), they can be found in liquid form (Fig. 11.6). Once exposed to higher temperatures, the methylcellulose and hydroxypropyl methylcellulose solutions form gels, between 40 to 50ºC and 75 to 90ºC, respectively (Ruel-Gariépy and Leroux 2004). Studies done by Sarkar (1979) demonstrated that the temperature at which the phase transition of either solution occurs decreases at first with increasing concentration, up to a critical concentration; above this value, temperature is faintly influenced by changes in concentration (Sarkar 1979). It was also shown that strength of the resulting gels is time dependent, that it increases with an increase in molecular weight and decreases with greater hydroxypropyl substitution (Sarkar 1979). A hydrophobically modified methyl cellulose (HMMC) with NaCl solution provided much faster gelation (Lee *et al.* 2005). Also by adjusting the concentration of HMMC and NaCl, Lee *et al.* (2005) were able to obtain a sol-gel transition at body temperature and a gel-sol transition at room temperature. Siepmann and Peppas (2001) have modeled different drug delivery systems consisting of hydroxypropyl methylcellulose. Cellulose derivatives have been used in various applications, which include substitutes for bone repair when mixed with biphasic calcium phosphate (Fellah *et al.* 2006) or as an injectable bone substitute for dental sockets (Weiss *et al.* 2007). Methylcellulose can also be combined with gelatin type A and chondroitin 6-sulfate to serve as a combination gel for protein drug delivery (Jin and Kim 2008).

Although this section was focused mainly on chitosan and cellulose derivatives, there are quite a few other naturally-occuring polymers used for medical applications. Xyloglucan, a polysaccharide which originates from tamarind seeds, shows thermally reversible gelation as its galactose side chains are partially degraded (Ruel-Gariépy and Leroux 2004). It has a broad gelation range, from 5 to 50ºC, and a morphology dependent on the hydrogel concentration (Nisbet *et al.* 2006). Xyloglucan has been used to coat layered double hydroxides for drug delivery (Ribeiro *et al.* 2009) as well as to obtain nanocomposites with hydrophobic matrices (Zhou *et al.* 2007). Gelatin is also used as a thermosensitive polymer as it is found in gel form below 25ºC and returns to its liquid form above 30ºC (Klouda and Mikos 2008). It is a collagen-derived protein; however, since it is found in liquid state at body temperature, studies have been performed to chemically crosslink gelatin to improve its gelation properties, such as crosslinking it with hyaluronan for extracellular matrix (Weng *et al.* 2008). Gelatin has also been used to serve as a scaffold for chondrogenic differentiation of adult stem cells (Awad *et al.* 2004).

11.2.4 Pluronics

Pluronics, also known as poloxamers, are a class of synthetic block copolymers which consist of hydrophilic poly(ethylene oxide) (PEO) and hydrophobic poly(propylene oxide) (PPO), arranged in an A-B-A triblock structure, thus giving PEO-PPO-PEO (Fig. 11.7) (Batrakova and Kabanov 2008). They can be found either as liquids, pastes or solids (Ruel-Gariépy and Leroux 2004). Due to their amphiphilic characteristics (presence of hydrophobic and hydrophilic components), pluronics possess surfactant properties which allow them to interact with hydrophobic surfaces and biological membranes (Batrakova and Kabanov 2008). Being amphiphilic also results in the ability of the individual block copolymers, known as unimers, to combine and form micelles in aqueous solutions. When the concentration of the block copolymers is below that of the critical micelle concentration (CMC), the unimers remain as molecular solutions in water. However, as the block copolymer concentration is increased above the CMC, the unimers will self-assemble and form micelles, which can take on spherical, rod-shaped or lamellar geometries. Their shapes depend on the length and concentration of the block copolymers (i.e. EO and PO), and the temperature (Kabanov *et al.* 2002). Micelles usually have a hydrophobic core, in this case the PO chains, and a hydrophilic shell, the EO chains.

The formation of micelles in Pluronics has lead to a plethora of studies in the field of drug delivery. Micelles have a feasible structure for drug loading, since drugs can be incorporated into the core of the micelle at high loads. A characteristic of micelle use is that the distribution of the drug from the drug-loaded micelles is not so much dependent on the drug itself, but rather on the size and surface properties of the micelles, which can be tailored with chemical techniques (Kataoka *et al.* 2001). By doing so, the solubility, metabolic activity and circulation time of the drug can be increased (Kabanov *et al.* 2002). Poloxamer 407 in conjuction with HPMC has been used for rectal delivery of quinine in children (Koffi *et al.* 2008). Use of poloxamer 188 as a membrane sealant on *in*

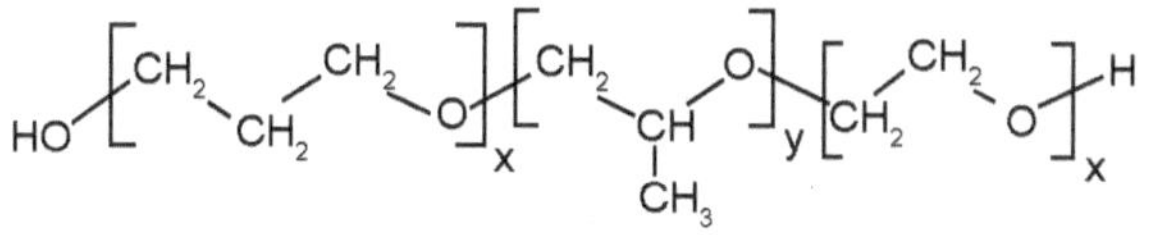

11.7 Poloxamer, poly(ethylene oxide)-poly(propylene oxide)-poly(ethylene oxide) (PEO-PPO-PEO).

vitro studies of cardiac myocytes showed signs of possible prevention of cardiomyopathy and heart failure in muscular dystrophy (Yasuda *et al.* 2005). A combination of poloxamer 407, poloxamer 188 and carbopol was utilized as an ophthalmic delivery system for puerarin, thus providing an alternative for longer-lasting drug availability to the precorneal area (Qi *et al.* 2007). Poloxamer 407 has also shown prolonged duration of the painkiller, lidocaine, at the injection site as well as sustained drug release and increased therapeutic efficacy (Ricci *et al.* 2005). Batrakova *et al.* (2006) investigated the use of Pluronic P85 with the antineoplastic drug, doxorubicin, and determined that presence of pluronic resulted in the inability of human breast cancer cells to grow. Other studies of pluronics involve use of Pluronic F127 for delivery of human growth hormone (Chung *et al.* 2008), combination of Pluronic F127 with chitosan as an injectable cell delivery carrier for cartilage regeneration (Park *et al.* 2009), and for enhanced transcription of reporter genes (Sriadibhatla *et al.* 2006).

11.2.5 Poly(ethylene glycol) (PEG)-poly(D,L-lactic acid co-glycolic acid) (PLGA)-PEG

Poly(ethylene glycol) (PEG) is quite a popular polymer in biomedical applications due to its hydrophilicity and biocompatibility. When PEG is copolymerized with poly(D,L-lactic acid co-glycolic acid) (PLGA) as a triblock copolymer (Fig. 11.8), the polymer was shown to possess biocompatibility, biodegradability and a sol-gel phase transition (Jeong and Gutowska 2002). At higher temperatures (around 45°C), the polymer can be found as a solution and therefore allows for loading of bioactive molecules. Once the polymer is injected at body temperature, the decrease in temperature allows the hydrogel to form a gel. The creation of a gel consisting of loaded bioactive molecules renders the system appropriate for sustained release of drugs from the matrix (Jeong and Gutowska 2002). Further work by Tarasevich *et al.* (2009) has demonstrated that alteration to the gelation temperature can be achieved by increasing the concentration of PEG in the copolymer. The study also concluded that the gelation temperature was also dependent on molecular weight of the polymer as well as concentration. The PEG-PLGA-PEG copolymer was also used for delivery of plasmid DNA in rat models and it was determined that the copolymer has the potential to improve gene delivery efficiency (Chang *et al.*

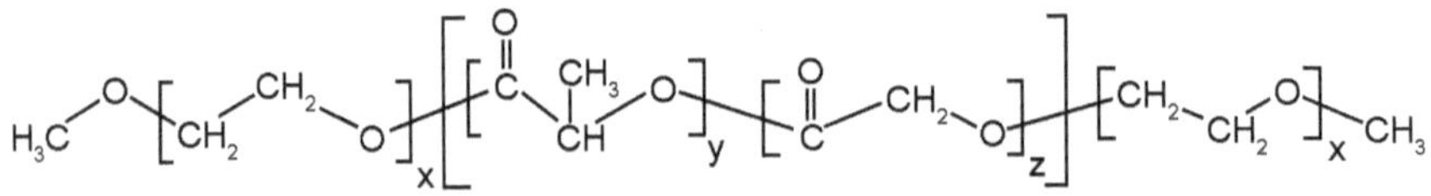

11.8 Thermo-sensitive copolymer PEG-PLGA-PEG, which consists of poly(ethylene glycol) (PEG) and poly(D,L-lactic acid co-glycolic acid) (PLGA).

2007). Lee *et al.* (2007) investigated the properties of the copolymer for wound dressing and scaffold of diabetic skin wounds. They witnessed an increase in engraftment of muscle-derived stem cells, which in turn allowed for better wound healing and collagen deposition. Poly(D,L-lactide-co-glycolide) (PLGA) microspheres dispersed within a PEG-PLGA-PEG gel were used for the sustained release of ganciclovir, an antiviral drug (Duvvuri *et al.* 2005). The group witnessed a decrease in the drug release rate from the microspheres within the gel, compared to the microspheres alone. They also developed a set of equations to describe the various phases of drug release from the microspheres, these stages being initial diffusion, matrix hydration and degradation (Duvvuri *et al.* 2005). By coating a PEGylated monoclonal antibody, which has high affinity for an antigen on prostate cancer cells, with PLGA-PEG-PLGA, an enhanced transfection efficiency and uptake of the plasmid was seen due to copolymer coating (Moffatt and Cristiano 2006).

11.3 Electrically sensitive polymers

11.3.1 Properties and models

Electrosensitive hydrogels have also shown their capabilities of serving as smart materials due to their response upon stimulation by an electric field. These hydrogels usually consist of polyelectrolytes as well as a polymer network which contains ionic particles (Kaewpirom and Boonsang 2006). Their potential in biomechanical and biosensory applications results from their low cost, biocompatibility, biodegradability, good response to stimuli and efficient permeability (Luo and Li 2009). It is only since 1982 that the existence of electrosensitive polymers has been known. Tanaka *et al.* (1982) discovered that phase transition in a polymer not only occurs through temperature or solvent properties, but also through application of an electric field across the gel. Through electrical stimulation, a stress gradient is created along the electric field lines of the gel. Below a particular stress level, the gel is found to be swollen, whereas above it, the gel collapses. The solvent properties and degree of ionization of the gel dictate the volume change at the transition point. They found that once they exposed their polyacrylamide gel to an electric field, a force was produced on the negative-charged acrylic acid groups, pulling it towards the positive electrode. A stress gradient is thus formed along the gel, with a maximum at the positive electrode and minimum at the negative electrode; this stress causes the gel to deform. With higher voltage values, more collapsing occurred in the gel. By removing the applied electric field, the gel transforms back from its collapsed state to its swollen state, rendering this process reversible. Doi *et al.* (1992) devised a semiquantitative theory to describe the swelling and deswelling of the gel under electric field, based on Flory's equation for equilibrium volume of a gel, given by:

$$\Pi_{\text{network}}(V) + RT \cdot \left[\sum_i (c_{is} - c_{ig})\right] = 0 \qquad 11.2$$

where the first term describes the osmotic pressure of the neutral gel prior to dissociation of the ionic groups, R is the gas constant, T is the absolute temperature, c_{is} is the ion concentration of species i in the solution and c_{ig} is the ion concentration in the gel. A neutral gel is characterized by two phenomena: the interaction between the polymer and the solvent which causes swelling and the elasticity of the network which opposes the expansion (Doi *et al.* 1992). Both of these are taken into account by the first term of Eqn. 11.2 and equilibrium volume is determined when this term is set to zero. In the case of an electrically charged gel, a difference occurs between the ion concentration inside and outside the gel. The second term of the equation relates this imbalance in ionic concentration with the variation in osmotic pressure, which causes the gel to swell.

From their theory derivations, they concluded that for a cationic gel exposed to an electric field, if the gel comes in contact with the anode, that particular side will undergo shrinking. However, if the gel is sufficiently separated from the anode, the side of the gel near the anode will first swell and then shrink (Doi *et al.* 1992). As for the cathode side, shrinking of the gel occurs regardless of contact.

More recently, Wallmersperger *et al.* (2004) have developed a chemo-electro-mechanical multi-field formulation for predictions on the swelling and deswelling behavior of polyelectrolyte gels. Chemical and electrical field equations were used to calculate the ion concentrations and electric field, while the mechanical equation described the swelling behavior of the gel (Wallmersperger *et al.* 2004). Their simulations were able to envisage not only the swelling/deswelling of the gel, but also the ion concentrations and the electric potential in the hydrogel as well as in the solution. Li *et al.* (2004) have generated a multi-effect-coupling electric-stimulus (MECe) model for transient simulation of the kinetics of an electrosensitive hydrogel. This elaborate model, which uses nonlinear coupled partial differential equations, efficiently simulated the concentration kinetics of the diffusive ions. It also determined parameters which are crucial to the swelling behavior of polyelectrolyte gels, mainly the applied electric voltage, the charge density and bath solution concentration, and the displacement of the hydrogel (Li *et al.* 2004).

11.3.2 Applications

Due to their sensitivity to electric stimulus, polyelectrolyte hydrogels have been investigated for their potential applications for electrically controlled drug delivery systems, electro-chemical actuators and sensors, as well as muscular actuators (Kaewpirom and Boonsang 2006). The set up for electrostimulation of polyelectrolyte gels can vary and thus can have different effects on the response. The gel can be in contact with one or both electrodes; if the gel is not in contact with the electrodes, a conducting medium is used, whereas in the case of contact, no conducting medium is necessary (Murdan 2003). A polyelectrolyte gel can have various responses to an electric field: swelling, deswelling or erosion. By utilizing an interpenetrating polymer network comprising PEG macromer and chitosan in a NaCl solution, once an electric field was applied, bending of the hydrogel occurred toward the cathode (Kaewpirom and Boonsang 2006). Bending did not take place in pure water, confirming this behavior is due to electrochemical reactions (see Fig. 11.9). The study concluded that the higher the voltage applied, the greater the ion concentration gradient and the more the gel bends. Liu *et al.* took advantage of the electrosensitive response of chitosan as well and incorporated montmorillonite (MMT), a clay-like mineral, to form a polymer-clay hydrogel. The negatively charged MMT was added to obtain a strong crosslinked hydrogel, resulting from its interaction with the positively charged chitosan (Liu *et al.* 2008). This hydrogel was then investigated for release of vitamin B_{12} under an electric field. The study concluded that drug release was influenced by the MMT concentration, which is related to the crosslinking density of the hydrogel. The release of vitamin B_{12} followed pseudo-zero-order kinetics and a change from diffusion-controlled to swelling-controlled release was witnessed with low MMT concentration (1 wt%). When the concentration was increased (>1 wt%), a decrease in the electrical stimulation response was observed. Additionally, the hydrogel demonstrated capabili-

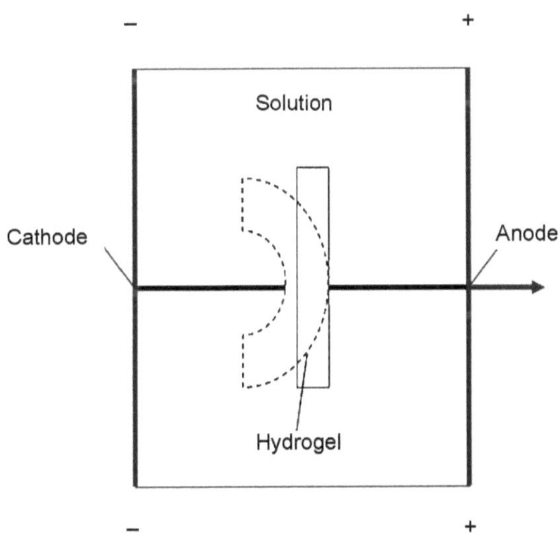

11.9 Schematic of a hydrogel within a bath solution under applied electric field; as can be seen, bending occurs in the hydrogel when subjected to an electric field (adapted from Li *et al.* 2007).

ties of withstanding fatigue. Polyacrylonitrile (PAN) fibers have also been examined for potential use as muscle actuators due to their contraction and elongation properties when exposed to acidic and caustic solutions, respectively (Choe and Kim 2006). Under electrostimulation, hydrogen ions are generated at the anode end and hydroxyl ions are generated at the cathode end. PAN fibers were observed to shrink at the anode and elongate at the cathode (Choe *et al.* 2006). When a 100 mm single strand of PAN fiber was placed under a voltage of 5 V, a force of 0.1 N was generated, which reached steady-state after approximately 10 minutes (Choe and Kim 2006). These results of the performance of the PAN fibers suggest their possible application as muscle actuators. A review by Kikuchi and Okano (2002) discussing various pulsatile drug release systems, including further studies on electric stimuli-responsive pulsatile release, is recommended for further reading.

11.4 pH-sensitive polymers

11.4.1 Properties

Polymers with pH sensitivity have gained popularity in biomedical uses since various pH levels are encountered throughout the human body, whether in the stomach, intestine, blood vessels, vagina or tumor sites. pH sensitive polymers are composed of ionizable groups and they undergo changes in the ionization degree and water-solubility at specific pHs (He *et al.* 2008). They can be classified as acidic weak polyelectrolytes or basic weak polyelectrolytes depending on whether they are proton donors or acceptors. Acidic polyelectrolytes usually contain carboxylic or sulfonic groups, and some examples of such polymers include poly(acrylic acid) (PAA), poly(methacrylic acid), or poly(L-glutamic acid) (He *et al.* 2008). Basic polyelectrolytes are typically made up of ammonium salts and such common polymers include poly(2-(dimethylamino)ethyl methacrylate) (PDMAEMA) and poly(2-(diethylamino)ethyl methacrylate) (PDEAEMA) from the poly(tertiary amine methacrylate) group, and poly(ethylene imine). The presence of ionic groups on a polymer chain causes electrostatic repulsion between the various charges on the polymer, which in turn causes swelling (Qiu and Park 2001). Since swelling results from the interaction between charged groups, it can be manipulated with pH, ionic strength or counterions, which will reduce this electrostatic repulsion. By using neutral comonomers, such as methyl methacrylate or maleic anhydride, the pH and swelling behavior can be altered. Below are chemical structures of poly(acrylic acid) and poly(*N,N'*-diethylaminoethyl methacrylate), anionic and cationic polyelectrolytes, respectively (Fig. 11.10). As can be seen, the anionic polymer (PAA) dissolves more readily and swells at a high pH whereas the cationic polymer (PDEAEMA) dissolves and swells at lower pH values. Studies done using a poly(tertiary amine methacrylate) in conjuction with PEO-PPO-

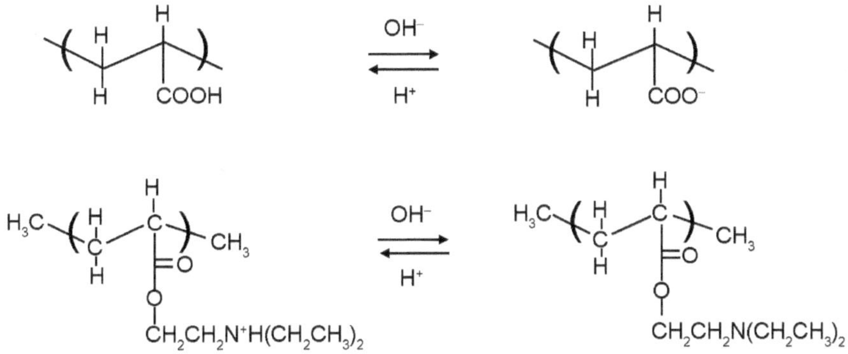

11.10 Representation of pH-dependent ionization of poly(acrylic acid) and poly(*N,N′*-diethylaminoethyl methacrylate) polyelectrolytes (adapted from Qiu and Park 2001).

PEO, a poloxamer, resulted in a pH-sensitive as well as a thermosensitive hydrogel. Determan *et al.* (2007) loaded this hydrogel with lysozyme and observed its release kinetics *in vitro*. They found that pH of the release media influenced the release rate of the lysozyme from the hydrogel, specifically in that an increase in pH resulted in a decrease in release rate (Determan *et al.* 2007).

11.4.2 Applications

Values of pH change from one physiological location to another. For example, gastric pH is around 2 whereas intestinal pH ranges from 7.4 to 7.8 (Jeong and Gutowska 2002). Polymers which can respond to changes in pH are highly useful for *in vivo* applications. One such system involves poly(methacrylic acid) (PMAA) and poly(ethylene glycol) (PEG). At low pH, hydrogen bonds are formed between the carboxylic acid group on PMAA and the ether group on PEG. A graft copolymer of PMAA and PEG has been studied for use as a carrier of calcitonin for oral delivery (Torres-Lugo and Peppas 1999). Since at low pH this graft copolymer remains collapsed, the loaded substance, whether drug, protein or peptide, is not easily released. Thus, PMAA-*g*-PEG loaded with calcitonin, a polypeptide hormone involved in calcium metabolism, was utilized as a potential oral administration route for various bone diseases. Due to its pH sensitivity, calcitonin can be protected from the acidic environments of the stomach and prevent its early release, and once it reaches the small intestine, the higher pH will cause the hydrogel to swell and release calcitonin (Torres-Lugo and Peppas 1999). Chao *et al.* (2008) also investigated PMAA with poly(caprolactone) (PCL) and PEG to study the hydrolytic degradation of this pH-sensitive hydrogel. They noted that with an increase in pH of the aqueous media, the swelling ratio of the hydrogel also increased due to the presence of carboxylic acid groups on PMAA (Chao *et al.* 2008).

With addition of sulfamethazine oligomers (SMO) to each end of a poly(ϵ-caprolactone-co-lactide) (PCLA) block copolymer, PCLA-PEG-PCLA, a pH and thermo-sensitive hydrogel was obtained (Kim *et al.* 2008; Shim *et al.* 2007). At the physiological pH of 7.4 and at body temperature (37ºC), a gel was formed; however, as the pH was slightly increased to 8 while remaining at the same temperature, the gel transformed into a solution. Thus, they encapsulated human mesenchymal stem cells (MSCs) and recombinant human bone morphogenetic protein-2 (rhBMP-2) during the solution phase and injected it subcutaneously into the back of mice to observe its properties. The solution formed a gel within 10 minutes of injection and remained in its gel shape over the course of the 7-week study, allowing release of rhBMP-2 and proliferation of MSCs (Kim *et al.* 2008). Shim *et al.* (2007), with the same block copolymer, determined the release of paclitaxel from the hydrogel and tested it *in vivo*. The drug underwent sustained release for the duration of the month without experiencing burst release and their immunohistology results showed good anti-tumor effects (Shim *et al.* 2007). Although mentioned in a previous section for its thermosensitive capabilities, chitosan has also been used in combination with other compounds to form pH-sensitive hydrogels (Chen *et al.* 2004; Lin *et al.* 2007). Chen *et al.* (2004) prepared *N,O*-(carboxymethyl) chitosan with alginate, using genipin for crosslinking, and loaded it with bovine serum albumin (BSA) to examine the release behavior in gastric and intestinal media. The release profiles indicated that at low pH (1.2), the amount of BSA released was low, whereas with high pH (7.4), BSA release increased significantly.

11.5 Light-sensitive polymers

11.5.1 Properties

Light-sensitive materials have been used, throughout the course of history, in different parts of the world for various therapeutic reasons, including vitiligo and psoriasis (Pervaiz and Olivo 2006). However, experimental results were not reported until 1900 by a medical student when he witnessed that the protozoan paramecium is at risk of survival at low concentrations of acridines and under light exposure (Pervaiz and Olivo 2006). Concluding that this was due to photosensitization, the reaction was termed a 'photodynamic reaction'. Nowadays, photosensitive polymers have been researched for applications such as ophthalmic drug delivery, gene therapy, and optical switches due to their localization abilities (Christie and Kompella 2008). Qiu and Park (2001) discuss that light-sensitive hydrogels can respond to either visible light or ultraviolet irradiation. Visible light has several practical advantages, in that it is resourceful, inexpensive, and safe. To produce hydrogels which respond to visible light, a chromophore, a chemical molecule which absorbs light and gives off color, is needed. An example of a chromophore is trisodium salt of copper chlorophyllin (Qiu and Park 2001). When

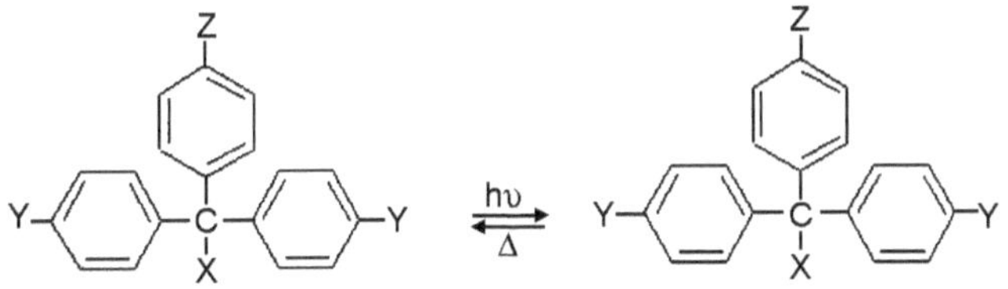

11.11 General structure of a light-sensitive leuco derivative (adapted from Irie and Kunwatchakun 1986).

exposed to light, the chromophore absorbs it and causes heat dissipation. This phenomenon increases the temperature of the hydrogel and in turn changes the swelling properties of the gel. An increase in light intensity and chromophore concentration causes an increase in the hydrogel temperature. To obtain UV light-induction, a leuco derivative molecule must be incorporated in the hydrogel, such as bis(4-di-methylamino)phenylmethyl leucocyanide (Qiu and Park 2001). The mechanism behind the function of triphenylmethane leuco derivatives involves a reversible dissociation of the photochromic molecule into ion pairs, which is triggered by UV irradiation and results in a colored triphenylmethyl cation (Irie and Kunwatchakun 1986), as shown in Fig. 11.11. Ultraviolet irradiation also induces swelling of the hydrogel due to the internal osmotic pressure build-up during ionization of the hydrogel (Suzuki and Tanaka 1990). By removal of UV light, the hydrogel equilibrium leans the system towards neutrality and causes a collapse in the gel. Since this process relies on photochemical ionization, it remains quite slow compared to visible light (Suzuki and Tanaka 1990). When NIPAAm and a leuco derivative, known as bis(4-(dimethylamino)phenyl)(4-vinylphenyl)methyl leucocyanide), were analyzed under UV irradiation, a discontinuous volume phase transition was observed as opposed to a sharp and continuous volume phase transition without light (Mamada *et al.* 1990). It was also noted that upon UV removal, the hydrogel underwent shrinking caused by the osmotic pressure of cyanide ions after photochemical ionization. When NIPAAm was also employed with a different leuco derivative, trisodium salt of copper chlorophyllin, they detected that without irradiation, the gel is swollen and once light is used, the gel collapses, with most of its shrinking occurring in its temperature transition phase (Suzuki and Tanaka 1990). They also were intrigued to find that the light-induced phase transition results in a change from a continuous to a discontinuous transition (as also mentioned by Mamada *et al.* 1990), as well as a decrease in the transition temperature.

11.5.2 Applications

A useful method of combining polymers and light sensitivity is through use of polymer micelles. By incorporating hydrophobic photosensitizers within the core of the micelle, the system can then be utilized for photodynamic therapy (PDT)

(Christie and Kompella 2008). PDT encompasses the systemic administration of photosensitizers with the local use of light to target specific diseased sites (Nishiyama *et al.* 2003). Ionic dendritic porphyrins mixed with PEG-*block*-poly(L-lysine) have thus been investigated for their potential application in PDT. Porphyrins are chromophores which can fluoresce and signal reaction occurrence (Pasternack *et al.* 1993). Upon photoirradiation, the dendritic porphyrin-loaded micelles showed similar oxygen consumption results as free dendritic porphyrin in phosphate buffered saline and BSA (Nishiyama *et al.* 2003). However, the micelles containing the porphyrin molecules underwent a drastic increase in photocytotoxicity when exposed to cells compared to the free porphyrin molecules.

Aside from polymeric micelles, hydrogels have also been investigated as light-sensitive systems. PEG in conjunction with cinnamic groups has been often used for photosensitive medical applications (Andreopoulos and Persaud 2006; Micic *et al.* 2003; Lendlein *et al.* 2005). Andreopoulos and Persaud (2006) utilized PEG and nitrocinnamate (NC) to release basic fibroblast growth factor (bFGF). Under UV irradiation, the release rate of bFGF could be controlled. With an increase in irradiation time, a decrease in the swelling of the hydrogel was observed, as well as a decrease in the release rate (Andreopoulos and Persaud 2006). Cell studies revealed that the hydrogel scaffold was not cytotoxic to human neonatal fibroblast cells while the bFGF maintained its activity and promoted proliferation of the fibroblasts. The advantage of the PEG-NC system is that its gelation upon photoradiation allows for easier handling of the gelation process *in situ*, especially for wound healing, surgical implants, tissue engineering and artificial muscles (Micic *et al.* 2003). Polymers with cinnamic groups have also shown shape-memory properties when induced by light (Lendlein *et al.* 2005). The photosensitive polymer systems can experience deformation and be manipulated to remain in pre-determined shapes under UV irradiation. The formed shapes are long-lasting and can be transformed back into their original shape only by being exposed to ambient temperature and by altering the wavelength of UV light (Lendlein *et al.* 2005). Andreopoulos *et al.* (1999), in a different study, immobilized the enzyme, organophosphorous hydrolase, in a PEG-cinnamylidene acetate hydrogel. They observed that the hydrogel, with an irradiation of 30 and 45 minutes at 300 nm, provoked the crosslinking of the gel and little enzyme escape was detected. The study also determined that the immobilization of the enzyme within the hydrogel led to longer enzyme activity and improved stability with PEGylation, as opposed to the native enzyme.

11.6 Biomolecular-sensitive polymers

11.6.1 Antigen-responsive

Use of biological molecules to stimulate a response in materials can be advantageous for biomedical applications for which previously discussed environmental stimuli may not be feasible. There are various methods by which antigen–antibody interactions can be explored in a hydrogel. These techniques include entrapment of the antigen or antibody in the hydrogel network, chemically conjugating the antibody or antigen to the polymer network, and using the antigen–antibody pair grafted to the hydrogel network to induce crosslinking (Lu *et al.* 2003). Due to their high specificity and incorporation in hydrogels, antigen-antibody interactions can be employed in applications such as immunoassays or biosensor technology (Lu *et al.* 2003). The idea of using an antigen to spark a change in behavior of a hydrogel was first elucidated by Miyata *et al.* (1999). The concept was pursued by developing a hydrogel composed of an antigen and antibody grafted to the polymer network. When the antigen binds to the antibody, a crosslink results. However, if free antigens are introduced into the system, competitive binding for the antibody takes place, causing crosslinks to dissociate (Fig. 11.12). This decrease in the crosslinking density leads to swelling of the hydrogel (Miyata *et al.* 1999). Once the free antigens are removed, the polymer network shrinks, demonstrating a reversible swelling process, as well as a shape-memory behavior. By alternating the antigen concentration, a pulsatile permeation of a protein into the network can

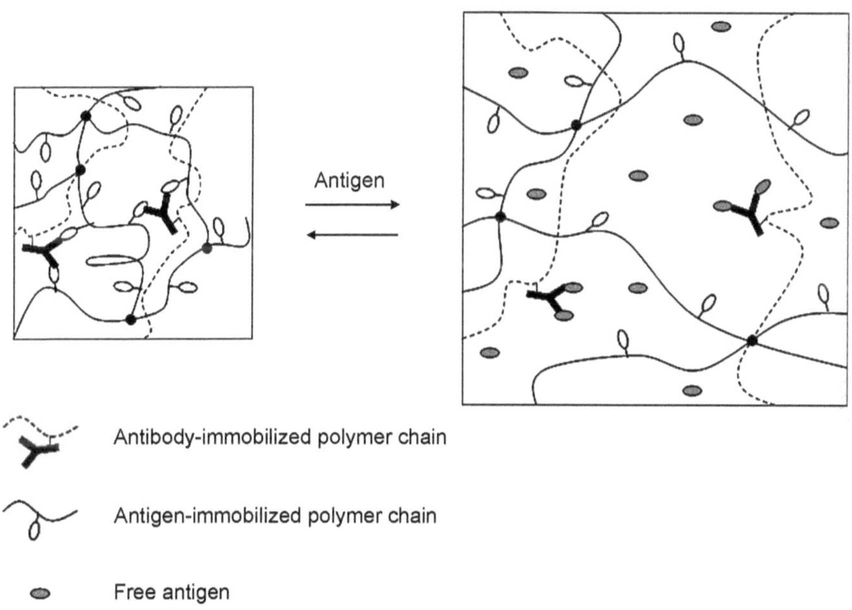

11.12 Representation of the swelling of a hydrogel containing antibody–antigen interactions and free antigens. It is suggested that interactions between immobilized antibodies and immobilized antigens on polymer chains result in crosslinks within the polymer network. However, as free antigens are introduced, competition occurs for binding to the antibody, leading to swelling of the hydrogel (adapted from Miyata *et al.* 1999).

be attained. In a separate study, antibody Fab′ fragment from a monoclonal anti-fluorescein BDC1 antibody was integrated within a poly(N-isopropylacrylamide) hydrogel network (Lu *et al.* 2003). With an increase in Fab′ content, a decrease in the thermosensitivity of the gel occurred. It was noted that the antigen response was triggered by changes in pH, temperature or Fab′ content. For example, at a pH value of 5 and an alternating incubation temperature of 33.7 and 36.8°C, a reversible volume change was witnessed (Lu *et al.* 2003). In addition, antigens can potentially be used as stimuli for liquid microlenses (Dong *et al.* 2006).

11.6.2 Glucose-sensitive

Glucose-sensitive materials are in high demand for insulin delivery applications. For patients suffering from diabetes mellitus, the time and amount of insulin required are important factors. By using hydrogels which contain a glucose sensor as well as an insulin delivering mechanism, more efficient treatments can be developed. These hydrogel systems usually crosslink from interactions between concanavalin A (ConA), a molecule with four glucose binding sites, and glucose molecules bound within a polymer network (Obaidat and Park 1997). Similarly to antigen competitive binding interactions, the hydrogel conforms to a solution as the polymer-bound glucose molecules and the free glucose molecules experience binding competition for ConA. By utilizing poly(hydroxyethyl methacrylate) membranes with polymer-bound glucose and ConA, a glucose-sensitive hydrogel membrane was developed and release of insulin was observed. The release rate of insulin through the glucose-sensitive hydrogel membrane relied on the concentration of free glucose molecules. It was also shown that by altering the concentration of glucose in the receptor chamber, the release rate of insulin could be adjusted (Obaidat and Park 1997). This system had a slow response, however, due to the difficult control over the glucose concentration present. Kim and Park (2001) noted that with an increase in the glucose concentration, an increase in the release rate of insulin was found. Of the three insulin delivery systems that they have configured, the diffusion controlled reservoir and diffusion-controlled matrix demonstrated efficient modulation of insulin release, whereas the erosion-controlled matrix provided for feasible long-term delivery (Kim and Park 2001). By crosslinking carboxymethyl dextran with ConA, a glucose sensitive hydrogel membrane was synthesized with no cytotoxic groups (Zhang *et al.* 2006). The permeability of the hydrogel membrane increased with changes in glucose concentration, demonstrating a reversible permeability with addition or removal of glucose. Insulin delivery has also been examined through use of glucose sensitive polymeric composite membranes consisting of glucose oxidase, catalase and a NIPAAm copolymer, with similar behavior of glucose concentration on gel permeability (Zhang and Wu 2002). A multi-effect coupling glucose stimulus model was developed to analyze the effects of pH, Young's modulus and enzyme catalysis (Li and Luo 2009; Luo *et al.* 2009). From the model, it was determined that a change in Young's modulus affects the enzyme-catalyzed chemical reaction and the equilibrium swelling ratio of the gel. Utilizing the model can assist the optimization of insulin delivery systems.

11.6.3 Enzyme-triggered

Hydrogels which respond to enzyme action comprise of a component that controls enzyme sensitivity and one that directs the interactions, causing changes in the overall transitions of the hydrogel (Ulijn 2006). Enzyme reactions can be used for either stimulation of a phase transition (sol-gel or gel-sol) in the hydrogel or a more localized event such as the opening of pores in a membrane (Ulijn 2006). Hydrogel microparticles made of PEG-acrylamide functionalized with branched peptide actuators were investigated for use as enzyme responsive hydrogels (McDonald *et al.* 2009). With enzymatic hydrolysis occurring causing a change in the charge balance of the hydrogel, the particles were seen to undergo swelling. When the particles were loaded with FITC-dextran, a release of the drug was observed at physiological ionic strength as they were exposed to the target enzyme (McDonald *et al.* 2009). Peptide actuators can also be designed to release a drug or protein as the charge on peptide actuator matches that of the drug/protein to be released (Thornton *et al.* 2008). In a similar system, biomolecules enzymatically attached to a PEG-based hydrogel illustrated a dual response at physiological conditions: through one enzymatic reaction, a polymer network was created and through another enzymatic reaction, degradation occurred (Ehrbar *et al.* 2007). These hydrogels have the potential to encapsulate cells for drug delivery or tissue engineering implants. Additionally, when an enzyme, urease, was trapped within a crosslinked hydrogel network made from a NIPAAm-copolymer, a change in the hydrogel particle size was instigated with the onset of the enzymatic reaction (Ogawa *et al.* 2001). These particles can then be loaded into cellulose membrane pores and allow liquid access through the membrane as the enzyme reaction occurs.

11.6.4 Thrombin-induced

Devices which would release antibiotics only upon microbial infection are in need and few studies have been conducted on the development of such systems. To provide the appropriate antibiotic concentration at the time and location of infection for *Pseudomonas aeruginosa* (PA), an antibiotic delivery system comprising of gentamicin bound to a PVA hydrogel using a peptide linker was investigated (Suzuki *et al.* 1998). Experiments showed that when a wound is infected with PA, the peptide linker is cleaved by the proteinase, allowing the release of gentamicin. With the accumulation of gentamicin in the wound area, a reduction in PA growth is observed (Suzuki *et al.* 1998). A similar delivery system was explored for *Staphylococcus aureus*, in which the release of gentamicin occurred only in infected fluid and diminished the bacteria number (Tanihara *et al.* 1999).

11.7 Other stimuli-sensitive polymers

11.7.1 Magnetic field-responsive

Polymers can be sensitive to applied fields, whether electric or magnetic, because of the presence of liquid as a swelling medium. When magnetoparticles are incorporated within the polymer network, two different responses can be observed when a magnetic field is applied: a field–particle interaction or a particle–particle interaction (Zrínyi 2000). The occurrence of either outcome depends on the uniformity of the magnetic field. In a nonuniform field, the field–particle interaction is likely to take place as the particles are subject to a magnetophoretic force which leads them to become attracted to higher magnetic field areas (Zrínyi 2000). This can result in changes in the molecular conformation and consequently, changes in shape. On the other hand, if a uniform magnetic field is applied, the field–particle interaction does not occur since no magnetic field gradient is present, and rather the particle–particle interaction dominates (Fig. 11.13). The field conjures a magnetic dipole, allowing particle interactions and can change the structure of the particle dispersion, resulting in an assembly similar to a pearl chain (Zrínyi 2000). Because magnetic particles respond to applications of magnetic fields externally over specific body locations, they have potential for numerous biomedical applications. Some of these applications include drug delivery, gene therapy, tissue engineering, isolation and purification of compounds, and blood detoxication (Brazel 2009).

Of the research done on magnetic field-responsive materials, most attention has been focused on magnetothermally responsive materials. Such systems are composed of magnetic nanoparticles, which can generate localized heat upon magnetic field application using an AC current source, and a polymer which can undergo a phase or conformation change under heat (Brazel 2009). Considering the demands, the popular thermo-sensitive polymer poly(N-isopropyl acrylamide) (NIPAAm) is feasible for the application. Many studies have been conducted on the use of NIPAAm with magnetic particles, most commonly magnetite (Fe_3O_4) (Zrínyi 2000; Zhang and Misra 2007; Satarkar and Hilt 2008; Ang *et al.* 2007; Wakamatsu *et al.* 2006; Deng *et al.* 2003). Zrínyi's study reported that when no magnetic field is applied, the magnetic beads within the NIPAAm hydrogel do not aggregate and no attraction between beads is witnessed (Zrínyi 2000). However, if a non-uniform magnetic field is applied, the beads aggregate to where the magnetic field intensity is highest, and if under a uniform magnetic field, the beads experience polarization and a magnetic

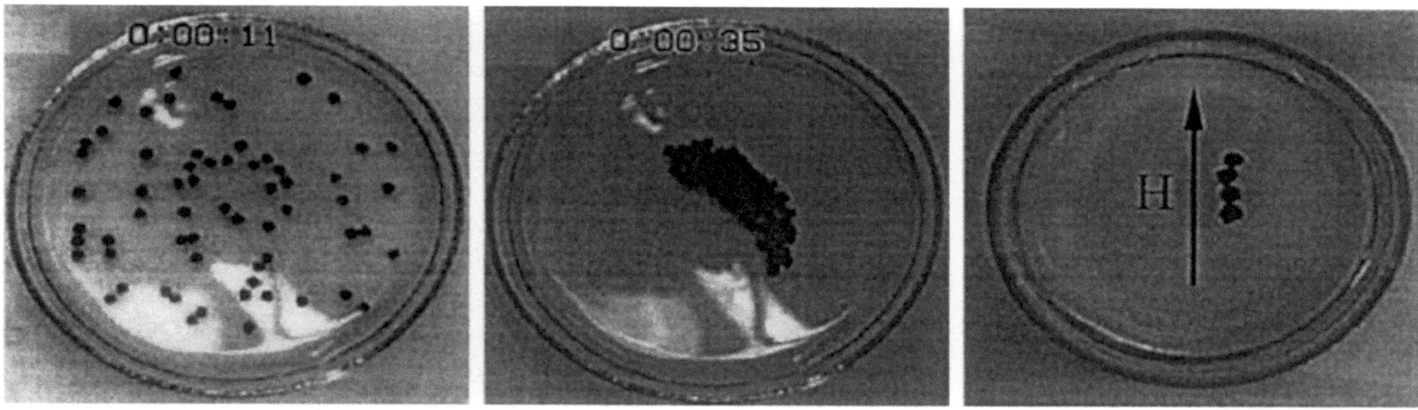

11.13 Effect of uniform and nonuniform magnetic field on poly(NIPAAm) gel beads. In the left panel, no magnetic field is applied; in the middle panel, a nonuniform magnetic field is applied; and in the right panel, a uniform magnetic field is applied with the arrow designating the field direction. With kind permission from Springer Science+Business Media: *Colloid and Polymer Science*, Intelligent polymer gels controlled by magnetic fields, 278, 2000, 100, M. Zrínyi, Fig. 1a–c.

moment which leads them to align in a chain, parallel to the applied magnetic field. The NIPAAm/magnetite system has also been investigated for drug delivery purposes. A magnetic drug-targeting carrier comprising functionalized magnetite and conjugated doxorubicin encapsulated in a dextran-NIPAAm copolymer was developed (Zhang and Misra 2007). At low temperature (20°C), a low drug release rate was observed; whereas at body temperature and higher, a drug burst release occurred. The polymer absorbs heat due to the magnetic particles which drives it to undergo a reversible hydrophilic–hydrophobic change (Wakamatsu *et al.* 2006). Similarly, with pulsatile exposure of magnetic field, heating arose in NIPAAm loaded with superparamagnetic particles which led to a faster collapse of the gel, and therefore, a faster release of the model drugs (vitamin B_{12} and methylene blue) (Satarkar and Hilt 2008). Since the magnetite particles absorb heat caused by the applied magnetic field, studies have been conducted on using the magnetothermal system for hyperthermia treatment of cancer (Ang *et al.* 2007; Zhang and Misra 2007; Satarkar and Hilt 2008; Brazel 2009; Wakamatsu *et al.* 2006; Frimpong *et al.* 2007). Hyperthermia involves the use of heat, in temperatures ranging from 42 to 45°C, to kill cancerous cells (Brazel 2009). Ang *et al.* (2007) analyzed the possible temperatures which can be reached by using magnetite particles in NIPAAm. Observations demonstrated that the maximum temperature which can be achieved relies on an increase in the concentration of the magnetic particles as well as the strength of the magnetic field. When comparing use of Fe_3O_4 versus Fe particles, the Fe_3O_4 particles obtained better results since they could attain the highest temperature (45C) (Ang *et al.* 2007).

Aside from use of NIPAAm, poly(vinyl alcohol) (PVA) with magnetite particles has also been examined. When PVA loaded with magnetite particles was suspended in water between the poles of a magnet, shortening of the gel occurred (Zrínyi 2000). Owing to the change in shape of the magnetic hydrogel and its contractile activity under magnetic field, this phenomenon can be investigated for use in mimicking muscle contraction (Zrínyi 2000). By on/off application of a magnetic field, the drug released from the PVA-magnetite network can be evaluated. When the magnetic field is applied, it was noticed that the model drug (vitamin B_{12}) loaded with PVA was released and remained around the gel. However, when the field application was stopped, the drug dispersed. The best sensitivity to the magnetic field was found in larger sized Fe_3O_4 particles (Liu *et al.* 2006). They concluded that by controlling the on/off mechanism and the duration, the system could have potential in drug delivery. Other investigations of magnetic field sensitive materials include use of a magnetic gelatin hydrogel for coating of stainless steel to control anti-thrombic drug release from stents under magnetic field (Huang and Yang 2007) as well as using luminescent semiconductors with magnetite particles in polymer capsules for marking and external manipulation by magnetic field for directed drug delivery (Gaponik *et al.* 2004).

11.7.2 Ionic strength-induced

Effect of ionic strength in hydrogels is highly interrelated to the pH. For a neutral hydrogel, ionic strength will not affect its swelling behavior. However, in a charged hydrogel, such as poly(N-isopropylacrylamide), a sharp volume phase transition occurs at a specific sodium chloride concentration in aqueous solution (Qiu and Park 2001). There is a correlation between the swelling and sodium chloride concentration below its lower critical solution temperature (LCST). At a critical sodium chloride concentration, the hydrogel experiences a collapse, which is also temperature-related (Qiu and Park 2001). Ionic strength and pH have shown to have an effect on poly(acrylic acid) (PAA) hydrogels in that they alter the chain conformation of the growing polymer chain (Elliott *et al.* 2004). This can lead to crosslinking or cyclization reactions. Cyclization occurs when the ends of the crosslinking agent combine in the same growing polymer chain, resulting in a loop-like structure (Elliott *et al.* 2004). With an increase in ionic strength, cyclization increased which developed a less crosslinked polymer. Crosslinking influences the swelling behavior of the polymer. Polyelectrolyte gels made of methacrylic acid and acrylonitrile monomers were also affected by ionic strength. An increase in ionic strength demonstrated a decrease in the swelling ratio of the gel due to the osmotic pressure between the ions in and outside the gel (Zhang *et al.* 2007).

Effects of ionic strength on hydrogels can be tailored to benefit drug delivery applications. Kozlovskaya *et al.* (2006) entrapped FTIC-dextran into poly(N-vinylpyrrolidone) (PVPON) and poly(methacrylic acid) (PMAA) and observed that at high pH, PVPON is released from the hydrogel and that the PMAA gel size depends on pH and ionic strength. The drug (FTIC-dextran) was released at high salt concentrations as the polycationic capsule wall dissociated. Diffusion of a protein lysozyme from a carboxy methyl dextran hydrogel was also shown to be affected by pH and ionic strength, revealing an increase in diffusion with an increase in the two factors (Zhang *et al.* 2005). However, once a critical ionic strength is reached, the gel deforms from a swollen to a compact matrix, resulting in a decrease in diffusion beyond that point. The assembly of peptides can also be manipulated with various ionic strengths. With a net peptide charge of zero, aggregates form; however, with a small net peptide charge, a gel results which changes into a fluid with a large net peptide charge (Carrick *et al.* 2007). These salt concentration-dependent self-assembled peptides are reported to be used as injectable lubricants for early stage knee joint osteoarthritis.

11.7.3 Pressure-sensitive

Studies on pressure-sensitive hydrogels are quite scarce. Pressure investigations were done on the following polymers: poly(N-isopropyl acrylamide), poly(N-n-propylacrylamide), and poly(N,N-diethylacrylamide), all of which are temperature-sensitive polymers (Zhong *et al.* 1996). Through examination of the excess enthalpy and excess volume of the gel-water systems during their volume phase-transitions, the gels underwent an increase in their lower critical solution temperature (LCST) with pressure. It was also determined that this pressure sensitivity occurs only around their respective LCSTs. In a separate study, model predictions demonstrated an increase in the gel volume caused by an increase in pressure (Lee *et al.* 1990). It was determined, however, that this volume change was more sensitive to temperature than pressure.

11.8 Conclusion and future trends

As seen in this work, hydrogels can be made to respond to various environmental stimuli. Temperature and pH are stimuli present in the body which can be employed to trigger changes in a hydrogel form. Owing to their amphiphilic nature, thermosensitive hydrogels undergo a sol-gel phase transition upon reaching a particular temperature (LCST/UCST). This characteristic allows them to be used for controlled drug delivery purposes, as this transition is reversible. Having polyelectrolyte properties, pH, ionic strength, light and electro-sensitive hydrogels experience swelling and shrinking behaviors upon stimulation. By controlling glucose concentration or magnetic field application, a modulated response can be obtained to achieve pulsatile release. With the diverse stimuli available for managing hydrogel characteristics, a plethora of biomedical applications can take advantage of these mechanisms. These include controlled drug delivery, bone regeneration, scaffolds for cell differentiation, enhanced gene transcription and therapy, muscle actuators, and lubricants for joint diseases, to name a few. These environmentally responsive hydrogels are advantageous in that they provide for easier drug administration, they do not use organic solvents, they enhance localization and specificity, as well as allow for a sustained drug release.

Although tremendous work has been accomplished in the field of stimuli-responsive materials, there is room for improvement in providing more suitable systems. Hydrogels need to possess faster gelation time and appropriate temperature and pH values to maintain homeostasis. Owing to their high water content, the mechanical strength of hydrogels can sometimes fall short of the required mechanical strength needed for physiological applications. Additionally, biocompatibility and biodegradability, when necessary, are essential components for success of a hydrogel. With degradable compounds, proper elimination from the body must be ascertained. Most of the complications with hydrogels listed above can be ameliorated via manipulation of copolymerization. By utilizing diverse copolymers, the hydrophobic–hydrophilic interactions can be altered, resulting in different mechanical strength, swelling behavior, and gelation temperature. The molecular weight of the copolymers can also be adjusted for better clearance from the body and the biocompatibility can also be amended for more feasible physiological applications.

For more information on particular aspects of this chapter, various review articles and journal articles can be consulted. Recommended reviews on temperature-sensitive systems are from Ruel-Gariépy and Leroux (2004) and Klouda and Mikos (2008). A good reference on biodegradable copolymers is written by Jeong *et al.* (1997). For pulsatile drug release from hydrogels, Kikuchi and Okano (2002) has a comprehensive review, as for enzyme responsive materials, a review by Ulijn (2006) is suggested for reading. Some papers discussing fundamentals in various stimuli fields also make for good reading. For electric field-sensitive gels, refer to Tanaka *et al.* (1982) as well as Murdan (2003), and for photosensitive gels, to Mamada *et al.* (1990) as well as Suzuki and Tanaka (1990). Zrínyi (2000) has a review on the effect of magnetic field on gels, with examples for muscle applications, and for emphasis on magnetothermal gels, Brazel (2009) can be consulted. For better understanding of free volume and entropy, particularly when applied to thermosensitive gels, Frank and Evans (1945) is advised.

11.9 References

Andreopoulos, F.M. & Persaud, I. 2006, 'Delivery of basic fibroblast growth factor (bFGF) from photoresponsive hydrogel scaffolds', *Biomaterials*, vol. 27, no. 11, pp. 2468–2476.

Andreopoulos, F.M., Roberts, M.J., Bentley, M.D., Harris, J.M., Beckman, E.J. & Russell, A.J. 1999, 'Photoimmobilization of organophosphorus hydrolase within a PEG-based hydrogel', *Biotechnology and Bioengineering*, vol. 65, no. 5, pp. 579–588.

Ang, K., Venkatraman, S. & Ramanujan, R.V. 2007, 'Magnetic PNIPA hydrogels for hyperthermia applications in cancer therapy', *Materials Science & Engineering C*, vol. 27, no. 3, pp. 347–351.

Awad, H.A., Quinn Wickham, M., Leddy, H.A., Gimble, J.M. & Guilak, F. 2004, 'Chondrogenic differentiation of adipose-derived adult stem cells in agarose, alginate, and gelatin scaffolds', *Biomaterials*, vol. 25, no. 16, pp. 3211–3222.

Bae, Y.C., Lambert, S.M., Soane, D.S. & Prausnitz, J.M. 1991, 'Cloud-point curves of polymer solutions from thermooptical measurements', *Macromolecules*, vol. 24, pp. 4403–4407.

Batrakova, E.V. & Kabanov, A.V. 2008, 'Pluronic block copolymers: evolution of drug delivery concept from inert nanocarriers to biological response modifiers', *Journal of Controlled Release*, vol. 130, no. 2, pp. 98–106.

Batrakova, E.V., Kelly, D.L., Li, S., Li, Y., Yang, Z., Xiao, L., Alakhova, D.Y., Sherman, S., Alakhov, V.Y. & Kabanov, A.V. 2006, 'Alteration of genomic responses to doxorubicin and prevention of MDR in breast cancer cells by a polymer excipient: pluronic P85', *Molecular Pharmaceutics*, vol. 3, no. 2, pp. 113–123.

Brazel, C.S. 2009, 'Magnetothermally responsive nanomaterials: combining magnetic nanostructures and thermally sensitive polymers for triggered drug release', *Pharmaceutical Research*, vol. 26, no. 3, pp. 644–656.

Carrick, L.M., Aggeli, A., Boden, N., Fisher, J., Ingham, E. & Waigh, T.A. 2007, 'Effect of ionic strength on the self-assembly, morphology and gelation of pH responsive β-sheet tape-forming peptides', *Tetrahedron*, vol. 63, no. 31, pp. 7457–7467.

Chang, C.W., Choi, D., Kim, W.J., Yockman, J.W., Christensen, L.V., Kim, Y.H. & Kim, S.W. 2007, 'Non-ionic amphiphilic biodegradable PEG–PLGA–PEG copolymer enhances gene delivery efficiency in rat skeletal muscle', *Journal of Controlled Release*, vol. 118, no. 2, pp. 245–253.

Chao, G.T., Qian, Z.Y., Huang, M.J., Kan, B., Gu, Y.C., Gong, C.Y., Yang, J.L., Wang, K., Dai, M. & Li, X.Y. 2008, 'Synthesis, characterization, and hydrolytic degradation behavior of a novel biodegradable pH-sensitive hydrogel based on polycaprolactone, methacrylic acid, and poly (ethylene glycol)', *Journal of Biomedical Materials Research Part A*, vol. 85, no. 1, pp. 36–46.

Chen, S.C., Wu, Y.C., Mi, F.L., Lin, Y.H., Yu, L.C. & Sung, H.W. 2004, 'A novel pH-sensitive hydrogel composed of N, O-carboxymethyl chitosan and alginate cross-linked by genipin for protein drug delivery', *Journal of Controlled Release*, vol. 96, no. 2, pp. 285–300.

Chenite, A., Chaput, C., Wang, D., Combes, C., Buschmann, M.D., Hoemann, C.D., Leroux, J.C., Atkinson, B.L., Binette, F. & Selmani, A. 2000, 'Novel injectable neutral solutions of chitosan form biodegradable gels *in situ*', *Biomaterials*, vol. 21, no. 21, pp. 2155–2161.

Choe, K. & Kim, K.J. 2006, 'Polyacrylonitrile linear actuators: chemomechanical and electro-chemomechanical properties', *Sensors & Actuators: A.Physical*, vol. 126, no. 1, pp. 165–172.

Choe, K., Kim, K.J., Kim, D., Manford, C., Heo, S. & Shahinpoor, M. 2006, 'Performance characteristics of electro-chemically driven polyacrylonitrile fiber bundle actuators', *Journal of Intelligent Material Systems and Structures*, vol. 17, no. 7, pp. 563–576.

Christie, J.G. & Kompella, U.B. 2008, 'Ophthalmic light sensitive nanocarrier systems', *Drug Discovery Today*, vol. 13, no. 3–4, pp. 124–134.

Chung, H.J., Lee, Y. & Park, T.G. 2008, 'Thermo-sensitive and biodegradable hydrogels based on stereocomplexed Pluronic multi-block copolymers for controlled protein delivery', *Journal of Controlled Release*, vol. 127, no. 1, pp. 22–30.

Cui, Z., Lee, B.H. & Vernon, B.L. 2007, 'New hydrolysis-dependent thermosensitive polymer for an injectable degradable system', *Biomacromolecules*, vol. 8, no. 4, pp. 1280–1286.

De Salamanca, A.E., Diebold, Y., Calonge, M., Garcia-Vazquez, C., Callejo, S., Vila, A. & Alonso, M.J. 2006, 'Chitosan nanoparticles as a potential drug delivery system for the ocular surface: toxicity, uptake mechanism and *in vivo* tolerance', *Investigative Ophthalmology & Visual Science*, vol. 47, no. 4, pp. 1416–1425.

Deng, Y., Yang, W., Wang, C. & Fu, S. 2003, 'A novel approach for preparation of thermosensitive polymer magnetic microspheres with core-shell structure', *Advanced Materials*, vol. 15, no. 20, pp. 1729–1732.

Denkbas, E.B. & Ottenbrite, R.M. 2006, 'Perspectives on: chitosan drug delivery systems based on their geometries', *Journal of Bioactive and Compatible Polymers*, vol. 21, no. 4, pp. 351–368.

Determan, M.D., Cox, J.P. & Mallapragada, S.K. 2007, 'Drug release from pH-responsive thermogelling pentablock copolymers', *Journal of Biomedical Materials Research Part A*, vol.81, no. 2, pp. 326–333.

Diebold, Y., Jarrín, M., Sáez, V., Carvalho, E.L.S., Orea, M., Calonge, M., Seijo, B. & Alonso, M.J. 2007, 'Ocular drug delivery by liposome–chitosan nanoparticle complexes (LCS-NP)', *Biomaterials*, vol. 28, no. 8, pp. 1553–1564.

Doi, M., Matsumoto, M. & Hirose, Y. 1992, 'Deformation of ionic polymer gels by electric fields', *Macromolecules*, vol. 25, no. 20, pp. 5504–5511.

Dong, L., Agarwal, A.K., Beebe, D.J. & Jiang, H. 2006, 'Adaptive liquid microlenses activated by stimuli-responsive hydrogels', *Nature*, vol. 442, no. 7102, pp. 551–554.

Duvvuri, S., Janoria, K.G. & Mitra, A.K. 2005, 'Development of a novel formulation containing poly (D,L-lactide-co-glycolide) microspheres dispersed in PLGA–PEG–PLGA gel for sustained delivery of ganciclovir', *Journal of Controlled Release*, vol. 108, no. 2–3, pp. 282–293.

Ehrbar, M., Rizzi, S.C., Schoenmakers, R.G., San Miguel, B., Hubbell, J.A., Weber, F.E. & Lutolf, M.P. 2007, 'Biomolecular hydrogels formed and degraded via site-specific enzymatic reactions', *Biomacromolecules*, vol. 8, no. 10, pp. 3000–3007.

Elliott, J.E., Macdonald, M., Nie, J. & Bowman, C.N. 2004, 'Structure and swelling of poly (acrylic acid) hydrogels: effect of pH, ionic strength, and dilution on the crosslinked polymer structure', *Polymer*, vol. 45, no. 5, pp. 1503–1510.

Feil, H., Bae, Y.H., Feijen, J. & Kim, S.W. 1993, 'Effect of comonomer hydrophilicity and ionization on the lower critical solution temperature of N-isopropylacrylamide copolymers', *Macromolecules*, vol. 26, pp. 2496–2500.

Fellah, B.H., Weiss, P., Gauthier, O., Rouillon, T., Pilet, P., Daculsi, G. & Layrolle, P. 2006, 'Bone repair using a new injectable self-crosslinkable bone substitute', *Journal of Orthopaedic Research*, vol. 24, no. 4, 628–635.

Frank, H.S. & Evans, M.W. 1945, 'Free volume and entropy in condensed systems. III. Entropy in binary liquid mixtures; partial molar entropy in dilute solutions; structure and thermodynamics in aqueous electrolytes', *The Journal of Chemical Physics*, vol. 13, no. 11, pp. 507–532.

Frimpong, R.A., Fraser, S. & Zach Hilt, J. 2007, 'Synthesis and temperature response analysis of magnetic-hydrogel nanocomposites', *Journal of Biomedical Materials Research Part A*, vol. 80, no. 1, pp. 1–6.

Fujimoto, K.L., Ma, Z., Nelson, D.M., Hashizume, R., Guan, J., Tobita, K. & Wagner, W.R. 2009, 'Synthesis, characterization and therapeutic efficacy of a biodegradable, thermoresponsive hydrogel designed for application in chronic infarcted myocardium', *Biomaterials*, vol. 30, pp. 4357–4368.

Gaponik, N., Radtchenko, I.L., Sukhorukov, B.G. & Rogach, A.L. 2004, 'Luminescent polymer microcapsules addressable by a magnetic field', *Langmuir*, vol. 20, pp. 1449–1452.

He, C., Kim, S.W. & Lee, D.S. 2008, '*In situ* gelling stimuli-sensitive block copolymer hydrogels for drug delivery', *Journal of Controlled Release*, vol. 127, no. 3, pp. 189–207.

Henderson, E., Lee, B.H., Cui, Z., McLemore, R., Brandon, T.A. & Vernon, B.L. 2008, '*In vivo* evaluation of injectable thermosensitive polymer with time-dependent LCST', *Journal of Biomedical Materials Research Part A*, vol. 90, no.4, pp. 1186–1197.

Huang, L.Y. & Yang, M.C. 2007, 'Behaviors of controlled drug release of magnetic-gelatin hydrogel coated stainless steel for drug-eluting-stents application', *Journal of Magnetism and Magnetic Materials*, vol. 310, no. 2–3, pp. 2874–2876.

Irie, M. & Kunwatchakun, D. 1986, 'Photoresponsive polymers. 8. Reversible photo-stimulated dilation of polyacrylamide gels having triphenylmethane leuco derivatives', *Macromolecules*, vol. 19, pp. 2476–2480.

Jeong, B. & Gutowska, A. 2002, 'Lessons from nature: stimuli-responsive polymers and their biomedical applications', *Trends in Biotechnology*, vol. 20, no. 7, pp. 305–311.

Jeong, B., Bae, Y.H., Lee, D.S. & Kim, S.W. 1997, 'Biodegradable block copolymers as injectable drug-delivery systems', *Nature*, vol. 388, no. 6645, pp. 860–862.

Jin, K.M. & Kim, Y.H. 2008, 'Injectable, thermo-reversible and complex coacervate combination gels for protein drug delivery', *Journal of Controlled Release*, vol. 127, no. 3, pp. 249–256.

Kabanov, A.V., Batrakova, E.V. & Alakhov, V.Y. 2002, 'Pluronic® block copolymers as novel polymer therapeutics for drug and gene delivery', *Journal of Controlled Release*, vol. 82, no. 2–3, pp. 189–212.

Kaewpirom, S. & Boonsang, S. 2006, 'Electrical response characterisation of poly (ethylene glycol) macromer (PEGM)/chitosan hydrogels in NaCl solution', *European Polymer Journal*, vol. 42, no. 7, pp. 1609–1616.

Kataoka, K., Harada, A. & Nagasaki, Y. 2001, 'Block copolymer micelles for drug delivery: design, characterization and biological significance', *Advanced Drug Delivery Reviews*, vol. 47, no. 1, pp. 113–131.

Kikuchi, A. & Okano, T. 2002, 'Pulsatile drug release control using hydrogels', *Advanced Drug Delivery Reviews*, vol. 54, no. 1, pp. 53–77.

Kim, H.K., Shim, W.S., Kim, S.E., Lee, K.H., Kang, E., Kim, J.H., Kim, K., Kwon, I.C. & Lee, D.S. 2008, 'Injectable *in situ*-forming pH/thermo-sensitive hydrogel for bone tissue engineering', *Tissue Engineering Part A*, vol. 15, no. 4, pp. 923–933.

Kim, J.J. & Park, K. 2001, 'Modulated insulin delivery from glucose-sensitive hydrogel dosage forms', *Journal of Controlled Release*, vol. 77, no. 1–2, pp. 39–47.

Kim, S.Y. & Lee, S.C. 2009, 'Thermo-responsive injectable hydrogel system based on poly (N-isopropylacrylamide-co-vinylphosphonic acid). I. Biomineralization and protein delivery', *Journal of Applied Polymer Science*, vol. 113, pp. 3460–3469.

Klouda, L. & Mikos, A.G. 2008, 'Thermoresponsive hydrogels in biomedical applications', *European Journal of Pharmaceutics and Biopharmaceutics*, vol. 68, no. 1, pp. 34–45.

Koffi, A.A., Agnely, F., Besnard, M., Kablan Brou, J., Grossiord, J.L. & Ponchel, G. 2008, '*In vitro* and *in vivo* characteristics of a thermogelling and bioadhesive delivery system intended for rectal administration of quinine in children', *European Journal of Pharmaceutics and Biopharmaceutics*, vol. 69, no. 1, pp. 167–175.

Kozlovskaya, V., Kharlampieva, E., Mansfield, M.L. & Sukhishvili, S.A. 2006, 'Poly (methacrylic acid) hydrogel films and capsules: response to pH and ionic strength, and encapsulation of macromolecules', *Chemistry of Materials*, vol. 18, no. 2, pp. 328–336.

Krauland, A.H., Guggi, D. & Bernkop-Schnürch, A. 2006, 'Thiolated chitosan microparticles: a vehicle for nasal peptide drug delivery', *International Journal of Pharmaceutics*, vol. 307, no. 2, pp. 270–277.

Kumar, M.N.V.R., Muzzarelli, R.A.A., Muzzarelli, C., Sashiwa, H. & Domb, A.J. 2004, 'Chitosan chemistry and pharmaceutical perspectives', *Chemical Reviews*, vol. 104, no. 12, pp. 6017–6084.

Lee, B.H. & Vernon, B. 2005, '*In situ*-gelling, erodible N-isopropylacrylamide copolymers', *Macromolecular Bioscience*, vol. 5, no. 7, pp. 629–635.

Lee, B.H., West, B., McLemore, R., Pauken, C. & Vernon, B.L. 2006, '*In-situ* injectable physically and chemically gelling NIPAAm-based copolymer system for embolization', *Biomacromolecules*, vol. 7, no. 6, pp. 2059–2064.

Lee, K.K., Cussler, E.L., Marchetti, M. & McHugh, M.A. 1990, 'Pressure-dependent phase transitions in hydrogels', *Chemical Engineering Science*, vol. 45, no. 3, pp. 766–767.

Lee, P.Y., Cobain, E., Huard, J. & Huang, L. 2007, 'Thermosensitive hydrogel PEG–PLGA–PEG enhances engraftment of muscle-derived stem cells and promotes healing in diabetic wound', *Molecular Therapy*, vol. 15, no. 6, pp. 1189–1194.

Lee, S.C., Cho, Y.W. & Park, K. 2005, 'Control of thermogelation properties of hydrophobically modified methylcellulose', *Journal of Bioactive and Compatible Polymers*, vol. 20, no. 1, pp. 5–13.

Lendlein, A., Jiang, H., Jünger, O. & Langer, R. 2005, 'Light-induced shape-memory polymers', *Nature*, vol. 434, no. 7035, pp. 879–882.

Li, H. & Luo, R. 2009, 'Modeling and characterization of glucose-sensitive hydrogel: effect of Young's modulus', *Biosensors and Bioelectronics*, vol.24, no. 12, pp. 3630–3636.

Li, H., Yuan, Z., Lam, K.Y., Lee, H.P., Chen, J., Hanes, J. & Fu, J. 2004, 'Model development and numerical simulation of electric-stimulus-responsive hydrogels subject to an externally applied electric field', *Biosensors and Bioelectronics*, vol. 19, no. 9, pp. 1097–1107.

Lin, Y., Chen, Q. & Luo, H. 2007, 'Preparation and characterization of N-(2-carboxybenzyl) chitosan as a potential pH-sensitive hydrogel for drug delivery', *Carbohydrate Research*, vol. 342, no. 1, pp. 87–95.

Liu, H.Y. & Zhu, X.X. 1999, 'Lower critical solution temperatures of N-substituted acrylamide copolymers in aqueous solutions', *Polymer*, vol. 40, no. 25, pp. 6985–6990.

Liu, K.H., Liu, T.Y., Chen, S.Y. & Liu, D.M. 2008, 'Drug release behavior of chitosan–montmorillonite nanocomposite hydrogels following electrostimulation', *Acta Biomaterialia*, vol. 4, no. 4, pp. 1038–1045.

Liu, T.Y., Hu, S.H., Liu, T.Y., Liu, D.M. & Chen, S.Y. 2006, 'Magnetic-sensitive behavior of intelligent ferrogels for controlled release of drug', *Langmuir*, vol. 22, no. 14, pp. 5974–5978.

Lu, Z.R., Kopeckova, P. & Kopecek, J. 2003, 'Antigen responsive hydrogels based on polymerizable antibody Fab' fragment', *Macromolecular Bioscience*, vol. 3, no. 6, pp. 296–300.

Luo, R. & Li, H. 2009, 'A modeling study of the effect of environmental ionic valence on the mechanical characteristics of pH–electrosensitive hydrogel', *Acta Biomaterialia*, vol. 5, no. 8, pp. 2920–2928.

Luo, R., Li, H. & Lam, K.Y. 2009, 'Modeling the effect of environmental solution pH on the mechanical characteristics of glucose-sensitive hydrogels', *Biomaterials*, vol. 30, no. 4, pp. 690–700.

Mamada, A., Tanaka, T., Kungwatchakun, D. & Irie, M. 1990, 'Photoinduced phase transition of gels', *Macromolecules*, vol. 23, pp. 1517–1519.

McDonald, T.O., Qu, H., Saunders, B.R. & Ulijn, R.V. 2009, 'Branched peptide actuators for enzyme responsive hydrogel particles', *Soft Matter*, vol. 5, no. 8, pp. 1728–1734.

Micic, M., Zheng, Y., Moy, V., Zhang, X.H., Andreopoulos, F.M. & Leblanc, R.M. 2003, 'Comparative studies of surface topography and mechanical properties of a new, photo-switchable PEG-based hydrogel', *Colloids and Surfaces B: Biointerfaces*, vol. 27, no. 2–3, pp. 147–158.

Miyata, T., Asami, N. & Uragami, T. 1999, 'A reversibly antigen-responsive hydrogel', *Nature*, vol. 399, no. 6738, pp. 766–769.

Moelbert, S. & De Los Rios, P. 2003, 'Hydrophobic interaction model for upper and lower critical solution temperatures', *Macromolecules*, vol. 36, no. 15, pp. 5845–5853.

Moffatt, S. & Cristiano, R.J. 2006, 'PEGylated J591 mAb loaded in PLGA-PEG-PLGA tri-block copolymer for targeted delivery: *In vitro* evaluation in human prostate cancer cells', *International Journal of Pharmaceutics*, vol. 317, no. 1, pp. 10–13.

Murdan, S. 2003, 'Electro-responsive drug delivery from hydrogels', *Journal of Controlled Release*, vol. 92, no. 1–2, pp. 1–17.

Nisbet, D.R., Crompton, K.E., Hamilton, S.D., Shirakawa, S., Prankerd, R.J., Finkelstein, D.I., Horne, M.K. & Forsythe, J.S. 2006, 'Morphology and gelation of thermosensitive xyloglucan hydrogels', *Biophysical Chemistry*, vol. 121, no. 1, pp. 14–20.

Nishiyama, N., Stapert, H.R., Zhang, G.D., Takasu, D., Jiang, D.L., Nagano, T., Aida, T. & Kataoka, K. 2003, 'Light-harvesting ionic dendrimer porphyrins as new photosensitizers for photodynamic therapy', *Bioconjugate Chemistry*, vol. 14, no. 1, pp. 58–66.

Obaidat, A.A. & Park, K. 1997, 'Characterization of protein release through glucose-sensitive hydrogel membranes', *Biomaterials*, vol. 18, no. 11, pp. 801–806.

Ogawa, K., Wang, B. & Kokufuta, E. 2001, 'Enzyme-regulated microgel collapse for controlled membrane permeability', *Langmuir*, vol. 17, no. 16, pp. 4704–4707.

Ougizawa, T., Inoue, T. & Kammer, H.W. 1985, 'Upper and lower critical solution temperature behavior in polymer blends', *Macromolecules*, vol. 18, pp. 2092–2094.

Park, K.M., Lee, S.Y., Joung, Y.K., Na, J.S., Lee, M.C. & Park, K.D. 2009, 'Thermosensitive chitosan–Pluronic hydrogel as an injectable cell delivery carrier for cartilage regeneration', *Acta Biomaterialia*, vol. 5, no. 6, pp. 1956–1965.

Pasternack, R.F., Bustamante, C., Collins, P.J., Giannetto, A. & Gibbs, E.J. 1993, 'Porphyrin assemblies on DNA as studied by a resonance light-scattering technique', *Journal of the American Chemical Society*, vol. 115, pp. 5393–5399.

Pervaiz, S. & Olivo, M. 2006, 'Art and science of photodynamic therapy', *Clinical & Experimental Pharmacology & Physiology*, vol. 33, no. 5–6, pp. 551.

Plummer, P.L.M. & Chen, T.S. 1983, 'A molecular dynamics study of water clathrates', *Journal of Physical Chemistry*, vol. 87, pp. 4190–4197.

Qi, H., Chen, W., Huang, C., Li, L., Chen, C., Li, W. & Wu, C. 2007, 'Development of a poloxamer analogs/carbopol-based *in situ* gelling and mucoadhesive ophthalmic delivery system for puerarin', *International Journal of Pharmaceutics*, vol. 337, no. 1–2, pp. 178–187.

Qiu, Y. & Park, K. 2001, 'Environment-sensitive hydrogels for drug delivery', *Advanced Drug Delivery Reviews*, vol. 53, no. 3, pp. 321–339.

Ribeiro, C., Arizaga, G.G.C., Wypych, F. & Sierakowski, M.R. 2009, 'Nanocomposites coated with xyloglucan for drug delivery: *in vitro* studies', *International Journal of Pharmaceutics*, vol. 367, no. 1–2, pp. 204–210.

Ricci, E.J., Lunardi, L.O., Nanclares, D.M.A. & Marchetti, J.M. 2005, 'Sustained release of lidocaine from Poloxamer 407 gels', *International Journal of Pharmaceutics*, vol. 288, no. 2, pp. 235–244.

Robb, S.A., Lee, B.H., McLemore, R. & Vernon, B.L. 2007, 'Simultaneously physically and chemically gelling polymer system utilizing a poly (NIPAAm-co-cysteamine)-based copolymer', *Biomacromolecules*, vol. 8, no. 7, pp. 2294–2300.

Ruel-Gariépy, E. & Leroux, J.C. 2004, '*In situ*-forming hydrogels – review of temperature-sensitive systems', *European Journal of Pharmaceutics and Biopharmaceutics*, vol. 58, no. 2, pp. 409–426.

Ruel-Gariépy, E., Chenite, A., Chaput, C., Guirguis, S. & Leroux, J.C. 2000, 'Characterization of thermosensitive chitosan gels for the sustained delivery of drugs', *International Journal of Pharmaceutics*, vol. 203, no. 1–2, pp. 89–98.

Ruel-Gariépy, E., Shive, M., Bichara, A., Berrada, M., Le Garrec, D., Chenite, A. & Leroux, J.C. 2004, 'A thermosensitive chitosan-based hydrogel for the local delivery of paclitaxel', *European Journal of Pharmaceutics and Biopharmaceutics*,

vol. 57, no. 1, pp. 53–63.
Sarkar, N. 1979, 'Thermal gelation properties of methyl and hydroxypropyl methylcellulose', *Journal of Applied Polymer Science*, vol. 24, no. 4, pp. 1073–1087.
Satarkar, N.S. & Hilt, J.Z. 2008, 'Magnetic hydrogel nanocomposites for remote controlled pulsatile drug release', *Journal of Controlled Release*, vol. 130, no. 3, pp. 246–251.
Shamji, M.F., Hwang, P., Bullock, R.W., Adams, S.B., Nettles, D.L. & Setton, L.A. 2008, 'Release and activity of anti-TNFá therapeutics from injectable chitosan preparations for local drug delivery', *Journal of Biomedical Materials Research Part B: Applied Biomaterials*, vol. 90, no. 1, pp. 319–326.
Shim, W.S., Kim, J.H., Kim, K., Kim, Y.S., Park, R.W., Kim, I.S., Kwon, I.C. & Lee, D.S. 2007, 'pH-and temperature-sensitive, injectable, biodegradable block copolymer hydrogels as carriers for paclitaxel', *International Journal of Pharmaceutics*, vol. 331, no. 1, pp. 11–18.
Siepmann, J. & Peppas, N.A. 2001, 'Modeling of drug release from delivery systems based on hydroxypropyl methylcellulose (HPMC)', *Advanced Drug Delivery Reviews*, vol. 48, no. 2–3, pp. 139–157.
Solis, F.J., Weiss-Malik, R. & Vernon, B. 2005, 'Local monomer activation model for phase behavior and calorimetric properties of LCST gel-forming polymers', *Macromolecules*, vol. 38, no. 10, pp. 4456–4464.
Southall, N.T., Dill, K.A. & Haymet, A.D.J. 2002, 'A view of the hydrophobic effect', *Journal of Physical Chemistry B – Condensed Phase*, vol. 106, no. 3, pp. 521–533.
Sriadibhatla, S., Yang, Z., Gebhart, C., Alakhov, V.Y. & Kabanov, A. 2006, 'Transcriptional activation of gene expression by pluronic block copolymers in stably and transiently transfected cells', *Molecular Therapy*, vol. 13, no. 4, pp. 804–813.
Suzuki, A. & Tanaka, T. 1990, 'Phase transition in polymer gels induced by visible light', *Nature*, vol. 346, no. 6282, pp. 345–347.
Suzuki, Y., Tanihara, M., Nishimura, Y., Suzuki, K., Kakimaru, Y. & Shimizu, Y. 1998, 'A new drug delivery system with controlled release of antibiotic only in the presence of infection', *Journal of Biomedical Materials Research*, vol. 42, pp. 112–116.
Tanaka, T., Nishio, I., Sun, S.T. & Ueno-Nishio, S. 1982, 'Collapse of gels in an electric field', *Science*, vol. 218, no. 4571, pp. 467–469.
Tanihara, M., Suzuki, Y., Nishimura, Y., Suzuki, K., Kakimaru, Y. & Fukunishi, Y. 1999, 'A novel microbial infection-responsive drug release system', *Journal of Phamaceutical Sciences*, vol. 88, no. 5, pp. 510–514.
Tarasevich, B.J., Gutowska, A., Li, X.S. & Jeong, B.M. 2009, 'The effect of polymer composition on the gelation behavior of PLGA-g-PEG biodegradable thermoreversible gels', *Journal of Biomedical Materials Research Part A*, vol. 89, no. 1, pp. 248–254.
Thornton, P.D., Mart, R.J., Webb, S.J. & Ulijn, R.V. 2008, 'Enzyme-responsive hydrogel particles for the controlled release of proteins: designing peptide actuators to match payload', *Soft Matter*, vol. 4, no. 4, pp. 821–827.
Torres-Lugo, M. & Peppas, N.A. 1999, 'Molecular design and *in vitro* studies of novel pH-sensitive hydrogels for the oral delivery of calcitonin', *Macromolecules*, vol. 32, no. 20, pp. 6646–6651.
Ulijn, R.V. 2006, 'Enzyme-responsive materials: a new class of smart biomaterials', *Journal of Materials Chemistry*, vol. 16, no. 23, pp. 2217–2225.
Vernengo, J., Fussell, G.W., Smith, N.G. & Lowman, A.M. 2008, 'Evaluation of novel

injectable hydrogels for nucleus pulposus replacement', *Journal of Biomedical Materials Research Part B: Applied Biomaterials*, vol. 84B, no. 1, pp. 64–69.

Vernon, B. & Martinez, A. 2005, 'Gel strength and solution viscosity of temperature-sensitive, *in-situ*-gelling polymers for endovascular embolization', *Journal of Biomaterials Science. Polymer Edition*, vol. 16, no. 9, pp. 1153–1166.

Vernon, B., Kim, S.W. & Bae, Y.H. 2000, 'Thermoreversible copolymer gels for extracellular matrix', *Journal of Biomedical Materials Research*, vol. 51, no. 1, pp. 69–79.

Wakamatsu, H., Yamamoto, K., Nakao, A. & Aoyagi, T. 2006, 'Preparation and characterization of temperature-responsive magnetite nanoparticles conjugated with N-isopropylacrylamide-based functional copolymer', *Journal of Magnetism and Magnetic Materials*, vol. 302, no. 2, pp. 327–333.

Wallmersperger, T., Kröplin, B. & Gülch, R.W. 2004, 'Coupled chemo-electro-mechanical formulation for ionic polymer gels – numerical and experimental investigations', *Mechanics of Materials*, vol. 36, no. 5–6, pp. 411–420.

Wang, C.C., Su, C.H. & Chen, C.C. 2008, 'Water absorbing and antibacterial properties of N-isopropyl acrylamide grafted and collagen/chitosan immobilized polypropylene nonwoven fabric and its application on wound healing enhancement', *Journal of Biomedical Materials Research Part A*, vol. 84, no. 4, pp. 1006–1017.

Weiss, P., Layrolle, P., Clergeau, L.P., Enckel, B., Pilet, P., Amouriq, Y., Daculsi, G. & Giumelli, B. 2007, 'The safety and efficacy of an injectable bone substitute in dental sockets demonstrated in a human clinical trial', *Biomaterials*, vol. 28, no. 22, pp. 3295–3305.

Weng, L., Pan, H. & Chen, W. 2008, 'Self-crosslinkable hydrogels composed of partially oxidized hyaluronan and gelatin: *in vitro* and *in vivo* responses', *Journal of Biomedical Materials Research Part A*, vol. 85, no. 2, pp. 352–365.

Wu, J., Wei, W., Wang, L.Y., Su, Z.G. & Ma, G.H. 2007, 'A thermosensitive hydrogel based on quaternized chitosan and poly (ethylene glycol) for nasal drug delivery system', *Biomaterials*, vol. 28, no. 13, pp. 2220–2232.

Yasuda, S., Townsend, D.W., Michele, D.E., Favre, E.G., Day, S.M. & Metzger, J.M. 2005, 'Dystrophic heart failure blocked by membrane sealant poloxamer', *Nature*, vol. 436, no. 7053, pp. 1025–1029.

Yun, K. & Moon, H.T. 2008, 'Inducing chondrogenic differentiation in injectable hydrogels embedded with rabbit chondrocytes and growth factor for neocartilage formation', *Journal of Bioscience and Bioengineering*, vol. 105, no. 2, pp. 122–126.

Zhang, J. & Misra, R.D.K. 2007, 'Magnetic drug-targeting carrier encapsulated with thermosensitive smart polymer: Core–shell nanoparticle carrier and drug release response', *Acta Biomaterialia*, vol. 3, no. 6, pp. 838–850.

Zhang, K. & Wu, X.Y. 2002, 'Modulated insulin permeation across a glucose-sensitive polymeric composite membrane', *Journal of Controlled Release*, vol. 80, no. 1–3, pp. 169–178.

Zhang, K., Luo, Y. & Li, Z. 2007, 'Synthesis and characterization of a pH-and ionic strength-responsive hydrogel', *Soft Materials*, vol. 5, no. 4, pp. 183–195.

Zhang, R., Tang, M., Bowyer, A., Eisenthal, R. & Hubble, J. 2005, 'A novel pH-and ionic-strength-sensitive carboxy methyl dextran hydrogel', *Biomaterials*, vol. 26, no. 22, pp. 4677–4683.

Zhang, R., Tang, M., Bowyer, A., Eisenthal, R. & Hubble, J. 2006, 'Synthesis and characterization of a D-glucose sensitive hydrogel based on CM-dextran and concanavalin A', *Reactive and Functional Polymers*, vol. 66, no. 7, pp. 757–767.

Zhong, X., Wang, Y.X. & Wang, S.C. 1996, 'Pressure dependence of the volume phase-transition of temperature-sensitive gels', *Chemical Engineering Science*, vol. 51, no. 12, pp. 3235–3239.

Zhou, Q., Rutland, M.W., Teeri, T.T. & Brumer, H. 2007, 'Xyloglucan in cellulose modification', *Cellulose*, vol. 14, no. 6, pp. 625–641.

Zrínyi, M. 2000, 'Intelligent polymer gels controlled by magnetic fields', *Colloid & Polymer Science*, vol. 278, no. 2, pp. 98–103.

12
Injectable nanotechnology

F. CELLESI and N. TIRELLI, University of Manchester, UK

Abstract: This chapter provides an overview of how nanotechnology has been applied to the design and engineering of advanced injectable biomaterials. Recent developments in the field of injectable nanoparticles are reviewed from the point of view of administration routes, applications (diagnostic, drug/gene delivery, cancer treatment, vaccine technologies) and material characteristics (inorganic/organic nanomaterial, morphology, etc.). The chapter then reviews the progress made in designing injectable hydrogel materials based on self-assembly of nano-scale building blocks and on nanocomposites, focusing on their promising applications in tissue engineering and drug delivery.

Key words: nanoparticles, nano-carriers, nanovaccines, *in vivo* diagnostics, self-assembled hydrogels, nanocomposites.

12.1 Introduction

12.1.1 Injectable formulations

Injectable formulations are fluids characterized by an internal complex structure and/or by the presence of heterogeneous phases that allow them, *inter alia,* to control the release of an active ingredient or to harden/gel in the presence of or within a biological system. In general, we recognize the presence of a carrier/matrix that can host one or more pharmacologically active principles, and/or control the mechanical and biological properties of the formulation. We will not include in the definition solid injectable materials, e.g. injectable monolithic implants such as Zoladex® (degradable poly(L,D-lactic acid) used for the release of goserelin acetate, a lutenizing hormone releasing hormone (LHRH) agonist used in the treatment of breast and prostate cancer).

In drug delivery, injectable systems can be administered systemically or topically, producing dosage forms that can have an extended circulation (dispersed systems) or provide a localized reservoir of an active ingredient (depot systems). Different combinations of route of administration and physical nature of the formulation can be used to spatially (biodistribution) and temporally (kinetics of release) control the concentration of the active principle and thus its bioavailability. For example, the characteristics of the administration (e.g. subcutaneous or intravenous) and the size of the carrier (e.g. capable or not of being transported by blood or of diffusing through interstitial fluids) would concur in determining the possibility of a long-range circulation, while the partition of a drug between carrier and biological fluids or the cellular uptake of the carrier would control the kinetics of delivery.

In tissue engineering, injectable systems are almost exclusively employed to generate *in situ* 3D matrices, which replace some or most of the functions of a tissue and possibly host cells and/or stimulate the regeneration of the tissue itself. These matrices are often referred to as scaffolds; the name suggests the presence of a solid 'skeleton', i.e. a fibrillar structure, but they may also be homogeneous in nature, as many *in situ* formed hydrogels are. The possibility to apply these formulations through an injection offers several advantages in comparison to the implantation of pre-formed scaffolds. For example, due to its viscous nature (it flows!) an injected, *in situ* gelling fluid can take the shape of the cavity produced by removing, e.g., a necrotic or decayed tissue, providing therefore a conformal implant. Furthermore, the injection of a fluid is a minimally invasive surgical operation which is easier for the patient than a solid implant.

12.1.2 Injectable nano-systems

In the last two decades nanotechnology has been extensively involved in the design and development of novel injectable biomaterials. The rationale is inherently biomimetic, since biology is based on systems that work at the nano-scale: carriers of insoluble compounds such as lipoproteins; membrane-based machinery such as pumps, channels, receptors, endocytic structures; even whole organisms such as viruses, etc. Therefore, an effective and biologically inspired approach to the delivery of active compounds and/or to the regeneration of a tissue must be based on concepts typical of this length scale. The term 'nanomedicine' has probably been abused and misused in press releases aiming to describe improbable scientific revolutions (see, for instance, the descriptions of nanoscopic machines that, once injected, roam through the body as miniature surgeons[1]). However, it is unequivocally true that innovative materials based on nanotechnology have now reached pre-clinical and even clinical stage, representing a real breakthrough in drug delivery and diagnostics. Nano-carriers (colloidal objects such as micelles, liposomes, organic and inorganic nano-particles) have been efficiently used as drug delivery systems *in vivo*. A number of molecular building blocks capable of nano-scale controlled aggregation (self-assembling peptides, block copolymers, nanoparticles) have shown promising results, e.g. as synthetic extracellular matrices for tissue engineering.

Nano-sized objects may be different in physical nature, e.g. perfectly elastic inorganic nanoparticles, viscoelastic polymeric nanoparticles, viscous micelles; however, all injectable nano-systems share a common macroscopic property: under the conditions employed during the application, they flow, i.e. they are dispersed in a water environment which allows a macroscopically viscous behaviour.

This chapter will provide an overview of how nanotechnology has been applied for the design and engineering of advanced injectable nanomaterials; we will mostly focus on nano-carriers used for diagnostic applications and for the delivery of 'drugs', including nucleic acids and vaccines, and on self-assembling nano-structures employed to generate macroscopic materials (scaffolds) for applications in tissue engineering and regenerative medicine. As the number of nanomaterials being tested *in vivo* or in clinical trials is rapidly growing, this chapter aims to be illustrative, but not exhaustive of these topics.

12.2 Route of administration and biodistribution of injectable nano-carriers

We will here focus on nanoparticles as a typical example of nano-carriers. Nanoparticles can be seen as sub-micron colloidal objects with a predominantly elastic mechanical behaviour (solid-like bodies), which can be loaded with therapeutically active compounds on their surface, in their bulk or both. Drug-loaded nanoparticles have been administered as nano-carriers in water-based dispersions through virtually all parenteral routes, i.e., intravenous, sub-cutaneous, intramuscular and also intraperitoneal, but they have also been used to prepare macroscopic materials *in situ* (Fig. 12.1).

In all cases, after injection the nanoparticles are diluted with physiological fluids, which have a roughly neutral pH (7.4), a temperature generally close to 37°C, and a relatively high ionic strength (130–150 meq/L).[2] These fluids also contain a variety of other colloidal objects; for example blood has proteins (albumin, fibrinogen, immunoglobulins, etc.) at a concentration of 50–70 mg/mL, 1–2 mg/mL of lipoproteins, $1.5–4.5 \times 10^8$/mL of platelets, etc.; in lymph, edema and other body fluids the colloidal content is generally lower, for example, in lymph the protein concentration is 10% to 80% that in blood.[3,4]

Local variations of these parameters (temperature, ionic strength, pH, presence of macromolecular compounds) may lead to the aggregation, flocculation and precipitation of the nanoparticles; for example, depletion interactions originating from high protein concentration may lead to the aggregation in larger colloidal objects, similarly to what happens to red blood cells in concentrated polymer solutions.[5] If such phenomena are to be avoided, because *inter alia* they may lead to embolization, the nanoparticles must be provided with sufficient colloidal stability; this is typically achieved using charged particles stabilized by electrostatic repulsion from (ζ-potential $\geq$ 20–30 mV),[6] or decorating the nanoparticle surface with hydrophilic polymer chains that confer a steric (or electrosteric, if the chains are charged) barrier against flocculation.[2]

Intravenous (IV) administration introduces nanoparticles directly into the blood stream. The carriers may remain within the blood circulation for a more or

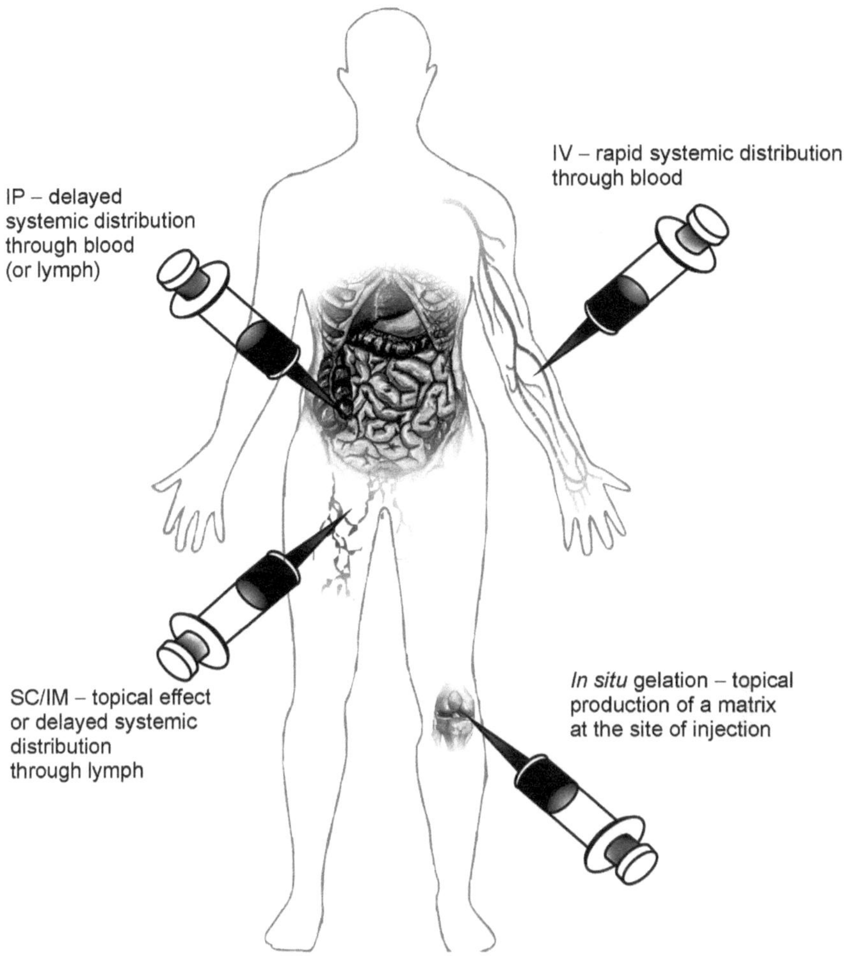

12.1 Most common routes of administration for injectable nano-systems.

less prolonged time, or accumulate in a target tissue or organ. There are major pharmacokinetic differences in the IV administration of nanoparticles vs. that of free drugs, most importantly in renal clearance: in absence of any specific accumulation, particles smaller than 5 nm are excreted through the kidneys,[7] but it has been proved, e.g. with using precisely sized quantum dots, that dimensions >15 nm quantitatively stop the eliminated through urine.[8] This theoretically allows a substantial prolongation of the circulation time for a nanoparticle-loaded drug and therefore an increase of its therapeutic window.

However, although blood-borne nanoparticles cannot be easily excreted, they may be removed from circulation either through capture by cells (clearance) or through accumulation in peripheral tissues (biodistribution); these phenomena are heavily dependent on the size and surface properties of the nanoparticles.[9]

For example, large or agglomerating particles with a size above 5 μm are quantitatively entrapped by fine capillary beds, embolizing them; although embolization may be a strategy for cutting the blood supply to a tissue (e.g. a tumour),[10] this is a generally a situation to avoid and, as a result, most nanoparticles are designed to have a size at least one order of magnitude smaller than this threshold (< 500 nm).

On the other hand, smaller nanoparticles may be able to pass through the walls of partially fenestrated blood vessels and/or can be captured by phagocytic sentinel cells. Correspondingly, nanoparticles accumulate with a kinetics that is size- and composition-dependent in organs characterized by the presence of extended and sometimes fenestrated capillary networks and of resident, blood-exposed phagocytes, i.e. liver, spleen, lungs, and to a lower degree also in the bone marrow.[11] In particular, cells of the mononuclear phagocytic system (MPS), also known as the reticulo-endothelial system (RES), have a central role in the rapid clearance of nanoparticles from the blood circulation; Kupffer cells (specialized macrophages resident in the liver) can quantitatively clear circulating objects within seconds, unless an appropriate surface composition is provided.[9] The clearance is indeed based on the recognition of the nanoparticles as foreign bodies, which is mediated by the adsorption of proteins on the nanoparticle surfaces. Proteins that can label foreign bodies and prepare them for phagocytosis are broadly called opsonins and their surface adsorption is generally referred to as opsonisation; most typically, they are complement proteins C3–C5, and immunoglobulins. In order to bypass the MPS and therefore prolong the blood circulation, nanoparticles (as much as micelles, liposomes and other nano-carriers) are often decorated with groups that hinder the adsorption of opsonins, thus providing the circulating object with invisibility or 'stealthness' to phagocytic cells. To achieve this effect, the 'golden standard' material is poly(ethylene glycol) (PEG), which is very well known to minimize opsonisation and prolong circulation to the objects it is grafted on.

Colloidal objects provided the means for an extended circulation, e.g. PEGylated nanoparticles, can still undergo accumulation in peripheral tissues, which can be used to target their action to specific sites. A classical example is offered by the enhanced permeability and retention (EPR) effect, which describes the diffusion of circulating colloids into solid tumours through their inherently leaky vascular walls and their accumulation due to the poor lymphatic drainage of those tissues;[12,13] this is a form of passive targeting that has been widely exploited for treating or imaging tumours of soft tissue and epithelial cell origin. A variety of active targeting strategies are possible too, with the common denominator that the presence of appropriate ligands on the nanoparticle surface allows their uptake in cells expressing specific cell receptors.[14]

The intraperitoneal (IP) injection is a less commonly utilized route of administration, which is advantageous when a slower liberation of nanoparticles in the blood stream is needed, although this use can also be envisaged as an alternative to IV in cases of low blood pressure. The peritoneal cavity is filled with about 50 mL of fluid; the transit from this environment into blood is already rather slow for low MW solutes and it is often mediated by the liver; while it is retarded for polymers and colloidal objects; most commonly, this route of administration is used for increasing the permanence time and decrease the clearance of antineoplastic drugs, possibly increasing also their efficacy towards tumours in the area. For nanoparticles, a quantitative evaluation of this retardation and of the mechanism of passage have been often overlooked, but the transfer to systemic circulation has been clearly demonstrated.[15,16] A possible complication of this approach, however, is that the nanoparticles may be transferred not only to blood circulation but also to the lymphatic system.[17]

In subcutaneous (SC) and intramuscular (IM) injections, on the other hand, the transfer of colloidal objects to blood is generally small and slow. Non-aggregating nanoparticles are retained in the interstitial fluid at the injection site until they: (a) are internalized by cells localized in the tissue, (b) are internalized by antigen-displaying cells (macrophages, dendritic cells) and carried to lymph nodes where their degradation products are presented to lymphocytes,[18] (c) migrate to the lymphatic system by simple drainage of the tissue,[19] or (d) are slowly degraded in the extracellular space.[11] The transfer to the lymphatic system[20] is particularly advantageous for the delivery of vaccines or for imaging, while the possibility of a localized action in a peripheral tissue is best exploited for the delivery of genetic material.

Finally, it is important to mention that the occurrence of aggregation and possibly of gelation phenomena allows topical production of materials at the site of injection; this approach has been widely employed for the *in situ* preparation of 3D matrices for regenerative medicine.

12.3 Diagnostic applications of injectable nano-carriers

In biomedical imaging most standard imaging probes and contrast agents are still chemical or radioactive agents used without a carrier structure; however, the advances in injectable nano-carriers have recently led to the development of a vast number of nano probes for non-invasive real-time imaging,[21] taking advantage, e.g., of the slow clearance or the reduced toxicity conferred by the encapsulation in a nano-carrier. Again, for sake of brevity we will mostly focus on nanoparticles, and some examples are provided in Table 12.1. As a common denominator for all nanoparticle-based agents, the imaging method allows their time-dependent biodistribution to be followed.

Magnetic resonance imaging (MRI) is one of the most powerful diagnostic tools available for high resolution biomedical imaging; it is thus considered the preferred imaging method for a number of soft tissues, e.g. the central nervous system, for assessing cardiac functions, and for tumour detection. MRI contrast

Table 12.1 Use of nanoparticles as contrast agents for biomedical imaging techniques

Technique	Detection	Nanoparticles	Applications
Magnetic resonance imaging (MRI)	Magnetic field	Magnetite (Fe_3O_4) or maghemite (γ-Fe_2O_3)[22–25]	Central nervous system imaging, cardiac functions, localization of tumours[22–25]
Computed tomography (CT)	X-rays	Au, Bi_2S_3 [26,27]	Vasculature, liver and lymph nodes[26,27]
Positron emission tomography (PET)	γ-rays	^{64}Cu-labelled single-walled carbon nanotubes (SWNTs)[28]	$\alpha v\beta 3$ integrin-positive tumors[28]
Single photon emission computed tomography (SPECT)	γ-rays	^{111}In-labelled iron oxide nanoparticles[29], integrin $\alpha v\beta 3$-targeted ^{111}In-labelled perfluorocarbon nanoparticles[30]	Breast cancer,[29] angiogenetic sites[30]
Optical imaging (OI)	Near infrared radiation (NIR)	Quantum dots (QDs),[31,32] Au[33]	Localization of tumours, lymph nodes[31,32]
Photoacoustic imaging (PAI)	Ultrasound	ICG-embedded ormosil nanoparticles,[34] Au-nanoshells[26,35,36]	Skin and other epithelia, breast cancer detection[35]

agents are designed to change the relaxation times T1 (spin-lattice/longitudinal relaxation time) and/or T2 (transverse relaxation time) of the protons in the vicinity of the agent; it is therefore possible to link the biodistribution of the agent to an image contrast (bright/dark), which allows then to highlight any alteration linked to a pathological situation.[24,25] Injectable superparamagnetic iron oxide nanoparticles (SPIO, size 50–500 nm) or ultra-small paramagnetic iron oxide nanoparticles (USPIO, size < 50 nm) are possibly the most popular T2 contrast agents, which allow negative contrast enhancement (darker images of the regions of interest) for liver, spleen and lymph nodes.[22–25] The crystalline magnetic core is generally composed of magnetite (Fe_3O_4) or maghemite (γ-Fe_2O_3) with a superficial coating of suitable hydrophilic polymers such as dextran or poly(ethylene glycol).[24,25] The use of these nanoparticles for functional imaging has drastically increase with the availability of vast number of different surface functionalizations iron oxide nanoparticles were synthesized which display functional groups such as peptides, conjugating proteins, antibodies, and oligonucleotides for procedures.[22,23]

In X-ray computed tomography (CT) the radioopacity of metallic nanoparticles (for example bismuth[27] and gold[26]) have been used to generate localized contrast in the imaging of blood vasculature, liver and lymph nodes.

In radionuclide-based imaging, nanoparticles labelled with low amounts of a radioisotope are used as *in vivo* tracers. Single photon emission computed tomography (SPECT) employs gamma ray-emitting radioisotopes, such as ^{111}In, reconstructing a 3D image from a series of planar pictures taken by a gamma camera. The introduction of the radionuclide on nanoparticles, possibly in combination with specific antibodies and 'stealth' surfaces, has been applied to the imaging of tumoural vasculature.[30] Positron emission tomography (PET) is based on nuclides, such as ^{64}Cu, which emit positrons that annihilate emitting gamma photons; compared to SPECT, it has a lower penetration, only up to few millimetres, and it is more expensive, but provides higher resolution. This has been used, often in conjunction with MRI, for imaging lymph nodes with high accuracy.[37]

Optical imaging, mostly with quantum dots (QDs) and gold nanoparticles, has been widely employed in animal studies and could be potentially used in clinic. QDs are fluorescent inorganic nanocrystals with tunable spectral properties (through their size and composition), high extinction coefficients and quantum yields, resistance to photobleaching and metabolic degradation, and possibility to be easily derivatized with targeting groups;[31,32] some concerns have been raised about their non-degradability and potential toxicity.[38] Gold nanoparticles are able to provide colorimetric contrast induced by surface plasmon resonance (SPR, tunable with size) and are highly resistant to photodecomposition and non-toxic. The main limitations to the *in vivo* use of fluorescence imaging are that living tissues often present autofluorescence and, more importantly, have high absorption and/or scattering in the visible region.

While the UV/Vis radiation presents therefore a penetration depth from a few micrometers to 1 mm, it is unsuitable for imaging internal organs. Near-infrared light (NIR, 650 to 900 nm, with a penetration up to a few cm) has been suggested as an alternative.

Photo-acoustic imaging is a promising new technique that combines spectral selectivity and penetration depth of laser light with the high resolution of ultrasound imaging. When short pulses of electromagnetic radiation illuminate a biological tissue, the thermoelastic effect generates an ultrasound wave at the point of interest, which can be detected for imaging. This technique is useful in the early detection of cancer and blood-rich lesions *in vivo*, due to the high optical absorption of haemoglobin which allows imaging of the blood vessels.[26] High photoacoustic contrast is provided by nanoparticles whose optical properties are based on surface plasmon resonance (SPR) or on NIR organic dyes. In the first case, gold nanoshells are used, with an absorption peak which can be tuned throughout the visible and near infrared (NIR) regions by controlling the size of the gold layer deposited on the nanoparticle surface.[26,35,36] In alternative NIR, organic dyes (such as the FDA-approved indocyanine green) can be introduced in virtually any nanoparticle structure but their photostability is a clear weakness.

12.4 Therapeutic applications of injectable nano-carriers

12.4.1 Cancer therapy

Most chemotherapic drugs suffer from poor efficiency in targeting a tumoural mass, essentially because of distribution and metabolism throughout off-target tissues; their preferential activity towards cancerous cells is overwhelmingly due to the higher proliferation rate of those cells. There is an overwhelming consensus that 'site-specificity' (→ increase of the drug concentration at the tumour site) and 'site-avoidance' (lower drug concentration and limited damages to healthy tissue) can be obtained in an incremental fashion by conjugating the drug molecules with appropriate structures. In a scale of growing complexity, a first approach is presented by the preparation of pro-drugs, i.e. low molecular weight compounds that are converted to active compounds by environmental conditions typical of a tumoural environment; a 'hot' example is offered by hypoxia-activated drugs.[39] A second approach consists in the conjugation of the drug with a targeting ligand (LTT, ligand-targeted therapeutics), which is most frequently an antibody or an antibody fragment, although other compounds such as folate, transferrin, and even RGD peptides can have similar actions.[40] The combination of these two strategies provides a further improvement: the systemic administration of a prodrug with an antibody + enzyme construct (ADEPT, antibody-directed enzyme prodrug therapy) allows the localization of the enzymatic prodrug-to-drug conversion by the use of a tumour-specific antibody.[41] The use of nano-carriers allows further possibilities:[42] if the nano-carriers are designed to avoid capture by the Mononuclear Phagocytic System and thus to have a prolonged systemic circulation,[43] then additional possibilities of targeting can be employed, such as the preferential accumulation of colloidal objects in tissues with leaky vasculature, which is indeed typical of solid tumours (the previously mentioned EPR effect), or the possibility of an enhanced targeting selectivity by modulating the ligand concentration and possibly clustering on the surface of the carrier. Last, but not least, nano-carriers' dimensions allow also the encapsulation of large (e.g. proteic) payloads or multiple types of drugs, thus different therapeutic approaches can be simultaneously applied in a controlled fashion.[44]

As a result, a vast number of nano-carriers have been used for the tumour-targeted delivery of active principles; they include liposomes,[44–46] micelles,[44–47] polymeric nanoparticles,[44–46,48] solid lipid nanoparticles (SLN),[49] dendrimers,[50] nanoshells,[51,52] and magnetic nanoparticles.[24,25] Examples of nano-carriers with proven clinical efficacy are reported in Table 12.2.

Liposomes have received most attention: their approval as nano-carriers for chemotherapeutic drugs dates from the mid-1990s.[44] The most significant achievement in the use of liposomes is probably the prolonged blood circulation which is obtained through their decoration with PEG chains, i.e. their PEGylation ('stealth' liposomes, e.g. Doxil), which reduces their unspecific uptake, e.g. in liver, lungs or spleen (the Reticulo-Endothelial System, RES). Due to their longer lifetime *in vivo*, PEGylated liposomes also allow better targetting through the presence of antibodies (immunoliposomes) or other agents (e.g. MBP-426 liposomes are decorated with transferrin in order to be preferentially internalized in cells overexpressing the transferring receptor). However, although liposomal formulations have clear advantages in reducing the toxicity and increasing the solubility of a number of drugs, it is still questioned whether they do provide a sound improvement in the clinically recorded antitumoral activity.[53]

Albumin-based nanoparticles (e.g. Abraxane) are extremely biocompatible and have been approved by FDA in 2005; although these nanoparticles showed a relatively high plasma clearance (albumin dissolve quickly upon administration into the circulatory system).[60] Other types of nano-carriers include polymeric micelles (Genexol-PM, NK911), and biodegradable polymeric nanoparticles (e.g. Xyotax, made of poly(glycolic acid)). Polymeric micelles show much higher accumulation and penetration in tumors than liposomes, due to their smaller size;[47] on the other hand, polymeric nanoparticles show a prolonged release profile regulated by the biodegradation of the polymeric constituent.

Despite the relatively large number of clinically tested nano-carriers, very few of them feature ligands for a targeted action; drawbacks that have hindered these carriers commonly include the expression of the targeted receptors by non-

Table 12.2 Examples of clinically tested injectable nano-carriers used for tumour targeting. All these formulations are administered intravenously[42,44–46,48,54–59]

Formulation	Carrier	Therapeutic agent	Targeting (receptor)	Tumour	Status
Doxil	Liposome	Doxorubicin	Passive	Breast, ovarian	FDA approved[44–46]
Daunoxome	Liposome	Daunorubicin	Passive	Kaposi sarcoma	FDA approved[44–46]
Abraxane	Albumin-based particles	Paclitaxel	Passive	Breast	FDA approved[44–46]
Genexol-PM	mPEG-PLA micelles	Paclitaxel	Passive	Breast, lung	Phase II clinical trials[44–46]
NK911	PEG–poly(aspartic acid) micelles	Doxorubicin	Passive	Various	Phase I clinical trials[44–46,57]
Xyotax	PGA nanoparticles	Paclitaxel	Passive	Lung, ovarian	Phase III clinical trials[44–46,48]
Mylotarg	Antibody–drug conjugate	Calicheamicin	Active (CD33)	Myeloid leukemia	FDA approved[44–46,55]
Ontak	Fusion protein	Diphtheria toxin fragment	Active (CD25)	T-cell limphoma	FDA approved[44–46,56]
Zevalin	Radiotherapeutic antibody	^{90}Yttrium	Active (CD20)	Non-Hodgkin lymphoma	FDA approved[44–46,54]
Bexxar	Radiotherapeutic antibody	^{131}Iodine	Active (CD20)	Non-Hodgkin lymphoma	FDA approved[44–46,54]
MBP-426	Liposome	Oxaliplatin	Active (Transferrin receptor)	Colon cancer	Phase I clinical trials[44,46,58]

tumoural tissues/organs (off-target action); immunorecognition or colloidal instability *in vivo*, which reduce the circulation time; the often unpredictable conformation of the ligand on the carrier, which may reduce the binding affinity to the target cells.[61]

Noteworthy is the use of metallic (e.g. gold[62]) or magnetic (e.g. iron oxide) nanoparticles for treating cancer by inducing hyperthermia, using, e.g., laser irradiation in the first case or an AC magnetic field of sufficient strength and frequency, and thus tissue necrosis. The threshold for these hyperthermia-based therapies is generally taken as a temperature of 42°C maintained for 30 min or more.[24,25]

12.4.2 Nucleic acid-based therapies

The delivery of nucleic acids (genetic material) is a promising treatment option for a vast number of diseases (including inherited disorders, some types of cancer, and certain viral infections), with a target that is generally the correction of genetic anomalies or gene activation paths that are responsible for the pathological condition. The direct injection of free DNA to a desired site is a simple but generally inefficient approach, because of the limited number of accessible sites (mostly skin and muscles) and of the easy degradation of the nucleic acids by the action of serum nucleases. A much higher efficiency can be obtained by encapsulating, protecting and finally releasing the nucleic acids with the use of nano-carriers, which are generally categorized as viral and non-viral ones.[63] Both these forms of carriers can be categorized as nanoparticles: indeed viruses can be seen as sophisticated, multifunctional nanoparticles, which are designed by nature to achieve the highest efficiency for gene delivery and expression. Viral carriers are generally categorized as: (a) retroviruses, i.e. RNA-containing viruses, which induce a transfected cell to produce an appropriate DNA sequence and integrate it in their genome; the lentivirus are likely the most popular sub-class of retrovirus, due to their capacity of transfecting also non-dividing cells; (b) adenoviruses, i.e. double stranded DNA viruses, that produce transient effects since their genome does not integrate with the host one and is therefore lost during mitosis; or (c) adeno-associated viruses, whose genome, differently form adenoviruses, integrate with the human one but always at the same chromosomal position and without disturbing any important gene. The clinical use of viral vectors, however, has to date been considerably limited by concerns about their safety and immunogenicity, which combine with the high costs of their preparation.[64,65]

Non-viral nano-carriers overwhelmingly consist of cationic polymers or cationic lipids; these compounds electrostatically bind negatively charged nucleic acids to form so-called polyplexes[66] and lipoplexes,[65] respectively. Poly(ethyleneimine) (PEI), poly(L-lysine) (PLL), polyamidoamine (PAMAM) dendrimers and chitosan are the most commonly used polycations, while lipoplex precursors are generally mixtures containing at least one amine-containing compound (e.g. N[1-(2,3-dioleyloxy) propyl]-N,N,N-trimethylammonium chloride (DOTMA)/1,2-dioleyl-sn-glycerol-3-phosphoethanolamine (DOPE); N-(2-hydroxyethyl)-N,N-dimethyl-2,3-bis(tetradecyloxy-1-propananium bromide) (DMRIE)/[N-(N0,N0-dimethylaminoethane)-carbamoyl] cholesterol; 1,2-dioleyl-3-trimethylammonium-propane (DOTAP)/cholesterol).

A significant limitation of polyplexes is their complex phase behaviour after complexation with nucleic acids, which lead to the transformation of liposomes into other lamellar or inverted hexagonal structures. There are also problems with the size of the carriers; first, the formation of both polyplexes and lipoplexes is essentially under kinetic control, which causes broad size distributions, and also a rather large variability in their average values (generally located from tens to hundreds of nanometers). Second, the frequent accumulation of both polyplexes and lipoplexes in the lungs, liver and spleen is often explained with their aggregation *in vivo*,[67] which is possibly mediated by protein adsorption. A futher limitation of non-viral vectors is their much lower transfection efficiency than viruses. However, non-viral vectors generally elicit considerably lower immune responses, their large-scale manufacture is possible and, although inefficient transfection and toxic responses have often hampered their clinical applications, the ease of chemical modification should eventually allow these problems to be minimized.[64,65,68]

For the above reasons, systems based on more stable nanoparticles, often presented PEGylated surfaces, have been developed.[65] For example, CAlAA-01, a complex nanoparticulate system based on four different components, has reached phase 1 in clinical trials. The formulation consists a duplex of synthetic siRNA, a cyclodextrin-containing polymer (CAL101), a PEG based stabilizing agent, and a targeting agent containing the human transferrin protein (Tf). These components assemble into highly multifunctional, targeted nanoparticles (approximately 100 nn in size) which are able to deliver siRNA for treating solid tumour cancers.[46]

12.4.3 Vaccines

Traditional vaccination methods consist of attenuated or heat-killed pathogens administered to healthy individuals; vaccines have been highly successful in preventing and eradicating a number of important global diseases, including smallpox and poliomyelitis. However, the search for an effective vaccine for several other widespread diseases such as malaria, tuberculosis and HIV has not produced sound results.[69] Therapeutic vaccines (i.e. designed to cure patients who are already infected or ill[70]) have also shown promising results against cancer, autoimmune diseases, as well as HIV, tuberculosis and hepatitis, although none of them are yet recognized as efficacious therapy in humans.[71] Vaccines currently have limitations with regard to two fundamental issues: (a) efficient delivery of the antigenic material to the antigen-presenting cells (APCs, mainly dendritic cells (DCs) and macrophages), and (b) subsequent APC activation to trigger adaptive immunity. APCs are efficient phagocytic cells, able to process and present peptidic antigens in form of both MHC (Major Histocompatibility Class) class I and class II molecules, which correspond to endogenous and exogenous antigens, respectively. Following antigen internalization and processing, these cells undergo activation (enhanced production of cytokines and chemokines, up-regulation of co-stimulatory signals which promote cell–cell interactions) and migration to lymph nodes for the purpose of activating antigen-specific T cells, i.e., the effector cells of the cell-mediated response.[72–74] Injectable nano-carriers have been used to deliver whole antigenic proteins, minimal peptide epitopes, or antigen-encoding DNA, into the MHC class I and II pathways of DCs.[75] These nano-carriers have been designed to prevent antigen degradation *in vivo*, sustain antigen release, and enhance DC targeting. A few examples follow.

Virosomes are liposomal carriers for antigens consisting of unilamellar vesicles with a mean diameter of 150 nm (approximately the size of a real virus); they are now commercially available for hepatitis and influenza vaccination.[76]

Virus-like particles (VLPs) are self-assembling particles ranging in size in the range 20–100 nm; they are composed of one or several viral proteins expressed *in vitro* through recombinant technologies.[77] A VLP-based vaccine for Hepatitis B is currently on the market,[77] as well as a prophylactic human papillomavirus (HPV) virus-like particle vaccine, which has shown clinical efficacy when administered intramuscularly.[78]

A number of more classical organic nanoparticles have also been used; for example poly(γ-glutamic acid) (γ-PGA) nanoparticles carrying ovalbumin (OVA) injected subcutaneously in mice induced significant expansion of OVA-specific $CD8^+$ T cells and antibody production without adverse effects.[79] Intradermal delivery of nanoparticles of dioleoylphosphatidylethanolamine (DOPE) and cholesterol, coated with an antigen-encoding pDNA, has shown efficacy in mice immunization.[80]

The efficacy of these particulate systems generally depends strongly on size and surface composition/charge, which determine likelihood and kinetics of their uptake in APCs, and on the way antigen is encapsulated or conjugated, which affects the antigen release profiles and the antigen processing pathway following uptake. Recent studies have shown the importance of nanoparticle size on the antigen trafficking to the draining lymph nodes near the injection site. In fact, large particles (>200–500 nm) generally limit the DC activation at the site of injection, whereas smaller particles were also found in lymph node-resident DC and macrophages, suggesting free drainage of these particles to the lymphatic system.[18]

Polymeric nanoparticles (Pluronic-stabilized poly(propylene sulphide) nanoparticles) with controlled size (20–40 nm) have been successfully delivered to the lymph nodes via interstitial flow, in order to target a large number of immature, lymph node-residing DCs.[72–74] This approach allows stimulation of cellular immunity without premature antigen presentation in peripheral tissues, which often leads to immune tolerance, and without inducing a strong inflammation for the recruitment of a sufficient number of peripheral DCs.

Since a large number of antigens are weak immunogens, unable to stimulate the necessary immune reaction,[81] vaccine formulations generally require co-administration of adjuvants, i.e. compounds that enhance antigen immunogenity with the effect of improving APC recruitment, migration and maturation. Injectable nanoparticulate vaccine systems can be designed to combine an efficient antigen presentation with adjuvant functions, for instance by co-loading or co-grafting antigens with 'danger signal', i.e. molecules which are able to activate the APCs (e.g. toll-like-receptor targeting by lipopolysaccharides, CpG DNA, etc.).[69,81] This additional adjuvant characteristic allows nanoparticles to trigger a more specific immune regulation and less non-specific (adverse) immune activation.

12.5 Injectable nanomaterials as matrix precursors

The *in situ* gelation of a fluid phase under physiological conditions of temperature and pH is a very promising approach for the preparation of 3D matrices for tissue engineering and drug delivery directly at the site of application. Such a procedure would be minimally invasive (to be compared to the implantation of a solid matrix) and its mild conditions would also allow for the safe incorporation of bioactive molecules or cells. Owing to biocompatibility requirements, the preparative processes cannot be based (solely) on the occurrence of chemical reactions, which often carry complications due to, e.g., temperature increase or presence of byproducts.[82] On the contrary, *in situ* gelling systems are often reliant on low-energy and physical (rather than chemical) self-assembly processes; these nano-scale aggregation phenomena yield structures that:

- are held together by attractive interactions and can be defined as nanostructured gels; they are characterized by multiple levels of order, bridging the (supra)molecular scale up to the microscopic one; often this corresponds to the production of fibrillar assemblies, which are directly inspired by or mimetic of natural structures.
- result from the arrest or the retardation of the dynamics of a system, and are often referred to as colloidal glasses and crystals. These structures are generally characterized by a lower or negligible degree of order at a molecular scale, and are often based on amphiphilic macromolecular compounds.

12.5.1 Self-assembled fibrillar hydrogels

Natural extra cellular matrices (ECMs) are characterized by a complex hierarchical organization centred at the nano scale. From a simplistic point of view, most ECMs are composed of fibrillar proteins (collagen and elastin) dispersed in a matrix of hydrated glycosaminoglycans; the fibre lateral size may range from tens to hundreds of nanometers.[83] This structure has inspired the design of fibrillar biomaterials as it is reasonable to expect that hydrogels with an ECM-mimetic morphology can show similarities in biomechanics and in the way they control cell adhesion, migration and proliferation. For instance, such an architecture provides resistance to tensile stresses through the fibrillar components and to compression through the hydrated glycosaminoglycan network. On the other hand, the aggregation of cell-adhesive molecules in fibres promotes cell ligand clustering that appears to be necessary for an effective adhesion to substrates.[84] For a long time, however, the *in situ* preparation of fibrillar materials has been essentially limited to the production of collagen gels.[85] The use of collagen has an important drawback, i.e. the necessity of maintaining a low pH to avoid its off-site gelation, which hinders its co-dispersion, e.g. with cells under non-gelling conditions. Additionally, concerns regarding the purity of animal products (presence of retrovirus, prion proteins, etc.) have always accompanied the use of collagen.

More recently, the issue of *in situ* forming fibrillar matrices has been tackled with the development of self-assembling synthetic peptides. Two main classes of such peptides can be recognized: the first one takes inspiration from the association properties of amyloid protein, with a self-assembly primarily based on the formation of β-sheets and on hydrophobic association;[86,87] this latter feature is often obtained by alternating ionic and hydrophobic aminoacidic residues,[88] although the presence of hydrophobic end-groups can promote similar effects.[89]

A second class of peptides takes the elastin $(VPGVG)_n$ motif as an inspiration to produce thermosensitive β-spirals, which allows a temperature-triggered formation of fibrillar hydrogels.[90,91]

The infinite possibilities that we have to synthesize a peptide sequence provide great versatility in designing the final structure and properties of the self-assembled hydrogel. However, unwanted immune responses when these gels are applied *in vivo* still remain a challenge.

12.5.2 Colloidal crystals and glasses

In soft matter, gels are commonly defined as materials kept together through attractive interactions. Strictly speaking, the materials described here, mostly derived from the self-assembly of macroamphiphiles, do not provide hydrogels but rather dynamically arrested colloidal systems with higher (crystals) or lower (glasses) degree of order.

A typical example is offered by Pluronics, i.e. triblock copolymers of PEG and poly(propylene glycol) (PPG); Pluronic suspensions, above a critical concentration, are typically liquid at room temperature, but undergo a very fast thermo-reversible gelation at body temperature, as a result of micellar ordering into mesoscopic crystalline phases.[92] The corresponding 'gels' have been widely used as injectable biomaterials to release *in vitro* and *in vivo* low MW therapeutics (sulindac, lidocaine, pilocarpine) as well as proteins (insulin, interleukin-2, chymotrypsin, and lactose dehydrogenase).[93] These systems suffer from major limitations arising from the weak noncovalent forces which hold together the polymeric micelles, e.g. weak mechanical strength, rapid dissolution in physiological fluids and correspondingly too fast drug release profiles. Some of these drawbacks can be overcome: for example, functional Pluronics can be first thermally gelled and then covalently cross-linked (e.g. under physiological conditions by Michael-type addition reactions[94]), irreversibly stabilizing the structure of the material. In alternative, Pluronic polymers can made be part of much larger colloidal structures, e.g. nanoparticles, that undergo similar sol-'gel' (vitrification) transitions, but due to their size show a much slower solubilization kinetics when placed in excess fluids.[95]

Pluronic-like block copolymers where PPG has been replaced by other hydrophobic blocks, such as poly(lactic-co-glycolic acid) (PLGA), have also been used as injectable biomaterials.[96] Similarly to Pluronics, these copolymers can undergo thermosensitive gel transition in the physiological range of temperatures, but the increased hydrophobicity and rigidity of the PLGA block improves mechanical strength and resistance to dilution in body fluids. These injectable hydrogels were capable of sustained release of various proteins (insulin, growth hormone, lysozyme, and calcitonin) and showed application potentials for cartilage regeneration.

12.5.3 Injectable inorganic/organic nanocomposites

Injectable nanocomposites are generally based on the use of an *in situ* gelling liquid dispersing an inorganic nano-sized material, most often of inorganic nature. Although the inorganic component can be used because, e.g., its radio-opacity allows a non-invasive imaging of the *in situ* produced material, these systems have been extensively used in the regeneration/replacement of hard tissues, where the presence of a mineralized component is essential to obtain the desired mechanical properties and possibly also to achieve optimal tissue morphogenesis: morphologicall, mineralized tissues such as bone or teeth are indeed inorganic/organic nanocomposites, where the nano-size of hydroxy-apatite crystals dispersed in a collagen matrix and their spatial organization contribute to the mechanical properties and functionality of the tissue[97] (see Fig. 12.2 for a pictorial sketch of this hierarchical organization).

A variety of nanocomposite materials designed to mimic the nanostructure and composition of natural bone have been proposed. The most common inorganic component is hydroxyapatite: it is the mineral component of bone and indeed it provides good osteoconductivity and adhesion to existing bone tissues.

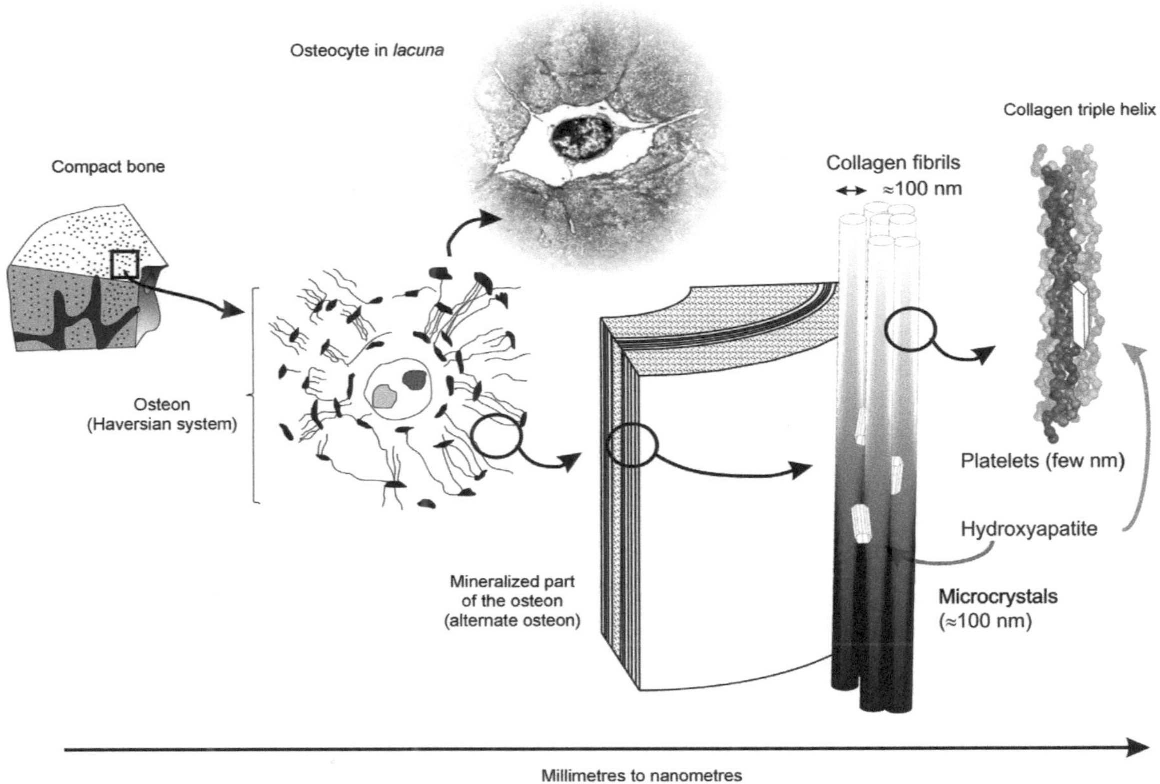

12.2 Bones offer a classical example of hierarchically organized architecture from nano-scale, where the collagen/hydroxyapatite nanocomposite is organized in fibrils, and fibrils are then laid in different textures, to the microscopic one where a regular organization of cells (osteocytes) and matrix around blood vessels constitutes the basic structure of compact bone (the so-called Haversian system or osteon).

The organic components (natural or synthetic polymeric matrices) must, on the contrary, provide structural continuity, porosity and possibility of remodelling which are necessary for cells to proliferate and differentiate.

In terms of composition, the most popular systems are those composed of collagen and of biodegradable polyesters/nano-hydroxyapatite, which have been widely used for bone regeneration *in vivo* with promising results. Compared to micron-sized hydroxyapatite, the incorporation of nano-hydroxyapatite offers a more biomimetic environment: the dimensions of hydroxyapatite crystals interdispersed with collagen fibrils are always in the nano range. Indeed the use of nano-hydroxyapatite generally results into an improved cell-mediated resorption during scaffold biodegradation.

Although these materials can be pre-fabricated in the lab and then implanted to the bone defect *in vivo*, injectable scaffolds are more suitable for treating irregularly shaped defects in applications such as vertebroplasty, bone cysts, and focal cartilage defects, where rigid scaffolds are clearly more difficult or even impossible to implant.[98] An ideal injectable precursor of a nanocomposite scaffold should be designed to exhibit suitable rheological properties for injection, maximum adhesion between the polymer and inorganic phase after gelation/solidification, to degrade concurrently *in vivo* to allow new hard tissue formation, and provide permeation and release bioactive agents. Taking into account these needs, aqueous dispersions of poly(L-lactide-*co*-ethylene oxide-*co*-fumarate) reinforced with nanosized hydroxyapatite particles have been proposed as injectable multiphasic polymer/ceramic nanocomposites,[98] with a peptide crosslinker which is degradable enzymatically by matrix metallo-proteinases. This nanocomposite has been shown to support attachment and migration of marrow stromal cells.

Thermoreversible gels of Pluronic conjugated with a hydroxyapatite binding peptide were used to template the growth of inorganic calcium phosphate in aqueous solutions.[82] This biomimetic approach was able to generate plate-like hydroxyapatite nanocrystals similar in size and shape to those present in the bone, thus showing promise as self-assembling, injectable nanocomposite biomaterials for orthopaedic applications.

12.6 Conclusions

The two main fields of application for nano-sized systems in injectable formulations are due to their capacities of:

- long-range circulation, which, coupled with the possibility of encapsulating, protecting and releasing a pharmacologically active payload, allows their use as nano-carriers. We here have illustrated some of the most important applications of nano-carriers in biomedicine, i.e. in imaging or in cancer, gene or vaccine therapies.

- producing solid-like matrices through mild and biologically acceptable processes, and with good control over their internal architecture. We have here illustrated the possible applications of these systems in regenerative medicine with examples of self-assembled peptide hydrogels, colloidal glasses and nanocomposites.

12.7 References

1. Hill, C.; Amodeo, A.; Joseph, J. V.; Patel, H. R. H., Nano- and microrobotics: how far is the reality? *Expert Review of Anticancer Therapy* **2008**, 8, 1891–1897.
2. Duran, J. D. G.; Arias, J. L.; Gallardo, V.; Delgado, A. V., Magnetic colloids as drug vehicles. *Journal of Pharmaceutical Sciences* **2008**, 97, (8), 2948–2983.
3. Haddy, F. J.; Grega, G. J.; Scott, J. B., Effects of histamine on lymph protein concentration and flow in dog forelimb. *American Journal of Physiology* **1972**, 223, (5), 1172–&.
4. Witte, C. L.; Witte, M. H.; Dumont, A. E.; Cole, W. R.; Smith, J. R., Protein content in lymph and edema fluids in congestive heart failure. *Circulation* **1969**, 40, (5), 623–&.
5. Neu, B.; Meiselman, H. J., Depletion-mediated red blood cell aggregation in polymer solutions. *Biophysical Journal* **2002**, 83, (5), 2482–2490.
6. Di Marco, M.; Sadun, C.; Port, M.; Guilbert, I.; Couvreur, P.; Dubernet, C., Physicochemical characterization of ultrasmall superparamagnetic iron oxide particles (USPIO) for biomedical application as MRI contrast agents. *International Journal of Nanomedicine* **2007**, 2, (4), 609–622.
7. Minchin, R., Sizing up targets with nanoparticles. *Nature Nanotechnology* **2008**, 3, (1), 12–13.
8. Choi, H. S.; Liu, W.; Misra, P.; Tanaka, E.; Zimmer, J. P.; Ipe, B. I.; Bawendi, M. G.; Frangioni, J. V., Renal clearance of quantum dots. *Nature Biotechnology* **2007**, 25, (10), 1165–1170.
9. Storm, G.; Belliot, S. O.; Daemen, T.; Lasic, D. D., Surface modification of nanoparticles to oppose uptake by the mononuclear phagocyte system. *Advanced Drug Delivery Reviews* **1995**, 17, (1), 31–48.
10. Vauthier, C.; Dubernet, C.; Fattal, E.; Pinto-Alphandary, H.; Couvreur, P., Poly(alkylcyanoacrylates) as biodegradable materials for biomedical applications. *Advanced Drug Delivery Reviews* **2003**, 55, (4), 519–548.
11. Kreuter, J., Nanoparticle-based drug delivery systems. *Journal of Controlled Release* **1991**, 16, (1–2), 169–176.
12. Brannon-Peppas, L.; Blanchette, J. O., Nanoparticle and targeted systems for cancer therapy. *Advanced Drug Delivery Reviews* **2004**, 56, (11), 1649–1659.
13. Maeda, H.; Wu, J.; Sawa, T.; Matsumura, Y.; Hori, K., Tumor vascular permeability and the EPR effect in macromolecular therapeutics: a review. *Journal of Controlled Release* **2000**, 65, (1–2), 271–284.
14. Tirelli, N., (Bio)responsive nanoparticles. *Current Opinion in Colloid & Interface Science* **2006**, 11, (4), 210–216.
15. Kim, J. S.; Yoon, T. J.; Kim, B. G.; Park, S. J.; Kim, H. W.; Lee, K. H.; Park, S. B.; Lee, J. K.; Cho, M. H., Toxicity and tissue distribution of magnetic nanoparticles in mice. *Toxicological Sciences* **2006**, 89, (1), 338–347.
16. Reddy, L. H.; Sharma, R. K.; Chuttani, K.; Mishra, A. K.; Murthy, R. S. R.,

Influence of administration route on tumor uptake and biodistribution of etoposide loaded solid lipid nanoparticles in Dalton's lymphoma tumor bearing mice. *Journal of Controlled Release* **2005**, 105, (3), 185–198.
17. Maincent, P.; Thouvenot, P.; Amicabile, C.; Hoffman, M.; Kreuter, J.; Couvreur, P.; Devissaguet, J. P., Lymphatic targeting of polymeric nanoparticles after intraperitoneal administration in rats. *Pharmaceutical Research* **1992**, 9, (12), 1534–1539.
18. Manolova, V.; Flace, A.; Bauer, M.; Schwarz, K.; Saudan, P.; Bachmann, M. F., Nanoparticles target distinct dendritic cell populations according to their size. *European Journal of Immunology* **2008**, 38, (5), 1404–1413.
19. Harisinghani, M. G.; Barentsz, J.; Hahn, P. F.; Deserno, W. M.; Tabatabaei, S.; van de Kaa, C. H.; de la Rosette, J.; Weissleder, R., Noninvasive detection of clinically occult lymph-node metastases in prostate cancer. *New England Journal of Medicine* **2003**, 348, (25), 2491–U5.
20. Nishioka, Y.; Yoshino, H., Lymphatic targeting with nanoparticulate system. *Advanced Drug Delivery Reviews* **2001**, 47, (1), 55–64.
21. Sharrna, P.; Brown, S.; Walter, G.; Santra, S.; Moudgil, B., Nanoparticles for bioimaging. *Advances in Colloid and Interface Science* **2006**, 123, 471–485.
22. Morawski, A. M.; Lanza, G. A.; Wickline, S. A., Targeted contrast agents for magnetic resonance imaging and ultrasound. *Current Opinion in Biotechnology* **2005**, 16, (1), 89–92.
23. Na, H. B.; Song, I. C.; Hyeon, T., Inorganic nanoparticles for MRI contrast agents. *Advanced Materials* **2009**, 21, (21), 2133–2148.
24. Pankhurst, Q. A.; Connolly, J.; Jones, S. K.; Dobson, J., Applications of magnetic nanoparticles in biomedicine. *Journal of Physics D – Applied Physics* **2003**, 36, (13), R167–R181.
25. Pankhurst, Q. A.; Thanh, N. K. T.; Jones, S. K.; Dobson, J., Progress in applications of magnetic nanoparticles in biomedicine. *Journal of Physics D – Applied Physics* **2009**, 42, (22).
26. Debbage, P.; Jaschke, W., Molecular imaging with nanoparticles: giant roles for dwarf actors. *Histochemistry and Cell Biology* **2008**, 130, (5), 845–875.
27. Rabin, O.; Perez, J. M.; Grimm, J.; Wojtkiewicz, G.; Weissleder, R., An X-ray computed tomography imaging agent based on long-circulating bismuth sulphide nanoparticles. *Nature Materials* **2006**, 5, (2), 118–122.
28. Liu, Z.; Cai, W. B.; He, L. N.; Nakayama, N.; Chen, K.; Sun, X. M.; Chen, X. Y.; Dai, H. J., *In vivo* biodistribution and highly efficient tumour targeting of carbon nanotubes in mice. *Nature Nanotechnology* **2007**, 2, (1), 47–52.
29. Natarajan, A.; Gruettner, C.; Ivkov, R.; DeNardo, G. L.; Mirick, G.; Yuan, A.; Foreman, A.; DeNardo, S. J., NanoFerrite particle based radioimmunonanoparticles: binding affinity and *in vivo* pharmacokinetics. *Bioconjugate Chemistry* **2008**, 19, (6), 1211–1218.
30. Hu, G.; Lijowski, M.; Zhang, H. Y.; Partlow, K. C.; Caruthers, S. D.; Kiefer, G.; Gulyas, G.; Athey, P.; Scott, M. J.; Wickline, S. A.; Lanza, G. M., Imaging of Vx-2 rabbit tumors with alpha v beta(3)-integrin-targeted In-111 nanoparticles. *International Journal of Cancer* **2007**, 120, (9), 1951–1957.
31. Michalet, X.; Pinaud, F. F.; Bentolila, L. A.; Tsay, J. M.; Doose, S.; Li, J. J.; Sundaresan, G.; Wu, A. M.; Gambhir, S. S.; Weiss, S., Quantum dots for live cells, *in vivo* imaging, and diagnostics. *Science* **2005**, 307, (5709), 538–544.
32. Rhyner, M. N.; Smith, A. M.; Gao, X. H.; Mao, H.; Yang, L. L.; Nie, S. M., Quantum dots and multifunctional nanoparticles: new contrast agents for tumor

imaging. *Nanomedicine* **2006**, 1, (2), 209–217.
33. Frangioni, J. V., *In vivo* near-infrared fluorescence imaging. *Current Opinion in Chemical Biology* **2003**, 7, (5), 626–634.
34. Kim, G.; Huang, S. W.; Day, K. C.; O'Donnell, M.; Agayan, R. R.; Day, M. A.; Kopelman, R.; Ashkenazi, S., Indocyanine-green-embedded PEBBLEs as a contrast agent for photoacoustic imaging. *Journal of Biomedical Optics* **2007**, 12, (4), 044020.
35. Xu, M. H.; Wang, L. H. V., Photoacoustic imaging in biomedicine. *Review of Scientific Instruments* **2006**, 77, (4), 041101.
36. Schultz, D. A., Plasmon resonant particles for biological detection. *Current Opinion in Biotechnology* **2003**, 14, (1), 13–22.
37. Cheon, J.; Lee, J. H., Synergistically integrated nanoparticles as multimodal probes for nanobiotechnology. *Accounts of Chemical Research* **2008**, 41, (12), 1630–1640.
38. Mancini, M. C.; Kairdolf, B. A.; Smith, A. M.; Nie, S. M., Oxidative quenching and degradation of polymer-encapsulated quantum dots: new insights into the long-term fate and toxicity of nanocrystals *in vivo*. *Journal of the American Chemical Society* **2008**, 130, (33), 10836–10837.
39. Brown, J. M.; William, W. R., Exploiting tumour hypoxia in cancer treatment. *Nature Reviews Cancer* **2004**, 4, (6), 437–447.
40. Allen, T. M., Ligand-targeted therapeutics in anticancer therapy. *Nature Reviews Cancer* **2002**, 2, (10), 750–763.
41. Kratz, F.; Muller, I. A.; Ryppa, C.; Warnecke, A., Prodrug strategies in anticancer chemotherapy. *Chemmedchem* **2008**, 3, (1), 20–53.
42. Ferrari, M., Cancer nanotechnology: opportunities and challenges. *Nat Rev Cancer* **2005**, 5, (3), 161–171.
43. Owens Iii, D. E.; Peppas, N. A., Opsonization, biodistribution, and pharmacokinetics of polymeric nanoparticles. *International Journal of Pharmaceutics* **2006**, 307, (1), 93–102.
44. Heath, J. R.; Davis, M. E., Nanotechnology and cancer. *Annual Review of Medicine* **2008**, 59, 251–265.
45. Lammers, T.; Hennink, W. E.; Storm, G., Tumour-targeted nanomedicines: principles and practice. *British Journal of Cancer* **2008**, 99, (3), 392–397.
46. Davis, M. E.; Chen, Z.; Shin, D. M., Nanoparticle therapeutics: an emerging treatment modality for cancer. *Nat Rev Drug Discov* **2008**, 7, (9), 771–782.
47. Sutton, D.; Nasongkla, N.; Blanco, E.; Gao, J. M., Functionalized micellar systems for cancer targeted drug delivery. *Pharmaceutical Research* **2007**, 24, (6), 1029–1046.
48. Boddy, A. V.; Plummer, E. R.; Todd, R.; Sludden, J.; Griffin, M.; Robson, L.; Cassidy, J.; Bissett, D.; Bernareggi, A.; Verrill, M. W.; Calvert, A. H., A phase I and pharmacokinetic study of paclitaxel poliglumex (XYOTAX), investigating both 3-weekly and 2-weekly schedules. *Clinical Cancer Research* **2005**, 11, (21), 7834–7840.
49. Joshi, M. D.; Muller, R. H., Lipid nanoparticles for parenteral delivery of actives. *European Journal of Pharmaceutics and Biopharmaceutics* **2009**, 71, (2), 161–172.
50. Tomalia, D. A.; Reyna, L. A.; Svenson, S., Dendrimers as multi-purpose nano-devices for oncology drug delivery and diagnostic imaging. *Biochemical Society Transactions* **2007**, 35, 61–67.
51. Fu, K.; Sun, J.; Bickford, L. R.; Lin, A. W. H.; Halas, N. J.; Yu, T. K.; Drezek, R. A., Measurement of immunotargeted plasmonic nanoparticles' cellular binding: a key factor in optimizing diagnostic efficacy. *Nanotechnology* **2008**, 19, (4), 045103.

52. Lowery, A. R.; Gobin, A. M.; Day, E. S.; Halas, N. J.; West, J. L., Immunonanoshells for targeted photothermal ablation of tumor cells. *International Journal of Nanomedicine* **2006**, 1, (2), 149–154.
53. Zamboni, W. C., Liposomal, nanoparticle, and conjugated formulations of anticancer agents. *Clinical Cancer Research* **2005**, 11, (23), 8230–8234.
54. Allen, T. M., Ligand-targeted therapeutics in anticancer therapy. *Nat Rev Cancer* **2002**, 2, (10), 750–763.
55. Bross, P. F.; Beitz, J.; Chen, G.; Chen, X. H.; Duffy, E.; Kieffer, L.; Roy, S.; Sridhara, R.; Rahman, A.; Williams, G.; Pazdur, R., Approval summary: Gemtuzumab ozogamicin in relapsed acute myeloid leukemia. *Clinical Cancer Research* **2001**, 7, (6), 1490–1496.
56. Kawakami, K.; Nakajima, O.; Morishita, R.; Nagai, R., Targeted anticancer immunotoxins and cytotoxic agents with direct killing moieties. *The Scientific World Journal* **2006**, 6, 781–790.
57. Matsumura, Y.; Hamaguchi, T.; Ura, T.; Muro, K.; Yamada, Y.; Shimada, Y.; Shirao, K.; Okusaka, T.; Ueno, H.; Ikeda, M.; Watanabe, N., Phase I clinical trial and pharmacokinetic evaluation of NK911, a micelle-encapsulated doxorubicin. *Br J Cancer* **2004**, 91, (10), 1775–1781.
58. Zamboni, W. C., Concept and clinical evaluation of carrier-mediated anticancer agents. *The Oncologist* **2008**, 13, 248–260.
59. Padera, T. P.; Stoll, B. R.; Tooredman, J. B.; Capen, D.; Tomaso, E. D.; Jain, R. K., Pathology: cancer cells compress intratumour vessels. *Nature* **2004**, 427, (6976), 695.
60. Sparreboom, A.; Scripture, C. D.; Trieu, V.; Williams, P. J.; De, T. P.; Yang, A.; Beals, B.; Figg, W. D.; Hawkins, M.; Desai, N., Comparative preclinical and clinical pharmacokinetics of a cremophor-free, nanoparticle albumin-bound paclitaxel (ABI-007) and paclitaxel formulated in cremophor (Taxol). *Clinical Cancer Research* **2005**, 11, (11), 4136–4143.
61. Nobs, L.; Buchegger, F.; Gurny, R.; Allemann, E., Current methods for attaching targeting ligands to liposomes and nanoparticles. *Journal of Pharmaceutical Science* **2004**, 93, 1980–1992.
62. Day, E. S.; Morton, J. G.; West, J. L., Nanoparticles for Thermal Cancer Therapy. *Journal of Biomechanical Engineering-Transactions of the Asme* **2009**, 131, (7), 074001.
63. El-Aneed, A., An overview of current delivery systems in cancer gene therapy. *Journal of Controlled Release* **2004**, 94, (1), 1–14.
64. Liu, F.; Huang, L., Development of non-viral vectors for systemic gene delivery. *Journal of Controlled Release* **2002**, 78, (1–3), 259–266.
65. Morille, M.; Passirani, C.; Vonarbourg, A.; Clavreul, A.; Benoit, J. P., Progress in developing cationic vectors for non-viral systemic gene therapy against cancer. *Biomaterials* **2008**, 29, (24–25), 3477–3496.
66. Wagner, E., Strategies to improve DNA polyplexes for *in vivo* gene transfer: will 'artificial viruses' be the answer? *Pharmaceutical Research* **2004**, 21, (1), 8–14.
67. Simberg, D.; Danino, D.; Talmon, Y.; Minsky, A.; Ferrari, M. E.; Wheeler, C. J.; Barenholz, Y., Phase behavior, DNA ordering, and size instability of cationic lipoplexes – relevance to optimal transfection activity. *Journal of Biological Chemistry* **2001**, 276, (50), 47453–47459.
68. Niidome, T.; Huang, L., Gene therapy progress and prospects: nonviral vectors. *Gene Therapy* **2002**, 9, (24), 1647–1652.
69. Gamvrellis, A.; Leong, D.; Hanley, J. C.; Xiang, S. D.; Mottram, P.; Plebanski, M.,

Vaccines that facilitate antigen entry into dendritic cells. *Immunology and Cell Biology* **2004**, 82, (5), 506–516.
70. Dawson, A., Therapeutic vaccines: a solution to the prevention problem? *Vaccine* **2005**, 23, (17–18), 2363–2366.
71. Melief, C. J. M.; van der Burg, S. H., Immunotherapy of established (pre) malignant disease by synthetic long peptide vaccines. *Nature Reviews Cancer* **2008**, 8, (5), 351–360.
72. Reddy, S. T.; Rehor, A.; Schmoekel, H. G.; Hubbell, J. A.; Swartz, M. A., *In vivo* targeting of dendritic cells in lymph nodes with poly(propylene sulfide) nanoparticles. *Journal of Controlled Release* **2006**, 112, (1), 26–34.
73. Reddy, S. T.; Swartz, M. A.; Hubbell, J. A., Targeting dendritic cells with biomaterials: developing the next generation of vaccines. *Trends in Immunology* **2006**, 27, (12), 573–579.
74. Reddy, S. T.; van der Vlies, A. J.; Simeoni, E.; Angeli, V.; Randolph, G. J.; O'Neill, C. P.; Lee, L. K.; Swartz, M. A.; Hubbell, J. A., Exploiting lymphatic transport and complement activation in nanoparticle vaccines. *Nature Biotechnology* **2007**, 25, (10), 1159–1164.
75. Perrie, Y.; Mohammed, A. R.; Kirby, D. J.; McNeil, S. E.; Bramwell, V. W., Vaccine adjuvant systems: enhancing the efficacy of sub-unit protein antigens. *International Journal of Pharmaceutics* **2008**, 364, (2), 272–280.
76. Couvreur, P.; Vauthier, C., Nanotechnology: intelligent design to treat complex disease. *Pharmaceutical Research* **2006**, 23, (7), 1417–1450.
77. Scheerlinck, J.-P. Y.; Greenwood, D. L. V., Virus-sized vaccine delivery systems. *Drug Discovery Today* **2008**, 13, (19–20), 882–887.
78. Schiller, J. T.; Castellsagué, X.; Villa, L. L.; Hildesheim, A., An update of prophylactic human papillomavirus L1 virus-like particle vaccine clinical trial results. *Vaccine* **2008**, 26, (Supplement 10), K53–K61.
79. Uto, T.; Wang, X.; Akagi, T.; Zenkyu, R.; Akashi, M.; Baba, M., Improvement of adaptive immunity by antigen-carrying biodegradable nanoparticles. *Biochemical and Biophysical Research Communications* **2009**, 379, (2), 600–604.
80. Cui, Z.; Baizer, L.; Mumper, R. J., Intradermal immunization with novel plasmid DNA-coated nanoparticles via a needle-free injection device. *Journal of Biotechnology* **2003**, 102, (2), 105–115.
81. Swartz, M. A.; Hubbell, J. A.; Reddy, S. T., Lymphatic drainage function and its immunological implications: from dendritic cell homing to vaccine design. *Seminars in Immunology* **2008**, 20, (2), 147–156.
82. Yusufoglu, Y.; Hu, Y.; Kanapathipillai, M.; Kramer, M.; Kalay, Y. E.; Thiyagarajan, P.; Akinc, M.; Schmidt-Rohr, K.; Mallapragada, S., Bioinspired synthesis of self-assembled calcium phosphate nanocomposites using block copolymer-peptide conjugates. *Journal of Materials Research* **2008**, 23, (12), 3196–3212.
83. Ma, Z.; Kotaki, M.; Inai, R.; Ramakrishna, S., Potential of nanofiber matrix as tissue-engineering scaffolds. *Tissue Engineering* **2005**, 11, (1–2), 101–109.
84. Lutolf, M. P.; Hubbell, J. A., Synthetic biomaterials as instructive extracellular microenvironments for morphogenesis in tissue engineering. *Nature Biotechnology* **2005**, 23, (1), 47–55.
85. Gillette, B. M.; Jensen, J. A.; Tang, B. X.; Yang, G. J.; Bazargan-Lari, A.; Zhong, M.; Sia, S. K., *In situ* collagen assembly for integrating microfabricated three-dimensional cell-seeded matrices. *Nature Materials* **2008**, 7, (8), 636–640.
86. Krysmann, M. J.; Castelletto, V.; Kelarakis, A.; Hamley, I. W.; Hule, R. A.; Pochan, D. J., Self-assembly and hydrogelation of an amyloid peptide fragment.

Biochemistry **2008**, 47, (16), 4597–4605.
87. Nagarkar, R. P.; Hule, R. A.; Pochan, D. J.; Schneider, J. P., *De novo* design of strand-swapped beta-hairpin hydrogels. *Journal of the American Chemical Society* **2008**, 130, (13), 4466–4474.
88. Kisiday, J.; Jin, M.; Kurz, B.; Hung, H.; Semino, C.; Zhang, S.; Grodzinsky, A. J., Self-assembling peptide hydrogel fosters chondrocyte extracellular matrix production and cell division: implications for cartilage tissue repair. *Proceedings of the National Academy of Sciences of the United States of America* **2002**, 99, (15), 9996–10001.
89. Smith, A. M.; Williams, R. J.; Tang, C.; Coppo, P.; Collins, R. F.; Turner, M. L.; Saiani, A.; Ulijn, R. V., Fmoc-Diphenylalanine self assembles to a hydrogel via a novel architecture based on pi-pi interlocked beta-sheets. *Advanced Materials* **2008**, 20, (1), 37–41.
90. Bellingham, C. M.; Lillie, M. A.; Gosline, J. M.; Wright, G. M.; Starcher, B. C.; Bailey, A. J.; Woodhouse, K. A.; Keeley, F. W., Recombinant human elastin polypeptides self-assemble into biomaterials with elastin-like properties. *Biopolymers* **2003**, 70, (4), 445–455.
91. Ma, M. L.; Kuang, Y.; Gao, Y.; Zhang, Y.; Gao, P.; Xu, B., Aromatic–aromatic interactions induce the self-assembly of pentapeptidic derivatives in water to form nanofibers and supramolecular hydrogels. *Journal of the American Chemical Society* **2010**, 132, (8), 2719–2728.
92. Mortensen, K., PEO-related block copolymer surfactants. *Colloids and Surfaces A – Physicochemical and Engineering Aspects* **2001**, 183, 277–292.
93. Branco, M.; Wagner, N.; Pochan, D.; Schneider, J., Release of model macromolecules from self-assembling peptide hydrogels for injectable delivery. *Biopolymers* **2009**, 92, (4), 318–318.
94. Cellesi, F.; Tirelli, N.; Hubbell, J. A., Materials for cell encapsulation via a new tandem approach combining reverse thermal gelation and covalent crosslinking. *Macromolecular Chemistry and Physics* **2002**, 203, (10–11), 1466–1472.
95. Missirlis, D.; Hubbell, J. A.; Tirelli, N., Thermally-induced glass formation from hydrogel nanoparticles. *Soft Matter* **2006**, 2, (12), 1067–1075.
96. Chung, H. J.; Park, T. G., Self-assembled and nanostructured hydrogels for drug delivery and tissue engineering. *Nano Today* **2009**, 4, (5), 429–437.
97. Wei, G. B.; Ma, P. X., Nanostructured biomaterials for regeneration. *Advanced Functional Materials* **2008**, 18, (22), 3568–3582.
98. Sarvestani, A. S.; Jabbari, E., Modeling and experimental investigation of rheological properties of injectable poly(lactide ethylene oxide fumarate)/hydroxyapatite nanocomposites. *Biomacromolecules* **2006**, 7, (5), 1573–1580.

13
Injectable biodegradable materials

B. JEONG, Ewha Womans University, South Korea

Abstract: During the last decade, there has been extensive research on injectable biodegradable materials that are to be used as an *in-situ* gelling depot system for sustained release of an incorporated drug. In this chapter, thermogelling biodegradable polymer aqueous solutions are reviewed. These are low-viscous sols at a low temperature and become gels at the body temperature of warm-blooded animals by heat induced sol-to-gel transition. Such a thermogelling polymer aqueous solution has been suggested to be a very promising biomaterial as a minimally invasive injectable system for drug delivery and tissue engineering applications. This chapter focuses on 'material characteristics' of the theromogelling biodegradable polymers developed so far, and 'perspectives' on the new material.

Key words: biodegradability, sol-gel transition, thermosensitivity, hydrogel, block copolymer, *in-situ* gelation, drug delivery system.

13.1 Introduction

A thermogelling polymer aqueous solution undergoes a sol-to-gel transition as the temperature increases. It is an aqueous solution at room temperature (20°C) or lower, and forms a semisolid gel at the body temperature (37°C). Recent reviews related to the current topic are cited in the references.[1–4] To show thermal gelation behavior, the polymer should have a balanced structure of hydrophobicity and hydrophilicity. Typically, polyesters, polyphosphazenes, poly(propylene glycol), polypeptides, polyorthoesters, polycarbonates, and polycyanoacrylates, and poly(N-hydroxypropylmehacrylamide-oligolactate) have been used as a biodegradable hydrophobic block and poly(ethylene glycol) have been used as a hydrophilic block.

13.2 Poly(ethylene glycol) (PEG) copolymers

Historically, the most extensively studied biodegradable polymer is based on poly(lactide), poly(glycolide) and their copolymers. To give the aqueous solubility to the poly(L-lactic acid-co-glycolic acid) (PLGA), poly(ethylene glycol) (PEG) was conjugated to form a PLGA/PEG block copolymer. PEG is a hydrophilic polymer that is approved by the Food and Drug Administration for

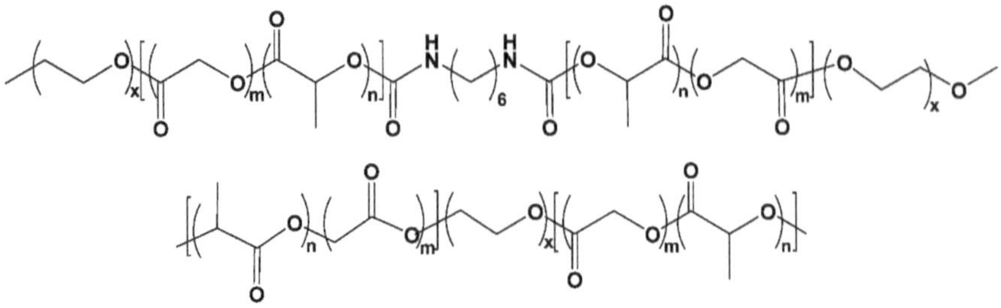

13.1 Structure of PEG/PLGA triblock copolymers. ABA type (top) and BAB type (bottom).

clinical uses in intravenous, intramuscular, topical, and oral applications.[5] Two water molecules are hydrogen bonded to an ethylene glycol repeating unit of the PEG, which are detached as the temperature increases, and finally the PEG is precipitate at its lower critical solution temperature (LCST).[6] LCST is dependent on its molecular weight. As the molecular weight of PEG increases, the LCST decreases.[7] Initially, PEG/poly(L-lactic acid) di- and triblock copolymers were reported as an injectable system.[8] When a short chain PEG was used to increase the hydrophobicity of polymer, the PEG/PLGA polymer aqueous solution showed sol-to-gel transition as the temperature increased.[9] PEG/PLGA triblock copolymers with ABA and BAB types were reported as a biodegradable thermogelling polymer (Fig. 13.1).[10–12] An *in-situ* formed gel of PEG-PLGA-PEG was degraded *in-vivo* (in rats) and *in-vitro* (in phosphate buffered saline) over 1–2 months. A tight aggregation of the PEG-PLGA-PEG and an increase in the hydrophobicity of the polymer during the degradation prolong the duration of PEG-PLGA-PEG gel, whereas a poly(ethylene glycol)-poly(propylene glycol)-poly(ethylene glycol) (PEG-PPG-PEG; Poloxamer® or Pluronic®) gel shows a few days of gel duration at best.[13]

A gel duration from a week to several months was realized by topological variation of the PEG/PLGA copolymer system. The PEG-g-PLGA showed one week of gel duration, whereas PLGA-g-PEG showed more than three months of gel duration, even though the composition of the two polymers was similar.[14,15] The topological structures of PEG-g-PLGA and PLGA-g-PEG are shown in Fig. 13.2.

The thermogelling PLGA is an amorphous polymer with a low glass transition temperature. Therefore, the PEG/PLGA copolymer systems of which

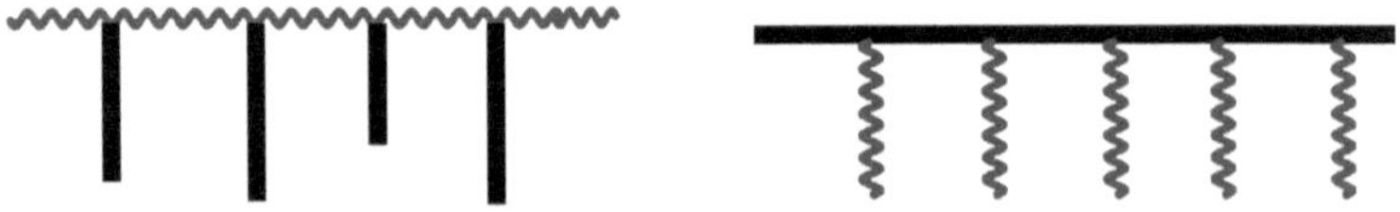

13.2 Schematic presentation of the structure of PLGA-g-PEG and PEG-g-PLGA. Thick black bars and wavy gray lines indicate the hydrophobic PLGA and hydrophilic PEG, respectively.

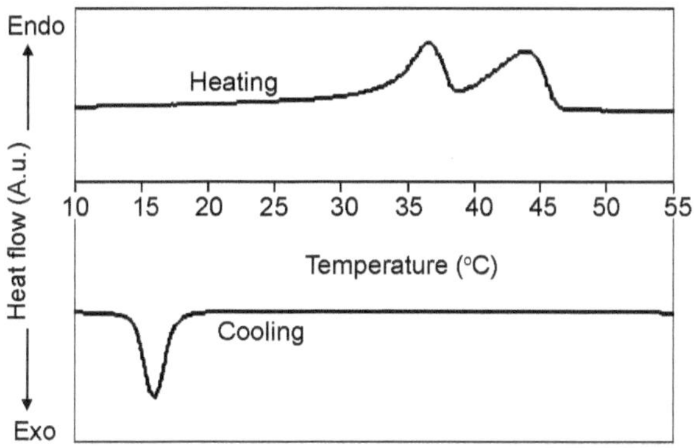

13.3 Differential scanning calorimeter thermogram of PEG-PCL-PEG (550-2100-550)[16] (with permission from American Chemical Society).

aqueous solution show thermal gelation properties has thick paste morphology at room temperature. It takes several hours to prepare a polymer aqueous solution (1.0 ml), as the aqueous solubility of the polymer decreases as the temperature increases. To solve these problems, biodegradable crystalline polycaprolactone (PCL) was introduced instead of amorphous PLGA in designing a thermogelling polymer. The PEG/PCL system shows a melting point of 40–50°C and powder morphology at room temperature (Fig. 13.3). Thus, the polymer is convenient to handle to weigh and transfer in a powder form. A homogeneous polymer aqueous solution can be prepared in a minute by heating the polymer suspension in water to the melting point of the polymer (40–50°C), followed by quenching the mixture into an ice-bath.[16,17]

However, a clear aqueous solution of PEG/PCL becomes turbid in 30 minutes at room temperature due to the crystallization of PCL block. The poly(caprolactone-co-trimethylene carbonate)-PEG-poly(caprolactone-co-trimethylene carbonate) (PCTC-PEG-PCTC) was prepared to prevent the crystallization of the PCL block.[18] A multiblock copolymer of $(PEG\text{-}PCL)_n$ with kinks in the hydrophobic block also decreases the crystallization of the PCL.[19] Aqueous solutions of poly(caprolactone-co-glycolic acid)-PEG-poly(caprolactone-co-glycolic acid) (PCGA-PEG-PCGA) were also reported.[20] Such systems keep the solution stability against crystallization-induced precipitation, while the gel modulus significantly decreased compared with PEG/PCL system. As an end group modification of the polymer, hydroxyl end groups of PLGA-PEG-PLGA were modified by acetyl, propionyl, and butanoyl groups.[20,21] In addition, hydroxyl end groups of poly(caprolactone-co-lactic acid)-PEG-poly(caprolactone-co-lactic acid) (PCLA-PEG-PCLA) were also modified by alkyl group.[22] The increase in the hydrophobicity of the polymer by the alkyl end groups decreased the thermal gelation temperature of the polymer aqueous solution. Star-shaped PEG/PLGA was developed as a thermogelling polymer. The star-shaped polymer showed a smaller micelle size and a higher critical gel concentration (CGC) than liner triblock copolymers.[23] An eight-armed star-shape was end-capped by hydrophobic cholesterol. The aqueous solutions of the cholesterol end-capped star shape poly(L-lactic acid)-PEG showed the CGC of 3 wt%. Such a decrease in the CGC is caused by the strong hydrophobic association of cholesterol groups in water.[24] Poly(propylene fumarate)-PEG-poly(propylene fumarate) has unsaturated double bonds that can be further crosslinked to modulate the mechanical properties and stability of an *in-situ* formed gel.[25,26] Poly(DL-3-methylene glycolide)-PEG-poly(DL-3-methylene glycolide) has an alternating structure of glycolic acid and lactic acid in the repeating unit. The aqueous solution of the polymer also showed thermal gelation, similar to the PLGA system.[27] Poly(L-lactic acid) (PLLA) and poly(D-lactic acid) (PDLA) can make a stereocomplex. Stereocomplex of PLLA-PEG-PLLA and poly PDLA-PEG-PDLA aqueous solutions showed thermal gelation, even though the aqueous solutions of each enantiomeric polymer did not show thermal gelation.[28]

A pH/temperature sensitive system was also reported as an injectable system. The pH sensitive units can complex with a protein drug with opposite charges to reduce the initial burst release of an incorporated drug.[29] Thermogelling PEG/PCGA, PEG/PCL, and PEG/PCLA were coupled to pH sensitive amine containing blocks to prepare pH/temperature sensitive gelling system.[30,31]

13.3 Poloxamer® and Pluronic® gels

Aqueous solutions of Poloxamer or Pluronic undergo sol-to-gel transition as the temperature increases (Fig. 13.4). However, the implanted gel of Poloxamer is quickly eroded and does not persist for more than a few days at most. To improve the system, end-group modified Poloxamers, and multiblock copolymers consisting of Poloxamer and biodegradable polymers have been developed. In addition, random multiblock copolymers consisting of PEG, PPG, and a biodegradable polymer were reported.

Even though modification of the hydroxyl end groups of Poloxamer by oligolactides (LA_6) and oligocaprolactones (CL_6) increases hydrophobicity of the polymer, the sol-to-gel transition temperature and critical gel concentration increased, compared with the unmodified Poloxamer.[32,33] The sol-to-gel transition of the Poloxamer aqueous solution is driven by the unimer-to-micelle transition, followed by packing of the micelles. The oligolactide and oligocaprolactone partition into the PPG micelle core and disturb the integrity and

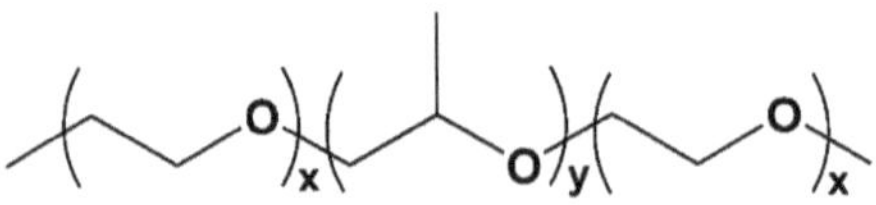

13.4 Structure of poloxamer.

density of the original micelles of the unmodified Poloxamer. Thus, the micelle packing mechanism for the sol-to-gel transition is interfered with. Poloxamer (F127) was modified by oligolactide (LA_8 or LA_{18}), and was then reacted with succinic anhydrides to prepare a carboxylic acid end-capped Poloxamer. The polymer showed sol-gel transition in a pH/temperature dependent manner. The ionization of carboxylic acid and the decrease in solubility of PEG at high pH were suggested to explain the phase behavior.[34,35] L-dihydroxyphenyalanine end-capped Poloxamer (F127) showed an increase in bioadhesion between the polymer and bovine mucin, an increase in the sol-to-gel transition temperature.[36]

Multiblock copolymers were prepared to improve gel properties such as gel duration and biodegradation. Poloxamers (F127) were coupled by hexa-methylene diisocyanate to prepare multiblock Poloxamer.[37] The drug release rate from the multiblock Poloxamer hydrogel was slower than from the unmodified Poloxamer hydrogel. PEG/PPG alternating multiblock copolymers showing thermogelling were reported.[38,39] In addition, PEG end-capped by oligocaprolactone or oligolactide and PPG were coupled to make PEG/PPG alternating biodegradable block copolymers.[40,41] As a ternary system, hydroxyl end groups of PEG, PPG, and poly(hydroxyl butyrate) (PHB) were reacted with hexamethylene diisocynate to give biodegradability and thermogelling properties of the resulting random multiblock copolymer of PEG/PPG/PHB. The polymer showed a CGC as low as 2.0 wt% and the gel persisted for more than six months.[42,43] Poloxamer was coupled by terephthalic anhydride to introduce the biodegradability as well as pH sensitivity.[35] Poloxamer was also coupled by disulfide to show glutathione sensitive degradation and drug release.[44] In addition, Poloxamer was end capped by L-oligolactide or D-oligolactide, then coupled to prepare the multiblock Poloxamer containing PLA. By mixing the L-isomer and D-isomer containing multiblock Poloxamer, a stereocomplex showing thermal gelation was prepared.[45]

Polyphosphazene is prepared by ring-opening polymerization of hexachloro-cyclotriphosphazene to make a poly(dichlorophosphazene), followed by nucleo-philic substitution reactions to poly(dichlorophosphazene) (Fig. 13.5). Biodegradability and hydrophilic/hydrophobic balance can be controlled by

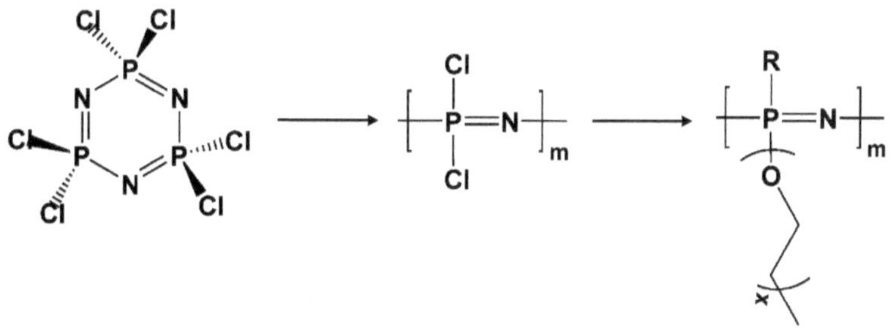

13.5 Synthetic scheme of polyphosphazene.

varying the substituent. PEGs with a molecular weight range of 350–750 daltons were used as a hydrophilic block. Hydrophobic blocks varying from single amino acid such as Ile, Leu, and Val to di-, tri-, and oligopeptides were used to control the sol-to-gel transition temperature and the gel modulus.[46] Increasing the molecular weight of PEG, the sol-to-gel transition temperature increased. The sol-to-gel transition temperature decreased as the hydrophobicity of the polyphosphazene increased. The sol-to-gel transition temperature of methoxy PEG/Gly-Phe-ethoxyLeu substituted polyphosphazene aqueous solution (10 wt%) was 15°C , which was lower than that of methoxy PEG/ Gly-Phe-ethoxyIle substituted polyphosphazene aqueous solution of 32°C.[47] By simple mixing the polyphosphazenes aqueous solutions with different sol-to-gel transition temperatures, the sol-to-gel transition temperature of the polymer aqueous solution could be controlled.[48] The degradation rate of polyphosphazene could be controlled by varying amino acid sequence, composition of the polypeptide, and molecular weight of PEG. When glycylglycolate was incorporated into the hydrophobic block, the degradation rate of the polyphosphazene was significantly accelerated.[49,50] The intra- and intermolecular catalyses by carboxylic acid generated by the hydrolysis of the glycylglycolate units were suggested as the enhancement mechanism of the degradation rate of the polyphosphazene.

The structure of chitosan is shown in Fig. 13.6. Chitosan/β-glycerol phosphate aqueous solutions undergo sol-to-gel transition as the temperature increases.[51] Chitosan is dissolved in acidic aqueous solution with a 1.5 wt%. Then, β-glycerol phosphate is slowly added up to 4.5 wt%, and the final pH of the solution is adjusted to 7.0. pK_as of chitosan and β-glycerol phosphate are 6.2 and 6.65, respectively, at 25°C.[52] As the temperature increases, the extent of protonation of chitosan slightly decreases, leading to a decrease in solubility of chitosan. On the other hand, the degree of ionization of β-glycerol phosphate significantly increases as the temperature increases.[53] The increased ionic strength of the aqueous solution screens the ionic repulsion of the chitosan, therefore, hydrophobic associations of chitosan are facilitated to

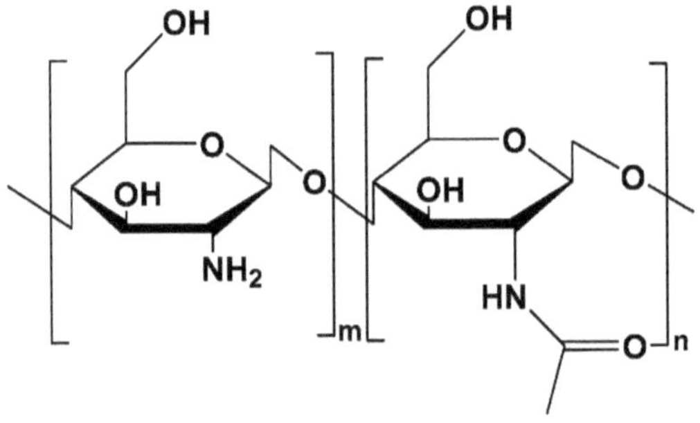

13.6 Structure of chitosan.

induce the sol-to-gel transition of the chitosan/β-glycerol phosphate aqueous solution.

Aqueous solutions of chitosan-g-PEG and hyarulonic acid-g-Poloxamer undergoing thermal gelation were reported.[54,55] Aqueous solutions of hydroxypropyl methylcellulose or methyl cellulose also show thermal gelation. The hydrophobic interactions were suggested as the sol-to-gel transition mechanism.[56] Aqueous solutions of the inclusion complexes between methylated α-cyclodextrin (α-CD) and PEG were reported as a thermogelling system.[57,58] The aggregation of methylated α-CD forms a cluster network in the gel state.[59]

13.4 Polypeptides

Owing to the well-defined stereochemistry, the diversities in choosing hydropbobic/hydrophilic amino acids, and specific secondary structures, polypeptides have been intensively investigated as a biomaterial.[60–67] Contrary to the random hydrophobically driven self-assembly of the most synthetic polymer, the secondary structures of the polypeptides such as α-helix , β-sheet, and random coil significantly affect the gelation behavior.

Aqueous solutions of natural polypeptides such as β-lactoglobulin and elastin-like polypeptide (ELP) showed thermal gelation. The dimeric form of β-lactoglobulin with antiparallel β-sheet structure at room temperature dissociates into monomeric forms as the temperature increases to above 65°C.[68] Then, they expose their hydrophobic groups (denaturation) and thiols, resulting in aggregate formation (aggregation). The exposed thiol/disulfide groups undergo thiol/ disulfide exchange reactions to induce gelation of the β-lactoglobulin (gelation) as the temperature increases.[69,70]

Elastin has a Val-Pro-Gly-Val-Gly (VPGVG) as a most prominent sequence. Poly(VPGVG) was synthesized as an elastin-like polypeptide. It undergoes random coil-to-β-sheet transition in water and shows sol-to-precipitation as the temperature increases. The VPGVG, (Pro-Hyp-Gly), poly(ethylene glycol), or L-polyhistidine were copolymerized to prepare a theromogelling polymer.[71,72] In addition, elastin-like (VPGVG) polypeptides and silk-like (Gly-Ala-Gly-Ala-Gly-Ser) polypeptides were connected to form a silk-elastin-like polymer.[73] As a purely synthetic polypeptides, a *de novo* synthesized polypeptide (Val-Lys-Val-Lys-Val-Lys-Tyr-Lys-Val-Pro-Pro-Tyr-Lys-Val-Lys-Tyr-Lys-Val-Lys-Val) was reported as a thermogelling polypeptide. It underwent a random coil to β-hairpin like transition in water as the temperature increased.[74] Thus, the polypeptide aqueous solution becomes a gel at high temperature.

MonomethoxyPEG-polyalanine (mPEG-PA), polyalanine-Poloxamer-polyalanine (PA-PLX-PA) and mPEG-poly(Ala-co-Phe) (mPEG-PAF) were reported as thermogelling polypeptides.[75–77] As the temperature increased, β-sheet conformation was partially strengthened and PEG dehydrated. The secondary structure of polypeptides plays a role in driving the sol-to-gel transition.

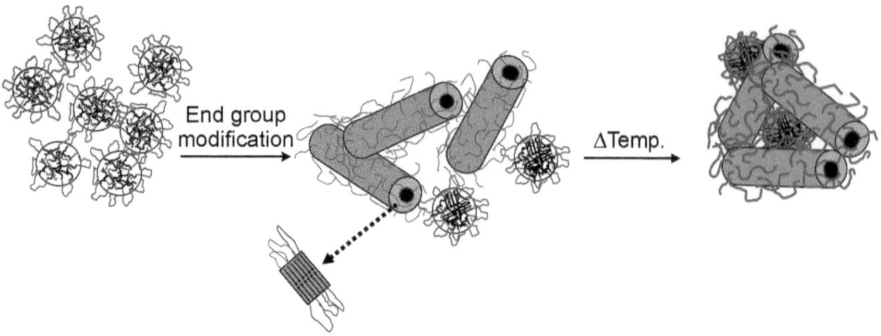

13.7 Schematic presentation of end group effects of R-PA-PLX-PA-R on sol-gel transition[80] (with permission from American Chemical Society).

When the polypeptides of mPEG-PA with a similar molecular weight were compared, the DL-isomer with a random coil conformation did not undergo sol-to-gel transition whereas the L-isomer with β-sheet structure showed sol-to-gel transition as the temperature increased. The well-organized secondary structure facilitates the molecular assembly in inducing sol-to-gel transition of the polymer aqueous solution. mPEG-PAF was developed as an enzymatically degradable thermogelling polypeptide. The polymer gel was quite stable in the phosphate buffered saline, whereas more than 90% of the gel disappeared when implanted in the subcutaneous layer of rats. The mPEG-PAF was proven to be degraded by cathepsin B, cathepsin C, and elastase that are present in the subcutaneous layer of mammals. The thermal gelation is not limited to an aqueous solution. When the PEG-polypeptide was dissolved in chloroform, the polymer solution also underwent sol-to-gel transition as the temperature increased.[78,79] The desolvation of the chloroform from the PEG is responsible for the transition. When the polypeptides have a mixed conformation of β-sheets and α-helixes in chloroform, the gel morphology tends to be a spherical micelles or short tubular structure, whereas the gel morphology tends to be a fibrous structure when the polypeptides dominantly form a β-sheet conformation in chloroform. End group modification of PA-PLX-PA by methyl, ethyl, and propyl group reduced the sol-to-gel transition temperature as well as induced a conformational change of the PA from random coil to β-sheet structure (Fig. 13.7).[80] The enhanced hydrophobic interactions of the alkyl groups recruit the PAs to effectively form a β-sheet structure and induce the sol-to-gel transition of the polymer aqueous solution. This system also emphasizes the importance of the secondary structure in thermal gelation of the polymer aqueous solution.

13.5 Other thermogelling polymers

Orthoester is the triether groups linked a carbon atom. Contrary to the ester that subject to acid-base catalyzed hydrolysis, orthoester is hydrolyzed faster under

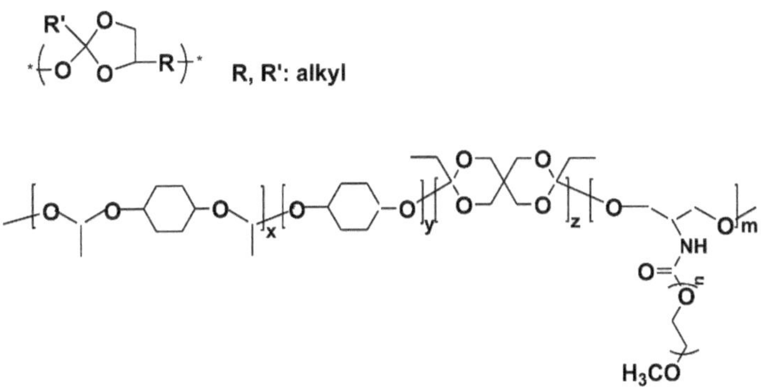

13.8 Structure of injectable polyorthoester: generation III (top) and V (bottom).

acidic conditions. Since the pioneering work of Choi and Heller on polyorthoester I, several generations (II, III, IV, and V) of the polyorthester were developed. As an injectable *in-situ* gelling system, polyorthoester III and V were developed (Fig. 13.8).[81] Polyorthoester III is an aliphatic low molecular weight polyorthoester prepared by condensation polymerization. It is an injectable semisolid material at room temperature. However, the polymer also suffers from reproducibility in molecular weight control. Polyorthoester V is a thermogelling polyorthoester based on PEG-polyorthoester block copolymers. The poly(acetal-co-orthoester) (PAO) form a hydrophobic block, whereas PEG form a hydrophilic block. The PAO-g-PEG aqueous solution underwent sol-to-gel transition as the temperature increased, and the gel degradation was accelerated under the acidic condition.[82]

mPEG-aliphatic polycarbonate diblock copolymers have been developed as a thermogelling biomaterial. In particular, poly(trimethylene carbonate) (PTMC) showed good biocompatibility. Contrary to the polyesters that produce carboxylic acid as a degradation product, polycarbonate is quite stable in phosphate buffered saline and degraded by reactive oxygen species and enzymes to produce carbon dioxide and alcohol. There is no significant change in pH during the degradation of the PTMC.[83] The mPEG-PTMC (550-2750) aqueous solution underwent sol-to-gel transition as the temperature increased (Fig. 13.9). The modulus of *in-situ* formed gel (G') was rather low and the gel could be injected through a 21-gauge syringe needle.[84] In the *in-vivo* experiments in the subcutaneous layer of rats, about 15% of the gel was lost over 20 days, whereas

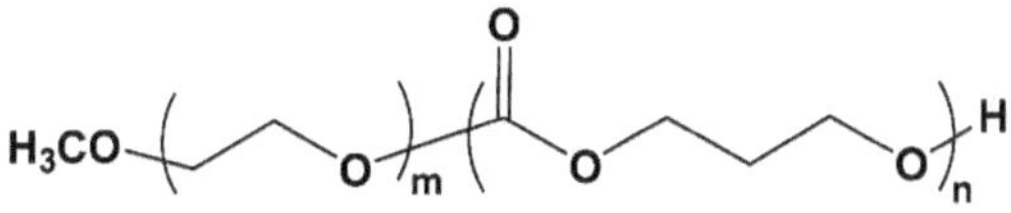

13.9 Structure of PEG-PTMC.

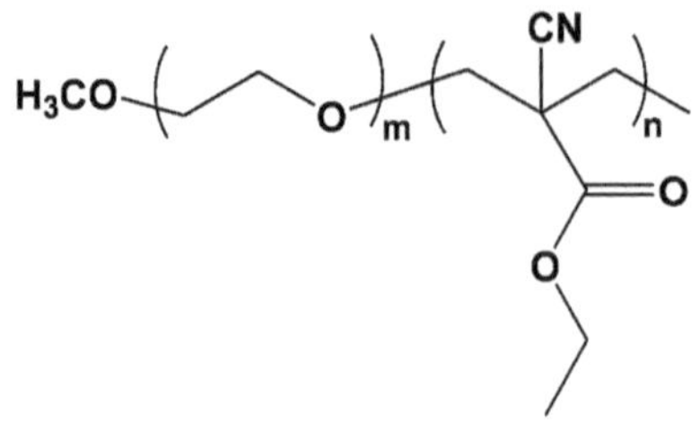

13.10 Structure of PEG-PEC.

it was quite stable in the *in-vitro* experiments in the phosphate buffered saline at pH = 7.4 and 37°C.

Thermogelling aqueous solutions of poly(ethylene glycol)-poly(ethyl-2-cyanoacrylate) (PEG-PEC) were reported (Fig. 13.10).[85] Polycyanoacrylate is degraded by esterases to cyanoacrylic acid. The PEG-PEC diblock copolymer aqueous solution showed a sol-to-gel-to-sol transition as the temperature increased as well as the concentration increased, thus, forming a closed-loop gel domain in the phase diagram.

Poly(N-(2-hydroxyproyl) methacrylamide (HPMAm)-oligolactate) (MW = 10–20 K Daltons) was linked to PEG (MW = 10 K Daltons) to show thermogelling polymer aqueous solution (Fig. 13.10).[86] The gel modulus could be controlled by the molecular weight of the poly(HPMAm-oligolactate) (Fig. 13.11).

Poly(N-isopropyl acrylamide) (PNIPAAm) is one of the most widely studied temperature sensitive polymers that undergoes clear solution to precipitation. However, its nonbiodegradability and concern for residual monomer toxicity limit the biomedical applications. To improve the problems, biodegradable

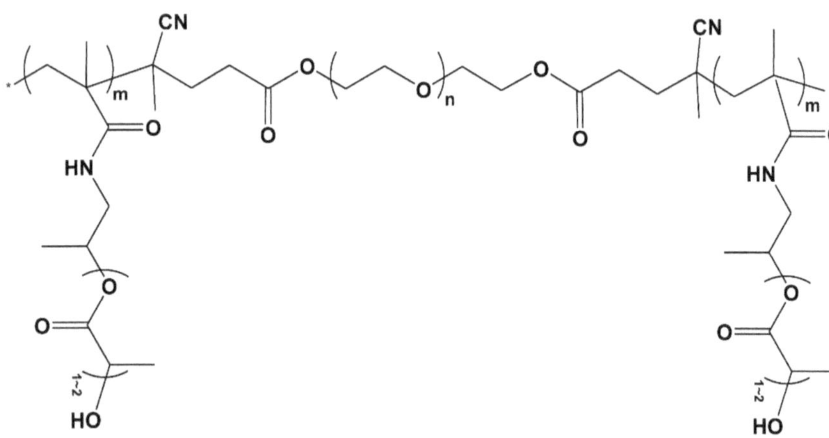

13.11 Structure of poly(HPMAm-oligolactate)-PEG-poly(HPMAm-oligolactate).

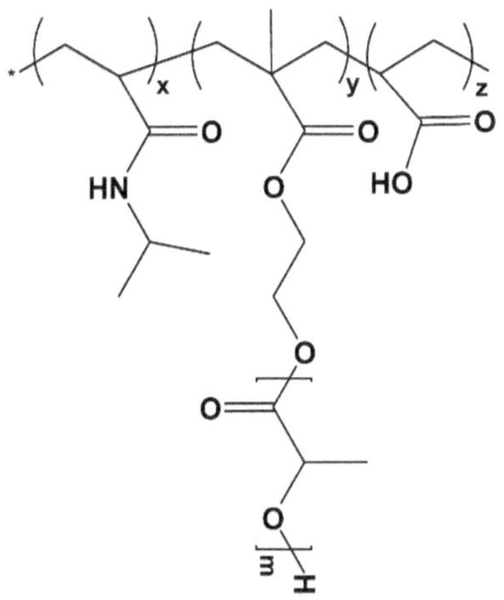

13.12 Structure of biodegradable NIPAAm copolymers.

NIPAAm copolymers have been developed as the thermogelling biodegradable polymers. Polylactide, and poly(dimethyl-γ-butyrolactone) were used to give the biodegradability of the copolymer (Fig. 13.12).[87–88] Due to the degradation the hydrophobic block with time, the polymer of which aqueous solutions underwent thermal gelation at 37°C becomes soluble at 37°C at a later stage of degradation.

13.6 Conclusions and future trends

In this chapter, biodegradable polymers whose aqueous solutions show thermal gelation have been reviewed. The polymer aqueous solution can be used as an *in-situ* gel forming drug delivery depot as well as cell growing matrix. The thermogelling system has several advantages including: non-surgical procedure is necessary to make an implant, no organic solvent is used in the fabrication of the implant system, and sterilization is simply done by syringe filtration in a sol state. With such advantages, Massachusetts Institute Technology (MIT) review reported in 2003 that injectable tissue engineering will be one of the most promising technologies in the future. In particular, a multiple-stimuli sensitive system can trigger gelation by pH, electric field, light, or biochemicals in addition to temperature. Such a system can be designed to improve the current temperature-sensitive thermogelling systems such as an initial burst of the loaded drug, gel modulus control, etc. Polypeptide-based systems are also promising due to the diversity of amino acids, the diversity of secondary structure of the polypeptide, and specific biological function of the polypeptide. We have already proved the significance of the secondary structure of polypeptide in inducing the sol-gel transition. In the case of three-dimensional cell culture systems, the matrix can be constructed based on the secondary structure of the polypeptide. The difference in the microenvironment might affect the cell growth and differentiation. The polypeptide system is also unique in that enzymatic degradability can be introduced. The polymer can be designed to be stable in an *in-vitro* system; however, it can be degradable just upon *in-vivo* application. Oligonucleotide also can be designed as a thermogelling material. The hydrophilic and hydrophobic balance can be achieved by selecting the base pairs or modification of the base-pair. Transition metal systems that can change a coordination number depending on a stimulus are also interesting, as in case of cobalt.[89] The change in the coordination number by varying temperature can induce a sol-to-gel transition of the polymer aqueous solution as the temperature increases.

To conclude, biodegradable injectable systems were reviewed, focusing on a thermogelling system. In designing a new thermogelling material, biodegradability, biocompatibility, and the control of an initial burst release of an incorporated drug, and reconstitution kinetics should be overcome in an actual application using an injectable drug delivery system. We are expecting an excellent system that solves the above issues to appear in the near future.

13.7 Acknowledgements

This work was supported by Mid-career Researcher Program through NRF of Korea grant funded by the MEST (Grant: 2010-0000832).

13.8 References

1. B. Jeong, S. W. Kim, and Y. H. Bae, *Adv. Drug Del. Rev.,* 2002, **54**, 37.
2. X. J. Loh, and J. Li, *Export Opin. Ther. Patents*, 2007, **17** (8), 965.
3. C. He, S. W. Kim, and D. S. Lee, *J. Controlled Rel.*, 2008, **127**, 189.
4. L. Liu, and J. Ding, *Chem. Soc Rev.*, 2008, **37**, 1473.
5. K. J. Zhu, X. Lin, and S. Yang, *J. Appl. Polym. Sci.* 1990, **39**, 1.
6. C. A. Finch, *Chemistry and technology of water soluble polymers.* Plenum Press, NY, 1983, pp. 157–178.
7. L. V. Mohite, and V. A. Juvekar, *Fluid Phase Equil.,* 2009, **278**, 41.
8. B. Jeong, Y. H. Bae, D. S. Lee, and S. W. Kim, *Nature*, 1997, **388**, 860.
9. B. Jeong, Y. K. Choi, Y. H. Bae, G. Zentner, and S. W. Kim, *J. Controlled Rel.*, 1999, **62**, 109.
10. B. Jeong, Y. H. Bae, and S. W. Kim, *Macromolecules*, 1999, **32**, 7064.
11. R. Rathi, G. Zentner, and B. Jeong, 2000, *US Patent* 6117949.
12. R. Rathi, G. Zentner, and B. Jeong, 2001, *US Patent* 6201072.
13. B. Jeong, Y. H. Bae, and S. W. Kim, *J. Biomed. Mater. Res.*, 2000, **50**, 171.
14. B. Jeong, M. R. Kibbey, J. C. Birnbaum, Y. Y. Won, and A. Gutowska, *Macromolecules,* 2000, **33**, 8317.
15. B. Jeong, L. Q. Wang, and A. Gutowska, *Chem. Commun.*, 2001, **16,** 1516.
16. M. J. Hwang, J. M. Suh, Y. H. Bae, S. W. Kim, and B. Jeong, *Biomacromolecules,* 2005, **6**, 885.

17. S. J. Bae, J. M. Suh, Y. S. Sohn, Y. H. Bae, S. W. Kim, and B. Jeong, *Macromolecuels,* 2005, **38**, 5260.
18. S. H. Park, B. G. Choi, M. K. Joo, D. K. Han, Y. S. Sohn, and B. Jeong, *Macromolecules,* 2008, **41**, 6486.
19. S. J. Bae, M. K. Joo, Y. Jeong, S. W. Kim, W. K. Lee, Y. S. Sohn, and B. Jeong, *Macromolecules,* 2006, **39**, 4873.
20. Z. Jang, Y. You, X. Deng, and J. Hao, *Polymer*, 2007, **48**, 4786.
21. L. Yu, H. Zhang, and J. Ding, *Angew Chem. Int. Ed.,* 2006, **45**, 2232.
22. S. Jo, J. Kim, and S. W. Kim, *Macrmol. Biosc.,* 2006, **6**, 923.
23. S. J. Lee, B. R. Han, S. Y. Park, D. K. Han, and S. C. Kim, *J. Polym. Sci. Polym. Chem.,* 2006, **44**, 888.
24. K. Nagahama, T. Ouchi, and Y. Ohya, *Adv. Funct. Mater.*, 2008, **18**, 1220.
25. E. Behravesh, A. K. Shung, S. Jo, and A. G. Mikos, *Biomacromolecules,* 2002, **3**, 153.
26. T. Vermonden, N. E. Fedorovich, D. V. Geemen, J. Alblas, C. F. V. Nostrum, W. J. A. Dhert, and W. E. Hennik, *Biomacromolecules*, 2008, **9**, 919.
27. Z. Zhong, P. J. Dijkstra, J. Feijen, Y. M. Kwon, Y. H. Bae, and S. W. Kim, *Macromol. Chem. Phys.*, 2002, **203**, 1797.
28. T. Fujiwara, T. Mukose, T. Yamaoka, H. Yamane, S. Sakurai, and Y. Kimura, *Macromol. Biosci.*, 2001, **1**, 204.
29. D. P. Huynh, M. K. Nguyen, B. S. Pi, M. S. Kim, S. Y. Chae, K. C. Lee, B. S. Kim, S. W. Kim, and D. S. Lee, *Biomaterials*, 2008, **29**, 2527.
30. W. S. Shim, J. S. Yoo, Y. H. Bae, and D. S. Lee, *Biomacromolecules*, 2005, **6**, 2930.
31. D. P. Huynh, W. S. Shim, J. H. Kim, and D. S. Lee, *Polymer*, 2006, **47**, 7918.
32. X. Y. Xiong, K. C. Tam, and L. H. Gan, *Polymer*, 2005, **46**, 1841.
33. X. Y. Xiong, K. C. Tam, and L. H. Gan, *J. Appl. Polym. Sci.*, 2006, **100**, 4163.
34. S. Y. Park, Y. Lee, K. H. Bae, C. H. Ahn, and T. G. Park, *Macromol. Rapid Commun.*, 2007, **28**, 1172.
35. J. M. Suh, S. J. Bae, and B. Jeong, *Adv. Mater.*, 2005, **17**, 118.
36. K. Huang, B. P. Lee, D. R. Ingram, and P. B. Messersmith, *Biomacromolecules*, 2002, **3**, 397.
37. D. Cohn, A. Sosnik, and A. Levy, *Biomaterials*, 2003, **24**, 3707.
38. A. Sosnik, and D. Cohn, *Biomaterials*, 2005, **26**, 349.
39. J. S. Ahn, J. M. Suh, M. Lee, and B. Jeong, *Polym. Int.*, 2005, **54**, 842.
40. D. Cohn, and A. Sosnik, *J. Mater. Sci.: Mater. Med.*, 2003, **14**, 175.
41. D. Cohn, G. Lando, A. Sosnik, S. Garty, and A. Levi, *Biomaterials*, 2006, **27**, 1718.
42. X. J. Loh, S. H. Goh, and J. Li, *Biomacromolecules*, 2007, **8**, 585.
43. X. J. Loh, S. H. Goh, and J. Li, *Biomaterials*, 2007, **28**, 4113.
44. K. H. Sun, Y. S. Shon, and B. Jeong, *Biomacromolecules*, 2006, **7**, 2871.
45. H. J. Chung, Y. Lee, and T. G. Park, *J. Controlled Rel.*, 2008, **127**, 22.
46. B. H. Lee, Y. M. Lee, Y. S. Sohn, and S. C. Song, *Macromolecules*, 2002, **35**, 3876.
47. J. Y. Seong, Y. J. Jun, B. Jeong, and Y. S. Sohn, *Polymer*, 2005, **46**, 5075.
48. G. D. Kang, J. Y. Heo, S. B. Jung, and S. C. Song, *Macrol. Rapid Commun.*, 2005, **26**, 1615.
49. B. H. Lee, and S. C. Song, *Macromolecules*, 2004, **37**, 4533.
50. S. B. Lee, S. C. Song, J. I. Jin, and Y. S. Sohn, *Macromolecules*, 1999, **32**, 7820.
51. A. Chenite, A. Chaput, D. Wang, C. Combes, M. D. Buscgmann, C. D. Hoemann, J. C. Leroux, B. L. Atkinson, F. Binette, and A. Selmani, *Biomaterials*, 2000, **21**, 2155.
52. J. Cho, M. C. Heuzey, A. Begin, and P. J. Carreau, *Carbohydrate Polym.,* 2006, **63**, 507.

53. J. Cho, M. C. Heuzey, A. Begin, and P. J. Carreau, *Biomacromolecules*, 2005, **6**, 3267.
54. F. Ganji, and M. J. Abdekhodaie, *Carbohydrate Polym.*, 2008, **74**, 435.
55. K. Y. Cho, T. W. Chung, B. C. Kim, M. K. Kim, J. H. Lee, W. R. Wee, and C. S. Cho, *Int. J. Pharm.*, 2003, **260**, 83.
56. S. Q. Liu, S. C. Joshi, Y. C. Lam, and K. C. Tam, *Carbohydrate Polym.*, 2008, **72**, 133.
57. M. Kidowaki, C. Zhao, T. Kataoka, and K. Ito, *Chem. Commun.*, 2006, 4102.
58. T. Karino, Y. Okumura, C. Zhao, M. Kidowaki, T. Kataoka, K. Ito, and M. Shibayama, *Macromolecules*, 2006, **39**, 9435.
59. T. Kataoka, M. Kidowaki, C. Zhao, H. Minamikawa, T. Shimizu, and K. Ito, *J. Phys. Chem. B.*, 2006, **110**, 24377.
60. D. W. Urry, C. H. Harris, and T. Parker, *Protein-based materials*, K. McGathm D. Kaplan, Eds., Birkhauser, Boston, 1977.
61. J. D. Hartgerink, E. Beniash, and S. I. Stupp, *Science*, 2001, **294**, 1684.
62. H. Yokoi, T. Kinoshita, and S. Zhang, *Proc. Natl. Acad. Sci. U. S. A.*, 2005,**102**, 8414.
63. W. A. Petka, J. L. Harden, K. P. McGrath, D. Wirtz, and D. A. Tirrell, *Science*, 1998, **281**, 389.
64. A. P. Nowak, V. Breedveld, L. Pakstis, B. Ozbas, D. J. Pine, D. J. Pochan, and T. J. Deming, *Nature*, 2002, **417**, 424.
65. A. Aggeli, M. Bell, N. Boden, J. N. Keen, P. F. Knowles, T. C. B. Mcleish, M. Pitkeathly, and S. E. Radford, *Nature*, 1997, **386**, 259.
66. H. A. Klok, *Angew. Chem. Int. Ed.*, 2002, **41**, 1509.
67. C. Wang, R. J. Stewart, and J. Kopecek, *Nature*, 1999, **397**, 417.
68. G. Palazolo, F. Rodriguez, B. Farruggia, G. Pico, and N. Delorenzi, *J. Agri. Food Chem.*, 2000, **48**, 3817.
69. N. Kitabatake, R. Wada, and Y. Fujita, *J. Agri. Food Chem.*, 2001, **49**, 4011.
70. M. A. M. Hoffmann, and P. J. J. M. van Mil, *J. Agri. Food Chem.*, 1997, **45**, 2942.
71. H. Reiersen, A. R. Clarke, and A. R. Rees, *J. Mol. Biol.*, 1998, **283**, 255.
72. E. R. Wright, and V. P. Conticello, *Adv. Drug. Del. Rev.*, 2002, **54**, 1057.
73. Z. Megeed, J. Cappello, and H. Ghandehari, *Adv. Drug. Del. Rev.*, 2002, **54**, 1075.
74. D. J. Pochan, J. P. Schneider, J. Kretsinger, B. Ozbas, K. Rajagopal, and L. Haines, *J. Am. Chem. Soc.*, 2003, **125**, 11802.
75. Y. Y. Choi, M. K. Joo, Y. S. Sohn, and B. Jeong, *Soft Matter,* 2008, **4**, 2383.
76. H. J. Oh, M. K. Joo, Y. S. Sohn, and B. Jeong, *Macromolecules*, 2008, **41**, 8204.
77. Y. Jeong, M. K. Joo, K. H. Bahk, Y. Y. Choi, H. T. Kim, Y. S. Sohn, H. J. Lee, and B. Jeong. *J. Controlled Rel.* 2009, **137**, 25.
78. Y. Jeong, M. K. Joo, Y. S. Sohn, and B. Jeong, *Adv. Mater.*, 2007, **19**, 3947. 2008.
79. Y. Y. Choi, Y. Jeong, M. K. Joo, and B. Jeong, *Macromol. Biosci.*, 2009, **9**, 869.
80. J. Y. Kim, M. H. Park, M. K. Joo, S. Y. Lee, and B. Jeong, *Macromolecules*, 2009, **42**, 3147.
81. J. Heller, J. Barr, S. Y. Ng, K. S. Abdellauoi, and R. Gurny, *Adv. Drug Del. Rev.*, 2002, **54**, 1015.
82. E. Schacht, V. Toncheva, K. Vandertaelen, and J. Heller, *J. Controlled Rel.*, 2006, **116**, 219.
83. Z. Zhangg, D. W. Grijpma, and J. Feijen, *J. Controlled Rel.*, 2006, **112**, 57.
84. S. Y. Kim, H. J. Kim, K. E. Lee, S. S. Han., Y. S. Sohn, and B. Jeong, *Macromolecules*, 2007, **40**, 5519.
85. B. G. Choi, Y. S. Sohn, and B. Jeong, *J. Phys. Chem. B.*, 2007, **111**, 7715.

86. T. Vermonden, N. A. M. Besseling, M. J. Van Steenbergen, and W. E. Hennink, *Langmuir*, 2006, **22**, 10180.
87. B. H. Lee, and B. Vernon, *Macromolecular Bioscience*, 2005, **5**, 629.
88. E. Handerson, B. H. Lee, Z. Cui, R. Mclemore, T. A. Brandon, and B. Vernon, *J. Biomed. Mater. Res. Part A*. 2009, **90A**, 1186.
89. K. Kuroiwa, T. Shibata, A. Takada, N. Nemoto, and N. Kimizuka, *J. Am. Chem. Soc.*, 2004, **126**, 2016.

14
Troubleshooting and hurdles to development of biomaterials

T. A. BECKER, Independent Medical Device Consultant, USA

Abstract: This chapter discusses common hurdles to developing a new injectable biomaterial along the path of new medical device creation. The first half of the chapter describes material characterization studies for consideration when attempting to develop a new device. The second half of the chapter describes the process of gaining device approval in the United States, and highlights options for funding a medical device development venture.

Key words: material characterization, rheology testing, biocompatibility testing, Food and Drug Administration (FDA), Investigational Device Exemption (IDE), Small Business Innovative Research (SBIR), device development.

14.1 Introduction

This chapter discusses common hurdles to developing a new injectable biomaterial along the path of new medical device creation. The first section describes the important mechanical characterization factors to consider when optimizing the biomaterial. Next, the common biocompatibility characterization studies needed to assess pre-clinical safety are highlighted. Throughout this chapter the injectable biomaterial, calcium alginate, will be referenced as an example of a material that has undergone all material characterization studies required by the Food and Drug Administration (FDA) in the United States. The FDA sets all guidelines and grants all the approvals required for a new material to be tested as a medical device in a clinical trial.

Once a new injectable biomaterial begins material characterization testing and begins to show promise as a new treatment option, the next step described in this chapter is patent protection. A strong patent with broad protection is the single most important tool for blazing a pathway that leads to translation of a technology from a laboratory setting to a marketable device that can ultimately be used in patients. The general medical device requirements to conduct a clinical trial in the United States, set by the FDA, are also described. Lastly, the stages of funding for a potential medical device are described with respect to the stage of injectable biomaterial development. The ultimate goal is to reach a level of progress and funding that will support a clinical trial that leads to premarket approval (PMA). PMA is the official FDA approval that labels an injectable biomaterial as a new biomedical device that can be sold in the United States.

14.2 Material development hurdles

The two most important areas of research when developing an injectable biomaterial for potential human use are: (1) material characterization and (2) biocompatibility testing. Material characterization requires extensive rheological testing to assess a material's delivery performance and mechanical stability. The following lists summarize the general material characterization tests required by the FDA.

Delivery performance of the injectable biomaterial:

- controllable delivery (consistent results)
- accurate placement of the injectable biomaterial
- adequate imaging of the injection (visualization during delivery)
- penetration of the injection to the intended location
- the injectable biomaterial's viscosity profile (relates to ease of injection).

Mechanical stability of the resulting biomaterial implant:

- strength
- fatigue resistance
- particulate generation
- migration
- solidification time (if applicable).

14.2.1 Delivery performance testing

Endovascular microcatheters are continually advancing and becoming more viable for use in complex vasculature and in areas with limited access by other surgical means. Therefore, microcatheter compatibility is often the major hurdle for an injectable biomaterial's ultimate success as a usable device. Microcatheters used to deliver injectable biomaterials to both the peripheral and cerebrovascular systems are rapidly becoming easier to navigate and control. As a result, these catheters are highly flexible, with an extremely small profile. Common microcatheters used in cerebrovascular applications are approaching inner diameters of 0.012″ (0.3 mm), outer diameters of 1.3 F (0.43 mm), and lengths typically greater than 150 cm. An injectable biomaterial intended for use in such a catheter is will have a limited effective flow rate that will require a reduced liquid viscosity profile and higher injection pressures. Most injectable biomaterials must be usable over a large flow rate range. High flows help penetrate and fill larger lesions in a timely manner, whereas low flows can provide higher control for treating smaller areas and avoiding overfilling. Therefore, it is important that new injectable biomaterials have flow properties and viscosity profiles that are compatible with current and future endovascular microcatheters.

Viscosity profile testing characterizes a biomaterial's injectability through modern medical microcatheters or equivalent delivery systems. As a specific example, calcium alginates underwent extensive studies for the minimally invasive occlusion of vascular defects in the brain via endovascular delivery (Becker *et al.*, 2005; 2007; Soja *et al.*, 2004; Becker and Kipke, 2002). The modern endovascular microcatheter has become a very small, flexible, and guidable tube that can access even the smallest and most tortuous vasculature of the brain. One-component systems delivered through a microcatheter typically require a viscosity below 1000 cP during injection, and before solidification, to ensure adequate delivery with injection pressures below the microcatheter's safety rating. Two-component systems, such as calcium alginate (calcium chloride and sodium alginate), delivered through a microcatheter in separate chambers (e.g. a concentric-tube configuration) typically require a viscosity below 250 cP to be delivered successfully and still maintain injection pressures below the microcatheter's safety rating (Becker and Kipke, 2002; Becker *et al.*, 2001a,b).

FDA testing and previous studies have verified that 150–250 cP is an ideal range for decreased sodium alginate injection resistance in many standard over-the-wire microcatheter systems and increased calcium alginate stability in gel form (Becker *et al.*, 2005; 2007). As for newer flow-directed microcatheter systems, an injectable biomaterial requires a lower alginate viscosity range (1–150 cP) to accommodate the microcather's minimal inner diameter.

Since many injectable biomaterials may show significant correlations between liquid viscosity and the resulting implant strength, it is important to investigate ways to maximize gel strength and minimize viscosity. Many hydrogels come in various molecular weights, so the determination of molecular weight ranges and their resulting stability is also important. Investigation of the combination of various molecular weight ranges can be an effective method to optimize implant strength and reduce injection viscosity (Kong *et al.*, 2002).

Controllable delivery and accurate placement of an injectable biomaterial is highly dependent on the ability to visualize the injection. Therefore, the molecular alteration or addition of imaging additives to a biomaterial can have significant tradeoffs that may include increased viscosity and decreased implant strength. Therefore, it is important to understand the maximum acceptable viscosity for delivery, the minimum acceptable imaging additive concentration for visualization during delivery, and the minimum acceptable strength of the resulting implant.

The viscosity of many liquid hydrogels and other injectable biomaterials is significantly affected when designed for optimal imaging and strength. In the case of calcium alginates, radiopacity (image density using angiographic instrumentation) is a critical aspect of the injectable material to ensure the end user can track and control the exact placement of the resulting implant. The two main types of radiographic materials are micrionized metallic particles and liquid contrast agents consisting of iodine attached to large organic molecules. The larger-molecule liquid contrast agents typically approach the osmolality of blood, but are also significantly more viscous than their smaller-molecule counterparts. Both forms of radiographic materials can significantly increase the injectable biomaterial's viscosity, increase the solidification rate, and decrease the resulting implant strength, when compared to the original material. Liquid contrast agents can also diffuse out of many forms of solidified hydrogels over time. Therefore the timeframe that the implant is considered radiopaque must be determined.

An appropriate guideline for the validation of radiopacity of devices used with angiography is the ASTM Standard Test Method for Radiopacity of Plastics for Medical Use (designation F 640-79). The standard describes using three aluminum sheets (1100 series) measuring 20 cm × 20 cm × 0.3 cm for background absorption. The injectable biomaterial or implant is placed on the plates in a simulated *in vivo* environment (e.g. placement in a container of Ringer's solution). An aluminum standard (1100 series, 3 cm × 10 cm × 0.3 cm) is placed next to the biomaterial to serve as a reference for image contrast comparison. Images can be recorded over time with an angiographic imaging system (e.g. a fluoroscope) and processed with image analysis software (e.g. NIH Image or Adobe Photoshop). The luminosity of the background, the standard, and the biomaterial samples are calculated and compared to determine radiopacity over time. A sample with an opacity greater (darker) than the standard, when compared to the background opacity, is considered radiopaque for medical use. If the radiopacity diffuses with time, then your effective timeframe for radiopacity equals the time point at which the sample image is no longer darker than the standard.

14.2.2 Mechanical stability testing

Mechanical strength can be effectively assessed with rheological testing. Many of these techniques have been described in this publication. This section will summarize and reference publications that discuss stability tests performed on the injectable biomaterial – calcium alginate (Becker and Kipke, 2002; Becker *et al.*, 2001a; 2001b). Ideally, implant strength and mechanical stability are optimized in a laboratory setting and verified in an *in vivo* model. Appropriate strength and stability profiles vary depending on the intended treatment area and can be challenging to determine. However, reference to the rheological data of normal tissues that the implant would mimic or replace is a good start. The FDA typically has no preset guidelines as to the required material characteristics of a potentially new injectable biomaterial. Rather, it is up to the researcher to provide repeatable data that justifies why a new material's strength profile is adequate for the intended application.

In the example of endovascular occlusion with calcium alginates, compressive strength and shear strength are the dominating forces seen from pulsatile blood flow, blood pressure, and muscoskeletal forces applied to the vessels. To estimate the strength profile required for a endovascular injectable biomaterial, the stress frequency sweep (rad/s) for an *in vivo* aneurysm system was calculated by estimating the range of blood flow velocities in vessels that can form aneurysms (υ), divided by the radius of calcium alginate gels (r), (gel radius equals the aneurysm radius, assuming 100% occlusion).

$$\text{Rad/s} = \upsilon / r \qquad 14.1$$

Cerebrovascular blood flow velocities can range from 100 to 300 mm/s and an aneurysm radius can vary from 3 to 20 mm (Lot *et al.*, 1999; Weir, 2002; Park *et al.*, 2003). Using the equation 14.1 as a guide, the result is a potential frequency sweep from 5 to 100 rad/s, with a typical value of 40 rad/s (average flow of 160 mm/s with a typical aneurysm radius of 4 mm).

Calcium alginate implant samples were prepared using an *in vitro* testing method that approximated injection and gelation via a microcatheter delivery system. One ml of ungelled alginate was injected at 1 ml/min through a 23-gauge needle into 1 ml of $CaCl_2$ contained in a 2 cm-diameter, 10 cc beaker. At least three gels were made for each test. The result was implant samples with consistent sizes and shapes for rheological testing. The shear strength was determined using a rheometer (RA 550, TA Instruments, New Castle, DE) with a 20 mm cylindrical parallel plate. Shear strength was tested at 40% and 60% compression and 37°C. At each compression level the gels underwent an oscillation procedure with a 1% strain and a frequency sweep from 1 to 100 rad/s. Adhesive sand paper (150 grit) was applied to the testing surfaces to minimize slip at the gel/plate interface. Shear strength was graphed as the complex moduli (G^*) of the samples at specific frequencies within the tested range (Becker *et al.*, 2001b; Nunamaker, 2006; Nunamaker *et al.*, 2007).

Calcium alginate testing resulted in a shear resistance of $>$10 kPa at 40% compression and $>$30 kPa at 60% compression at 40 rad/s (Becker *et al.*, 2005). This testing was completed on the optimized version of the calcium alginate implant and resulted in statistically significant results. Therefore, this data would be submitted to the FDA as part of the device specification for acceptable implant strength. An injectable biomaterial that passes all device specifications accepted by the FDA could then be released for use in a clinical trial under an approved Investigational Device Exemption (IDE).

In vitro modeling and ultimately *in vivo* testing are the final hurdles in the optimization of an injectable biomaterial. Model testing provides a complete picture of the injectability, control, and implant material characteristics. Can the material be delivered and controlled at the set viscosity? Can the injection be tracked and delivered consistently within a required time frame? Is the strength and fatigue resistance adequate to maintain stability without migration or particulation? With calcium alginate, the initial data that helped answer these material characterization questions was obtained from a sophisticated *in vitro* flow model that simulated the *in vivo* environment during microcatheter delivery. The resulting implants were cycled under simulated endovascular flows and pressures for up two weeks and monitored for migration or particulation. The implants were then be retrieved at the end of the cycle period and tested rheologically for strength and fatigue resistance (Becker *et al.*, 2003). Once a material is tested, modified, and retested in an *in vitro* model, then the next step is application in an appropriate animal model. To gain IDE approval, the FDA will require proof of safety and efficacy in standardized biocompatibility tests as well as in peer-reviewed and accepted *in vivo* models.

14.2.3 Biocompatibility testing

There is a battery of testing, leading up to advanced *in vivo* modeling, that is required by the FDA to ensure the injectable biomaterial's safety and efficacy. Biocompatibility testing must be performed on all components of the device that may come in contact with the patient. For example, both components of the two-component calcium alginate system (calcium chloride and sodium alginate) were tested along with the final implant in instances where the components may contact the endovascular or tissue space before complete gelation.

The majority of biocompatibility testing must be performed to Good Laboratory Practice (GLP) standards, especially those tests with standardized procedural and evaluation criteria. Therefore, it is often beneficial to contract these studies to an outside laboratory that specializes in biocompatibility testing (e.g. Toxikon, Bedford, MA; NAMSA, Northwood, OH). Several GLP tests are required by the FDA to assess an injectable biomaterial's purity, toxicity profile, irritation and sensitization profile, tissue and blood reactivity, and mutagenic profile. These tests are required on the final device as well as any components of the device that may come in contact with human tissues or fluids. Table 14.1 summarizes the *in vitro* testing requirements expected for a new injectable biomaterial, as disclosed in the FDA's IDE preparation documents (FDA, 2009).

Purity of the injectable biomaterial is characterized by protein content, heavy metal content, and endotoxin content. Leachable testing determines the chemical compatibility of the injectable biomaterial with the delivery device (e.g. microcatheters) and whether the injectable biomaterial may act as a solvent, extracting impurities from the delivery device during implantation. Cytotoxicity gives an initial glimpse of the biomaterial's biological reactivity and genotoxicity tests assess whether bacterial mutations may occur or whether chromosomal damage or increased metabolic activation can be detected in mouse cells. Finally,

Table 14.1 FDA-required GLP *in vitro* biocompatibility testing

Test name	Test host	Required result
Endotoxin (Kinetic-Chromogenic LAL) • Bacterial toxins	Limulus amebocyte lysate (LAL)	< 0.5 EU/ml peripheral < 0.06 EU/ml intrathecal
Heavy metal content	ICP spectroscopy	< 5 ppm total < 0.2 ppm Pb < 0.015 ppm Hg
Protein content	Varies	Overall $\leq$ 0.1%
Leachables from delivery catheter • Volatile and semi-volatile organic compounds	FTIR, gas chromatography, mass spectometry	Difference of 0, control vs. sample
Cytotoxicity (MEM elution)	Mammalian L929 cells	No reactivity (Grade 0)
Genotoxicity		
• Bacterial reverse mutation (Ames)	Bacteria	95% confidence, control = sample
• Sister chromatid exchange assay	Mouse lymphoma L5178Y cells	95% confidence, control = sample
Hemocompatibility		
• *In vitro* hemolysis	Rabbit blood	$\leq$ 5% hemolysis
• C3a complement activation assay	Human blood	95% confidence, control = sample
• Lee-White clotting times	Human blood	coagulation within 8–15 min.

hemocompatibility tests detect blood cell hemolysis, changes in blood count, and effects on blood clotting time that may be attributable to the injectable biomaterial.

Table 14.2 summarizes the *in vivo* testing requirements expected for a new injectable biomaterial, as disclosed in the FDA's IDE preparation documents (FDA, 2009).

In vivo biocompatibility studies further characterize an injectable biomaterial's reactivity and immune response. Sensitization and Pyrogen testing help assess a device's tendency to cause an allergic reaction or fever in a patient. Intracutaneous reactivity testing can detect tissue irritation from the device, whereas acute and subchronic toxicity studies can determine any transient toxic effects from single or multiple doses of the extract from a device. The immunogenic test is performed in an attempt to detect whether the implant can initiate a systemic immune response (T-cell activation), which could lead to a larger inflammatory response. Muscle implantation is a general test to assess the extent of a local immune response caused by the implant.

Table 14.2 FDA-required GLP *in vivo* biocompatibility testing

Test name	Test host	Required result
Sensitization test (Kligman Maximization)	Guinea pigs	Non-sensitizing (Grade I)
Intracutaneous reactivity	Rabbits	Difference ≤ 1, control vs. sample
Acute systemic toxicity	Mice	Difference of 0, control vs. sample
Subchronic toxicity – 14-day IV dosing study	Mice	95% confidence, control = sample
Pyrogen test	Rabbits	Temp rise $< 0.5°C$
Immunogenic potential and cytokine release	CSF	Difference of 0, control vs. sample
Genotoxicity (Micronucleus cytogenic assay)	Mice	95% confidence, control = sample
*Muscle implantation test – 7 and 30 days	Rabbits	Non-reactive tissue irritant

* Note: Muscle implantation is the initial survival implant study required by the FDA. Testing in a more representative model for the device, as well as long-term survival studies in an *in vivo* model appropriate for the injectable biomaterial (survivals ranging from 3 months to 1 year), are also required.

In many cases, the implant studies suggested by the FDA may not be appropriate or adequate to gain a complete picture of an injectable biomaterials immune response and resulting biocompatibility. In the example of calcium alginate, the standard muscle implantation test for 7 and 30 days was not an appropriate test for assessing reactivity of a material intended for cerebral endovascular implantation. Therefore, under the guidance of the FDA, alternative studies were designed to assess calcium alginate placed in direct contact with dura and brain tissue for up to two weeks. The FDA also requested implantation in sophisticated large-animal models that more accurately assessed vascular size, flow properties, and vascular malformations that could be surgically created, treated, and survived for up to one year. It is important to design survival animal models that can complement *in vitro* material characterization studies. In the case of calcium alginates, *in vitro* material characterization studies of strength, fatigue resistance, migration, penetration, particulation, and degradation are considered preliminary data by the FDA. Verification of calcium alginate's material characteristics *in vivo* is the best way to approximate a new device's potential benefit in a patient. The FDA has moved towards *in vivo* studies with longer survival times (up to one year) in an attempt to obtain conclusive evidence of a material's stability and biocompatibility before granting IDE approval.

Standard biocompatibility testing procedures should be done in a GLP-certified laboratory when applicable. However, it is possible to conduct the larger-animal, longer-term biocompatibility tests in a non-GLP facility, as long as the study is in accordance with Institutional Animal Care and Use Committee (IACUC) review, the Animal Welfare Act, the NIH Guide, and institutional guidelines. In addition, all study traceability documents, (signed-off surgical logs, data recording paperwork, lab-book entries, and animal traceability data) must be provided to the FDA in lieu of institutional GLP certification. Typically, study disclosure by a non-GLP facility would be acceptable only if the testing procedure is not standardized or the model could not be adequately created without the specific surgical expertise or specialized equipment provided by the non-GLP facility. Many non-GLP facilities within teaching hospitals or within peer-review driven institutions can provide these specialized services. As long as the facility can provide all of the documentation that would be required for a typical GLP study, then in these specific instances, the study can be conducted at a non-GLP facility and still be acceptable to the FDA.

14.3 Device development hurdles

Engaging the end-user in the early stages of a new injectable biomaterial's development into a device is a crucial step. In the example of injectable biomaterials for vascular applications, the end-user is not the patient, but rather the interventional cardiologist or interventional neuroradiologist. A major hurdle for any researcher is seeing beyond the technical challenges of a new material and maintaining a vision of a useable end product. Constant communication with the end-user throughout the development process is beneficial in three ways:

1. The end-user helps maintain a practical and focused vision of the technology and can help prevent losing sight of the final device's applicability.
2. The end-user can help the researcher understand the broad applications of the technology, which is important for submitting broad and all-encompassing patent claims for the current treatment focus or future treatment options.
3. A strong relationship with the end-user can evolve into a qualified advocate for the device. Someone with credibility in the field of application that can speak to the device's utility during pre-IDE and PMA meetings with the FDA, and also attest to the device's benefits during funding pitches, partnership discussions, and acquisition opportunities.

14.3.1 Patent protection

The most important component for bringing a promising material from the basic research stage to a potential biomedical device is patent protection. Once a material has shown promise in the laboratory and has undergone some preliminary *in vitro* and *in vivo* optimization studies, a patent disclosure should be filed. A strong patent filing contains both a large breadth of knowledge on the technical side of the injectable biomaterial as well as a broad coverage of applications beyond just the current treatment focus. The technical knowledge comes from extensive material characterization studies and optimization of the material, which leads to applicable formulation ranges that can be patented. An ironclad patent comes from a detailed technical knowledge of the material and a knowledge of the current and future potential fields of use of the device. A strong patent portfolio is the basis for any successful device development effort. A medical device start-up company cannot compete, much less exist, without adequate patent protection for their potential device.

14.3.2 Focus on the device

Transitioning a promising material into a medical device can be a challenge in itself. The researcher's focus to optimize and perfect a material must also be mitigated by a focus to create a complete package that can become a user-friendly device. A usable device is an all-inclusive system that can be taken out of a 'box' and is ready for the patient. Is the device compatible with delivery systems that the end-user already uses? Can the device be deployed in a manner that is similar or easier than current technologies? These questions are great engineering challenges in themselves, and yet can be as important as the material characteristics of the device. If the end-user is ultimately not confident or comfortable with the new device, then it will never gain support over existing patient treatment options.

14.3.3 Investigational device exemption (IDE) submission

As summarized by the FDA, an investigational device exemption (IDE) allows a device to be used in a clinical study to collect safety and effectiveness data required to support a PMA application or a Premarket Notification [510(k)] submission to FDA. All clinical evaluations of investigational devices must have an approved IDE before a clinical study can be initiated. An approved IDE permits a device to be shipped lawfully for the purpose of conducting investigations of the device without complying with other requirements of the Food, Drug, and Cosmetic Act that would apply to devices in commercial distribution (FDA, 2009).

The IDE submission is the crucial hurdle and major milestone that transitions a promising material into a viable and testworthy medical device. The IDE's format is a testament to this transformation. The first half of the submission is a detailed report of the injectable biomaterial's evolution and optimization – including all background data and all reports of prior investigation. This section includes the history of the material, all current mechanical and chemical testing, *in vitro* and *in vivo* modeling, and biocompatibility results. The second half of the submission, however, focuses on the injectable biomaterial as a device. This section can be a major hurdle for a researcher to complete because the device section must include all validation studies, traceability reports, manufacturing procedures, clinical trial procedures, and release requirements of a final packaged device for patient use. This device section of the IDE is outlined below.

Formulate a complete device description:

- Describe all components of the injectable device.
- Verify availability and approvals of all components.
- Define all specifications required to release the device for human use.

Create all necessary manufacturing standard operating procedures (SOPs):

- Ensure all device specifications are met and documented.
- Track all components and vendors used in creating the device.
- Maintain traceability for acceptance or rejection of manufactured lots.
- Conduct shipping, stability, and shelf-life testing of the final device.
- Have all labeling, packaging, and device components approved by the FDA.

Investigational plan:

- Outline the clinical trial protocol under Good Clinical Practices (GCP) guidelines.
- Create patient disclosure and consent forms for enrollment in the clinical trial.
- Identify clinical investigators and obtain Institutional Review Board (IRB) approvals.
- Create a training protocol for the clinical trial doctors and support staff.
- Identify clinical support monitors for clinical data acquisition, storage, and interpretation.

(***http://www.fda.gov/cdrh/devadvice/ide/index.shtml)

If the device also includes a drug component, then additional testing beyond the IDE may be required by the Center For Drug Evaluation and Research (CDER). However, if the drug is already approved, then the additional testing focuses on the interaction and compatibility of the drug with the injectable biomaterial.

It is important to maintain fluid communication with the FDA when applying for an IDE. The application process can take over a year or more and often more than one round of responses and requests for additional data on both sides of the submission. At the same time, the FDA provides the guidance needed to ensure complete disclosure of the device before its use in a patient. The process is a learning experience for both the FDA and the applicant company. Ultimately the FDA and the applicant company have the same goal: creation of a reliable device that will ensure safety and efficacy when used in a patient.

In the example of a research institution's technology development, the execution of required biocompatibility testing, manufacturing, and clinical setup requirements for an IDE submission is often beyond the scope of most institutions. In many cases, such development actions may represent a conflict of interest to the research institution and its employees. Therefore, it is important that a company (either a small business start up or a partnering company) transfer the material knowledge, and operate separately to develop a device submission to the FDA. Working with the technology transfer department of the research institution that originating the technology university will allow for the transition of any patents and technical knowledge to the company. The research institution will likely take a small equity and patent royalty position in the company for reimbursement of patent filing costs and for the transfer of the material technology.

14.4 Funding challenges

Many promising technologies have their origins on university campuses in a small corner of a research lab. An obvious hurdle to development of this new technology is adequate funding. Initial funding typically begins with the traditional university route, such as research startup funds or research grants from national institutions. Many funding options also exist outside the arena of basic research grants and where, in the case of product development, such external funding is a necessity. The following section highlights opportunities to help overcome the hurdle of funding translational research for creating an injectable biomaterial device.

14.4.1 Material development funding

The push by state and federal governments to bolster the economy in general and advance biotechnology in particular has led to grant opportunities that are ideal for small business startup in the medical device field. The first step to funding translational research is to apply for federal funding for small business. The Small Business Innovative Research initiative (SBIR) is an established division of the National Institutes of Health (NIH) and the National Science Foundation (NSF) that offers competitive grants for startup technology companies. These funds are geared towards the final stages of material development (Phase I) and device development towards a clinical trial (Phase II). SBIRs require no payback and no equity share in the company granted to the government. However, the majority of these funds are mandated for technological investments only and the award amounts can be small relatively small in Phase I (US$100 000 to US$250 000). Only 7% of the awarded amount (called a fixed fee) can be used for administrative or business development costs (capitalization) (NIH, 2009). Phase I SBIR are first-round grants that typically run for six months to one year, so rotating in new funding applications one to two times per year can help sustain a company during the material development stage.

However, as with most federal grants, the turnaround time from application to approval process can initially take one to two years. Sustaining a high rate of Phase I SBIR grant applications per year to fund a startup can be very time consuming, and often spreads the research effort too thin. A common result is a company with multiple funded projects, but none that advance beyond the material development stage. Phase I SBIR grants are a good starting point, but the company should remain focused on the second round of funding as well: Phase II SBIR grants and state economic stimulus funding.

The next hurdle is attaining the second round of funding to help propel a fledgling device company into a productive business and technology venture. Second-round funds come in three basic forms: angel investors, venture capitalists, and state and federal funding. Angel investors are individuals, or small groups of individuals that can contribute small amounts of capital as an investment for a small share of company equity. In the area of biomedical devices, buy-in from doctors in the field where your device will be used is the best link to angel investors. Other likely angel groups include university contributors that are supporting their Alma Mater. Typically, it may take dozens of angel investors to support a company's second round of funding, meaning the equity share in the company held by angel investors can become significant.

The second form of investor is the venture capitalist (VC). VCs are organized groups that represent a large number of investors that are looking for high yields on their money in a relatively short period of time. VCs typically have their own administrative staff and will often transplant their own operational staff into a company in which they invest. VCs are unlikely to show interest in a material that is still in development. VCs typically look to companies with devices that have FDA approvals to start clinical trials, or have already begun the trial. VCs are strongly focused on the business leadership of the startup and the market potential of the device. If a VC were to invest in a startup at an earlier stage, they would typically require an 80+% equity share and would take over business leadership. For this reason, it is important to work with VCs that have in-depth experience in the startup's device market. Venture capitalists are typically looking for ten times return on their money, therefore, they are not the first major investors in most companies. Often small startups that feel they need a large initial investment are passed over by VC groups because the risk is too high. Conversely, these same startups that manage to grow and build a validated technology portfolio without VC investment will often gain the interest of VC groups. However, by this stage, the startup no longer needs the VC investment.

The third form of second-round investment, and the most appealing to most biomedical startups, is Phase II SBIR grants and state economic funding. The next section will highlight the benefits of state and government funding for device development.

14.4.2 Device development funding

Once Phase I SBIR funding has been attained, opportunities for Phase II SBIR funding and local State economic development funding are available. Phase II SBIR grants are continuations of successful Phase I grants and must be applied for. Phase II grants can provide as much as US$1.25 million of second-round funding, typically over two years, with no payback or equity share granted to the government. This money is ideal for funding device development activities such as running GLP-required biocompatibility testing, paying for long-term and large-animal FDA survival studies, paying consultants that assist in IDE preparation and submission, and for device manufacture and release. SBIR Phase II funds still do not allow for company capitalization (beyond the seven per cent fixed fee) and the SBIR program will not pay for an approved clinical trial. The intention of the SBIR program is to fund the technical development to a point where the device is appealing to larger, private funding sources such as partnerships with or acquisitions by established biomedical companies.

Another appealing second-round funding source for pushing a company into device development, company capitalization, and clinical trial setup is through State economic development grants and loans. These funds are intended to grow new companies in the State that will ultimately bring in strong revenues and create jobs for the local economy. The funds are competitive like SBIR grants and typically have minimal payback or equity requirements. Small startups that are not yet funded will often be required to give up a small share of equity to the State in the form of a small stock position (typically less than 10%) and milestone payments. In many cases, state funds are given as loans. The payback percentage is often much lower than a bank loan, and qualification is based on business potential and technical merit (much like a government grant) rather than secured by company assets. Repayment is also not required for several years or until a major milestone is reached (i.e. market approval of the device, acquisition of additional funding, or acquisition by a larger company).

They key to small startup success in the biomedical industry is to remain focused on one's predicate device, develop a sound technology background, obtain broad and strong patent protection, and focus on a lucrative market niche. One proven model for growing a biomedical device startup company and creating significant valuation is to first gain seed funding through a first-round of SBIR Phase I competitive grants or select angel investors that require little or no equity. Follow up with a second round of funding from State economic competitive funding and competitive Phase II SBIRs, which will allow the company to advance its technology quickly, capitalize the company for growth, and maintain a competitive advantage (NIH, 2009).

Biomedical device development is a fast-paced industry with large competitors that release new devices every few years. It is unlikely a small startup company can keep pace, even with strong patent protection and a novel product, if a company does not focus on its highest potential technologies and works to fund them all the way through device development. Once funding is attained to ensure completion of FDA submissions for the predicate device, then further seed funding (back to Phase I SBIRs) should be pursued to research other uses and technical modifications. These further studies can open pathways to other technologies and market niches, which can increase the chance of gaining interest from a potential partner, an acquiring company, or some other form of additional investment (third-round of investment). Hopefully, once this third round is attained, all necessary resources will be in place to propel the new device through a full clinical trial and on the path to FDA PMA approval. The result would be commercialization of a new injectable biomaterial device to provide an alternative treatment option for patients.

14.5 References

Becker T A and Kipke D R (2002), 'Flow properties of liquid calcium alginate polymer when injected through medical microcatheters for endovascular embolization', *J Biomed Mater Res*, 61, 533–540.

Becker T A, Collins V E and Kipke D R (2001a), 'Method for forming an endovascular occlusion', US Patent 6592566.

Becker T A, Kipke D R, Brandon T (2001b), 'Calcium alginate gel: a biocompatible and mechanically stable polymer for endovascular embolization', *J Biomed Mater Res*, 54, 76–86.

Becker T A, Kipke D R and Brakora K M (2003), 'Endovascular embolization of aneurysms with ALGEL®: an *in vitro* study of delivery techniques and resulting gel stability', 25th Annual international Conference of the IEEE-EMBS, Cancun, Mexico.

Becker T A, Preul M C, Bichard, W D, Kipke D R and McDougall C G (2005), 'Calcium alginate gel as a biocompatible material for endovascular AVM embolization: six-month results in an animal model', *Neurosurgery*, 56, 793–801.

Becker T A, Preul M C, Bichard, W D, Kipke D R and McDougall C G (2007), 'Preliminary investigation of calcium alginate gel as a biocompatible material for endovascular aneurysm embolization *in vivo*', *Neurosurgery*, 60, 1119–1128.

FDA US Food and Drug Administration, 2009. Available from: http://www.fda.gov/MedicalDevices/DeviceRegulationandGuidance/HowtoMarketYourDevice/InvestigationalDeviceExemptionIDE/default.htm (updated 10 July 2009).

Kong H J, Lee Y L and Mooney D (2002), 'Decoupling the dependence of rheological/mechanical properties of hydrogels from solids concentration', *Polymer*, 43, 6239–6246.

Lot G, Houdart E, Cophignon J, Casasco A and George B (1999), 'Combined management of intracranial aneurysms by surgical endovascular treatment. Modalities and results from a series of 395 cases', *Acta Neurochir (Wien)*, 141, 557–562.

NIH National Institutes of Health, 2009. Office of Extramural Research. Available from: http://grants.nih.gov/grants/funding/sbir.htm (updated 23 June 2009).

Nunamaker E A (2006), 'Alginate as a novel material for duraplasty: Investigation of the material properties, *in vivo* stability, and sealing capabilities', Doctoral dissertation, University of Michigan.

Nunamaker E A, Purcell E K and Kipke D R (2007), '*In vivo* stability and biocompatibility of implanted calcium alginate disks, *J Biomed Mater Res Part A*, 83, 1128–1137.

Park H, Horowitz M, Jungreis C, Kassam A, Koebbe C, Genevro J, Dutton K and Purdy P (2003), 'Endovascular treatment of paraclinoid aneurysms: experience with 73 patients', *Neurosurgery*, 18, 43–44.

Soja Y, Preul M C, Furuse M, Becker T and McDougall C G (2004), 'Calcium alginate provides a high degree of embolization in aneurysm models: a specific comparison to coil packing', *Neurosurgery*, 55, 1401–1409.

Weir B (2002), 'Unruptured intracranial aneurysms: a review', *J Neurosurg*, 96, 3–42.

15

Biocompatibility of injectable materials

S. A. GUELCHER, Vanderbilt University, USA

Abstract: Injectable biomaterials present significant advantages relative to implants, such as the ability to conform to complex anatomical defects and to be administered using minimally invasive techniques. However, injectable biomaterials also present additional biocompatibility challenges beyond the basic requirements for implantable devices. This chapter reviews the unique biocompatibility challenges presented by injectable biomaterials that are currently being investigated and developed as therapies for tissue engineering and regenerative medicine.

Key words: *in situ* polymerizable biomaterials, controlled biodegradation, non-cytotoxic degradation products, environmentally responsive biomaterials.

15.1 Introduction

Biomaterials considered for use in regenerative medicine must possess certain basic requirements, including biocompatibility, biodegradation at a controlled rate to non-toxic breakdown products, support of cellular infiltration and tissue ingrowth, mechanical properties consistent with the requirements of the host tissue, and handling properties that facilitate ease of use in a clinical environment. Injectable biomaterials present significant advantages relative to implants, such as the ability to conform to complex anatomical defects and to be administered using minimally invasive techniques. For example, in the field of orthopedics, injectable biomaterials are of interest for a number of clinical indications, including filling of defects in trabecular bone at sites that are not weight-bearing and in contained defects where the structural bone is intact.[1] However, injectable biomaterials also present additional challenges beyond the basic requirements for biomedical implants described above. A primary concern is the toxicity and ultimate fate of reactive intermediates that are not incorporated in the final cured product. Additionally, the injected material may have adverse effects on surrounding host tissue due to the reactivity of specific components or to the release of heat through a reaction exotherm. In some cases, the viscosity of the injected material may be too low, resulting in extravasation of the material into surrounding tissues where it has an adverse effect.

This chapter reviews the unique biocompatibility challenges presented by injectable biomaterials that are currently being investigated and developed as

Table 15.1 Schematic illustrating the four classes of injectable biomaterials reviewed in this chapter. Materials are divided into those that gel *in situ* due to physical forces and those that cure by formation of chemical bonds

Physical forces	Chemical bonds
Environmentally responsive Set *in situ* in response to pH, temperature, or other stimulus	**Calcium phosphate cements (CPCs)** Set *in situ* by an acid/base reaction
Poly(NIPAAm) PEO-PPO block co-polymers	Brushite and hydroxyapatite cements Composite CPCs incorporating a porogen
Self-assembling Set *in situ* in response to phase-separation of hydrophilic and hydrophobic domains	***In situ* polymerizable** Set *in situ* by crosslinking of reactive monomers and macromers to form a network
Amphiphilic peptides Ionically crosslinked micro- and nano-spheres Biotinylated microspheres	Photopolymerizable hydrogels Thermally activated crosslinked gels Two-component polyurethanes Alginates

therapies for tissue engineering and regenerative medicine. As shown in Table 15.1, several classes of biomaterials will be highlighted, including: (a) self-assembling and environmentally responsive materials that undergo gelation due to physical forces, (b) calcium phosphates that set via an acid/base reaction, and (c) *in situ* polymerizable materials that undergo a chemical reaction to form crosslinks. These classes of biomaterials were selected to highlight different approaches that are commonly used or are promising in their potential for future use as injectable scaffolds and delivery systems for tissue regeneration. While the specific biocompatibility issues associated with injectability will be emphasized for each class of biomaterials, the relative advantages and disadvantages of each class will also be discussed in terms of handling, mechanical properties, and tissue remodeling.

15.2 Environmentally responsive biomaterials

Environmentally responsive biomaterials undergo physical gelation in response to changes in the tissue microenvironment after injection, such as temperature, pH, chemical composition, or an applied external field (e.g., electrical or magnetic).[2–4] One of the most extensively investigated classes of responsive biomaterials comprises thermogels, which after injection undergo phase-separation driven by the increase in temperature from ambient (~ 20–25°C) to physiological (37°C) conditions.[5] Since phase-separation occurs at temperatures above the lower critical solution temperature (LCST), preferred polymers are soluble in water and exhibit an LCST close to but below normal body temperature. Poly(N-isopropylacrylamide) (PNIPAAm), the most well-known thermoresponsive polymer, has an LCST of 32°C. By co-polymerizing N-isopropylacrylamide with biocompatible hydrophilic monomers or macromers, thermo-responsive polymers with LCSTs closer to body temperature have been prepared.[6,7] Other thermo-responsive polymers have also been investigated as injectable biomaterials for tissue engineering,[2] including poly(ethylene oxide)-poly(propylene oxide) block co-polymers,[8] poly(ethylene glycol)-poly(propylene fumarate) co-polymers,[9] and natural polymers (e.g., chitosan).[10,11]

Environmentally responsive injectable biomaterials are reviewed in detail in Chapter 11. In contrast to chemically or photo-crosslinked biomaterials that polymerize to form a solid *in situ*, responsive biomaterials are generally injected as aqueous polymer solutions, not as reactive monomers or macromers. Challenges associated with the biocompatibility of reactive intermediates, catalysts, solvents, and other additives are largely avoided, thereby rendering environmentally responsive biomaterials suitable for encapsulation of viable cells and growth factors.[2] However, since gelation is induced by relatively weak physical forces, the mechanical properties of environmentally responsive gels are typically rather low. To address this limitation, physical and chemical gelation techniques have been used in combination to prepare biomaterials with enhanced mechanical properties.[12]

15.3 Self-assembling biomaterials

Self-assembling injectable biomaterials also undergo gelation or phase-separation without chemical crosslinking reagents as described previously for environmentally responsive materials.[2] Phase-separation of either hydrophobic bulk material or hydrophobic domains of amphiphilic molecules is a frequently applied mechanism by which self-assembly proceeds.

In the bulk phase-separation approach, an organic solution of a polymer dissolved in a water-miscible solvent is injected into the tissue defect.[2] After injection, the solvent diffuses away from the injection site, resulting in precipitation of the water-insoluble polymer. Selection of an appropriate solvent, which must be non-cytotoxic and not harmful to host tissue, is a key factor for success of the bulk phase-separation system. Two solvents that meet these criteria are N-methyl-2-pyrrolidone (NMP) and dimethyl sulfoxide (DMSO). In recent years, improved strategies for removal of the solvent and release of growth factors have been active areas of investigation.[13] However, the requirement of a solvent to induce phase separation of the polymer limits the scale at which this approach can be applied *in vivo*. Even for relatively biocompatible solvents such as NMP and DMSO, injection of large volumes is anticipated to adversely affect host tissue, as well as the ability to eliminate the solvent from the body.

In recent years, self-assembly of amphiphiles with hydrophobic and hydrophilic domains has been investigated to create micro- and nano-structured biomaterials. Functionalization of amphiphiles such as peptides facilitates self-assembly of biomimetic materials without the use of crosslinkers, catalysts, solvents, and other agents. By modifying peptide amphiphiles (PA) with RGDS sequences, materials that support enhanced cellular adhesion have been prepared.[14,15] As shown in Fig. 15.1, B16 cells expressing green fluorescent protein-labeled integrin were observed to form focal adhesions in response to peptide amphiphiles (PA) modified with RGD epitopes. By varying the type of PA and the number of RGDS sequences, self-assembled nanoparticles with varying structures can be prepared (Fig. 15.1G–J). Functionalized self-assembling peptides that induce mineralization under physiological conditions have also been reported.[16,17] In an alternative approach, *in situ* crosslinking of nano- and micro-spheres used for drug delivery has been investigated to improve the structural integrity and mechanical properties of the delivery system. Negatively and positively charged nano-[18] and micro-[19] spheres that self-assemble to form crosslinks based on ionic interactions have been synthesized to create injectable biomaterials with tunable sustained release kinetics and mechanical properties. Self-assembling microsphere networks based on biotin-avidin binding have also been reported.[20] In this study, biotinylated PLA-PEG microspheres exhibited a three-fold increase in shear modulus in the presence of avidin. A significant advantage of these amphiphilic systems is that crosslinking and self-assembly can be achieved via physical forces to yield scaffolds displaying interconnected pores and tunable mechanical properties without the need for chemical reagents. However, as noted for environmentally responsive materials, the mechanical properties are typically lower than can be achieved with chemically crosslinked systems.

15.4 Calcium phosphate bone cements

Calcium phosphate cements (CPCs) have been investigated extensively as injectable bone replacement biomaterials due to their similar chemical composition to the mineral component of bone. A limitation of CPCs is their brittle mechanical properties and slow degradation *in vivo*.[2] Therefore, enhancing the mechanical properties, injectability, and rate of cellular infiltration and remodeling of CPCs while preserving their favorable biocompatibility is an important and active area of research. While ceramic biomaterials are discussed in greater detail in Chapter 2, the biocompatibility of conventional CPCs, as well as the implications of recent advancements on the biocompatibility of these biomaterials, will be reviewed in this chapter.

CPCs are nontoxic to cells, biocompatible, and osteoconductive. Furthermore, CPCs are biologically active such that they remodel and incorporate in host bone, and thus do not induce a foreign-body response.[21] These biomaterials set at a physiological pH with minimal reaction exotherm, and do not release toxic monomers or solvents.[22,23] There are two primary classes of CPCs: (a)

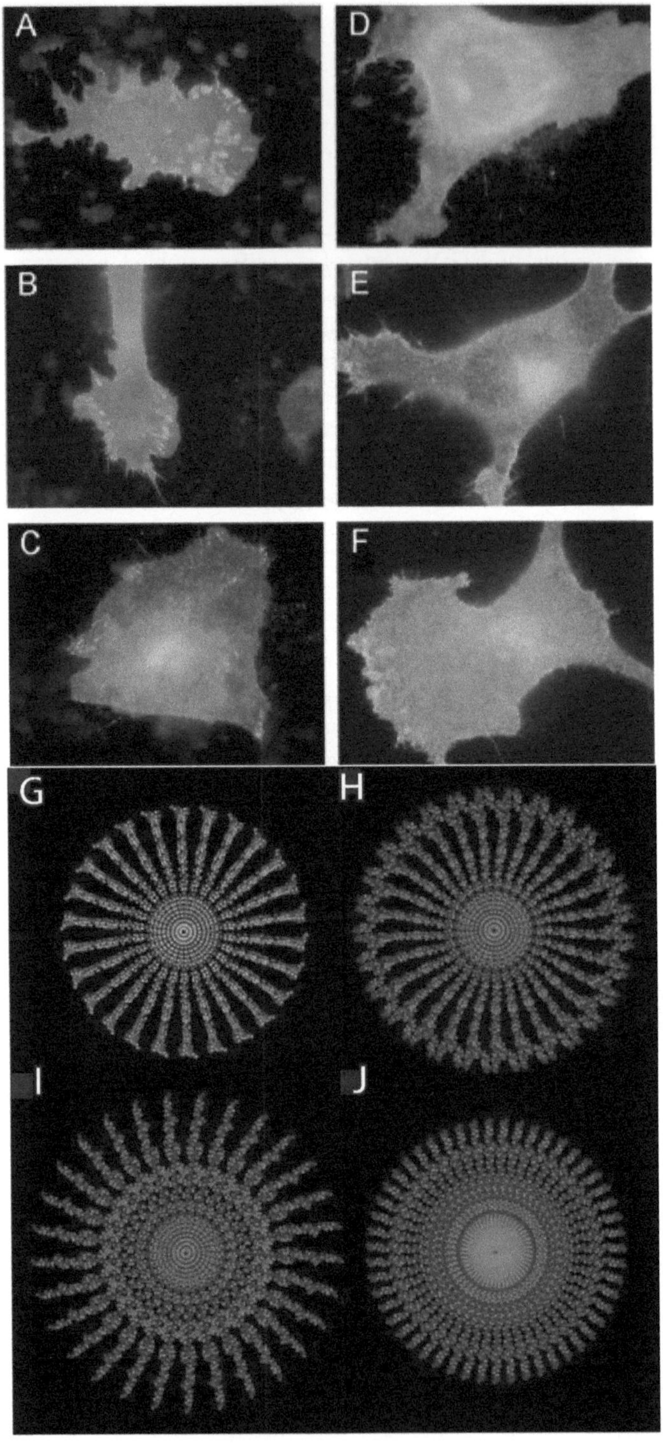
A
D
B
E
C
F
G
H
I
J

15.1 (opposite) Observation of focal adhesion formation for B16 cells expressing green fluorescent protein-labeled integrin in response to peptide amphiphiles (PA) modified with RGD epitopes. (A)–(F) B16 cells expressing GFP-β3 integrin cultured on coverslips coated with (A) branched PA with one cyclic RGDS, (B) branched PA with two RGDS, (C) branched PA with one RGDS, (D) branched PA with one RGDS, (E) linear PA with one RGDS, and (F) linear PA with one RGD showing punctate fluorescene (arrowheads) indicative of focal adhesion (FA) formation. (G)–(J) Cross-sections of PA nanofibers formed from branched and linear PA molecules. (G) Branched PA with one cyclic RGDS epitope, (H) branched PA with two RGDS epitopes, (I) branched PA with one RGDS epitope, and (J) linear PA with one RGDS epitope. Figure reproduced from Storrie *et al.*, Supramolecular crafting of cell adhesion, *Biomaterials* 28: 4608–4618, 2007.

apatite, which has a low solubility and resorbs more slowly, and (b) brushite, which has a higher solubility than apatite and resorbs more rapidly.[24] *In vivo*, brushite cements may be resorbed or may hydrolyze to hydroxyapatite and remain stable. CPCs set by an acid/base reaction, which can reduce the pH of the paste to values as low as 3.[25] While such low pH values immediately after setting of the CPC are anticipated to have a toxic effect on cells, a number of *in vivo* studies have reported favorable host responses after setting,[26,27] which suggests that the *in vivo* microenvironment has an extensive functional buffering capacity. In a recent study, the mechanism of cell-mediated degradation of brushite CPCs was investigated by culturing RAW264.7 cells on the cements *in vitro*.[28] The RAW264.7 cells differentiated to macrophages and multinucleated giant cells, as well as osteoclast-like cells, on the brushite CPCs. SEM analysis of the ultra-structure of osteoclast-like cells revealed characteristics associated with the osteoclast phenotype, such as formation of a sealing zone and ruffled border. Furthermore, osteoclast-like cells were observed to penetrate deep into the interior of the cements, which suggests that brushite CPCs are demineralized by osteoclast-mediated resorption *in vivo* (Fig. 15.2). Other studies have investigated the effects of nanometer-scale calcium phosphate (CaP) crystals on cellular interactions. Coating of mesenchymal stem cells with CaP nanorods has been reported to exhibit enhanced osteoblastic differentiation and production of extracellular matrix relative to uncoated cells,[29] which suggests that nanoscale injectable CPCs may be desirable carriers for stem cells.

The primary limitations of CPCs restricting their use in the clinic are brittle mechanical properties, which lead to low shear strength and fracture toughness, and the small pore size (0.1–10 μm), which results in slow infiltration.[21,30] Inadequate porosity and small pore size in CPCs do not facilitate ingrowth of new bone and have been suggested as a root cause for the failure of CPCs in periodontal bone repair.[31] Other studies have suggested that pulsatile forces from the dura induce failure and total fragmentation of CPCs in cranioplasty applications after a few months, thereby requiring a revision surgery to remove

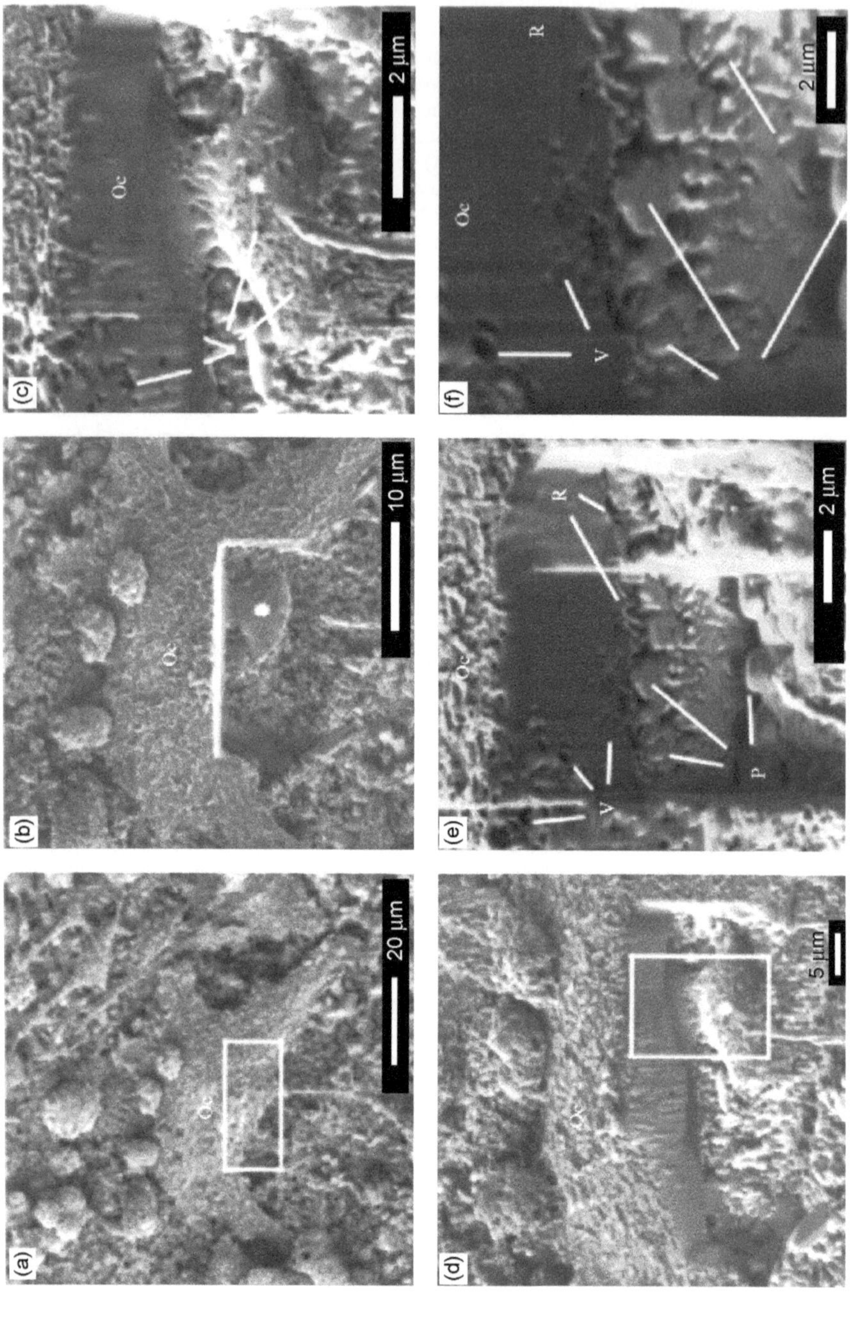

(a)
20 µm
Oc
(b)
10 µm
Oc
(c)
2 µm
Oc
V
(d)
5 µm
Oc
(e)
2 µm
Oc
R
V
P
(f)
2 µm
Oc
R
V

15.2 (opposite) Focused ion beam electron images showing the interface between an osteoclast-like cell and a β-TCP cement: (a) shows the area on an osteoclast-like cell chosen for milling; (b) the chosen area after milling, the part of cell labeled with a white star penetrating into the cement; (c) the sample tilted by 45° to highlight the cell penetration and the cell part and cell–material interface; (d) an additional area of interest selected for milling; (e) following milling of (c) the remaining cell organelles were removed and the interface between cell and material was exposed; and (f) a higher magnification of (e) to highlight the ruffled-border of the cells. Oc, osteoclast-like cells; V, vesicles within the osteoclast-like cells; P, cement particles; and R, the ruffled border of the osteoclast-like cells. Figure reproduced from Xia *et al.*, *In vitro* degradation of three brushite calcium phosphate cements by a macrophage cell line. *Biomaterials* 27: 4557–4565, 2006.

the fragments.[32] Therefore, recent investigations have focused on improving the mechanical and cellular infiltration properties of CPCs in order to improve their performance in clinical applications.

Macropores > 50 μm are essential for promoting ingrowth of new bone into the CPC.[33,34] In order to preserve the excellent biocompatibility of CPCs, adjuvants added to create macropores must be non-cytotoxic and biocompatible. A number of strategies have been investigated for generating macropores in CPCs *in situ*, including use of foaming agents (e.g., hydrogen peroxide solution,[35] hydrophobic liquids,[36] and degradable polymer microspheres (e.g., poly(lactic-co-glycolic acid), PLGA[37]). Other biocompatible and degradable porogens that have been investigated with injectable CPCs include poly(tri-methyl carbonate) and gelatin microparticles.[38,39] An additional advantage of CPCs incorporating degradable porogens is their potential for release of drugs or growth factors.[40] While incorporation of PLGA microspheres in CPCs has been suggested to improve the initial strength of the composites, the strength decreases upon dissolution of the microspheres and does not increase until new bone starts to grow into the macropores.[41] To improve the injectability of CPC incorporating 30 wt% PLGA microspheres, sodium citrate was added to the aqueous solution, which reduced the viscosity of the paste. Injectable composite CPCs incorporating a porogen have significant advantages compared to CPCs without a porogen, and it has been suggested that when these composite CPCs obtain regulatory approval they will be considered a preferred choice for healing of bony defects.[2] In an alternative approach, CaP granules suspended in aqueous solutions of hydroxy-propylmethyl-cellulose promoted faster initial ingrowth of new bone at the surface of the material relative to macroporous CPCs.[42,43] It has been suggested that the observed early apposition of new bone could potentially enhance the interfacial bonding between host bone and the CPC, thus reinforcing the material for weight-bearing applications.[2]

15.5 *In situ* polymerizable and crosslinkable biomaterials

In situ polymerizable materials comprise reactive monomers and/or macromers that are injected into the tissue defect in liquid form where they cure *in situ* to form a solid polymer. The cured polymer or gel forms by crosslinking of reactive monomers and macromer chains to form a polymer network. Depending on the crosslinking mechanism, various classes of materials can be prepared, including photopolymerized gels, chemically crosslinked thermosets, and ion-mediated gels.[44] Each of these types of biomaterials will be reviewed in this section.

15.5.1 Photopolymerization using ultraviolet light-activated initiators

There are several advantages to photopolymerization relative to other techniques, including control over the polymerization in space and time, curing rates on the order of seconds to minutes at physiological temperatures, and minimal reaction exotherms.[45] In the photopolymerization process, an initiator is activated by ultraviolet light to produce free radicals that react with the double bonds present in vinyl or acrylic groups, resulting in crosslinking *in situ* and enhanced mechanical properties of the scaffold. Hydrogels can be formed *in situ* from aqueous precursors using photopolymerization, which facilitates their use as injectable biomaterials. However, limitations include the need to polymerize at physiological pH and temperature, as well as the toxicity of the monomers, solvents, and initiators. In recent years, suitable photopolymerization systems that can be applied in the presence of cells and tissues have been identified.[45] Initiators that have been used to synthesize acrylated PEG hydrogels include acetophenone derivatives, such as 2,2-dimethoxy-2-phenyl acetophenone.[46] Isopropyl thioxanthone has also been reported to be a cytocompatible photoinitiator.[47] Owing to the cytotoxicity of monomers typically used in conventional photopolymerization processes, injectable photopolymerizable hydrogels are typically prepared from water-soluble macromers with two or more reactive groups, such as PEG acrylate derivatives, PEG methacrylate derivatives,[48] polyvinyl alcohol (PVA) derivatives,[49] and modified polysaccharides such as hyaluronic acid derivatives.[50] In order to promote cell adhesion, peptides incorporating adhesion domains of matrix proteins, such as KQAGDV (derived from fibronectin) and YIGSR (derived from laminin), have been covalently bound to hydrogels.[51,52] Proteolytically degradable hydrogels have also been prepared by incorporating peptide sequences in the gel that are recognizable by targeted proteases.[46]

Poly(propylene fumarate) (PPF) networks, which are formed by the reaction of PPF with a crosslinker and initiator, have been investigated as an injectable orthopedic biomaterial. While a number of crosslinkers, such as N-vinyl pyrrolidone (NMP) and poly(ethylene glycol) dimethacrylate, have been investigated, PPF-diacrylate (PPF-DA) has emerged as a preferred crosslinker due to its degradability.[53] The photoinitiator bis(2,4,6-trimethylbenzoyl) phenylphosphine oxide (BAPO), which is activated by long-wavelength ultraviolet light, has been reported to effectively crosslink PPF networks.[54] In a study investigating the effects of the PPF/PPF-DA double bond ratio on cytotoxicity *in vitro*, the leachable products from the reactive mixture were observed to adversely affect cell viability, and the toxicity increased with increasing fraction of PPF-DA.[53] This study underscores the challenges presented by the potential toxicity of the reactive intermediates prior to final cure of an injectable biomaterial. In a recent study, injectable porous PPF scaffolds were fabricated via a gas-foaming process using an NVP crosslinker and benzoyl peroxide initiator.[55] Scaffolds with 50% porosity and an elastic modulus of 20–40 MPa were fabricated. While the porosity and mechanical properties are promising, the effects of the solvents and initiator on *in vivo* biocompatibility are not known.

15.5.2 Thermosets

In many cases, the defect site has minimal light penetration, which limits the utility of the photopolymerization approach. Chemical or thermal initiation thus offers a significant advantage, since the polymerization can proceed throughout the bulk of the material in the absence of light. Thermoset polymers flow readily and conform to the desired shape when initially mixed, which renders these materials advantageous for injection. Final cure to a solid polymer is accomplished through the application of heat or a catalyst. An advantage of thermosets is that the polymer chains are covalently crosslinked, resulting in tunable mechanical properties ranging from rubbery elastomers to hard glassy plastics by controlling the crosslink density.[56,57] However, there are challenging limitations that have hindered the development of the technology.[58] The *in vivo* environment severely constrains the acceptable range of polymerization conditions, which is characterized by moderate temperatures, nontoxic monomers and catalysts, short gel and cure times, and the need to achieve final cure in a moisture-rich environment.[58,59] For example, cyanoacrylate glues that polymerize in the presence of blood have been investigated as liquid embolics for percutaneous filling of vascular spaces.[60] However, the toxicity of the reactants, as well as the heat released from the exothermic polymerization, has been reported to induce a significant acute and chronic inflammatory response.[61,62] Thus due to the adverse effects of the polymerization on host tissue, *in situ* thermosetting polymers have not been investigated extensively.[44]

Injectable, thermosetting biodegradable polyesters synthesized from D,L-lactide or L-lactide and ϵ-caprolactone have been investigated as biomedical devices for prosthetic implants and drug delivery systems.[63,64] In this system, OH-functional liquid polyols are first prepared by ring-opening polymerization of L-lactide and/or ϵ-caprolactone using a hydroxyl-functional initiator and a peroxide catalyst. The liquid polyols are subsequently converted to acrylic ester-terminated prepolymers. Prior to injection, the liquid prepolymers are mixed with a either a benzoyl peroxide or N,N-dimethyl-p-toluidene catalyst to promote cure, which requires 5–30 minutes. A significant advantage of the polyester technology is its simple injectability through a standard syringe. However, the disadvantages include a burst (~20%) release of drug due to its higher diffusivity in the reactive polymer prior to final cure and a reaction exotherm approaching 90°C. In addition, generation of free radicals by the benzyol peroxide catalyst potentially induces the formation of tumors.[65]

Thermally activated crosslinking, wherein an initiator first creates free radicals that subsequently react with unsaturated bonds present in the monomers or macromers, has also been investigated. As an example, a biocompatible and water-soluble thermal radical initiation system comprising an ammonium persulfate/N,N,N′,N′-tetramethylethylenediamine (APS/TEMED) initiator, a oligo(poly(ethylene glycol) fumarate) (OPF) macromer, and a poly(ethylene glycol)-diacrylate crosslinker has been applied to prepare cell/OPF hydrogel constructs with gel times < 10 min at 37°C.[66] While the initiator is non-cytotoxic at low concentrations, high concentrations are toxic to cells encapsulated in the gel, which limits the acceptable concentration range of the initiator. In this system, the viability of marrow stromal cells (MSCs) was > 90% for initiator concentrations < 100 mM, but at concentrations exceeding 100 mM, MSC viability was substantially reduced. The final pH and the extent of radical formation were found to significantly impact cell viability, thus requiring extensive testing of various initiators to identify suitable conditions that optimize both cell viability and other important parameters, such as gel and cure times and final mechanical properties.[2]

Polyurethanes comprise a class of thermosetting polymers that have recently been investigated as injectable biomaterials and drug delivery systems using the approach of two-component reactive liquid molding.[67–71] By mixing a polyisocyanate with a polyol and a tertiary amine or metal catalyst, a reactive liquid mixture is formed that subsequently cures to form a solid porous elastomeric scaffold within 10–15 minutes *in situ*.[72] The reaction between the polyisocyanate and polyol yields a urethane crosslink, while the reaction between the polyisocyanate and amine (or water, which can be added to generate pores) yields a urea crosslink. Polyurethanes have tunable degradation rates, which have been shown to be highly dependent on the choice of polyol and polyisocyanate components,[72–74] and tunable mechanical properties ranging from rubbery elastomers to hard glassy plastics.[68,75] Furthermore, two-component polyurethane scaffolds can be combined with a biological, such as an antibiotics or growth factor, prior to injection.[72,76–79] However, for these thermosetting biomaterials to be of use in the clinic, challenges associated with the toxicity of the polyisocyanate and catalyst components, as well as the adverse effects of the reaction exotherm must be addressed.

In an early study, a reactive putty comprising a lysine methyl ester diisocyanate (LDI) prepolymer and a calcium phosphate filler exhibited good integration with host tissue, cellular infiltration, and ingrowth of new blood vessels when implanted in rats.[70] This initial study introduced two key approaches to improving the biocompatibility of injectable two-component polyurethanes. Lysine-derived polyisocyanates, such as LDI and lysine triisocyanate (LTI), which are synthesized by phosgenation of amine-terminated lysine esters,[73,80,81] possess low vapor pressures (e.g., 0.00075 mm Hg at 25°C for LTI[80]) compared to aliphatic polyisocyanates (e.g., hexamethylene diisocyanate (HDI)). Since most polyisocyanates are toxic by inhalation, the low vapor pressure of LDI and LTI presents handling advantages by reducing the risk of exposure to an inhalation hazard. Another advantage of lysine-derived polyisocyanates is their biodegradation to non-toxic breakdown products such as lysine.[82] Reaction of the monomeric polyisocyanate with a polyol to form an isocyanate-terminated prepolymer further reduces the toxicity associated with monomeric polyisocyanates.[71,83]

In a recent study, two-component polyurethanes with and without calcium phosphate fillers were injected into 6 × 12 mm bilateral diaphyseal cortical defects in the femurs of skeletally mature Merino wether sheep.[75] The prepolymer was synthesized by capping pentaerythritol with lysine ethyl ester diisocyanate (ELDI) to yield a viscous liquid with isocyanate functionality, which was combined with a poly(glycolic acid) polyol and stannous octoate catalyst, mixed, and injected into the defects. For some of the materials, either water was included in the formulation to generate pores or calcium phosphate particles were added to reinforce mechanical properties. The yield strength varied from 6 to 13 MPa and the modulus from 270 to 580 MPa, which are comparable to the properties of trabecular bone. Free amine breakdown products were reported for *in vitro* degradation experiments in saline at 37°C, suggesting hydrolysis of urethane and urea bonds to lysine. At 6 weeks, there was no observable degradation of the polymer and no adverse acute or chronic inflammatory tissue response. Direct apposition of new bone onto the surface and into the pores of the material was observed. At 12 weeks, extensive degradation of the polymer and active bone formation were observed on the surface and within the pores of the materials. Some of the materials exhibited reactive cellular activity, which was conjectured to result from degradation of the polymer. Small pockets of neutrophils and lymphocytes were observed for some of the samples, and by 24 weeks only one specimen showed a small region of neutrophils. Thus both the reactive mixture comprising the prepolymer, poyol, and stannous octoate catalyst, as well as the breakdown products from the cured polymer, exhibited a mild inflammatory response and appeared to be well-tolerated. However, the potential long-term toxicity associated with the accumulation of stannous octoate in the body was not evaluated in this study.

In an alternative approach, two-component reactive polyurethane/allograft bone composites were injected into femoral plug defects in rats.[83] The pre-polymer was synthesized by capping poly(ethylene glycol) (PEG, 200 g/mol) with lysine triisocyanate (LTI) to yield a viscous liquid with isocyanate functionality, which was combined with a poly(ϵ-caprolactone-*co*-glycolide-*co*-lactide) polyol and triethlyene diamine catalyst, mixed, and injected into the defects. Tertiary amine catalysts exhibit significant advantages relative to heavy metals, including lower acute and chronic toxicity and elimination of the amine or its metabolites from the body in the urine.[84] The injectable composites incorporated particulated (e.g., >100 μm) allograft bone particles and had tunable (e.g., 30–70%) porosities. The initial dynamic viscosity was 220 Pa·s at clinically relevant shear rates (40 s^{-1}) and the wet compressive strength ranged from < 1–13 MPa. By adjusting the concentration of triethylene diamine catalyst, working times of 3–8 min and setting times of 10–20 min were achieved, which are comparable to the properties of calcium phosphate bone cements. The composites supported cellular infiltration, allograft resorption, collagen deposition, and new bone formation at three weeks when injected into femoral plug defects in athymic rats (Fig. 15.3). No adverse inflammatory response was observed. Other studies have shown that reactive two-component polyurethane scaffolds are effective delivery systems for antibiotics[76,85] and recombinant human (rh) growth factors, such as rhBMP2[78] and rhPDGF.[72,77] Despite the potential for active hydrogen (e.g., amine and hydroxyl) groups in the protein to reactive with the polyisocyanate, growth factors encapsulated in reactive two-component polyurethanes undergo sustained release from the scaffold with largely preserved bioactivity. Taken together, these studies show that injectable two-component polyurethanes can be safely administered to yield materials that cure *in situ* to polymers that elicit a minimal inflammatory response, support sustained release of biologics, and exhibit mechanical properties comparable to those of trabecular bone.

15.5.3 Ion-mediated gels

Ion-mediated gelation can be accomplished using polymers that form gels in the presence of ions.[44] Alginates, a class of naturally derived polysaccharide co-polymers of 1-4 linked β-D-mannuronic acid (M) and α-L-guluronic acid (G) that form gels in the presence of divalent ions (e.g., Ca^{2+}), have been investigated as a cell delivery vehicle and extracellular matrix analog.[86–88] The cations bind between the guluronic acid blocks of adjacent alginate chains, resulting in crosslinks between chains.[89] In the cell microencapsulation approach, cells that secrete therapeutic products are immobilized and immunoprotected within a biocompatible device, such as an alginate microsphere.[90] An important first step toward developing encapsulation devices is to evaluate the immunogenicity of the alginates used to fabricate the microcapsules as well as the biocompatibility

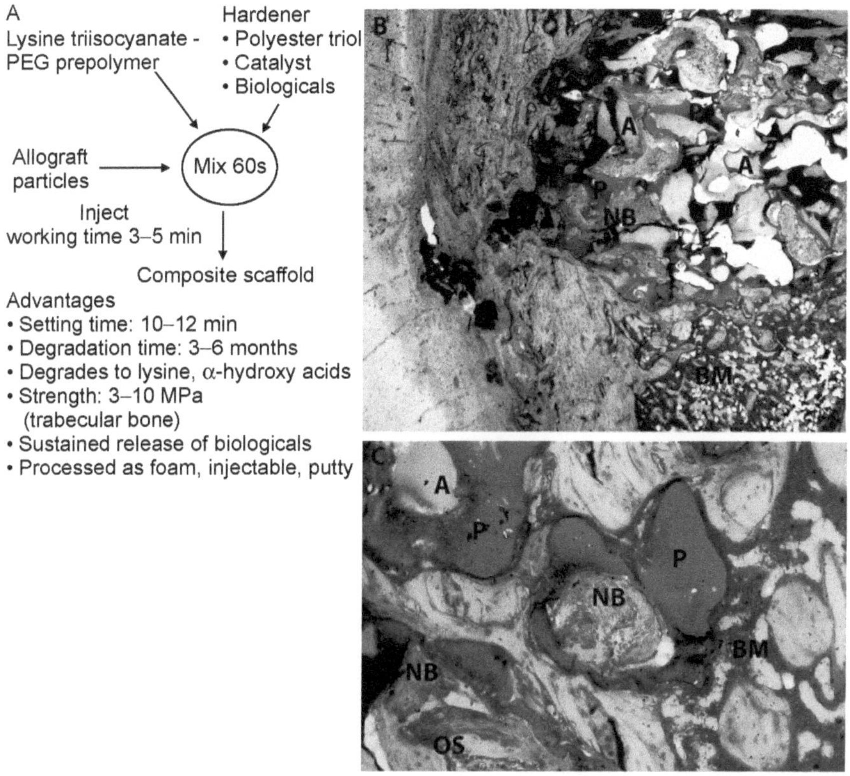

15.3 Injection of reactive polyurethane (PUR)/allograft bone particle composites in plug defects in rat femora. (A) Schematic of the mixing and injection process. (B) Low magnification (1.25×) images of histological sections taken at 3 weeks of composites injected into the plug defects showing host bone marrow (BM), allograft bone particles (A), new bone (NB), and residual polymer (P). New bone is formed at the composite/host bone interface, as well as in the interior of the composite. (C) Higher magnification (20×) images of histological sections showing allograft resorption, cellular infiltration, and remodeling. Osteoid (OS) is also observed along the surface of the remodeling bone.

of the microcapsule system. A key limitation of the use of alginate in the clinic is contamination due to impurities present in the seaweed from which it is extracted, as well as contamination resulting from industrial processing. Potential impurities include endotoxins, proteins, and polyphenols, which can be removed by chemical extraction[91] and electrophoresis.[92]

Both the purity and the composition of alginates affect their biocompatibility.[93] Alginates that have high β-D-mannuronic acid (M) content have been reported to induce an inflammatory response by stimulating monocytes to secrete interleukin (IL)-1, IL-6, and tumor necrosis factor (TNF), which has been suggested to occur through binding to CD14.[94,95] In support of this observation, another study has shown that antibodies to alginates were observed for transplanted high-M alginates but not for G-alginates.[96] A recent definitive study has investigated the effects of both alginate composition (M/G ratio) and purity on its *in vitro* and *in vivo* biocompatibility.[93] While contaminants present in the alginate more significantly impacted the inflammatory response compared to the alginate composition, the degree of contamination was related to the composition of the alginate. Specifically, it was observed that alginates high in M content also incorporated a higher concentration of polyphenol, endotoxin, and protein impurities. It has been suggested that development of standards for high-G and high-M alginates, as well as purity standards for the monomeric units, would contribute to the understanding of the effects of impurities and alginate composition on the immune response.[97] Understanding the mechanism of interaction between alginates and inflammatory cells in an attempt to improve their biocompatibility is an active area of investigation.

15.6 Future trends

Injectable biomaterials are generally injected as a liquid that sets *in situ* to form a solid scaffold. Setting can result from physical forces, as observed for self-assembling and environmentally responsive biomaterials, or from the formation of chemical bonds, as observed for calcium phosphate cements, photo-polymerizable gels, and thermosets. Physical gelation systems offer substantial biocompatibility advantages by avoiding the need to inject toxic reactive monomers and catalysts, but the mechanical properties of the resulting scaffolds are typically weak. Thus future research is anticipated to focus on the development of physically crosslinked systems with enhanced mechanical properties. Hybrid systems incorporating both physical and chemical crosslinks are a potentially effective approach to prepare biomaterials with both desirable physical crosslinking kinetics and enhanced mechanical properties.[12] Self-assembling peptides comprise a flexible biomimetic technology platform wherein cellular outcomes, mechanical properties, and nanostructure of the scaffold can be tuned to physiological requirements. Injectable biomaterials that support the delivery of viable stem cells are also anticipated to be an active area of future research.

While chemically crosslinked systems exhibit higher mechanical properties relative to physically crosslinked materials, the *in vivo* environment severely constrains the choice of reagents that can be used. Another challenge is the generation of defined pores that facilitate transport of cells and metabolites throughout the scaffold. Future research is thus anticipated to focus on the development of new injectable chemically crosslinking technologies that yield porous scaffolds after cure and are compatible with physiological conditions.

15.7 Sources of further information and advice

Several review papers on injectable biomaterials may be of interest to the reader, including Kretlow *et al.*, *Advanced Materials* 21: 3368, 2009; Khan *et al.*, *J Bone Joint Surg Am* Suppl 1:36, 2008; and Low *et al.*, *J Biomed Mater Res B Appl Biomater* Mar 24 2010.

15.8 References

1. Khan Y, Yaszemski MJ, Mikos AG, Laurencin CT. Tissue engineering of bone: material and matrix considerations. *J Bone Joint Surg Am* 2008; 90 Suppl 1: 36–42.
2. Kretlow JD, Young S, Klouda L, Wong M, Mikos AG. Injectable biomaterials for regenerating complex craniofacial tissues. *Adv Mater Deerfield* 2009; 21(32–33): 3368–3393.
3. Qiu Y, Park K. Environment-sensitive hydrogels for drug delivery. *Adv Drug Deliv Rev* 2001; 53(3): 321–339.
4. Galaev IY, Mattiasson B. 'Smart' polymers and what they could do in biotechnology and medicine. *Trends Biotechnol* 1999; 17(8): 335–340.
5. Klouda L, Mikos AG. Thermoresponsive hydrogels in biomedical applications. *Eur J Pharm Biopharm* 2008; 68(1): 34–45.
6. Hacker MC, Klouda L, Ma BB, Kretlow JD, Mikos AG. Synthesis and characterization of injectable, thermally and chemically gelable, amphiphilic poly(N-isopropylacrylamide)-based macromers. *Biomacromolecules* 2008; 9(6): 1558–1570.
7. Ohya S, Nakayama Y, Matsuda T. Thermoresponsive artificial extracellular matrix for tissue engineering: hyaluronic acid bioconjugated with poly(N-isopropylacrylamide) grafts. *Biomacromolecules* 2001; 2(3): 856–863.
8. Sosnik A, Cohn D. Ethoxysilane-capped PEO-PPO-PEO triblocks: a new family of reverse thermo-responsive polymers. *Biomaterials* 2004; 25(14): 2851–2858.
9. Fisher JP, Jo S, Mikos AG, Reddi AH. Thermoreversible hydrogel scaffolds for articular cartilage engineering. *J Biomed Mater Res A* 2004; 71(2): 268–274.
10. Bhattarai N, Ramay HR, Gunn J, Matsen FA, Zhang M. PEG-grafted chitosan as an injectable thermosensitive hydrogel for sustained protein release. *J Control Release* 2005; 103(3): 609–624.
11. Bhattarai N, Matsen FA, Zhang M. PEG-grafted chitosan as an injectable thermoreversible hydrogel. *Macromol Biosci* 2005; 5(2): 107–111.
12. Robb SA, Lee BH, McLemore R, Vernon BL. Simultaneously physically and chemically gelling polymer system utilizing a poly(NIPAAm-co-cysteamine)-based copolymer. *Biomacromolecules* 2007; 8(7): 2294–2300.
13. Tae G, Kornfield JA, Hubbell JA. Sustained release of human growth hormone from *in situ* forming hydrogels using self-assembly of fluoroalkyl-ended poly(ethylene glycol). *Biomaterials* 2005; 26(25): 5259–5266.
14. Storrie H, Guler MO, Abu-Amara SN, Volberg T, Rao M, Geiger B, *et al.* Supramolecular crafting of cell adhesion. *Biomaterials* 2007; 28(31): 4608–4618.
15. Guler MO, Hsu L, Soukasene S, Harrington DA, Hulvat JF, Stupp SI. Presentation of RGDS epitopes on self-assembled nanofibers of branched peptide amphiphiles. *Biomacromolecules* 2006; 7(6): 1855–1863.
16. Kirkham J, Firth A, Vernals D, Boden N, Robinson C, Shore RC, *et al.* Self-assembling peptide scaffolds promote enamel remineralization. *J Dent Res* 2007; 86(5): 426–430.

17. Firth A, Aggeli A, Burke JL, Yang X, Kirkham J. Biomimetic self-assembling peptides as injectable scaffolds for hard tissue engineering. *Nanomedicine (Lond)* 2006; 1(2): 189–199.
18. Singh M, Berkland C, Detamore MS. Strategies and applications for incorporating physical and chemical signal gradients in tissue engineering. *Tissue Eng Part B Rev* 2008; 14(4): 341–366.
19. Van Tomme SR, van Steenbergen MJ, De Smedt SC, van Nostrum CF, Hennink WE. Self-gelling hydrogels based on oppositely charged dextran microspheres. *Biomaterials* 2005; 26(14): 2129–2135.
20. Salem AK, Rose FRAJ, Oreffo RO, Yang X, Davies MC, Mitchell JR, *et al.* Porous polymer and cell composites that self-assemble *in situ*. *Adv Mater* 2003; 15(3): 210–213.
21. Low KL, Tan SH, Zein SH, Roether JA, Mourino V, Boccaccini AR. Calcium phosphate-based composites as injectable bone substitute materials: a review. *J Biomed Mater Res B Appl Biomater* 2010; 94B(1), 273–286.
22. Liu C, Wang W, Shen W, Chen T, Hu L, Chen Z. Evaluation of the biocompatibility of a nonceramic hydroxyapatite. *J Endod* 1997; 23(8): 490–493.
23. Fernandez E, Ginebra MP, Boltong MG, Driessens FC, Ginebra J, De Maeyer EA, *et al.* Kinetic study of the setting reaction of a calcium phosphate bone cement. *J Biomed Mater Res* 1996; 32(3): 367–374.
24. Bohner M. Calcium orthophosphates in medicine: from ceramics to calcium phosphate cements. *Injury* 2000; 31(Supplement 4): S-D37–47.
25. Bohner M, Van Landuyt P, Merkle HP, Lemaitre J. Composition effects on the pH of a hydraulic calcium phosphate cement. *J Mater Sci Mater Med* 1997; 8(11): 675–681.
26. Frayssinet P, Gineste L, Conte P, Fages J, Rouquet N. Short-term implantation effects of a DCPD-based calcium phosphate cement. *Biomaterials* 1998; 19(11–12): 971–977.
27. Constantz BR, Barr BM, Ison IC, Fulmer MT, Baker J, McKinney L, *et al.* Histological, chemical, and crystallographic analysis of four calcium phosphate cements in different rabbit osseous sites. *J Biomed Mater Res* 1998; 43(4): 451–461.
28. Xia Z, Groverb LM, Huang Y, Adamopoulosa IE, Gbureck U, Triffitt JT, *et al. In vitro* biodegradation of three brushite calcium phosphate cements by a macrophage cell-line. *Biomaterials* 2006; 27: 4557–4565.
29. Gonzalez-McQuire R, Green DW, Partridge KA, Oreffo RO, Mann S, Davis SA. Coating of human mesenchymal cells in 3D culture with bioinorganic nanoparticles promotes osteoblastic differentiation and gene transfection. *Adv Mater* 2007; 19(17): 2236–2240.
30. Shindo ML, Costantino PD, Friedman CD, Chow LC. Facial skeletal augmentation using hydroxyapatite cement. *Arch Otolaryngol Head Neck Surg* 1993; 119(2): 185–190.
31. Brown GD, Mealey BL, Nummikoski PV, Bifano SL, Waldrop TC. Hydroxyapatite cement implant for regeneration of periodontal osseous defects in humans. *J Periodontol* 1998; 69(2): 146–157.
32. Goldberg CS, Antonyshyn O, Midha R, Fialkov JA. Measuring pulsatile forces on the human cranium. *J Craniofacial Surgery* 2005; 16(1): 134–139.
33. Livingston T, Ducheyne P, Garino J. *In vivo* evaluation of a bioactive scaffold for bone tissue engineering. *J Biomed Mater Res* 2002; 62(1): 1–13.
34. Pilliar RM, Filiaggi MJ, Wells JD, Grynpas MD, Kandel RA. Porous calcium polyphosphate scaffolds for bone substitute applications – *in vitro* characterization. *Biomaterials* 2001; 22(9): 963–972.

35. Almirall A, Larrecq G, Delgado JA, Martinez S, Planell JA, Ginebra MP. Fabrication of low temperature macroporous hydroxyapatite scaffolds by foaming and hydrolysis of an alpha-TCP paste. *Biomaterials* 2004; 25(17): 3671–3680.
36. Bohner M. Calcium phosphate emulsions: possible applications. *Key Eng Mater* 2001; 192–195: 765–768.
37. Link DP, van den Dolder J, Jurgens WJ, Wolke JG, Jansen JA. Mechanical evaluation of implanted calcium phosphate cement incorporated with PLGA microparticles. *Biomaterials* 2006; 27(28): 4941–4947.
38. Habraken WJ, de Jonge LT, Wolke JG, Yubao L, Mikos AG, Jansen JA. Introduction of gelatin microspheres into an injectable calcium phosphate cement. *J Biomed Mater Res A* 2008; 87(3): 643–655.
39. Habraken WJ, Zhang Z, Wolke JG, Grijpma DW, Mikos AG, Feijen J, *et al.* Introduction of enzymatically degradable poly(trimethylene carbonate) microspheres into an injectable calcium phosphate cement. *Biomaterials* 2008; 29(16): 2464–2476.
40. Ruhe PQ, Boerman OC, Russel FG, Spauwen PH, Mikos AG, Jansen JA. Controlled release of rhBMP-2 loaded poly(DL-lactic-co-glycolic acid)/calcium phosphate cement composites *in vivo*. *J Control Release* 2005; 106(1–2): 162–171.
41. Martin RB, Chapman MW, Holmes RE, Sartoris DJ, Shors EC, Gordon JE, *et al.* Effects of bone ingrowth on the strength and non-invasive assessment of a coralline hydroxyapatite material. *Biomaterials* 1989; 10: 481–488.
42. Trojani C, Boukhechba F, Scimeca JC, Vandenbos F, Michiels JF, Daculsi G, *et al.* Ectopic bone formation using an injectable biphasic calcium phosphate/Si-HPMC hydrogel composite loaded with undifferentiated bone marrow stromal cells. *Biomaterials* 2006; 27(17): 3256–3264.
43. Gauthier O, Muller R, von Stechow D, Lamy B, Weiss P, Bouler JM, *et al. In vivo* bone regeneration with injectable calcium phosphate biomaterial: a three-dimensional micro-computed tomographic, biomechanical and SEM study. *Biomaterials* 2005; 26(27): 5444–5453.
44. Chitkara D, Shikanov A, Kumar N, Domb AJ. Biodegradable injectable *in situ* depot-forming drug delivery systems. *Macromol Biosci* 2006; 6(12): 977–990.
45. Nguyen KT, West JL. Photopolymerizable hydrogels for tissue engineering applications. *Biomaterials* 2002; 23(22): 4307–4314.
46. Mann BK, Gobin AS, Tsai AT, Schmedlen RH, West JL. Smooth muscle cell growth in photopolymerized hydrogels with cell adhesive and proteolytically degradable domains: synthetic ECM analogs for tissue engineering. *Biomaterials* 2001; 22(22): 3045–3051.
47. Bryant SJ, Nuttelman CR, Anseth KS. Cytocompatibility of UV and visible light photoinitiating systems on cultured NIH/3T3 fibroblasts *in vitro*. *J Biomater Sci Polym Ed* 2000; 11(5): 439–457.
48. Kim IS, Jeong YI, Kim SH. Self-assembled hydrogel nanoparticles composed of dextran and poly(ethylene glycol) macromer. *Int J Pharm* 2000; 205(1–2): 109–116.
49. Martens P, Anseth KS. Characterization of hydrogels formed from acrylate modified poly(vinyl alcohol) macromers. *Polymer* 2000; 41: 7715–7722.
50. Bulpitt P, Aeschlimann D. New strategy for chemical modification of hyaluronic acid: preparation of functionalized derivatives and their use in the formation of novel biocompatible hydrogels. *J Biomed Mater Res* 1999; 47(2): 152–169.
51. Mann BK, Tsai AT, Scott-Burden T, West JL. Modification of surfaces with cell adhesion peptides alters extracellular matrix deposition. *Biomaterials* 1999; 20(23–24): 2281–2286.

52. Hern DL, Hubbell JA. Incorporation of adhesion peptides into nonadhesive hydrogels useful for tissue resurfacing. *J Biomed Mater Res* 1998; 39(2): 266–276.
53. Timmer MD, Shin H, Horch RA, Ambrose CG, Mikos AG. *In vitro* cytotoxicity of injectable and biodegradable poly(propylene fumarate)-based networks: unreacted macromers, cross-linked networks, and degradation products. *Biomacromolecules* 2003; 4(4): 1026–1033.
54. Fisher JP, Dean D, Mikos AG. Photocrosslinking characteristics and mechanical properties of diethyl fumarate/poly(propylene fumarate) biomaterials. *Biomaterials* 2002; 23(22): 4333–4343.
55. Kim CW, Talac R, Lu L, Moore MJ, Currier BL, Yaszemski MJ. Characterization of porous injectable poly-(propylene fumarate)-based bone graft substitute. *J Biomed Mater Res A* 2008; 85(4): 1114–1119.
56. Timmer MD, Ambrose CG, Mikos AG. *In vitro* degradation of polymeric networks of poly(propylene fumarate) and the crosslinking macromer poly(propylene fumarate)-diacrylate. *Biomaterials* 2003; 24(4): 571–577.
57. Timmer MD, Ambrose CG, Mikos AG. Evaluation of thermal- and photo-crosslinked biodegradable poly(propylene fumarate)-based networks. *J Biomed Mater Res A* 2003; 66(4): 811–818.
58. Hatefi A, Amsden B. Biodegradable injectable *in situ* forming drug delivery systems. *J Control Release* 2002; 80(1–3): 9–28.
59. Burkoth AK, Anseth KS. A review of photocrosslinked polyanhydrides: *in situ* forming degradable networks. *Biomaterials* 2000; 21(23): 2395–2404.
60. Jordan O, Doelker E, Rufenacht DA. Biomaterials used in injectable implants (liquid embolics) for percutaneous filling of vascular spaces. *Cardiovasc Intervent Radiol* 2005; 28(5): 561–569.
61. Kerber CW, Wong W. Liquid acrylic adhesive agents in interventional neuroradiology. *Neurosurg Clin N Am* 2000; 11(1): 85–99, viii–ix.
62. Vinters HV, Galil KA, Lundie MJ, Kaufmann JC. The histotoxicity of cyano-acrylates. A selective review. *Neuroradiology* 1985; 27(4): 279–291.
63. Moore LA, Norton RL, Whitman SL, Dunn RL. An injectable biodegradable drug delivery system based on acrylic terminated poly ϵ-caprolactone. Annual Meeting of the Society of Biomaterials; 1995.
64. Dunn RL, English JP, Cowsar DR, Vanderbelt DD, inventors. Biodegradable *in-situ* forming implants and methods for producing the same. US Patent 5,340,849, 1994.
65. Zhao J, Lahiri-Chatterjee M, Sharma Y, Agarwal R. Inhibitory effect of a flavonoid antioxidant silymarin on benzoyl peroxide-induced tumor promotion, oxidative stress and inflammatory responses in SENCAR mouse skin. *Carcinogenesis* 2000; 21(4): 811–816.
66. Temenoff JS, Shin H, Conway DE, Engel PS, Mikos AG. *In vitro* cytotoxicity of redox radical initiators for cross-linking of oligo(poly(ethylene glycol) fumarate) macromers. *Biomacromolecules* 2003; 4(6): 1605–1613.
67. Guelcher S, Srinivasan A, Hafeman A, Gallagher K, Doctor J, Khetan S, *et al.* Synthesis, *in vitro* degradation, and mechanical properties of two-component poly(ester urethane)urea scaffolds: Effects of water and polyol composition. *Tissue Eng* 2007; 13(9): 2321–2333.
68. Gorna K, Gogolewski S. Preparation, degradation, and calcification of biodegradable polyurethane foams for bone graft substitutes. *J Biomed Mater Res* 2003; 67A: 813–827.
69. Zhang J-Y, Beckman EJ, Piesco NJ, Agarwal S. A new peptide-based urethane polymer: synthesis, biodegradation, and potential to support cell growth *in vitro.*

Biomaterials 2000; 21: 1247–1258.
70. Bennett S, Connolly K, Lee DR, Jiang Y, Buck D, Hollinger JO, *et al.* Initial biocompatibility studies of a novel degradable polymeric bone substitute that hardens *in situ*. *Bone* 1996; 19(1, Supplement): 101S–107S.
71. Bonzani IC, Adhikari R, Houshyar S, Mayadunne RTA, Gunatillake PA, Stevens MM. Synthesis of two-component injectable polyurethanes for bone tissue engineering. *Biomaterials* 2007; 28: 423–433.
72. Hafeman A, Li B, Yoshii T, Zienkiewicz K, Davidson J, Guelcher S. Injectable biodegradable polyurethane scaffolds with release of platelet-derived growth factor for tissue repair and regeneration. *Pharm Res* 2008; 25(10): 2387–2399.
73. Storey RF, Wiggins JS, Puckett AD. Hydrolyzable poly(ester-urethane) networks from L-lysine diisocyanate and D,L-lactide/ϵ-caprolactone homo- and copolyester triols. *J Polym Sci, Part A: Polym Chem* 1994; 32(12): 2345–2363.
74. Skarja GA, Woodhouse KA. Structure-property relationships of degradable polyurethane elastomers containing an amino acid-based chain extender. *J Appl Polym Sci* 2000; 75: 1522–1534.
75. Adhikari R, Gunatillake PA, Griffiths I, Tatai L, Wickramaratna M, Houshyar S, *et al.* Biodegradable injectable polyurethanes: synthesis and evaluation for orthopaedic applications. *Biomaterials* 2008; 29(28): 3762–3770.
76. Li B, Brown KV, Wenke JC, Guelcher SA. Sustained release of vancomycin from polyurethane scaffolds inhibits infection of bone wounds in a rat femoral segmental defect model. *J Control Release* 2010; 145(3): 221–230.
77. Li B, Davidson JM, Guelcher SA. The effect of the local delivery of platelet-derived growth factor from reactive two-component polyurethane scaffolds on the healing in rat skin excisional wounds. *Biomaterials* 2009; 30(20): 3486–3494.
78. Li B, Yoshii T, Hafeman AE, Nyman JS, Wenke JC, Guelcher SA. The effects of rhBMP-2 released from biodegradable polyurethane/microsphere composite scaffolds on new bone formation in rat femora. *Biomaterials* 2009; 30(35): 6768–6779.
79. Hafeman A, Carney E, Litzner B, Zienkiewicz K, Hochhauser L, Davidson J, *et al.* Release of antibiotic from injectable, biodegradable polyurethane scaffolds for enhanced fracture healing. Orthopaedic Research Society Annual Meeting; March 2–5, 2008; San Francisco, CA.
80. Kitai M, Ryuutou H, Yahata T, Hara Y, Iwane H, Soejima Y, inventors. Aliphatic triisocyanate compound, process for producing the same, and polyurethane resin made from the compound. US Patent No. 20020123644 A1, 2002.
81. Yamasaki K, Iwasa T, Nihonmatsu T, Hisamura K, inventors. Lysine ester triiscyanate and method for production thereof. US Patent No. US2006/0167303 A1, 2006.
82. Guelcher S. Biodegradable polyurethanes: synthesis and applications in regenerative medicine. *Tissue Eng B* 2008; 14(1): 3–17.
83. Dumas JE, Zienkiewicz K, Tanner SA, Prieto EM, Bhattacharyya S, Guelcher S. Synthesis and characterization of an injectable allograft bone/polymer composite bone void filler with tunable mechanical properties. *Tissue Eng Part A* 2010; 16(8): 2505–2518.
84. Ballantyne R. Toxicology update: Bis[2-(dimethylamino)ethyl]ether. *J Appl Toxicol* 2005; 25: 260–269.
85. Hafeman AE, Zienkiewicz KJ, Carney E, Litzner B, Stratton C, Wenke JC, *et al.* Local delivery of tobramycin from injectable biodegradable polyurethane scaffolds. *J Biomater Sci: Polym Ed* 2009; DOI: 10.1163/156856209X410256.

86. Orive G, Tam SK, Pedraz JL, Halle JP. Biocompatibility of alginate-poly-L-lysine microcapsules for cell therapy. *Biomaterials* 2006; 27(20): 3691–3700.
87. Boontheekul T, Kong HJ, Mooney DJ. Controlling alginate gel degradation utilizing partial oxidation and bimodal molecular weight distribution. *Biomaterials* 2005; 26(15): 2455–2465.
88. Kretlow JD, Klouda L, Mikos AG. Injectable matrices and scaffolds for drug delivery in tissue engineering. *Adv Drug Del Rev* 2007; 59: 263–273.
89. Rowley JA, Madlambayan G, Mooney DJ. Alginate hydrogels as synthetic extracellular matrix materials. *Biomaterials* 1999; 20(1): 45–53.
90. Orive G, Hernandez RM, Gascon AR, Calafiore R, Chang TM, De Vos P, *et al.* Cell encapsulation: promise and progress. *Nat Med* 2003; 9(1): 104–107.
91. Zimmermann U, Thurmer F, Jork A, Weber M, Mimietz S, Hillgartner M, *et al.* A novel class of amitogenic alginate microcapsules for long-term immunoisolated transplantation. *Ann NY Acad Sci* 2001; 944: 199–215.
92. Zimmermann U, Klock G, Federlin K, Hannig K, Kowalski M, Bretzel RG, *et al.* Production of mitogen-contamination free alginates with variable ratios of mannuronic acid to guluronic acid by free flow electrophoresis. *Electrophoresis* 1992; 13(5): 269–274.
93. Orive G, Ponce S, Hernandez RM, Gascon AR, Igartua M, Pedraz JL. Biocompatibility of microcapsules for cell immobilization elaborated with different type of alginates. *Biomaterials* 2002; 23(18): 3825–3831.
94. Espevik T, Otterlei M, Skjak-Braek G, Ryan L, Wright SD, Sundan A. The involvement of CD14 in stimulation of cytokine production by uronic acid polymers. *Eur J Immunol* 1993; 23(1): 255–261.
95. Otterlei M, Ostgaard K, Skjak-Braek G, Smidsrod O, Soon-Shiong P, Espevik T. Induction of cytokine production from human monocytes stimulated with alginate. *J Immunother* 1991; 10(4): 286–291.
96. Kulseng B, Skjak-Braek G, Ryan L, Andersson A, King A, Faxvaag A, *et al.* Transplantation of alginate microcapsules: generation of antibodies against alginates and encapsulated porcine islet-like cell clusters. *Transplantation* 1999; 67(7): 978–984.
97. Orive G, Hernandez RM, Rodriguez Gascon A, Calafiore R, Chang TM, de Vos P, *et al.* History, challenges and perspectives of cell microencapsulation. *Trends Biotechnol* 2004; 22(2): 87–92.

16

Future applications of injectable biomaterials: the use of microgels as modular injectable scaffolds

R. SCOTT, Saint Louis University, USA and
R. KUNTZ WILLITS, The University of Akron, USA

Abstract: This chapter seeks to overview the fabrication and characterization of polymeric microgels and their current and potenial uses for injectable drug delivery and tissue engineering. As these materials can be formed with a wide range of functionalities, microgels can be utilized in a wide range of applications, including as building blocks for scaffold design.

Key words: microgel, dispersion polymerization, precipitation polymerization, p(NIPAm), PEG.

16.1 Introduction

In seeking out new technologies for biomedical applications, researchers tend to look to advances in adjacent fields such as materials science, electrical engineering, or nanotechnology. This review is focused on one such area: the investigation of microgels for injectable tissue engineering and drug delivery modalities. Microgels and nanogels are polymeric particles that range in size from 1 nm to 100 μm (IUPAC 1997) and the polymerization methods to form these gels have been the topics of excellent reviews, including solution (Arshady 1992), suspension (Arshady 1992; Vivaldo-Lima, Wood *et al.* 1997), emulsion (Arshady 1992), precipitation (Pelton 2000; Pich and Richtering 2010), or dispersion (Barrett 1975) polymerizations. Thorough coverage of all of these polymerization techniques is a book in itself, therefore this review will focus on microgels formed from precipitation and dispersion reactions. As dispersion reactions are essentially precipitation reactions with a surfactant, these terms will be used interchangably throughout the text. Section 16.2 includes both a history of the technology and how microgels are fabricated and characterized. Section 16.3 seeks to orient the reader to the current usage of microgels in biomedical applications. Finally, Section 16.4 serves to propose future trends with these materials. The reader should keep in mind that these particles can be formed with many polymers, with this review serving as a jumping off point for novel potential applications for injectable biomaterials.

16.2 Background

16.2.1 History of microgels

As chip technology has improved, the biomedical industry has shown a desire to capture those methodologies and utilize them to improve medical devices. In the same manner, the use of micro- and nano-materials in tissue engineering and drug delivery applications has become increasingly popular due to the development of polymer particulates, allowing for a reduction in system, and sub-system sizing. Structurally, polymer microgels consist of crosslinked colloidal particles; microgels are generally defined as particulates ranging in size from 0.1 to 100 μm (IUPAC 1997), while nanogels are typically less than 100 nm in size (Alemán, Chadwick *et al.* 2007). These colloid systems can be produced with a variety of methods and materials, making them interesting candidates for use in tissue engineering and drug delivery applications.

Microgel particles were first prepared in 1935 by Staudinger and Husemann via suspension polymerization; poly(divinyl benzene) (DVB) microparticles were polymerized in organic solvents at a high dilution (Staudinger and Husemann 1935). Although the term 'microgel' was not introduced until nearly 15 years later (Baker 1949), these first colloid particles provided a foundation upon which a new branch of scientific exploration was founded. Since its discovery, microgel research has become progressively more popular due to the large array of potential applications. However, a major explosion in polymer colloids fabrication occurred following the discovery of microgel particles formed from poly(N-isopropylacrylamide) (pNIPAm) in 1986 (Pelton and Chibante 1986). In recent years, a large amount of work has been performed toward the development of novel microgel systems in addition to the on-going investigation of older systems using newer techniques or methods.

Historically, the development of techniques for the preparation of colloid polymer particles has been driven predominantly by the surface coatings industry (Barrett 1975). In order to achieve durable paint films, surface coatings were generally required to be composed of a polymer of high molecular weight. However, as the concentration or the molecular weight of the polymer used in solution was increased, the viscosity of the solutions also increased. As most surface coatings were applied by brush or spray, an increased solution viscosity caused application limitations. To avoid such limitations, lower concentration polymeric solutions were used; however, this technique required a number of separate layers of polymer solution to be applied in order to build up a coating of adequate thickness. To overcome the disadvantages exhibited by conventional methods of paint application, surface coatings were formulated using solutions of polymer dispersions. This technique, originally developed by the rubber industry (Whitby and Katz 1933), allowed for the preparation of dispersions of high molecular weight polymers in solutions of low viscosity. These polymer dispersions proved not only to be attractive for surface coatings, but also for use in the printing industry. In addition to their excellent surface coating characteristics, polymer microgels offered a high surface-to-volume ratio and were able to be functionalized to yield photo-crosslinkable particles. The increased surface area, provided by these functionalized microparticle systems, allowed the colloids to be used as printing offset plates, creating high-resolution, water-resistant images (Sasa and Yamaoka 1994).

Similarly, the use of microparticles in the biomedical industry has shown great promise. Currently, microgels formed from dispersion or precipitation reactions are used in a number of applications: immunoassays (Kamyshny and Magdassi 2000), affinity chromatography (Tuncel, Ecevit *et al.* 1996; Zhang and Rassi 1999; Spegel, Schweitz *et al.* 2001), controlled drug delivery (Herrmann and Bodmeier 1995; Morishita, Lowman *et al.* 2002; Yenice, Cali *et al.* 2002; Silva, Costa *et al.* 2005), and tissue engineering (Serpe, Yarmey *et al.* 2005; Nolan, Gelbaum *et al.* 2006; Scott, Nichols *et al.* 2010). These microgels are produced using straightforward protocols, with excellent control over particle size due to the nature of the polymerization. The synthesis of microgels is highly versatile, where production can occur in a variety of solvents, including ethanol (Kaneda and Vincent 2004), acetonitrile (Bai, Yang *et al.* 2004; Lime and Irgum 2009), or water (Nolan, Reyes *et al.* 2005; Scott, Nichols *et al.* 2010). Of these techniques, the fabrication of microspheres in water has proven most valuable to biomedical applications due to the high biocompatibility levels that these water-swollen microgels exhibit. In addition, microgels can be further enhanced by modifying the particulates with the addition of functional groups such as acrylic acid (AAc) (Kratz, Hellweg *et al.* 2000) or vinylacetic acid (Hoare and Pelton 2004) among others.

16.2.2 Fabrication of microgels

The preparation of micron-sized polymer particles has been achieved through the use of a variety of polymerization techniques, including emulsion, suspension, dispersion, and precipitation polymerization. Although the focus of this review is on dispersion and precipitation polymerization, a brief description of emulsion and suspension is included below to be able to compare the different mechanisms.

The preparation of microparticles by emulsion polymerization, originally developed in the synthetic rubber industry (Whitby and Katz 1933), allows for the formation of microparticles with a narrow distribution of sizes. In this technique, a monomer is dispersed in a solution of surfactant and water where the surfactant creates micelles in the water. Low solubility of the monomer in water is required, such that the addition of the polymer creates large droplets of the monomer within the water. Small amounts of monomer diffuse through the water into the surfactant micelles. To begin the polymerization process, water-soluble initiator is added to the solution, propagating the monomer to form polymer chains in the micelles, thus creating microparticles. The formation of microparticles via this technique can create polymer chains of high molecular weight, while the particle size is often small, on the nano-scale (Loxley and Vincent 1997; Sisson, Steinhilber *et al.* 2009). Removal of the particles from the continuous phase is often achieved by freeze-drying. The microgels can then be resuspended in a good solvent, which will cause them to swell.

In the process of suspension polymerization, the monomer, which is relatively insoluble in aqueous solutions, is dispersed into small droplets using a steric stabilizer and vigorous stirring. The main difference between emulsion and suspension polymerization involves the initiator; in emulsion techniques, the initiator is soluble in water; however, in suspension techniques, it is soluble in the monomer. The size of the monomer droplets is controlled by the interfacial tension, the agitation rate, and the design of the stirrer/reactor system (Vivaldo-Lima, Wood *et al.* 1997). Generally, microspheres from 10 μm to 5 mm in diameter are produced using this method (Vivaldo-Lima, Wood *et al.* 1997), causing a high polydispersity of microgels produced via this technique (Hunkeler, Candau *et al.* 1994).

In contrast to suspension polymerization, the fabrication of microspheres using dispersion polymerization produces colloid particles with a low polydispersity (Arshady 1992). In this process, the monomers, steric stabilizers, and initiators are soluble in a solvent as a continuous phase. Polymerization occurs initially within the homogeneous reaction mixture. Ultimately, it is the insolubility of formed polymer particles in the continuous phase that allows for the collection of these microspheres. The colloid particles formed using this technique are held together with the help of a colloidal stabilizing agent (Arshady 1992).

Similar to dispersion polymerization, precipitation polymerization occurs when monomer and initiator are soluble in the continuous phase. Polymerization occurs as the growing polymer chains phase separate from the continuous medium, via enthalpic or entropic precipitation (Bai, Yang *et al.* 2004). The newly formed polymer chains then aggregate to form polymer particulates. Using this technique, a variety of microparticles have been fabricated from various polymeric materials including: poly(ethylene glycol) (PEG) (Nolan, Reyes *et al.* 2005; Nichols, Scott *et al.* 2009; Scott, Nichols *et al.* 2010), poly(methacrylic acid) (PMAA) (Thomas, Tingsanchali *et al.* 2007), DVB (Lime and Irgum 2009), and pNIPAm (Chen, Zhang *et al.* 2008). This polymerization method is unique in the fact that stabilizers and surfactants are not required to produce microspheres of uniform size and shape. Due to the high amount of initiator utilized, microparticles fabricated using this polymerization technique are self-stabilized. However, while these microspheres are characteristically stable without the use of surfactant, precipitation polymerization must often be performed at high temperatures. It is only when a polymer solution reaches a critical temperature, the lower critical solution temperature

(LCST), that the polymer chains are able to collapse and phase separate to form the microparticles. To reduce the LCST, several groups have investigated the use of kosmotrophic salts, allowing formation of colloid particles at more relevant, physiological temperatures (Bailey and Callard 1959; Bai, Yang *et al.* 2004; Nichols, Scott *et al.* 2009; Scott, Nichols *et al.* 2010).

While all of the mechanisms described above have been used to produce microgels under various conditions, microgels fabricated via precipitation reaction have been an important area of particulate research over the last several decades. The polymer, pNIPAm, has been increasingly examined for microgel applications and will be used as an example of the precipitation reaction here. A significant advantage of utilizing a precipitation reaction is that the formed gels have low polydispersity (Bai, Yang *et al.* 2004; Zhang, Sun *et al.* 2004; Ju, Liu *et al.* 2009; Lime and Irgum 2009). PNIPAm is an interesting material as microgels fabricated from this polymer have been shown to undergo reversible volume-phase transitions, exhibiting changes in particle size, surface charge density, and water content over a small temperature range (Pelton and Chibante 1986). While the thermal sensitivity of these pNIPAm microgels is attractive for a variety of biomedical applications, researchers have been attempting to incorporate other monomers into the gels to further enhance the particles. In order to alter pNIPAm microparticles to suit the application, these microgels have been copolymerized with other materials, including dextran (Zhang, Sun *et al.* 2004), acrylic acid (Kratz, Hellweg *et al.* 2000), vinylacetic acid (Hoare and Pelton 2004), PEG (Gan and Lyon 2002; Nolan, Reyes *et al.* 2005), and benzo-18-crown-6-acrylamide (BCAm) (Ju, Liu *et al.* 2009), among others. With the addition of functional groups, the physical nature of the microparticles can be altered. Hoare and Pelton demonstrated that the addition of microgels fabricated from pNIPAm and vinylactic acid, acrylic acid, or methacrylic acid created microspheres with increased hydrodynamic diameters as compared to non-functionalized pNIPAm microgels (Hoare and Pelton 2004), indicating that particle size is not only dependent on conditions of the reaction, but also by the monomers utilized.

The vast magnitude of applications for these microgel systems is indicative of the nature of their intramolecular structure. The physical and chemical characteristics of the microspheres are greatly affected by external stimuli. Merely changing the ambient conditions, such as pH (Hoare and Pelton 2004; Thomas, Tingsanchali *et al.* 2007; Nichols, Scott *et al.* 2009), temperature (Kratz, Lapp *et al.* 2002; Hoare and Pelton 2004; Nolan, Reyes *et al.* 2005; Nichols, Scott *et al.* 2009), ionic strength (Neyret and Vincent 1997), or quality of the solvent (Kaneda and Vincent 2004; Pich, Lu *et al.* 2004; Lime and Irgum 2009), have been to found alter the overall characteristics of the colloid particle. While investigating the effects of pH on the formation of PEG microgels, the Elbert group found the size of their microparticles was increased from 4.9 to 8.8 μm as the pH of the reaction decreased (Nichols, Scott *et al.* 2009). The hydrodynamic radius of pNIPAm microgels could be altered simply by changing the crosslinker used during the fabrication process (Kratz, Lapp *et al.* 2002). Temperature of the reaction altered PEG microsphere size, where smaller microgels were produced as the temperature of the precipitation reaction was increased (Nichols, Scott *et al.* 2009). Similarly, DVB microgels increased from 1.1 and 3.4 μm as the concentration of monomer increased (Bai, Yang *et al.* 2004). Therefore, it is possible to finely tune the size of the microparticles given simple reaction conditions.

The crosslinked nature of the polymer microspheres causes their physical characteristics to fall between those of classical 'hardsphere colloids' and ultrasoft colloids exhibited by dilute polymer solutions (Heyes and Branka 2009). It is the intramolecular crosslinked structure that separates the microgels from other polymer particle systems. As demonstrated in literature, the monomers within the polymer colloids are crosslinked by either chemical or physical bonds; however, as this review focuses upon dispersion and precipitation polymerization, only microgels formed by chemical bonds will be discussed. Chemically crosslinked microgels are formed by homogeneous nucleation (Pelton 2000); the soluble monomers grow, reaching a critical chain length and then collapse to form microparticles. Typically, chemically crosslinked particles are formed by free-radical (Bromberg and Alakhov 2003) or condensation (Pelton 2000) polymerization. In order to achieve stable microparticles, the use of surfactants and/or electrostatic stabilization from the ionic groups associated with the initiator is often required. Microgels formed with chemical crosslinking have been achieved using a variety of monomers, including DVB (Lime and Irgum 2009), PEG (Nolan, Reyes *et al.* 2005; Nichols, Scott *et al.* 2009; Scott, Nichols *et al.* 2010), pNIPAm (Kratz, Hellweg *et al.* 2000; Nolan, Reyes *et al.* 2005), and PMAA (Morishita, Lowman *et al.* 2002). Again, the fundamental idea behind all of these syntheses is the reduced solubility of the polymer in the system during the polymerization and although the technique may differ between polymers, most take advantage of the LCST.

16.2.3 Characterization of microgels

Microgels have been extensively characterized physically (size, swelling, and mechanical properties) and chemically. Various forms of microscopy and dynamic light scattering (DLS) have been utilized to determine size and swelling information; mechanical properties are primarily determined via rheology, and excellent reviews are available for mechanical characterization of colloid systems (Russel 1980; Chen, Wen *et al.* 2010). Finally, chemical characterization is briefly discussed below, primarily to give readers a sampling of the techniques that have been used to study these gels.

Size

Several groups have utilized DLS to determine the size of their microgels (Kratz, Hellweg *et al.* 2000; Hoare and Pelton 2004; Tan, Tam *et al.* 2005; Sorrell and Lyon 2008; Hantzschel, Hund *et al.* 2009; Ju, Liu *et al.* 2009; Nichols, Scott *et al.* 2009). This technique has efficiently measured radii of microgels with diameters as large as 34 μm (Nichols, Scott *et al.* 2009) and as small as 50 nm (Zhou, Wang *et al.* 2008). While DLS has been found to be an efficient technique for measuring the size of individual microgels, it cannot provide accurate results for microgels that aggregate during formation. The size of microgels has also been examined via scanning electron microscopy (SEM) (Fig. 16.1A) (Kratz, Hellweg *et al.* 2000; Bai, Yang *et al.* 2004; Zhang, Sun *et al.* 2004; Hantzschel, Hund *et al.* 2009; Janczewski, Tomczak *et al.* 2009; Ju, Liu *et al.* 2009; Lime and Irgum 2009; Zhang, Pan *et al.* 2009) and the images can be utilized to measure the polydispersity of particulates (Lime and Irgum 2009; Zhang, Pan *et al.* 2009). Other microscopy techniques, such as transmission electron microscopy (TEM) (Hoare and Pelton 2004; Hantzschel, Hund *et al.* 2009; Janczewski, Tomczak *et al.* 2009; Wang, Zhao *et al.* 2009) and atomic force microscopy (AFM) (Singh and Lyon 2008; Zhou, Wang *et al.* 2008), can also give insight into the size of microgels (Fig. 16.1B–C). As the microgels have been dried in order to use these microscopy techniques, the hydrodynamic radii of the swollen gel cannot be accurately measured. For example, using AFM, the Hu research lab reported their pNIPAm particles to be approximately 50 nm in size (Zhou, Wang *et al.* 2008). However, the size of these same nanogels from DLS had an average hydrodynamic radius of 85 nm at 21°C (Zhou, Wang *et al.* 2008). The size of microgels has been can be investigated using phase-contrast microscopy (Nichols, Scott *et al.* 2009). This technique is very appealing as most bioengineering and biotechnology research groups have access to this type of microscopy (Fig. 16.1D); however, nanoparticles may not be able to be resolved using traditional phase-contrast microscopy. Addition of fluorescence to the microparticles may enhance their ability to not only be resolved by microscopy, but also to have measurement be automated.

Swelling

The volume and swelling capacity of the microgels have also proven interesting to researchers. Not only has DLS been used in the sizing of microgels, but it has allowed several research groups to measure the hydrodynamic radii of pNIPAm microgels in both the swollen and shrunken state to give a sense of swelling capacity (Kratz, Hellweg *et al.* 2000; Gan and Lyon 2002; Debord and Lyon 2003; Nolan, Reyes *et al.* 2005; Serpe, Yarmey *et al.* 2005; Singh and Lyon 2008; Hantzschel, Hund *et al.* 2009; Ju, Liu *et al.* 2009; Wang, Zhao *et al.* 2009;

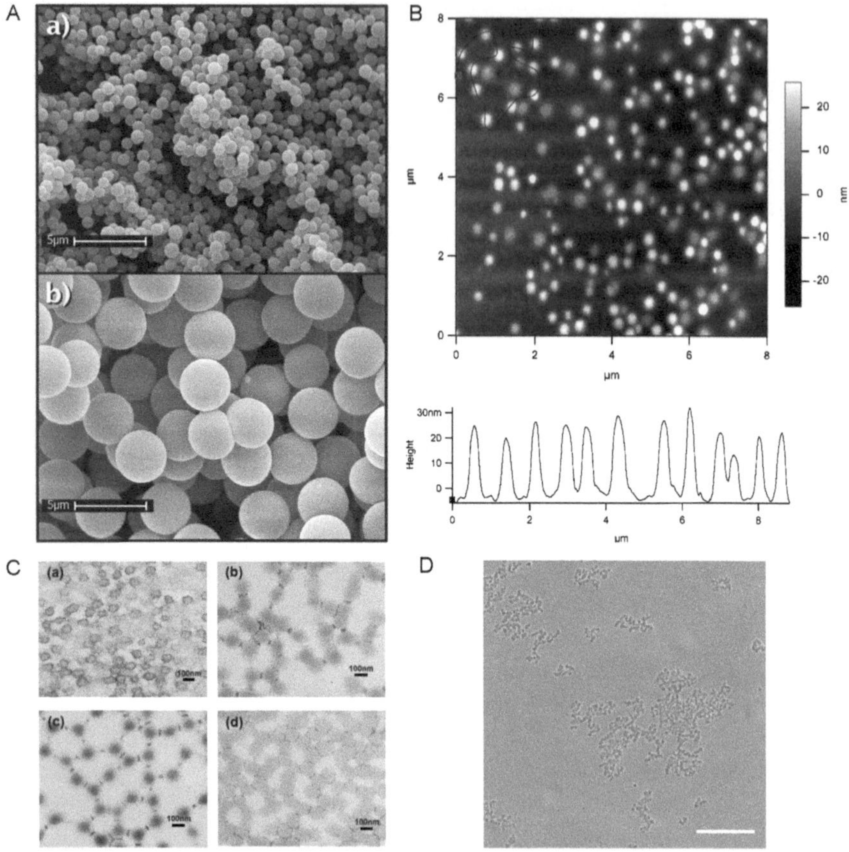

16.1 Characterization of microgels has been completed with various types of microscopy including: (A) SEM, where images of DVB microparticles polymerized in (a) acetonitrile and (b) acetonitrile with 10% tetrahydrofuran were utilized for sizing (Lime and Irgum 2009); (B) AFM, where both the topology (top) and line image (bottom) indicated the morphology and height of pNIPAm-Fmoc particles (Singh and Lyon 2008); (C) TEM, where images of pNIPAm microparticles functionalized with (a) vinylacetic acid, (b) acrylic acid, and (c) methacrylic acid were compared to (d) nonfunctionalized microgels (Hoare and Pelton 2004); and (D) phase-contrast microscopy, where images of PEG-DA microgels functionalized with PEG-glycine were used for sizing (Scott and Willits, unpublished data). All published figures were reproduced with permission.

Zhang, Pan *et al.* 2009). This technique has enabled researchers to successfully investigate the effect of various parameters, including crosslinker chain length and concentration, on the overall phase transition behavior of pNIPAm microgels (Fig. 16.2A) (Nolan, Reyes *et al.* 2005). Swelling and deswelling kinetics of microgels have also been examined using time-course UV-vis spectrography (Fig. 16.2B) (Chi, Cai *et al.* 2009; Wang, Zhao *et al.* 2009). This

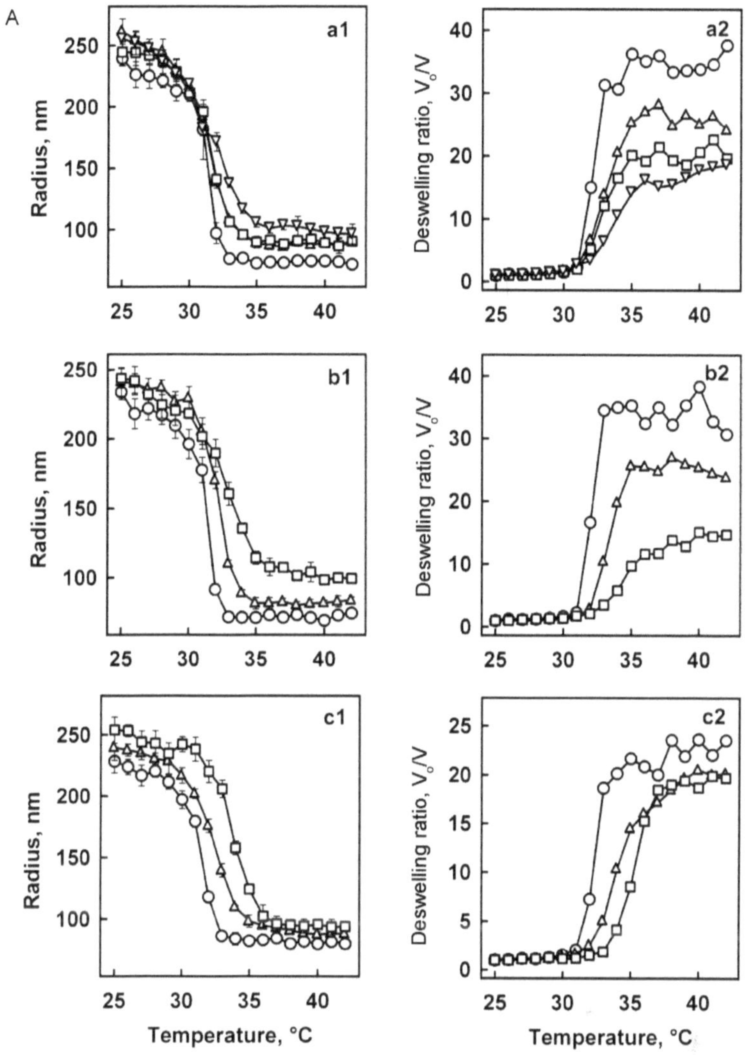

16.2 To further characterize microgels, sizing and swelling characteristics have been measured. (A) Temperature-dependent DLS determined hydrodynamic radii (panel 1) and deswelling ratios (panel 2) of pNIPAm microgels crosslinked with (a) PEG 200, (b) PEG 575, and (c) PEG 700 with 0.2 (filled circles), 1 (upward triangles), 2 (squares), and 5 (downward triangles) mol% crosslinker concentrations (Nolan, Reyes *et al.* 2005). Figures reproduced with permission.

method enabled the Yang group to characterize the swelling/deswelling process of their pNIPAm-co-acrylamide nanogels by examining the transmittance measurement of their microgels over a range of temperatures (Wang, Zhao *et al.* 2009).

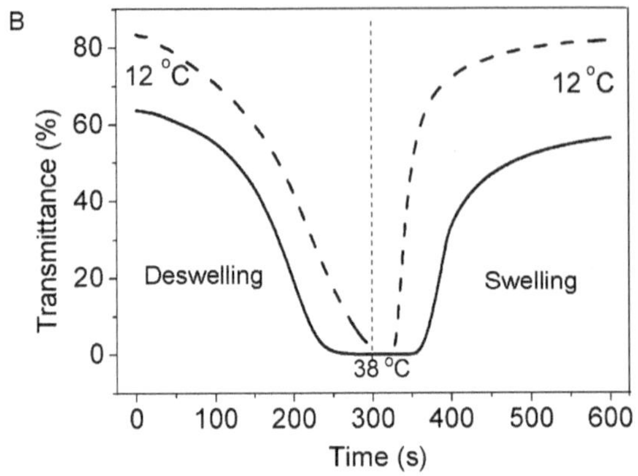

16.2 Continued (B) UV-vis spectroscopy revealed the influence of dispersion concentration on the swelling/deswelling kinetics of pNIPAm-co-acrylamide microgels with solutions containing 77 mg/mL (solid line) and 13 mg/mL (dashed line) microgel dispersions (Wang, Zhao *et al.* 2009). Figures reproduced with permission.

Mechanical properties

In order to further examine microgel structure, research groups have investigated the viscoelastic properties of microparticles using rheological measurements. The Graessley lab utilized rheological measurements to determine that Carbopol microgel solutions exhibited solid-like behavior in solutions above 1 wt% (Ketz, Prud'homme *et al.* 1988). Likewise, the Hu research group reported that the dynamic modulus of pNIPAm-co-poly(acrylic acid) microgel solutions increased with increasing solution concentration (Zhou, Wang *et al.* 2008). The dynamic modulus was also found to increase with temperature, as the pNIPAm microgels deswell with increased temperature, creating less viscous solutions (Zhou, Wang *et al.* 2008). Alternatively, the Tan group utilized rheoogy to investigate the relative viscosity of methacrylic acid-co-ethyl acrylate microgels formed from varying concentrations of crosslinker. It was reported that as the concentration of crosslinker utilized to form the microgels increased, the relative viscosity of the solution also increased (Tan, Tam *et al.* 2005). Ultimately, the results from these rheological testings have shown good agreement with colloidal soft sphere models (Tan, Pelton *et al.* 2010).

Density

One method for examining the relative density of swollen microgels is through isopycnic density gradient centrifugation (Nolan, Reyes *et al.* 2005). Using this technique, researchers were able to verify that a denser particle network was formed when a higher concentration of crosslinker was used; however, the actual density of the microgels was not determined. It may be possible to utilize a carefully planned density gradient of sucrose or dextran to ascertain the density of the microgels. As the density of the gradient layers can be easily calculated, the density of the microgels can be determined based on their relative position in the gradient post-centrifugation. Alternatively, the Sapurina group examined the density of microparticles, fabricated using varying mixtures of stabilizer, weighing dried samples in both air and decane (Stejskal, Sulimenko *et al.* 2000). By specifically selecting the composition of the stabilizing mixture, the density of the polyaniline microparticles could be altered from 1.345 to 1.858 g/cm^3 (Stejskal, Sulimenko *et al.* 2000).

Chemical composition

Chemical composition of microgels has been examined using a variety of spectroscopy techniques. To characterize the structural composition of microgels, Fourier transform infrared (FT-IR) spectroscopy has been performed by many groups (see, for example, Ju, Liu *et al.* 2009; Zhang, Pan *et al.* 2009). This technology has been used to verify that the copolymerizations of pNIPAm and BCAm (Ju, Liu *et al.* 2009) or 3-methacryloxypropyltrimethoxysilane (MPTMS) (Zhang, Pan *et al.* 2009) were successful. In addition, the Peppas group utilized FT-IR spectroscopy to show that PEG chains could be grafted to PMAA microparticles in order to functionalize the particles for mucoadhesion in the small intestine (Thomas, Tingsanchali *et al.* 2007). While this characterization method does verify the chemical composition of the microgel, the amount of copolymerization within the particle cannot be confirmed. To determine the amount of copolymerization acheived during synthesis, nuclear magnetic resonance (1H NMR) has been utilized (Gan and Lyon 2002; Debord and Lyon 2003; Nolan, Reyes *et al.* 2005; Singh and Lyon 2008; Janczewski, Tomczak *et al.* 2009). By examining the ratio of the integration values obtained from the peaks, the Lyons group was able to determine the composition of the pNIPAm-co-PEG microgels, even when small quantities of PEG, as low as 0.2 mole % PEG (MW 200 Da), was incorporated into the system (Nolan, Reyes *et al.* 2005). This technique allowed for an accurate detection of relatively small polymers in larger microgel systems. In addition, the removal of protective groups from the microgel has also been confirmed using 1H NMR (Singh and Lyon 2008). In addition to NMR, x-ray photoelectron spectroscopy (XPS) can demonstrate copolymer incorporation into microgels (Zhang, Pan *et al.* 2009). Upon examination of the XPS spectra, the incorporation of MPTMS into the pNIPAm microgels is discernable. However, the intensity of the signal of the sample was low and, therefore, Si-O and Si-C peaks from the MPTMS were indistinguishable from one another. The amount of MPTMS in the microgels was calculated using the XPS spectra, indicating that a small amount of MPTMS was actually incorporated into the particles, further explaining the small signal on the spectra.

Demonstrating the versatility of microscopy, it has also been utilized to examine chemical composition. The availability of functional groups on the surface of pNIPAm microgels has been examined via fluorescence spectroscopy (Singh and Lyon 2008), although the availability was not quantified. The relative composition of microgels has been examined via confocal microscopy through the mixing of fluorescently labeled components of the microgel (Nichols, Scott *et al.* 2009). TEM has also been utilized to determine the incorporation of functional groups to microgels (Hoare and Pelton 2004; Chastek, Wadajkar *et al.* 2010). The Pelton group has successfully utilized this technique, examining pNIPAm microgels copolymerized with vinylacetic acid, acrylic acid, or methacrylic acid, where the functional groups were selectively stained and imaged (Hoare and Pelton 2004). While this method does show that the functional groups were effectively incorporated into the microgels, the amount of incorporation is indiscernible.

16.3 Potential applications of microgels

An interesting feature of microgels is their ability to form modular, off-the-shelf, scaffolds. As these materials are pre-processed without cells, chemical interactions to make the microgels, which might normally limit the ability of a material to be a cellular scaffold, would be completed *a priori*. These microgels would then be mixed for design and cells can be encapsulated as the scaffold (or macrogel) is formed. The question then becomes: how can we take advantage of these microgel systems for tissue engineering and drug delivery applications? In their colloidal form, aqueous microgels are readily injectable. As with most colloid systems, as the concentration of the particles increases, the viscosity of the system increases (Ketz, Prud'homme *et al.* 1988; Tan, Tam *et al.* 2005). In addition, study of the formation of macrogels from the crosslinking of microgels has been investigated and could add another dimension to their injectability. This section will review the microgels as potential drug delivery and tissue engineered systems.

16.3.1 Drug delivery applications

The application of microgels as controlled drug delivery devices is a key area of study in current research. The low viscosity of the microparticle solutions, as shown by the surface coatings industry, makes them ideal for use as drug delivery systems. Small molecules can be incorporated into the microspheres and then released, as the microgels transition between states of increased and decreased swelling. In addition, changes in pH, ionic strength, and temperature have been shown to alter microparticle structure and these changes could be combined with biological components to cause drug release. Functionalization of the microparticle surface with receptor-specific proteins enables selective drug delivery to a specific site, effectively allowing targeted drug release to treat a localized area.

This ability to functionalize the microgels has been demonstrated to provide a means of cellular uptake with both poly(ethylene oxide)- (PEO) and polyglycerol-based microgels. The uptake of RGD-functionalized PEO microgels was increased over non-functionalized gels and was directed through clatherin-coated pits (Siegwart, Srinivasan *et al.* 2009). Functionalization with azide of polyglycerol microgels provided a site for conjugation of a fluorescent molecule to demonstrate the uptake by endocytosis, but with a variety of possible functionalizations to the glycerol, direct targeting can be envisioned (Fig. 16.3) (Sisson, Steinhilber *et al.* 2009). In addition to functionalization that enhances or targets cellular uptake, microgels have been modified with silver nanoparticles to enhance antibacterial properties (Hantzschel, Hund *et al.* 2009). However, to fully utilize the functionalization of these microgels with respect to drug delivery vehicles, encapsulation efficiency and release characteristics must be determined.

A variety of studies have examined encapsulation of relevant drug delivery molecules into these microgels. The ability to encapsulate molecules, and more importantly, active molecules, is dependent upon the reaction conditions to form the microgels. As described above, many microgels can be made with low polydispersity in mild conditions, making them ideal candidates for delivery vehicles. One of the primary methods to encapsulate agents is via swelling, as seen with N-vinylcaprolactam microgels (Imaz and Forcada 2010) and pNIPAm microgels (Foss, Goto *et al.* 2004; Serpe, Yarmey *et al.* 2005; Das, Mardyani *et al.* 2006; Wang, Zhao *et al.* 2007; Chen, Zhang *et al.* 2008; Lapeyre, Ancla *et al.* 2008; Liu, Yu *et al.* 2009). Researchers demonstrated that pNIPAm microgels, loaded with the anticancer drug doxorubicin (DX) via swelling, provided direct delivery of the drug to HeLa cancer cells and increased cancer cell mortality (Das, Mardyani *et al.* 2006). In addition, the Yang group found that pNIPAm-co-acrylamide microgels were able to release BLM, an anticancer drug, over a sustained period of 10 days (Wang, Zhao *et al.* 2007). While swelling is a viable option for lab scale operations, it is not practical at the production scale and other options, such as encapsulation during fabrication (Fig. 16.4), need further exploration and optimization.

In addition to microgel suspensions, research groups have utilized drug delivery technology from microgels fabricated into thin films (Nolan, Serpe *et al.* 2004; Serpe, Yarmey *et al.* 2005; Wang, Wang *et al.* 2008). The release of DX from thin films fabricated from pNIPAm-co-AAc microgels and poly(allylamine hydrochoride) (PAH) was shown to increase with thermal cycling, due to the deswelling of the film (Serpe, Yarmey *et al.* 2005). Similarly, exposing these pNIPAm-co-AAc microgel films to thermal cycling has caused insulin, previously loaded into the films, to release (Nolan, Serpe *et al.* 2004). The amount of insulin released from the films was shown to increase with

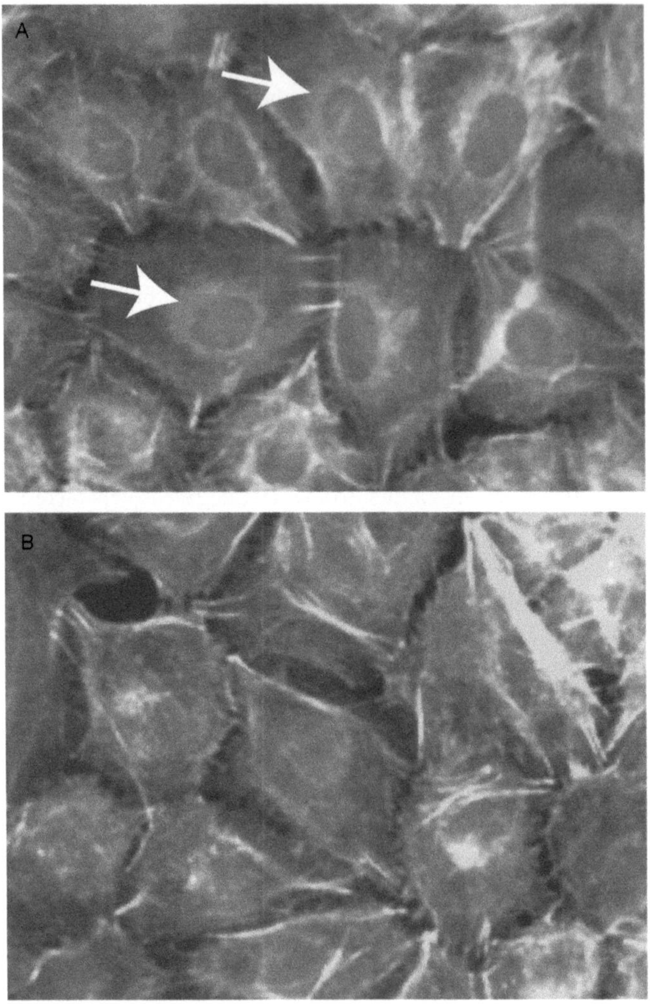

16.3 Culture of human lung cancer cell line A549 incubated with ICC-labeled PG microgels for 4 h at (A) 37°C and (B) incubated with control dye at 37°C (Sisson, Steinhilber *et al.* 2009). The labeled microgels are noted with white arrows in A, and are seen as localized in the perinuclear region. Although the control dye is much smaller in size than the microgel, the cell has appreciably more uptake of the microgels than the dye. Figure reproduced with permission.

increased film thickness and time. The Sun group fabricated multi-layer films composed of poly(styrene sulfonate) layered with PAH-co-dextran microgels that were found to reversibly load and release negatively charged dyes such as methyl orange (Wang, Wang *et al.* 2008). The dye was successfully loaded into the films at a density of 0.75 g/cm^3 and then was show to release from the films at a slow rate (Wang, Wang *et al.* 2008). As functionalization of the microgel particles can provide an easy mechanism of film formation, these suspensions

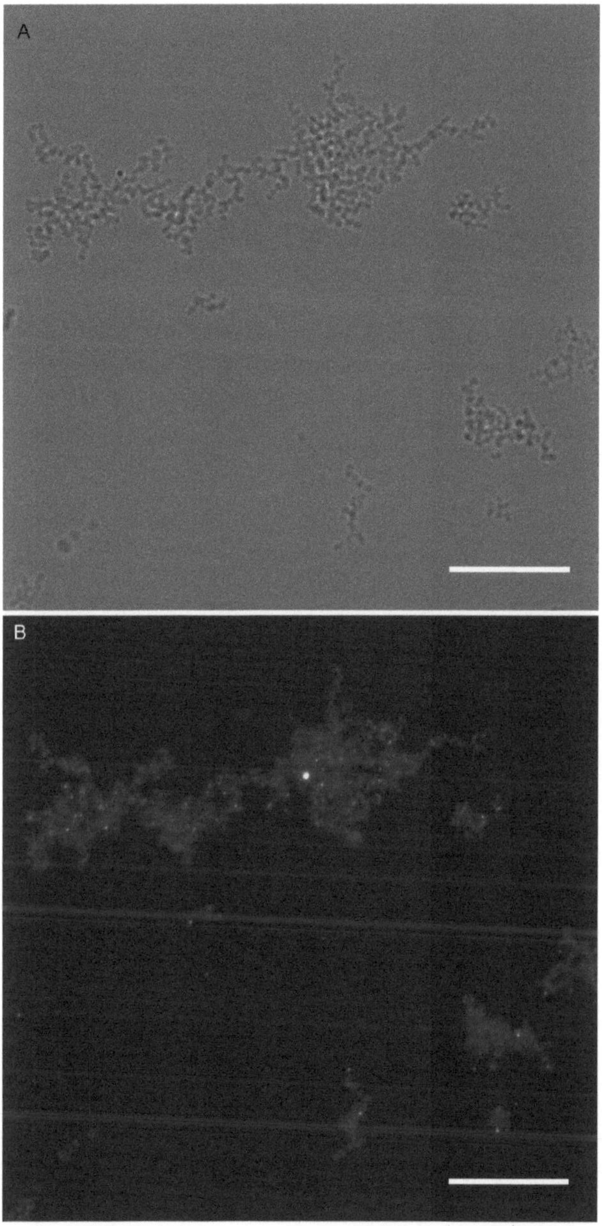

16.4 While a variety of gels have been used for drug delivery, most molecules are encapsulated after fabrication using swelling techniques. This image demonstrates the feasibility of encapsulating molecules during the microgel fabrication process, where AlexaFluor 555-ovalbumin was adding during the precipitation of PEG microgels (Stukel and Willits, unpublished data). Prior to imaging, gels were washed three times with buffer. This method of encapsulation needs to be further examined with other, more relevant, molecules to determine encapsulation percent and release profiles.

can be injected *in situ* and crosslinked into films to provide longer drug delivery profiles.

16.3.2 Tissue engineering applications

The utility of microgels has been demonstrated for a variety of applications; however, these materials have been only minimally investigated for tissue engineered applications. While pNIPAm microgels have been investigated for use in biomedical applications since their introduction in 1986 (Pelton and Chibante 1986), the study and use of other microgel materials for tissue engineering has only been introduced over the past five years. As the discovery of new functionalities enhance the capabilites of these materials, it is worthwhile to explore what has been done and look forward to the possibilities of microgels for tissue engineering.

As microgels

Spherical systems, in general, are desirable for some tissue engineering applications as they provide a high surface area to volume ratio for cellular interaction compared to two-dimensional systems. Nanogels or microgels, therefore, are potentially highly desireable for cell-based scaffolds, yet have not been extensively explored for tissue applications. One study has investigated poly(ethylene terephthalate) surfaces that have been tethered to pNIPAm-co-PEG microgels to block cellular adhesion (Singh, Bridges *et al.* 2007). Macrophage adhesion was significantly reduced when the PET surfaces were modified with microgels. As functionalized microgels have the capability to perform in tissue engineering applications, it may be more useful to speculate on how to take advantage of these functionalized spheres as building blocks for scaffolds.

16.5 (opposite) By fabricating a variety of different microgels, these materials can be used as a bottom-up method of building scaffolds for tissue engineering. Scott *et al.*'s protocol is demonstrated using this cartoon. (A) Eight-arm PEG-vinylsulfone (PEG_8-VS) was reacted with eight-arm PEG-amine (PEG_8-amine) in PBS. A similar strategy was followed with eight-arm PEG-acrylate (PEG_8-acrylate) and PEG_8-amine to produce porogenic microspheres. Microspheres were produced for the delivery of sphingosine 1-phosphate (S1P) to promote endothelial cell migration by reacting PEG_8-VS with bovine serum albumin (BSA). (B) Microspheres with different functionalities were mixed with HepG2 hepatoma cells, centrifuged for 10 min at 1000*g*, and allowed to crosslink overnight at 37°C. Within 48 h, PEG_8-acrylate/PEG_8-amine microspheres dissolved to form macroporous scaffolds. Endothelial cells seeded on the scaffolds adhered via RGD peptide incorporated in the non-degradable microspheres (Scott, Nichols *et al.* 2010). Figure reproduced with permission.

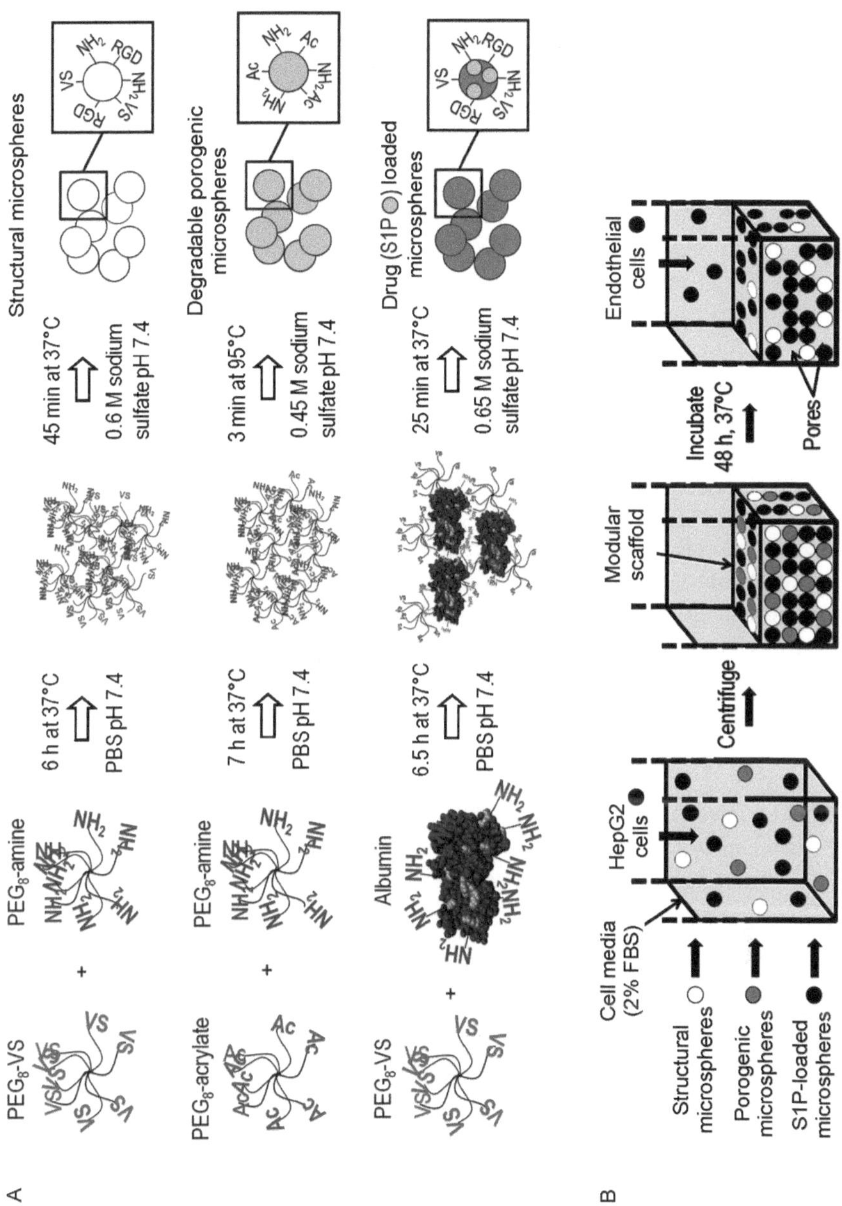
A
PEG8-VS
PEG8-amine
6 h at 37°C
PBS pH 7.4
45 min at 37°C
0.6 M sodium sulfate pH 7.4
Structural microspheres
PEG8-acrylate
PEG8-amine
7 h at 37°C
PBS pH 7.4
3 min at 95°C
0.45 M sodium sulfate pH 7.4
Degradable porogenic microspheres
PEG8-VS
Albumin
6.5 h at 37°C
PBS pH 7.4
25 min at 37°C
0.65 M sodium sulfate pH 7.4
Drug (S1P) loaded microspheres
B
Structural microspheres
Porogenic microspheres
S1P-loaded microspheres
Cell media (2% FBS)
HepG2 cells
Centrifuge
Modular scaffold
Incubate 48 h, 37°C
Pores
Endothelial cells

As macrogels

As functionalization of traditional polymers has become increasingly popular and more sophisticated, scientists have made the next leap into crosslinking the microgels into a macrogel. The initial studies presented here have demonstrated some of the possibilites of these materials and their interactions with cells. The Weitz research group has fabricated responsive macrogel scaffolds through the assembly of allylamine functionalized pNIPAm microgels and poly(acrylic acid) chains (Cho, Kim *et al.* 2007). Due to the hydrophobic properties exhibited by these scaffolds, these pNIPAm macrogels will take the shape of any slightly hydrophilic container in which they are formed and respond more quickly than bulk gels of similar composition (Cho, Kim *et al.* 2007), which could be very useful for tissue-engineered scaffolds. Crosslinked, PEG-functionalized pNIPAm microgels reduced protein adhesion and cellular attachment; increasing the molecular weight of the PEG crosslinker increased the materials ability to resist protein deposition in both the swollen and de-swollen states (Nolan, Reyes *et al.* 2005). Further demonstrating the modular capabilities of these materials, the Elbert group fabricated PEG microgels with vinylsulfone, acrylate, or amines as their interaction points (Fig. 16.5) and demonstrated that HepG2 cells within these modular macrogels were viable for at least three weeks and endothelial cells migrated faster when S1P-loaded microgels were incorporated into the macrogel (Scott, Nichols *et al.* 2010). PEG microgels have also been formed in the authors' laboratory from PEG-diacrylate (PEG-DA) and functionalized by incorporating acrylic acid or acryl-PEG-glycine into the precipitation. The carboxyl groups can be readily activated to form macrogels and these materials have been investigated for use with neural cultures such as DRG (Fig. 16.6A) and PC12 cells (Fig. 16.6B), as the low stiffness of these macrogels is relevant for neural tissue. And, as there is no need for harsh crosslinking agents or external stimuli, these microgels may be injected and crosslinked *in situ* to form macrogels.

16.4 Conclusions

While microgels have been utilized for years in the coatings industry, researchers have more recently demonstrated their potential utility for a variety of uses in drug delivery and tissue engineering applications. The ability to characterize microgels in both a physical and chemical manner has been thoroughly demonstrated in literature via a variety of techniques. Microgels are easily fabricated by many protocols and can be modified to suit the intended purpose. As the viscosity of colloidal systems lend them to be easily injectable, the ability to functionalize microgels can further direct these materials to release drugs or form scaffolds *in situ*. In addition, as they are readily formed from a variety of polymer systems using precipitation or dispersion reactions, many of

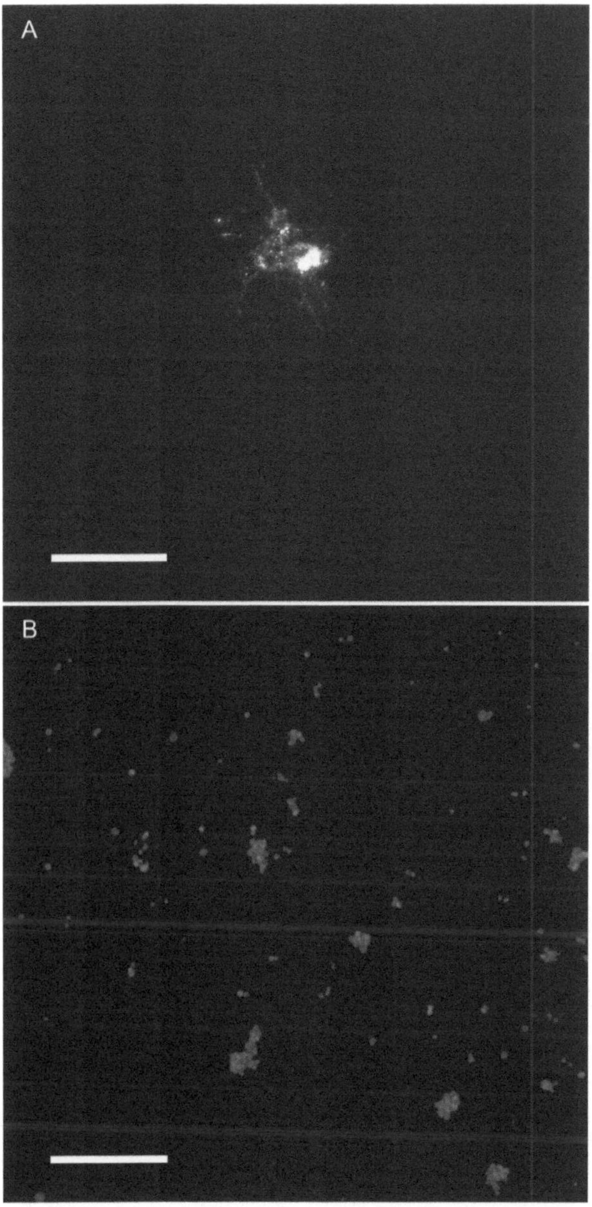

16.6 As macrogels formed from microgels generally have a lower stiffness than their bulk counterparts, these macrogels have been investigated for possible neural tissue engineering scaffolds. PEG macrogels from microgels that are approximately 1.6 μm in diameter were crosslinked with collagen to encapsulate (A) embryonic chick dorsal root ganglia (DRG) or (B) PC12 cells (Scott and Willits, unpublished data). After 4 days of culture, the DRG had neural extensions and PC12 cells were forming aggregates. Scale bars are 100 μm for (A) and 200 μm for (B).

the bulk hydrogel systems today could be formed using a building block or modular technique that the microgels offer, with well controlled sizing and commonly used analysis techniques.

16.5 Sources of further information and advice

As this topic contains such a rich history of microgel and nanogel preparation, it is difficult to choose a few key references. Therefore, this section will overview some of the current texts and reviews available to deepen the knowledge on the topics presented here. Two textbooks were excellent in their ability to delineate differences between the types of reactions and the basic characteristics for these polymerizations, including Barrett's *Dispersion Polymerization in Organic Media* (Barrett 1975) and Barton's *Radical Polymerization in Disperse Systems* (Barton and Capek 1994). Several recent reviews on microgels are also excellent resources for general information on the technologies including Karg and Hellweg (2009), Saunders, Laajam *et al.* (2009), and Pelton (2000). The characterization methods of microgels have also been described in detail in Pelton (2000) and Pich and Richtering (2010). Many of these reviews also touch on biomedical applications for the microgels and can be used as further references for those topics also.

16.6 References

Alemán, J., A. V. Chadwick, *et al.* (2007). 'Definitions of terms relating to the structure and processing of sols, gels, networks, and inorganic-organic hybrid materials (IUPAC Recommendations 2007).' *Pure and Applied Chemistry* **79**(10): 1801–1829.

Arshady, R. (1992). 'Suspension, emulsion, and dispersion polymerization: a methodological survey.' *Colloid & Polymer Science* **270**(8): 717–732.

Bai, F., X. Yang, *et al.* (2004). 'Synthesis of narrow or monodisperse poly(divinylbenzene) microspheres by distillation precipitation polymerization.' *Macromolecules* **37**(26): 9746–9752.

Bailey, F. and R. W. Callard (1959). 'Some properties of poly(ethylene oxide) in aqueous solution.' *Journal of Applied Polymer Science* **1**(1): 56–62.

Baker, W. O. (1949). 'Microgel, a new macromolecule.' *Industrial & Engineering Chemistry* **41**(3): 511–520.

Barrett, K. (1975). *Dispersion Polymerization in Organic Media*. New York, Wiley-Interscience.

Barton, J. and I. Capek (1994). *Radical Polymerization in Disperse Systems*. New York, Ellis Horwood.

Bromberg, L. and V. Alakhov (2003). 'Effects of polyether-modified poly(acrylic acid) microgels on doxorubicin transport in human intestinal epithelial Caco-2 cell layers.' *Journal of Controlled Release* **88**(1): 11–22.

Chastek, T., A. Wadajkar, *et al.* (2010). 'Polyglycol-templated synthesis of poly(N-isopropyl acrylamide) microgels with improved biocompatibility.' *Colloid & Polymer Science* **288**(1): 105–114.

Chen, D. T. N., Q. Wen, *et al.* (2010). 'Rheology of soft materials.' *Annual Review of Condensed Matter Physics* **1**(1).

Chen, H., J. Zhang, *et al.* (2008). '*In vivo* non-invasive optical imaging of temperature-sensitive co-polymeric nanohydrogel.' *Nanotechnology* **19**(18): 185707.

Chi, C., T. Cai, *et al.* (2009). 'Oligo(ethylene glycol)-based thermoresponsive core-shell microgels.' *Langmuir* **25**(6): 3814–3819.

Cho, E. C., J. W. Kim, *et al.* (2007). 'Highly responsive hydrogel scaffolds formed by three-dimensional organization of microgel nanoparticles.' *Nano Letters* **8**(1): 168–172.

Das, M., S. Mardyani, *et al.* (2006). 'Biofunctionalized pH-responsive microgels for cancer cell targeting: rational design.' *Advanced Materials* **18**(1): 80–83.

Debord, J. D. and L. A. Lyon (2003). 'Synthesis and characterization of pH-responsive copolymer microgels with tunable volume phase transition temperatures.' *Langmuir* **19**(18): 7662–7664.

Foss, A. C., T. Goto, *et al.* (2004). 'Development of acrylic-based copolymers for oral insulin delivery.' *European Journal of Pharmaceutics and Biopharmaceutics* **57**(2): 163–169.

Gan, D. and L. A. Lyon (2002). 'Synthesis and protein adsorption resistance of PEG-modified poly(N-isopropylacrylamide) core/shell microgels.' *Macromolecules* **35**(26): 9634–9639.

Hantzschel, N., R. D. Hund, *et al.* (2009). 'Hybrid microgels with antibacterial properties.' *Macromol Biosci* **9**(5): 444–449.

Herrmann, J. and R. Bodmeier (1995). 'The effect of particle microstructure on the somatostatin release from poly(lactide) microspheres prepared by a W/O/W solvent evaporation method.' *Journal of Controlled Release* **36**(1–2): 63–71.

Heyes, D. and A. Branka (2009). 'Interactions between microgel particles.' *Soft Matter* **5**: 2681–2685.

Hoare, T. and R. Pelton (2004). 'Highly pH and temperature responsive microgels functionalized with vinylacetic acid.' *Macromolecules* **37**(7): 2544–2550.

Hunkeler, D., F. Candau, *et al.* (1994). Heterophase polymerizations: a physical and kinetic comparison and categorization: *Theories and mechanism of phase transitions, heterophase polymerizations, homopolymerization, addition polymerization*, Springer, Berlin/Heidelberg: 115–133.

Imaz, A. and J. Forcada (2010). '*N*-vinylcaprolactam-based microgels for biomedical applications.' *Journal of Polymer Science Part A: Polymer Chemistry* **48**(5): 1173–1181.

IUPAC (1997). *Compendium of Chemical Terminology*, 2nd edn (the 'Gold Book'). Oxford, Blackwell Scientific Publications.

Janczewski, D., N. Tomczak, *et al.* (2009). 'Introduction of quantum dots into PNIPAM microspheres by precipitation polymerization above LCST.' *European Polymer Journal* **45**(7): 1912–1917.

Ju, X. J., L. Liu, *et al.* (2009). 'Dual thermo-responsive and ion-recognizable monodisperse microspheres.' *Polymer* **50**(3): 922–929.

Kamyshny, A. and S. Magdassi (2000). 'Fluorescence immunoassay based on fluorescer microparticles.' *Colloids and Surfaces B: Biointerfaces* **18**(1): 13–17.

Kaneda, I. and B. Vincent (2004). 'Swelling behavior of PMMA-g-PEO microgel particles by organic solvents.' *Journal of Colloid and Interface Science* **274**(1): 49–54.

Karg, M. and T. Hellweg (2009). 'New smart poly (NIPAM) microgels and nanoparticle microgel hybrids: properties and advances in characterisation.' *Current Opinion in Colloid & Interface Science* **14**(6): 438–450.

Ketz, R. J., R. K. Prud'homme, *et al.* (1988). 'Rheology of concentrated microgel solutions.' *Rheologica Acta* **27**(5): 531–539.

Kratz, K., T. Hellweg, *et al.* (2000). 'Influence of charge density on the swelling of colloidal poly(N-isopropylacrylamide-co-acrylic acid) microgels.' *Colloids and Surfaces A: Physicochemical and Engineering Aspects* **170**(2–3): 137–149.

Kratz, K., A. Lapp, *et al.* (2002). 'Volume transition and structure of triethyleneglycol dimethacrylate, ethylenglykol dimethacrylate, and N,N′-methylene bis-acrylamide cross-linked poly(N-isopropyl acrylamide) microgels: a small angle neutron and dynamic light scattering study.' *Colloids and Surfaces A: Physicochemical and Engineering Aspects* **197**(1–3): 55–67.

Lapeyre, V., C. Ancla, *et al.* (2008). 'Glucose-responsive microgels with a core-shell structure.' *J Colloid Interface Sci* **327**(2): 316–323.

Lime, F. and K. Irgum (2009). 'Preparation of divinylbenzene and divinylbenzene-co-glycidyl methacrylate particles by photoinitiated precipitation polymerization in different solvent mixtures.' *Macromolecules* **42**(13): 4436–4442.

Liu, Y. Y., Y. Yu, *et al.* (2009). 'Preparation and properties of cyclodextrin/PNIPAm microgels.' *Macromol Biosci* **9**(5): 525–534.

Loxley, A. and B. Vincent (1997). 'Equilibrium and kinetic aspects of the pH-dependent swelling of poly(2-vinylpyridine-co-styrene) microgels.' *Colloid & Polymer Science* **275**(12): 1108–1114.

Morishita, M., A. M. Lowman, *et al.* (2002). 'Elucidation of the mechanism of incorporation of insulin in controlled release systems based on complexation polymers.' *Journal of Controlled Release* **81**(1–2): 25–32.

Neyret, S. and B. Vincent (1997). 'The properties of polyampholyte microgel particles prepared by microemulsion polymerization.' *Polymer* **38**(25): 6129–6134.

Nichols, M. D., E. A. Scott, *et al.* (2009). 'Factors affecting size and swelling of poly(ethylene glycol) microspheres formed in aqueous sodium sulfate solutions without surfactants.' *Biomaterials* **30**(29): 5283–5291.

Nolan, C. M., M. J. Serpe, *et al.* (2004). 'Thermally modulated insulin release from microgel thin films.' *Biomacromolecules* **5**(5): 1940–1946.

Nolan, C. M., C. D. Reyes, *et al.* (2005). 'Phase transition behavior, protein adsorption, and cell adhesion resistance of poly(ethylene glycol) cross-linked microgel particles.' *Biomacromolecules* **6**(4): 2032–2039.

Nolan, C. M., L. T. Gelbaum, *et al.* (2006). '1H NMR investigation of thermally triggered insulin release from poly(N-isopropylacrylamide) microgels.' *Biomacromolecules* **7**(10): 2918–2922.

Pelton, R. (2000). 'Temperature-sensitive aqueous microgels.' *Advances in Colloid and Interface Science* **85**(1): 1–33.

Pelton, R. H. and P. Chibante (1986). 'Preparation of aqueous latices with N-isopropylacrylamide.' *Colloids and Surfaces* **20**(3): 247–256.

Pich, A. and W. Richtering (2010). Microgels by precipitation polymerization: synthesis, characterization, and functionalization, *Advances in Polymer Science*, Spinger, Berlin: 1–37.

Pich, A., Y. Lu, *et al.* (2004). 'Thermo-sensitive poly(N-vinylcaprolactam-co-acetoacetoxyethyl methacrylate) microgels. 3. Incorporation of polypyrrole by selective microgel swelling in ethanol-water mixtures.' *Polymer* **45**(4): 1079–1087.

Russel, W. B. (1980). 'Review of the role of colloidal forces in the rheology of suspensions.' *Journal of Rheology* **24**(3): 287–317.

Sasa, N. and T. Yamaoka (1994). 'Surface-activated photopolymer microgels.' *Advanced Materials* **6**(5): 417–421.

Saunders, B., N. Laajam, *et al.* (2009). 'Microgels: from responsive polymer colloids to biomaterials.' *Advances in Colloid and Interface Science* **147**: 251–262.

Scott, E. A., M. D. Nichols, *et al.* (2010). 'Modular scaffolds assembled around living cells using poly(ethylene glycol) microspheres with macroporation via a non-cytotoxic porogen.' *Acta Biomaterialia* **6**(1): 29–38.

Serpe, M. J., K. A. Yarmey, *et al.* (2005). 'Doxorubicin uptake and release from microgel thin films.' *Biomacromolecules* **6**(1): 408–413.

Siegwart, D. J., A. Srinivasan, *et al.* (2009). 'Cellular uptake of functional nanogels prepared by inverse miniemulsion ATRP with encapsulated proteins, carbohydrates, and gold nanoparticles.' *Biomacromolecules* **10**(8): 2300–2309.

Silva, G. A., F. J. Costa, *et al.* (2005). 'Entrapment ability and release profile of corticosteroids from starch-based microparticles.' *Journal of Biomedical Materials Research Part A* **73A**(2): 234–243.

Singh, N. and L. Lyon (2008). 'Synthesis of multifunctional nanogels using a protected macromonomer approach.' *Colloid & Polymer Science* **286**(8): 1061–1069.

Singh, N., A. W. Bridges, *et al.* (2007). 'Covalent tethering of functional microgel films onto poly(ethylene terephthalate) surfaces.' *Biomacromolecules* **8**(10): 3271–3275.

Sisson, A. L., D. Steinhilber, *et al.* (2009). 'Biocompatible functionalized polyglycerol microgels with cell penetrating properties.' *Angew Chem Int Ed Engl* **48**(41): 7540–7545.

Sorrell, C. D. and L. A. Lyon (2008). 'Deformation controlled assembly of binary microgel thin films.' *Langmuir* **24**(14): 7216–7222.

Spegel, P., L. Schweitz, *et al.* (2001). 'Molecularly imprinted microparticles for capillary electrochromatography: studies on microparticle synthesis and electrolyte composition.' *Electrophoresis* **22**(17): 3833–3841.

Staudinger, H. and E. Husemann (1935). *Ber* **68**: 1618.

Stejskal, J., T. Sulimenko, *et al.* (2000). 'Polyaniline dispersions 10. Coloured microparticles of variable density prepared using stabilizer mixtures.' *Colloid & Polymer Science* **278**(7): 654–658.

Tan, B. H., K. C. Tam, *et al.* (2005). 'Microstructure and rheology of stimuli-responsive microgel systems – effect of cross-linked density.' *Advances in colloid and interface science* **113**(2–3): 111–120.

Tan, B. H., R. H. Pelton, *et al.* (2010). 'Microstructure and rheological properties of thermo-responsive poly(N-isopropylacrylamide) microgels.' *Polymer* **51**(14): 3238–3243.

Thomas, J. B., J. H. Tingsanchali, *et al.* (2007). 'Dynamics of poly(ethylene glycol)-tethered, pH responsive networks.' *Polymer* **48**(17): 5042–5048.

Tuncel, A., K. Ecevit, *et al.* (1996). 'Nonswellable and swellable ethylene glycol dimethacrylate-acrylic acid copolymer microspheres.' *Journal of Polymer Science Part A: Polymer Chemistry* **34**(1): 45–55.

Vivaldo-Lima, E., P. E. Wood, *et al.* (1997). 'An updated review on suspension polymerization.' *Industrial & Engineering Chemistry Research* **36**(4): 939–965.

Wang, L., X. Wang, *et al.* (2008). 'Layer-by-layer assembled microgel films with high loading capacity: reversible loading and release of dyes and nanoparticles.' *Langmuir* **24**(5): 1902–1909.

Wang, Q., Y. Zhao, *et al.* (2007). 'Thermosensitive phase behavior and drug release of *in situ* gelable poly(N-isopropylacrylamide-co-acrylamide) microgels.' *Colloid & Polymer Science* **285**(5): 515–521.

Wang, Q., Y. Zhao, *et al.* (2009). 'Thermosensitive phase transition kinetics of poly(N-isopropylacryl amide-co-acrylamide) microgel aqueous dispersions.' *Journal of*

Applied Polymer Science **113**(1): 321–326.

Whitby, G. S. and M. Katz (1933). 'Synthetic rubber.' *Industrial & Engineering Chemistry* **25**(12): 1338–1348.

Yenice, I., S. Cali, *et al.* (2002). 'Biodegradable implantable teicoplanin beads for the treatment of bone infections.' *International Journal of Pharmaceutics* **242**(1–2): 271–275.

Zhang, J.-T., C.-J. Pan, *et al.* (2009). 'Monodisperse, temperature-sensitive microgels crosslinked by Si-O-Si bonds.' *Macromolecular Materials and Engineering* **294**(6–7): 396–404.

Zhang, M. and Z. E. Rassi (1999). 'Capillary electrochromatography with novel stationary phases: II. Studies of the retention behavior of nucleosides and bases on capillaries packed with octadecyl-sulfonated-silica microparticles.' *Electrophoresis* **20**(1): 31–36.

Zhang, X. Z., G. M. Sun, *et al.* (2004). 'Temperature sensitive dendrite-shaped PNIPAAm/Dex-AI hybrid hydrogel particles: formulation and properties.' *European Polymer Journal* **40**(9): 2251–2257.

Zhou, J., G. Wang, *et al.* (2008). 'Viscoelastic behavior and *in vivo* release study of microgel dispersions with inverse thermoreversible gelation.' *Biomacromolecules* **9**(1): 142–148.

Index

MIX
Papier | Fördert gute Waldnutzung
FSC® C083411

Kolibri 360 GmbH
Ferdinand-Jühlke-Straße 7
99095 Erfurt, Deutschland
produktsicherheit@kolibri360.de